# Maitland's Vertebral Manipulation

*For Butterworth-Heinemann:*

*Senior Commissioning Editor:* Heidi Harrison
*Development Editor:* Siobhan Campbell
*Project Manager:* Andrew Palfreyman
*Design Direction:* George Ajayi and Judith Wright
*Illustrations Manager:* Bruce Hogarth
*Illustrator:* Cactus Design and Illustration Ltd
            Chartwell

# Maitland's Vertebral Manipulation

## Seventh Edition

**Geoffrey D Maitland** MBE, AUA, FCSP, TACP, SASP Mapplsc

*Edited by*

**Elly Hengeveld** MSc, BPT, PTOMT, SVOMP, IMTA Member

*Senior Teacher, International Maitland Teacher's Association, Oberentfelden, Switzerland*

**Kevin Banks** BA, MMACP, MCSP, SRP, IMTA Member

*Chartered Physiotherapist, Rotherham, UK*

**Kay English** Dip Tech (Physio), Grad Dip (Adv MT), MMPAA, MAPA

*Private Practitioner, Medindie, South Australia, Australia*

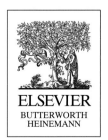

ELSEVIER
BUTTERWORTH
HEINEMANN

EDINBURGH  LONDON  NEW YORK  OXFORD  PHILADELPHIA  ST LOUIS  SYDNEY  TORONTO  2005

**ELSEVIER**
BUTTERWORTH
HEINEMANN

First published 1964
Second edition 1968
Third edition 1973
Fourth edition 1977
Fifth edition 1986
Sixth edition 2001
Seventh edition 2005
    Reprinted 2006, 2007 (twice), 2009

ISBN: 978–0–7506–8806–2

**British Library Cataloguing in Publication Data**
A catalogue record for this book is available from the British Library

**Library of Congress Cataloguing in Publication Data**
A catalogue record for this book is available from the Library of Congress

**Note**
Medical knowledge is constantly changing. As new information becomes available, changes in treatment, procedures, equipment and the use of drugs become necessary. The authors and the publishers have taken care to ensure that the information given in this text is accurate and up to date. However, readers are strongly advised to confirm that the information, especially with regard to drug usage, complies with the latest legislation and standards of practice.

*The Publisher*

your source for books, journals and multimedia in the health sciences
**www.elsevierhealth.com**

Working together to grow libraries in developing countries
www.elsevier.com | www.bookaid.org | www.sabre.org
ELSEVIER  BOOK AID International  Sabre Foundation

The publisher's policy is to use **paper manufactured from sustainable forests**

Printed in China

# Contents

# Preface to the seventh edition

Physiotherapists are being called upon increasingly by medical practitioners to help patients recover from episodes of uncomplicated or simple/mechanical spinal disorders. Manipulative Physiotherapy, it is clear, has an important role to play within the recovery and rehabilitation process.

The ability to identify and deal with spinal segmental mobility impairment, neurodynamic dysfunction and muscle imbalance, for example, requires finely tuned skills of clinical examination, clinical reasoning and technically accurate and effective treatment techniques.

The Maitland Concept has been one of the cornerstones of modern manipulative physiotherapy. Those who have been privileged enough to see Geoff Maitland at work will know how much thought and detail goes into the application of each individual technique of examination, mobilisation or manipulation. Having the opportunity to see and practice techniques performed in an expert way can only serve to help any clinician to understand and apply manipulative physiotherapy methods more effectively in the clinical setting.

Whilst textbooks can never substitute the real-time acquisition of manipulative skills, they can act as a standard and a platform from which the clinician can continue to improve. With this in mind, the revised 7th edition of *Vertebral Manipulation*, although having exactly the same text and description of techniques, is now enhanced by stills photographs and a DVD showing video clips of all relevant techniques. This should help the reader to see and apply more clearly aspects of each technique such as starting positions, localisation of forces and application of forces

If these dynamic additions allow students of manipulative physiotherapy to enhance their skills and experts to check and refine their skills and in turn apply such skills clinically to help maximise patient recovery, then the aim of this revised edition will have been achieved.

Elly Hengeveld – *Oberenfelden, Switzerland*
Kevin Banks – *Rotherham, UK*

# Preface to the first edition

Manipulation of the spine is associated so often with false diagnosis and 'hit or miss' methods of brute force. These associations have resulted in the exclusion of manipulative treatment from routine physical medicine. The cautious and apprehensive attitude towards this treatment would be largely eliminated if it were recognized that most patients can be relieved by the gentler procedures.

There are two ways of manipulating the conscious patient. The first, better thought of as mobilization, is the gentler coaxing of a movement by passive rhythmical oscillations performed within or at the limit of the range; the second is the forcing of a movement from the limit of the range by a sudden thrust. The difference between these two techniques may seem negligible when comparing a strongly applied mobilization with a gentle manipulative thrust, but there is an important difference. The patient can always resist the mobilization if it should become too painful, whereas the suddenness of the forceful manipulation prevents any control by the patient.

The practical approach to the use of manipulation is to relate treatment to the patient's symptoms and signs rather than to diagnoses. Such a plan avoids both the confusion caused by diagnostic titles calling to mind different symptoms to different people, and the controversy over pathology. Indeed, it is often impossible to know what the true pathology is. Also it will be agreed that under the umbrella of one diagnostic title, for example, 'disc lesion', symptoms and signs may vary widely and require different treatments.

Only the spinal joints from the occiput to the sacrum are discussed in this book, and the text has been planned to lead the reader in logical sequence from the examination of the different intervertebral levels to the techniques of mobilization applicable in each case. The way is then prepared for further development into the more forceful manipulative procedures and their application. Guiding principles of treatment follow and are then applied to specific case histories in the final chapter. It should be understood that all treatment in this book when done by physiotherapists is only carried out on medical referral.

To the many people who have contributed so much towards the final presentation of this book I am unable to express my gratitude adequately. Without the constructive help of those concerned with the typing and posing for the diagrams, my work would have been much more difficult.

Particular people were asked to undertake the task of reading and criticizing the manuscript in detail, so that it might meet as nearly as possible the needs for which it was undertaken; and I am sure that they will be able to see how invaluable their guidance has been. In particular I wish to express my sincere thanks to Miss M. J. Hammond, AUA, MCSP (Teachers Cert.), Miss J.-M. Ganne, MCSP (Teachers Cert.), Miss M. Martin-Jones, MCSP (Teachers Cert.), Dr A. W. Burnell, D Phys Med, Mrs H. S. Culshaw, BA, Dip Ed, Mr Lansell Bonnin, MCh (Orth), FRCS and Dr Bryan Gandevia, MD, BS (Melb), MRACP (Consultant Editor, *Australian Journal of Physiotherapy*). These persons by their individual comments and criticisms gave considerable guidance concerning different aspects of the work, namely the teaching of physiotherapy students, medical acceptance and composition. My thanks are due also to my wife who so painstakingly produced all the drawings.

I am most grateful for the courtesy extended to me during a recent study tour in Great Britain, the United States of America and Canada.

*Adelaide*                                                    G. D. Maitland

# Biography

## Geoffrey Douglas Maitland MBE, AUA, FCSP, FACP (Monograph), FACP (Specialist Manipulative Physiotherapist), MAppSc (Physiotherapy)

G. D. Maitland (1924–), was born in Adelaide, Australia, trained as a physiotherapist from 1946 to 1949 after serving in the RAAF during the second World War in Great Britain.

His first job was at the Royal Adelaide Hospital and the Adelaide Children's Hospital, with a main interest in the treatment of orthopaedic and neurological disorders. Later he continued working part-time in the hospital and part-time in his own private clinic. After a few years he became a part-time private practitioner and part-time clinical tutor at the School of Physiotherapy in the South Australian Institute of Technology, now the University of South Australia. He continuously studied and spent half a day each week in the Barr–Smith Library and the excellent library at the Medical School of the University of Adelaide.

He immediately showed an interest in careful clinical examination and assessment of patients with neuro-musculo-skeletal disorders. In those days assessment and treatment by specific passive movements were under-represented in physiotherapy practice. G. D. Maitland learned techniques from osteopathic, chiropractic and bonesetter books as well as from medical books such as those of Marlin, Jostes, James B. Mennell, John McMillan Mennell, Alan Stoddard, Robert Maigne, Edgar Cyriax, James Cyriax and many others.

As a lecturer, he emphasized clinical examination and assessment. He stimulated students to write treatment records from the very beginning, as he felt that 'one needed to commit oneself to paper to analyse what one is doing'. In 1954 he started with manipulative therapy teaching sessions.

In 1961 he received an award from a special studies fund, which enabled him and his wife Anne to go overseas for a study tour. They visited osteopaths, chiropractors, medical doctors and physiotherapy colleagues whom they had heard and read about and corresponded with in the preceding years. In London, Geoff had interesting lunchtime clinical sessions and discussions with James Cyriax and his staff. From this tour G. D. Maitland established a friendship with Gregory P. Grieve from the UK. They had extensive correspondence about their clinical experiences and this continued for many years.

Maitland delivered a paper, in 1962, to the Physiotherapy Society of Australia entitled 'The Problems of Teaching Vertebral Manipulation', in which he presented a clear differentiation between manipulation and mobilization and became a strong advocate of the use of gentle passive movement in the treatment of pain, in addition to the more traditional forceful techniques used to increase range of motion. In this context it may be suitable to quote James Cyriax, a founder of orthopaedic medicine and of major influence on the development of manipulative therapy provided by physiotherapists:

> ... more recently Maitland, a physiotherapist from Australia, has been employing repetitive thrusts of lesser frequency but with more strength behind them. They are not identical with the mobilizing techniques that osteopaths misname 'articulation', nor are they as jerky a chiropractors' pressures. The great virtue of Maitland's work is its moderation. He has not expanded his manipulative techniques into a cult; he claims neither autonomic effects nor that they are a panacea. Indeed, he goes out of his way to avoid theoretical arguments and insists on the practical effect of manipulation .... The patient is examined at frequent intervals during the session, to enable the manipulator to assess the result of his treatment so far. He continues or alters his technique in accordance with the change, or absence of change, detected. These mobilizations clearly provide the

*physiotherapist with a useful addition to those of orthopaedic medicine and, better still, with an introduction to them. She gains confidence from using gentle manoeuvres and, if the case responds well . . . need seek no further.*

Cyriax J (1984) Textbook of Orthopaedic Medicine. Part II – Treatment by Manipulation, Massage and Injection. 11th Edition. (Ballière-Tindall, London. Pages 40–41)

G. D. Maitland became a substantial contributor to the *Australian Journal of Physiotherapy* as well as to other medical and physiotherapy journals worldwide. On the instigation of Monica Martin-Jones, OBE, a leader of the Chartered Society of Physiotherapy in Great Britain, Maitland was asked to publish his work, which resulted in the first edition of *Vertebral Manipulation* in 1964, which was followed by a second edition in 1968. The first edition of *Peripheral Manipulation* was published in 1970, in which the famous 'movement diagram' was introduced, an earlier co-production with Ms Jennifer Hickling in 1965.

Over all the years of lecturing and publishing, Maitland kept treating patients as the clinical work remained his main source of learning and adapting ideas. Geoff treated patients in his private practice for over 40 years and although he closed his practice in 1988, he remained active in treating patients until 1995.

In 1965, one of Maitland's wishes came true; with the help of Ms Elma Caseley, Head of the Physiotherapy School, South Australian Institute of Technology and the South Australian Branch of the Australian Physiotherapy Association, the first three months course on Manipulation of the Spine was held in Adelaide. In 1974 this course developed into the one year postgraduate education 'postgraduate diploma in manipulative physiotherapy' at the South Australian Institute of Technology, now a Masters degree course at the University of South Australia.

He was one of the co-founders, in 1974, of the International Federation of Orthopaedic Manual Therapy (IFOMT), a branch of the World Confederation of Physiotherapy (WCPT).

Only in 1978, while teaching one of his first courses in continental Europe in Bad Ragaz, Switzerland, did he recognize, through discussion with Dr Zinn, Director of the Medical Clinic and the Postgraduate Study Centre in Bad Ragaz, that in fact his work and ideas were a specific concept of thought and action rather than a method of applying manipulative techniques. The Maitland Concept of Manipulative Physiotherapy as it became known emphasizes a specific way of thinking, continuous evaluation and assessment and the art of manipulative physiotherapy ('know when, how and which techniques to perform, and adapt these to the individual situation of the patient') and a total commitment to the patient.

Maitland has held a long and extensive commitment to various professional associations:

- Australian Physiotherapy Association (APA) where he was on the State branch committee for 28 years in various capacities and a State Delegate to Federal Council for 11 years. In conjunction with others, he was responsible for the revision of the constitution of APA in 1964–1965 In 1977, he put forward a submission regarding Specialization in Manipulative Physiotherapy, a concept which was subsequently accepted in modified form.
- Inaugural President of the Australian College of Physiotherapists for six years and a member of the council for a further six years.
- Member of the Physiotherapy Registration Board of South Australia for 22 years.
- Chairman of the Expert Panel for Physiotherapy for Australian Examining Council for Overseas Physiotherapists (AECOP) for 11 years.
- Australian delegate to IFOMT for five years and a member of its academic standards committee for another five years.

For his work he was honoured with several awards:

- Member of the Order of the British Empire in 1981.
- Fellowship of the Australian College of Physiotherapists by Monograph in 1970, with a further Fellowship by specialization in 1984.
- Honorary Degree of Master of Applied Science in Physiotherapy from the University of South Australia in 1986.
- Honorary Fellow of the Chartered Society of Physiotherapy (GB).
- Honorary life memberships of the South African Society of Physiotherapy, including the Group of Manipulative Physiotherapy, Manipulative Physiotherapy Association of Australia (MPAA), Swiss Association of Manipulative Physiotherapy (SVOMP), German Association of Manual Therapy (DVMT) and the American Physical Therapy Association (APTA).
- He received an award from IFOMT in appreciation of his service and leadership from its foundation.
- Mildred Elson Award by the World Confederation of Physical Therapy (WCPT) for his life's work in 1995.

In 1992 in Zurzach, Switzerland, the International Maitland Teachers' Association (IMTA) was founded, of which G. D. Maitland is a founding member and inaugural President.

All this work would not have been possible without the loving support of his wife Anne, the mother of their two children John and Wendy. Anne did most of the graphic arts in Maitland's publications, kept notes, made manuscripts and videotaped many of his courses. Their continuous feedback discipline is one of the very strengths of the Maitlands, who are practically inseparable since they met in England during the second World War. Anne was awarded the protectoress of the Dutch Association of Orthopaedic Manipulative Therapy (NVOMT).

Maitland's work, especially through the mode of thinking and the process of continuous assessment, has laid the foundation for the development of contemporary definitions and descriptions of the physiotherapy process.

Within this context it seems suitable to conclude with a quote from Professor Lance Twomey, Vice Chancellor, Professor of Physiotherapy, Curtin University of Technology, Perth, Australia:

> . . . Maitland's emphasis on very careful and comprehensive examination leading to the precise application of treatment by movement and followed in turn by the assessment of the effects of that movement on the patient, form the basis for the modern clinical approach. This is probably as close to the scientific method as is possible within the clinical practice of physical therapy and serves as a model for other special areas of the profession.
>
> Foreword in Refshauge K & Gass E (1995) *Musculoskeletal Physiotherapy*. Butterworth-Heinemann, Oxford. Page IX

Earlier in 1987, Twomey, having suggested Maitland should write about his contribution said:

> In my view, the Maitland approach to treatment differs from others, not in the mechanics of the technique, but rather in its approach to the patient and his particular problem. Your attention to detail in examination, treatment and response is unique in physical therapy, and I believe is worth spelling out in some detail:
>
> - the development of your concepts of assessment and treatment;
> - your insistence on sound foundations of basic biological knowledge;
> - the necessity for high levels of skill;
> - the evolution of the concepts. It did not 'come' to you fully developed, but is a living thing, developing and extending;
> - the necessity for detailed examination and for the examination/treatment/re-examination approach.

This area is well worth very considerable attention because, to me, it is the essence of 'Maitland'.

Twomey, L. T. and Taylor, J. R. (1987) The Maitland Concept: Assessment, Examination, and Treatment by Passive Movement. Eds *Physical Therapy of the Lower Back*. Churchill Livingstone.

Elly Hengeveld
Kay English
Kevin Banks

# Glossary

**ACCESSORY MOVEMENTS**. (a) Passive accessory intervertebral movements, PAIVM; (b) Passive intercostal movements, PAICM.

**ASSESSMENT**. This term has three definitions:

1. Assessment of the findings of the examination of a patient which gives the examiner the information required to make a diagnosis. Some countries use the term EVALUATION for this aspect.

2. Assessment of the changes which take place as a result of the use of a technique, to prove the effect of the technique on the disorder: also to determine the effect of the treatment techniques and the treatment sessions on the disorder.

3. ANALYTICAL assessment is an assessment made during treatment or at the conclusion of treatment. It takes into account all details of the patient's past and present history, the diagnostic details and the responses to the different treatments which will have been administered. This collection of information is analysed so as to allow understanding of the likely future of the patient's disorder.

**ASTERISKS**. The use of asterisks in the recording of each patient's examination findings and treatment effects has only one purpose; it is to *highlight* the main elements found. Their use saves recording time and makes the therapist quickly aware of essential points when making assessments.

**COMPRESSION**. This is the approximation of opposing joint surfaces, either in a position or during a movement, to assess the source of symptoms and to be used as a treatment technique.

**DIFFERENTIATION**. This applies to examination procedures that assess which joint or structure is the source of symptoms when more than one joint or structure is involved in a movement.

**DISORDERS**. Because a specific diagnosis is an area of determination which is frequently very difficult to make, the descriptive term such as 'the patient's disorder' is used in many places in the text of this book. The reason for using such a term is deliberate; it is meant to leave the reader's mind free to absorb the other essentials of the associated text. The alternative is to talk in diagnostic terms, but this can become counterproductive by clouding the impact of the related text thus losing the key of that related text.

**EVALUATION**. This term is not used in the text of this book, but it is understood to mean a form of Assessment (*see* Assessment).

**GRADES OF MOVEMENT**. See Movement.

**HYPERMOBILITY**. See Instability. Hyper-mobility is an excessive range of movement (examples being hyperextension of the elbow or knee) for which there is complete muscular control thus providing stability.

**INSTABILITY**. This term is used only to mean an excessive range of abnormal movement for which there is no protective muscular control.

**IRRITABILITY**. Irritability means that a little activity causes a lot of pain that takes a relatively long time to settle. In many cases this is an indication that caution is required during examination and treatment procedures.

1. Its susceptibility to become painful.
2. How painful it becomes.
3. The length of time this pain takes to recover (*see* pages 5, 116–117).

**JOINT**. This word refers to all the intra-articular structures, the capsule and all the non-contractile tissues that move during every passive and active movement. INTRA-ARTICULAR refers to the structure(s) (a) from the subchondral bone to the subchondral bone of adjacent joint surfaces, and (b) including everything within the joint space, including the inner capsule. PERI-ARTICULAR refers to structures outside the joint, adjacent to and including the outer capsule.

**LATENT PAIN**. See Pain.

**LIST**. See Protective Deformity.

**MANIPULATION**. This term is used in two distinct ways:

1. It can be used loosely to refer to any kind of 'passive movement' used in examination or treatment (*see* Passive Movement, and Mobilization).
2. In a restricted definition, it is used to mean a small-amplitude rapid movement (not necessarily performed at the limit of a range of movement), which the patient cannot prevent taking place.

**MANIPULATIVE PHYSIOTHERAPISTS**. This term includes manual therapists, clinicians and therapists.

**MOBILIZATION**. This is another 'passive movement' but its rhythm (*see* pages 5, 176, 179) and grade (*see* pages 5, 176) are such that the patient (or model) can prevent its being performed.

**MOVEMENT**. This is synonymous with the term MOTION which is used in some English-speaking countries. GRADES OF MOVEMENT: RHYTHMS OF MOVEMENT: These two terms serve only one purpose, that is they describe in an abbreviated form the quality of passive treatment movement being used. The terms are not essential to the practice of passive movement treatment, they are merely used as a means of quick recording and communication.

**MOVEMENT DIAGRAMS**. These are explained in detail in the appendices. They are not essential to the practice of treatment. They do, however, have the distinct advantage of forcing the therapist to analyse what she finds when passively moving a joint. Thus they are a self-learning process, a teaching medium and a means of communication.

**NATURE OF A DISORDER**. This refers to aspects of a problem that require consideration in examination and treatment procedures. It may include the pathobiological processes underlying the disorder, contributing factors such as osteoporosis, stage of healing, stage and stability of the disorder, and certain personal features such as the fear of moving.

**NEURAL MOVEMENTS**. This term is still not clearly defined, and is an unfortunate term because it can be misunderstood and provide fuel for the disbelievers. It refers to nerves and their infrastructure as well as to the connective tissue that supports them and through which they pass:

1. Vertebral canal
   a) dura
   b) other meninges
2. Foraminal canal
3. Peripheral tissues
   a) nerves
   b) interstitial tissues
   c) supportive tissues
   d) osseofibrous tunnels, etc.
4. Upper limb tension tests, ULTT. This is the commonly used term, but can be confused with other structures' tests involving movements. At this stage it would be better and more accepted by medical practitioners if 'upper limb neural movement tests' or 'upper limb neural tests', ULNT, were used.

**OVER-PRESSURE**. Every joint has a passive range of motion, which exceeds its active range. Further normal movement can be added to this passive range by a stretching application of over-pressure. This over-pressure range can cause a degree of discomfort or pain, and should be assessed before declaring a joint movement to be normal.

**PAIN**. This is used in this book to represent many kinds of pain and even includes other sensations such as discomfort, awareness of, abnormality, heaviness, etc. LATENT PAIN, of which there are many presentations (*see* pages 166, 167, 190–192), refers to pain and the other sensations which do not come on immediately a movement occurs, but rather occur at varying times after the movement, or after a position is sustained. REFERRED PAIN: any pain, discomfort or other sensation which is felt at a place which is *distant* from its source. RADICULAR PAIN: this is a term related to a referred pain which is generally recognized (rightly or wrongly) to be a clearly defined area related to a nerve root. THROUGH-RANGE PAIN: this is a pain which is first felt very early in an available range of movement and which continues until the limit of the range is reached. END OF RANGE PAIN: this differs from the above in that the pain is felt only when a movement has reached, or almost reached, its limit of range. An AFTER EFFECT is quite common, and if present is indicative of a disc disorder. What is meant by the 'after effect' is that, having performed activities in an unfavourable manner, the patient may not be aware of its having any effect BUT will know all about it by the following morning.

**PASSIVE MOVEMENT**. Any movement of a mobile segment which is produced by any means other than the particular muscles related to that particular segment's movement is a passive movement. It includes both mobilization and manipulation.

**PHYSIOLOGICAL MOVEMENTS**. These are active and passive functional movements. Passive physiological intervertebral movement (or inter-segmental movements) is abbreviated to PPIVM.

**PRODUCE/REPRODUCE**. The aim of physical examination is to provoke, with test movements, either an abnormal response in an appropriate site or, when suited to the disorder, reproduction of the symptoms.

**PROTECTIVE DEFORMITY**. A common 'protective deformity' in the cervical spine is the 'WRY NECK', and in the lumbar spine is a 'SCIATIC SCOLIOSIS'. SCIATIC SCOLIOSIS is an inexact term because the scoliosis (protective deformity) can occur without 'sciatic' pain. Better terms are LIST or SHIFT (*see* pages 131–132 and 350).

**RADICULAR PAIN**. See Pain.

**REFERRED PAIN**. See Pain.

**SCIATIC SCOLIOSIS**. See Protective Deformity.

**SEVERITY**. A symptom is defined as severe if the activity that causes the pain needs to be interrupted and stopped because of the intensity of the pain. In many cases this is an indication that caution is needed with examination and treatment procedures.

**SHIFT**. See Protective Deformity.

# Chapter 1

# Introduction

Manipulation is NOT, as many would have us believe, an 'empirical' treatment. This is largely due to advances in modern technology, particularly with the capabilities of modern computers. Although most authors on the subject describe techniques and techniques only, the *concept* of this book is aligned with the following quotation:

> *Despite its pathology often being something of a 'black box', much can be done to alleviate the distress. Manipulative therapists usually approach the treatment of low back pain by observing the outputs (signs and symptoms) of the 'black box', then carefully and methodically applying their skills (inputs), to bring about a favourable outcome. The hypothesis of what happens inside the 'black box' becomes less relevant except in those instances where reliable pathological data exists.*
> (*Low Back Pain. Prevention, Treatment, Research Symposium*, The Manipulative Physiotherapists' Association of Australia (MPAA), March, 1984)

**Although this book is oriented almost entirely to treatment by manipulation (i.e. passive movement), it** **does not mean that that manipulation is 'the be all and end all' in the overall management of patients with vertebral disorders**. However, the scope of application and the skills of manipulation are *not* sufficiently well appreciated by many doctors and physiotherapists. It is important, therefore, that manipulation should be given extra emphasis so that the appropriate readers, the teachers and the users, will use manipulation in its proper context and to its fullest extent.

Manipulation is not like a game of golf (*Figure 1.1*) where the player uses a technique to hit a ball in the direction he wants it to go, although most people tend to use techniques of manipulation in this way.

Manipulation is more like a game of chess (*Figure 1.2*) where different 'pieces' can be moved in many different and specific ways, and where plans are made and destroyed and changed until the goal is achieved.

An even better analogy is the game of Contract Bridge (*Figure 1.3*). Here *communication*, in the 'bidding', plays an important role, as also does the assessment of where important key cards are likely to be. In the game, the technique of playing the cards requires

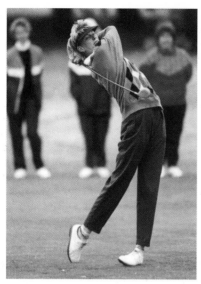

Figure 1.1 The technique of golf

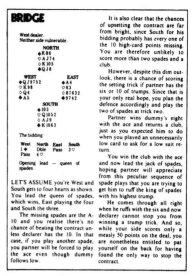

Figure 1.3 Contract Bridge

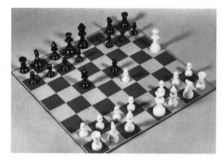

Figure 1.2 Chess

considered, thoughtful planning. Each facet is important to the whole, and each needs to be integrated with the others with knowledge, skill and experience.

The 'concept', as it has come to be known, of manipulative treatment embraced in this text is based, subject of course to diagnosis, upon the symptom response (its site, its quality and its behaviour) to movements and positions. It is the movement/pain response that is half of the concept's keystone, the other half being analytical assessment. It is the analytical assessment that reveals the changes in the pain/movement responses during treatment.

Keystones of the 'concept':

- Assessment
- Movement/pain response and its adaptation in treatment to the patient's current episode
- Specific mode of thinking when dealing with a given diagnosis

The growth and expansion of manipulation within routine orthodox medical care is most encouraging for the patient, particularly as government-accredited postgraduate courses are conducted in manipulative physiotherapy, and also as there is now a 'specialty qualification' within the physiotherapy profession in Australia. Even the word 'manipulation' is accepted by more medical practitioners. This greater awareness of the place of manipulation within the conservative management of patients with neuromusculoskeletal disorders has come about by a growth in the skills and the application of them, together with a growth in the ability to relate the prognosis to the degree of the patient's disability.

There are three main features about the ways in which manipulation is performed today that have made for its more ready acceptance:

1. The realization by the medical profession of the emphasis the manipulative physiotherapist places on the **continuous analytical assessment** before, during and after the application of each technique during each treatment session, from session to session throughout treatment, and when treatment is discontinued.

2. The gentleness of the initial treatment techniques, with stronger techniques being used only when the initial techniques have been progressed gradually and judiciously.

3. The demonstrable effect of such treatment and the refined information it can provide in terms of differential diagnosis and prognosis.

The increasing acceptance of manipulation is due to:

- Continuous analytical assessment
- Gentleness of initial treatment techniques
- Effects of the treatment which can give refinement to differential diagnosis and prognosis

The general acceptance of manipulation has nevertheless been slow, and manipulation is still far from being used to its fullest potential. There are two reasons for this. First, the diagnostic titles used by some manipulators, on which they have based their manipulative treatment, are unacceptable to the majority of the medical profession. The second reason is that some manipulations have been performed injudiciously, resulting in disasters – the literature provides the evidence. However, such incidents should be seen in their right context. To quote Brewerton (1964):

> Despite the worry of these cases, they must be kept in proportion; it is easy to sympathize with the argument that only five such cases appeared in the American literature over a period of 10 years. During this time there were 16 000 manipulators working regularly in the country who could be relied upon to manipulate at least one neck each day; and this would make an incidence of 1 in 10 000 000 manipulations.

More than 40 years on, this is still relatively unchanged.
    Disasters can be avoided by adhering to the following three rules:

1.  Continuous analytical assessment must be carried out during the performance of a technique and throughout treatment.
2.  The initial application of a technique must be gentle.
3.  The symptomatic responses, both during and after application of treatment, must be assessed and analysed before progressing. There must be an awareness of latent exacerbations that were not evident at the time of the initial consultation and must be clarified before selecting treatment techniques.

Before embarking on the 'concept' of manipulative treatment, which this book aims to describe, there are terms related to the word 'manipulation' which require clarification.

## PASSIVE MOVEMENT

**Passive movement** means any movement of any part of one person which is performed on that person by another person or piece of equipment. Passive movement may refer to the joint's accessory movements or its physiological movements. **Physiological movements** are those movements that patients can perform actively by themselves; **accessory movements** are those movements of their joints that individuals cannot perform actively, but which can be performed on them by another person. For example, it is impossible to rotate any interphalangeal joint actively, but it can be rotated by somebody else. Therefore, rotation of the interphalangeal joint is an accessory movement for that joint. Any of these movements can be performed slowly or at speed, gently or vigorously and through large or small amplitudes and still be called passive movements.

Passive movement may refer to the joints' accessory or physiological movement

## MANIPULATION

The word 'manipulation' can be used in many ways. Medically, it can be used loosely to mean passive movement of any kind. There are English dictionary definitions of manipulation, and medical dictionary definitions. Medical definitions vary from practitioner to practitioner and from school to school. Manipulation, mobilization and passive movement can be, and often are, used synonymously. Nevertheless, the manipulative physiotherapist is in a position to suggest precise definitions for terms used. In this book, the word 'manipulation' will be used in two ways:

1.  As a general term to cover any form of passive movement technique of any structure as a form of treatment for neuromusculoskeletal disorders. In this use it will cover all forms of passive movement listed above, as well as the specific definition of manipulation which follows.

2.  A technique performed at a *speed* such that it has taken place before the person on whom it is performed is able to prevent it is a *manipulative* technique. Such techniques are often gentle, always small in range, and rarely forceful (*see* Preface to First Edition).

The term manipulation embraces all kinds of passive movement, or can be viewed more specifically as a small amplitude manipulative thrust technique performed with speed

## MOBILIZATION

Mobilization is passive movement performed in such a manner (particularly in relation to the speed of the movement) that it is at all times within the ability of the patient to prevent the movement if he or she so chooses (*see* Preface to First Edition).

> Mobilizations are performed in such a manner that they can be prevented by the patient

The two types of mobilization are:

1.  Passive movements performed for the purpose of relieving pain and restoring full-range, pain-free, functional movements. These are of two kinds:
    a) **Passive oscillatory movements** performed slowly (one in 2 seconds) or quickly (three per second), smoothly or staccato, with small or large amplitude, and applied in any part of the total range of movement. These movements may be performed while the joint surfaces are distracted or compressed. Distraction is the separation of opposing joint surfaces and compression is the approximation, or squeezing together, of the opposing joint surfaces.
    b) **Sustained stretching** passive movements may be performed with tiny amplitude oscillations at the limit of the range.
2.  Passive movements performed for the purpose of maintaining a functional range of movement in patients who are unconscious or who have an active joint disease such as rheumatoid arthritis.

> Passive movements serve different purposes, for example relieving pain or restoring full-range and pain-free functional movement.
> They can be performed in an oscillatory manner or as sustained stretching

## MANIPULATIVE THERAPY

When people talk about 'manipulative treatment' it seems impossible to avoid the problem of their putting inordinate emphasis on the techniques, even comparing those used by different practitioners and authors. This is most unfortunate, because it prevents their seeing the *whole picture* of a treatment concept. Even surveys or research projects sometimes miss the point when trying to weigh up the value of a particular group of techniques. It is because of this misconception that this introductory chapter sets out to explain the concept of total management, with the techniques and their adaptability being given their correct relationship to the whole. In fact, the concept places great emphasis on pain and other allied symptoms. This emphasis is explained, together with the other aspects of the concept, under the separate headings that follow.

## THE RELATIONSHIP BETWEEN TECHNIQUES AND ASSESSMENT

Manipulative treatment can be divided into four main parts:

1.  Examination of the patient
2.  Mode of thinking and planning
3.  Treatment techniques
4.  Assessment.

Omitting the 'mode of thinking' part at this stage of discussion, the first feature of the 'concept' relates to understanding the relative importance that the parts of manipulative treatment bear to each other. Though skill in each area is important, the degree of the skill required for each is not equivalent. Every manipulative physiotherapist must always remember that the *best* treatment cannot be given without perfectly performed examination and treatment techniques. However, techniques are the least important of all the parts. **Continuous analytical assessment** heavily outweighs the others. Those who seek to copy any particular person's techniques, merely to use them on their patients, has a totally wrong idea of manipulative treatment, and anyone conducting courses that consist mainly of techniques should be vigorously censured.

These four parts, along with years of conscious experience and learning based on the mode of thinking and assessment, combine to provide effective and informative treatment.

The four main areas are depicted in *Figure 1.4* to demonstrate their relative importance to each other.

Manipulative treatment should never be administered without accurate examination (which involves both mental and manual skills). Without accurate examination, precise assessment is not possible.

**Assessment** involves evaluating the changes in the patient's symptoms and movement signs that occur as a result of the treatment technique(s), and it is this assessment that is the keystone of informative treatment. Assessment (discussed in full on pp. 53–83) is not an easy skill to master, and it is the area where most manipulators lose their effectiveness in treatment and their value in making prognoses.

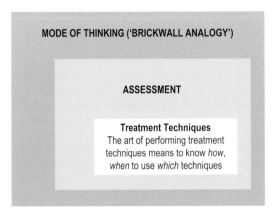

MODE OF THINKING ('BRICKWALL ANALOGY')

**ASSESSMENT**

**Treatment Techniques**
The art of performing treatment
techniques means to know *how*,
*when* to use *which* techniques

**Figure 1.4** The relative importance of treatment techniques, examination of the patient, assessment and the mode of thinking

## TECHNIQUES

Treatment techniques are discussed in relation to their importance, and to the fact that some people are always looking for new techniques rather than understanding how and when they should be modified and used. *Figure 1.4* demonstrates the relevance of techniques in relation to the total concept of treatment.

Techniques, as they apply to the concept proposed in this book, are never ending and they never will have an ending. So long as patients present with different symptoms and examination signs, there will have to be changes in techniques to free the patients of those symptoms.

Cyriax (1978a) said that the mobilization techniques included in the text of this book were first practised in France (Recamier, 1838), and it is certain that the 'bonesetters' of centuries ago (Cyriax, 1978b) have also practised them. We must always acknowledge that 'there is no new thing under the sun' (Ecclesiastes 1:9), and that all we do is 'walk the road made by another' (Chinese proverb).

If records of all the different techniques that have been described over the centuries were piled one atop another, the height of the pile would be astounding. Even then, all the possibilities would not have been exhausted. There is an immeasurable number of different techniques, and each one has an inexhaustible number of variations.

It has sometimes been said during a demonstration treatment of a patient, 'You didn't teach us that technique last year'. The reply has sometimes been, 'I couldn't, I've never done it like this before'. This is because the technique has been (and must always be) adapted to suit the examination findings.

Although there are basic techniques that must be taught, the **concept** is that manipulative physiotherapists' minds must be so open that they modify their technique until they achieve their intention. The basic treatment techniques must include every movement of which a structure is capable, the physiological movements and the accessory movements, plus all possible combinations. When it comes to selecting the technique for treatment, it is first necessary to know the passive movements or positions that provoke or relieve the patient's symptoms. When the symptoms are easily reproduced, the **technique** chosen may be either the movement that relieves the symptoms or the movement that provokes the symptoms. This choice depends on the 'nature' of the disorder, the 'severity' of the symptoms and the 'irritability' of the disorder!

### A technique is the brainchild of ingenuity

There are no set or invariable techniques; statements such as 'you must *never* do it this way' or 'you must *never* do that' have no place in our thinking or teaching. The only MUST is that the technique *must* achieve its intention, both while it is being performed and when it has been performed. Therapists' minds must always be open; *they must never be dogmatic.*

Primarily, the 'concept' demands knowing how to relate the rhythm, the speed, the position in the range, the amplitude and the strength of the technique to the examination findings.

Because the style of movement that can be used as a treatment technique can be of different amplitudes and in different parts of the available range, GRADES OF MOVEMENT become essential to the concept. They are essential for three reasons:

1. They form the best basis for teaching and communication.
2. They force the manipulator to think in much finer detail about the technique being performed.
3. They form an essential method of abbreviation when recording treatment. Their use saves time and they also, in forcing the manipulative physiotherapist to commit the technique to paper, make the therapist analyse the technique much more clearly.

Grades of movement are essential:

- As a basis for teaching and communication
- For detailed thinking about the technique and for assessing progress
- In recording treatment

THE RHYTHM OF THE TECHNIQUE is another factor to be considered in relation to a passive movement treatment technique. For the patient who has a very painful disorder, it is likely that physical examination will reveal a pain-through-range situation. Under these circumstances, the technique will need to be performed:

- slowly and smoothly
- probably in either the painless range available, or
- taking the movement into only a small degree of discomfort, certainly not into pain.

This brings us to the next factor to be considered in relation to a technique. Where should the slow, smooth technique be performed? If we consider the very painful disorder, it should initially be performed in as large a range of movement as is possible without the patient being able to feel any discomfort whatsoever. At the other end of the scale, if the patient has a chronic disorder which is only provoked by movement at the end-of-range stretch position, it will probably require a stretching, end-of-range, small amplitude movement, performed, perhaps, as a staccato rhythm. The movement would be considerably faster than the smooth, slow technique suggested above. This means that the technique (whether a palpatory type of direct technique or an indirect [localized] technique) would aim to be fast enough to make the spinal segment being treated reach its end-of-range position before the adjacent segments begin their movement.

> The rhythm in which the technique is performed is essential for the quality of the technique. It may vary from 'gentle–smooth' to 'stretching–staccato', depending on the clinical condition of the patient

When performing any technique, manipulative physiotherapists must become as intimately involved with what they are doing as do soloists performing with an orchestra and its conductor's interpretation of the concerto, which is the brainchild of the composer.

## THE MODE OF THINKING: THE PRIMACY OF CLINICAL EVIDENCE

### DEALING WITH PROBLEMS OF DIAGNOSIS (THE 'BRICK WALL')

The problems associated with diagnosis and **diagnostic titles** are difficult problems with which to come to terms. Even within medicine, many diagnostic titles are sometimes inadequate, incorrect, or may be merely linked with patterns of symptomatology; they may even be based on suppositions. In relation to treatment, many *medical* treatments are initially administered empirically; only later, as the science of medicine catches up, does the theory become known.

Within medicine today there is much that is clearly known and understood. There is also much that is being discovered day by day as science progresses, and there is still much that is as yet unknown. Also, there is a related facet that must be considered – there is much we THINK we know; yet as medical science progresses, the thought may be proved wrong. A perfect example of this is the changing knowledge of the neuro-physiology of pain, as is evidenced in the 'gate theory'. Another area of difficulty is indicated in *Gray's Anatomy*:

> the detailed mechanics of many individual joints still await resolution.

These facts alone demand that one should not be dogmatic or rigid in one's thinking when examining, treating, or making judgements about patients. In addition to the things we know and the things we think we know, there are things about which we can make speculations or suggest a hypothesis.

In summary then:

1. There is much we *do* know.
2. There is much we *think* we know.
3. There is much more we do *not* know.
4. We can make *speculations*.
5. We can propose *hypotheses*.

The four main areas of medical knowledge that are particularly applicable to treatment by manipulative physiotherapy are anatomy, physiology, biomechanics and pathology. In all of these, scientific investigation continues to make discoveries. All of the four areas of medical knowledge contain elements of knowns and unknowns, speculations and hypotheses. A diagnosis is arrived at by relating the clinical examination of a patient to the knowledge in these four main areas of medical knowledge.

It is sometimes difficult to relate a patient's history and the examination findings to a precise and meaningful **diagnosis**, as well as arriving at a clear understanding of both the state and stage of pathological changes and the relevant biomechanical implications. An example of this is given by Macnab (1971). Of 842 patients operated on for disc pathology, 68 were found during surgical exploration to have discs that were not abnormal in the way anticipated. As a result of this series of patients, five reasons other than disc herniation were determined for these patients' symptoms. This example means that a patient who on clinical examination presents with a set of symptoms and

Table 1.1    A single clinical presentation may have several diagnostic titles

| Diagnostic title | Clinical presentation |
|---|---|
| One-disc herniation<br>Macnab two<br>Macnab three<br>Macnab four<br>Macnab five<br>Macnab six | History (H)<br>Symptoms (S)<br>and Signs (S) |

Table 1.2    A single diagnostic title may mean several clinical presentations

| Diagnostic title | Clinical presentation | | |
|---|---|---|---|
| | $H_1$ | $S_1$ | $S_1$ |
| 'Disc herniation with nerve | $H_2$ | $S_2$ | $S_2$ |
| root irritation' | $H_3$ | $S_3$ | $S_3$ |
| | $H_4$ | $S_4$ | $S_4$ |

signs indicating nerve root irritation may have a disorder with one of at least six different diagnostic titles (*Table 1.1*).

The problem also occurs in the reverse order. That is, a patient who has a disorder that is diagnosed as 'disc herniation with nerve root irritation' may present clinically with one of many different sets of symptoms and signs and with one of many patterns of onset of the symptoms (*Table 1.2*).

It becomes apparent that if one is to base treatment on diagnosis alone, one must be aware of the real difficulties associated with making it precise and therefore meaningful. So, what can the physiotherapist rely on? It is usually possible to determine:

- that no *disease* process is involved; and
- whether there is a physical neuromusculo-skeletal problem present that may be suitable for treatment by a physiotherapist using passive movement.

Within this context the manipulative physiotherapist, understanding the pathological and biomechanical changes that may be present, is able to base treatment techniques, and subsequent changes to them, on analytical assessment of changes in the patient's symptoms and signs. Bearing this in mind, while also remembering the limitations of our scientific knowledge, it is helpful for the physiotherapist to split the thinking process into two compartments (*Table 1.3*); that is, one part comes under the general heading, 'theoretical and speculative', and the other under the general heading 'history and clinical presentation'.

Table 1.3    Division of thinking in diagnosis and the clinical presentation to the physiotherapist

| Theoretical/speculative | | | Clinical presentation |
|---|---|---|---|
| Anatomy<br>Physiology<br>Biomechanics<br>Pathology | Known<br>Thought<br>known<br>Unknown<br>Speculation<br>Hypothesis | Diagnostic<br>title | History<br>Symptoms<br>Signs |

There are three important reasons for employing this feature of two-compartment thinking:

1. It enables manipulative treatment to be used, even if the diagnosis is not precise, provided it is known that the symptoms are arising from a neuromuscu-loskeletal disorder and not from serious pathology.

2. It makes possible the use of manipulation and analytical assessment to assist differential diagnoses.

3. It enables the referring doctors and the physiotherapists to discuss their ideas on how manipulation works, without the speculations or hypotheses being interpreted as dogmatic certainties. It is essential that there should always be unrestricted avenues for discussion. This will lead to better surveys and research programmes being conducted. The liaison between the two compartments, the clinical compartment and the theoretical compartment, is vital for the growth of useful knowledge. Clinicians may speculate and hypothesize, while theoretical practitioners are often too far removed from the clinical situation to assist them. It can also be harmful when clinicians believe their hypotheses dogmatically.

There is considerable space for error in the theoretical compartment, whereas there can be no errors in the clinical compartment other than those caused by the examiner's lack of skill. Seldom do examination findings belie the patient's true physical condition. For a theoretical statement to be correct, it must fit the clinical situation. If it does not fit, it is the theoretical statement that must be wrong because the clinical presentation cannot be wrong.

This separating of one's mental processes into two linked compartments is commonly referred to metaphorically as the 'symbolic semi-permeable brick wall'. The dividing line between the 'theoretical/speculative' compartment and the 'clinical' compartment is the 'brick wall'. It is not a solid wall; it has many

**Table 1.4** The 'permeable brick wall'

| Theoretical/speculative | Clinical presentation |
| --- | --- |
| Diagnostic title | History, Symptoms and Signs |

openings to allow thoughts to flow from one compartment to the other (*Table 1.4*).

## THEORY

*Table 1.3* illustrates the relationship between the 'theoretical' knowledge and the 'clinical' knowledge. The next feature of the **concept** of this text rests with the statement, 'We must not get diverted by the theoretical aspects of a patient's disorder such that it is to the detriment of the clinical aspect'. There is still an enormous amount we do not know, and the theory must be seen in a balanced way. Two examples follow. The first emphasizes excessive attention being focused on the radiographs and not relating these findings to the history of a woman's symptoms (6 weeks). The second example demonstrates how the **theoretical implications** of a cervical radiograph may not fit the **clinical situation**.

> The 'symbolic semi-permeable brick wall' is a model that guides physiotherapists in their mode of thinking. In this way they can keep their thoughts, reflections, impressions, hypotheses and knowledge in two separate but independent compartments. At the same time information should be free to flow from one side to the other. One compartment should contain all theoretical information, known and speculative, including the precautions and possible contraindications for treatment. The other compartment should contain all the clinical evidence (history, signs and symptoms) to be assessed and evaluated. The advantage of thinking in this way is that theoretical knowledge does not have to limit or bias clinical thinking

### Example A – shoulder

A 74-year-old healthy woman, because of 'shoulder weakness and discomfort', had been unable either to comb her hair or reach far enough behind her back to do up her brassiere for 6 weeks. She was told that the only options open to her were 'major surgery' or to 'put up with it'. She refused surgery, preferring to put up with it. Because her sister, who 'had had exactly the same problem', was 'cured by physiotherapy', she pressed for the same treatment. The diagnosis was

'marked osteoarthritis'. She certainly did have gross joint changes, which were obvious both clinically and radiologically. Physically, she had a 35 per cent reduction in range, pain on stretching, and considerable painless dry crepitus during active movements. When moved passively with the glenohumeral joint surfaces compressed, crepitus was increased and discomfort (not pain) was provoked. Prior to the onset of symptoms 6 weeks previously, although she knew she had an arthritic shoulder, she did not consider she had any real disability. The 'major surgery' option was based on the radiological findings, which were interpreted academically. It would be unrealistic to think that these radiological changes could have occurred over the 6-week period, and in fact they were more likely to be very long-standing although her symptoms were relatively recent. On clinical examination, her problem was an 'end-of-range' problem rather than a 'through-range' (gross osteoarthritis) problem. Her shoulder responded quite satisfactorily to mobilization, regaining its pre-exacerbation state.

### Example B – cervical spine

*Figure 1.5* shows the radiograph of the cervical spine of a woman aged 73 years, who had neck symptoms following a fall 3 weeks previously. She had not had any neck symptoms, not even one day of neck stiffness, prior to this incident. She also responded very favourably to passive movement treatment. This must mean that a person can develop gross radiological changes and have no pain. Conversely, it can also be said that a person can have severe symptoms without having any radiological changes.

> A person can have gross radiological changes but have no pain and the converse is also true

The cervical spine report was as follows:

*The cervical spine is curved convex to the right. There is quite marked anterior angulation at C4–5 with slight anterior subluxation of C4 on C5. With flexion there is also anterior subluxation of C3 on C4. There is narrowing of all the intervertebral disc spaces below C2, but this is most pronounced at C5–6 and C6–7. Osteoarthritic changes are evident in the uncovertebral joints below the level of C2 bilaterally. There is encroachment on the intervertebral foramina on the left side at C2–3, C3–4 and C4–5, C5–6. There is some asymmetry of the superior facet of C2; this is particularly accounted for by rotation*

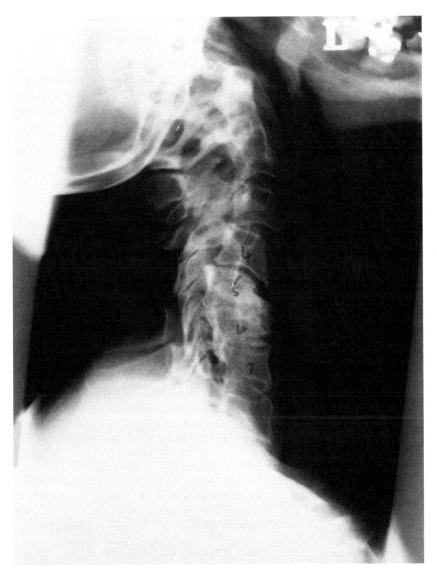

Figure 1.5  Radiograph of cervical spine in Example B. *Cervical spine*

*and the curvature of the cervical spine.* Impression: *Severe degenerative changes in the cervical spine as described. Was there any previous injury?*

## APPROPRIATE WORDING

To *speak* or *write* in *wrong* terms means to *think* in *wrong* terms.

The plan of relating theoretical knowledge to a patient's presenting symptoms and signs places another *demand* on the manipulative physiotherapist, who must employ a special pattern of thinking which requires very careful selection of the words and phrases used when speaking or recording in writing. The phraseology one uses shows clearly the way one is thinking, and therefore if, for example, the spoken phrases are collated wrongly, the thinking behind them must also be wrong.

> It is essential to select the appropriate wording, as this will influence the thinking process of the physiotherapist

A simple example may help to make this point clear. Imagine a physiotherapist presenting a patient, Mr X., at a clinical seminar. The patient, on being asked to demonstrate his **area of pain**, places his hand over the sacroiliac joint. The physiotherapist may, in ensuing discussion, refer to Mr X's 'sacroiliac pain'. To be true to the concept – that is, to be true to the separated 'theoretical/speculative' and 'clinical presentation' compartments – she should say 'pain *in this area*' while demonstrating on her own body. To have used the words 'sacroiliac pain' indicates that she COULD be thinking that the pain IS caused by some disorder of the sacroiliac joint. Obviously it does not mean that she MUST be thinking this way, but it does mean that she COULD, and is in fact highly likely to, be thinking this way. If, on the other hand, she refers to 'pain in this area', it is quite impossible for her to be thinking that the pain IS caused by a disorder of the sacroiliac joint. And this is the important element, and an essential one of the concept.

Many readers may believe that attention to this kind of detail is quite unnecessary. Quite the opposite is true: if the correct choice of words is made with care and with the right pattern in mind, then the thinking process must be right. And when this is so, the whole process of examination, treatment and interpretation must be the best that is possible.

A second example concerns a student being questioned by her teacher following the student's examination of a patient. The student has found that the patient's left buttock and posterolateral thigh pain are provoked by left lateral flexion and extension, and that on forward flexion he feels an arc of central back pain with a simultaneous arc of contralateral list. In the standing position, the left buttock pain is reproduced by rotation of the trunk to the left when it is performed in a position of roughly 30° of trunk flexion. The ranges of both straight leg raising and the slump test are normal, and there are no neurological changes. Gentle PA pressure on both L4 and L5 provoke deep central back pain.

One of the questions the student may be asked by the teacher is, 'What do you think is wrong with the patient?' If the teaching is oriented around diagnosis and pathology, the answer might be something like this:

A1.   The L4/5 intervertebral disc is bulging posteriorly on the left side, causing irritation of the fifth lumbar nerve root.

This demonstrates a very limited approach. The next question might be: 'What would you do in an attempt to make him better?'.

A2.   I would use movements to try to centralize the disc lesion and reduce the bulge.

If the same question were asked of an exponent of the 'concept' of the text, the student would answer in this fashion to question 1:

A1.   He has referred non-radicular pain in his left buttock and posterolateral thigh, which is linked with his arc of contralateral list on forward flexion.

And the answer to question 2 would be:

A2.   I would initially use painless passive movement techniques in an effort to improve his arc on flexion, and improve ranges of left lateral flexion and rotation. At the same time I would hope for a reduction in the severity of the referred pain. Continual assessment will provide me with the answer. If my thoughts in relation to the phase and present stability of the disorder are correct, I will probably finish up with movement techniques which move into provoking directions.

## LISTENING

It is extraordinary how often doctors and physiotherapists (in fact all people who deal with people) do not listen, nor listen carefully enough, nor listen sensitively enough, nor listen at sufficient depth, to their patients.

*Listening is itself, of course, an art: that is where it differs from merely hearing. Hearing is passive; listening is active. Hearing is involuntary; listening demands attention. Hearing is natural; listening is an acquired discipline.*   (The Age, 21 August 1982)

There is so much to learn about patients' problems, if only we will listen. This is especially relevant when it is believed that the patients' bodies can tell them things that we can only discover by listening to their comments. Our minds have to be free flowing, able to be directed, redirected or influenced by subtle comments that the patient may make as a passing remark. We must be good listeners, and we must *believe* patients' subtle comments or remarks. Also, when such a remark has been made, which influences our thinking, the relevance of the remark must be confirmed by asking other related questions. It is totally unfair to patients to make academic judgements on what should be done to help them, in preference to making a clinical judgement based on factual information from the patients and tempering this with what is known academically. Obviously, to listen involves communication of both the verbal and the non-verbal kind, picking up 'key words' and knowing how to establish good rapport. This subject is dealt with in detail in Chapter 3.

Assessment and understanding are assisted by asking questions based on believing that their body can inform patients about aspects of their disorder that cannot be found by examination. For example:

1. 'Is it "the thing that is wrong" which is sore, or is it just soreness from my treatment?'

2. 'No, it's not a silly question to ask whether your back problem could have any connection with headaches. What have you noticed that gives you this feeling?'

3. 'We both agree that your movements look better, but you obviously feel that your symptoms aren't any better. Are you able to say *why* it doesn't feel better, or in what way it isn't better?'

Information gained by such questioning can reveal invaluable information. *We must listen, we must search, and we must believe.*

## EXAMINATION

Greater detail and depth of examination is demanded by this **concept** than that with which the majority of clinicians are familiar. For example, in the following list of aspects important to examination, two (numbers 1 and 2) are not commonly used to their fullest value.

1. The precise **site and kind** of patients' symptoms (which can so often indicate from which structures the symptoms are NOT coming, as well as vice versa).
2. **Functional movements** that patients can demonstrate to reproduce their symptoms.
3. The standard test movements of joints and vertebral canal and neural structures.
4. Coupling different movements, sequences and positions.
5. Differentiation tests to determine which structure or movement component is involved with the painful movement.
6. The accessory movements and palpation findings (the tissues and joint movements) that have an effect on the symptoms.

The manipulative physiotherapist, during and following examinations, then has the task of collating the information gathered on examination to make it meaningful. This information can then be used to apply the appropriate treatment techniques. Grieve (1988), throughout his text, gives proper emphasis to palpation examination as expounded herein.

Sometimes the only signs that can be found on examination are palpation signs, while all physiological and functional movements are negative.

*Movement diagrams* – Movement diagrams have been included in the text of this book as an appendix rather than as a particular chapter of the book. This was done for the precise reason that movement diagrams should not be considered as a mandatory exercise for the manipulative physiotherapist. However, every effective manipulator goes through the process of movement diagrams, although this may be done quite instinctively. In teaching the concept that this book portrays, movement diagrams become an essential part of the learning process. This learning process includes both a teacher teaching students, and also the teaching of oneself as one continues to practise and learn from experience. Thinking purely superficially, it is understandable that a person may say that movement diagrams are unnecessary jargon, which serve only to complicate the learning. However, this is quite a false interpretation; their value is inestimable and can be fully appreciated only when an individual becomes totally conversant with, and involved in, the forming of movement diagrams and relating them to the selection of the grade and rhythm of treatment techniques when applied to a patient's presenting symptoms and signs.

It is a mandatory rule that in testing a movement of any kind, **range** plus its **symptomatic response** must always be related:

- Never think of range without thinking of symptomatic response.
- Never think of symptoms without thinking of range of movement.

> Never think of pain without thinking of range.
> Never think of range without thinking of pain

A detailed examination seeks to reveal the smallest changes in the behaviour of the symptoms and the resistance with each direction of movement. For example, can pain or discomfort be felt throughout the range, or is it painful only at the end of the range? Does the behaviour of the pain with movement match the behaviour of the resistance to movement within the available range? And so on. Appreciating the fine differences in the behaviour of the abnormal elements of the movements is imperative to the application of this 'concept of treatment', which illustrates the value of movement diagrams.

Another feature of examination, perhaps the most important feature, is knowing how much change in the examination findings certain treatment techniques should effect: 'You treat as gently as you can but as hard as the disorder requires' (Evjenth, O., unpublished observations). This is true, but many manipulative physiotherapists do not appreciate how gentle 'gentle' can be while still being effective (*see* the reference to the 'fly', p. 176), nor do they realize how strongly the techniques sometimes need to be performed even though they may be very uncomfortable for the patient. Teaching and using these extremes is an important element.

Yet another feature is the manner in which the active and passive test movements are examined and related to those of the patient's activities that are limited because they provoke symptoms. For example, a patient may have his left thoracic symptoms only when he reaches the fourteenth hole in a round of golf. His standard of golf is then reduced for the next four holes. Because this is the only time he has pain, and the pain always goes by the next day, the physical examination and the assessment of improvement from treatment will hinge around the golf-swing movements, and the behaviour of the symptoms from the fourteenth hole onwards. The aim of the physical examination will be to find a movement or combination of movements that produces pain comparable with the disorder.

**Differentiation tests** are special tests that are used when a passive test movement, involving simultaneous movement of at least two joints or other movement components such as neural structures, reproduces a patient's symptoms. The method is, when the test movement is at the point in the range of reproducing the pain, further movement is produced in one of the two components involved while at the same time the movement is reduced in the other component. The test is then performed in the reverse manner. The symptomatic response (i.e. increase, decrease) confirms which component is at fault (*see* pp. 162–163 for a clarifying example).

## RELATING TREATMENT TO THE HISTORY, SYMPTOMS AND SIGNS

Information known from the 'theoretical, speculative' compartment together with the 'history and clinical presentation' side of the 'brick wall' of the patient's disorder will indicate to the physiotherapist the stage of the pathological changes (assuming there is pathology) causing the disorder. This influences the interpretation of assessments of the changes in a patient's symptoms and signs during treatment. This linking yet separating of the two compartments, while at the same time assessing the effect of treatment based on changes in the patient's symptoms and signs, is a primary feature of this concept of treatment. Assessment of changes effected by a technique is made in each of the different physical components of a patient's disorder. The 'joint-movement/pain-response' component, the muscle spasm component, and the restricted neural movement component are each considered separately (*see* Chapter 4).

> Knowledge about pathology helps with the interpretation of the changes in symptoms and signs through detailed assessment. Thus both compartments of the 'symbolic semi-permeable brick wall' are linked together in the thinking of the therapist

A patient's pain can *present* in a seemingly never-ending number of different ways, and the pain can also *behave* in a never-ending number of different ways. To understand that moving a joint in a particular manner can produce an ache is just one aspect of understanding pain responses. Another aspect is to know what the different responses indicate. The important part of the concept is to know how to modify the treatment in response to the changes in the 'symptoms and signs'. Knowing and understanding the patient's pain – its site, its behaviour, its responses to positions, its responses during movements of examination and of treatment, as well as its response following treatment – is the clear-cut, positive information that forms the prime basis for treatment by this method. Even having used the word 'pain' restricts its importance because many patients do not have what they call pain, so the words *discomfort*, an *awareness of heaviness*, or a *feeling of 'difference'* at a particular site are equally important. Perhaps the word *discomfort* should be used throughout the text to emphasize the important role that symptoms play.

Recording the treatment session is a vital part of the treatment. It must be recorded in such a manner as to indicate the effect of the previous treatment, the pain responses during a treatment technique and the immediate effect of the technique (pp. 75, 108–109, 225).

## ASSESSMENT AND ANALYTICAL ASSESSMENT

Assessment has always been the keystone of this text, even during the writing of the first edition in 1962. Assessment will always be the keystone of progression.

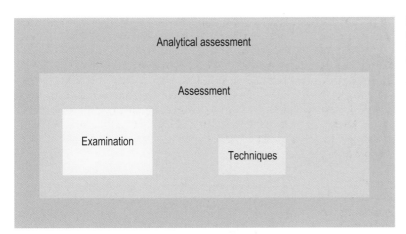

**Figure 1.6** The relative importance of analytical assessment, assessment, treatment techniques and examination of the patient

Assessment demands of the manipulative physiotherapist a mind that is:

1. Agile and open to receive information.
2. Plastic and innovative in the analysis of the information.
3. Disciplined, methodical and logical in its use of information.

Why is there a need for 'assessment' and 'analytical assessment'? Aren't they the same? No, they are different, although they are both assessment. While assessment involves proving the value of a technique, analytical assessment covers a wider field of investigation and assessing (*Figure 1.6*) and can be considered under a general heading of 'making features fit'. When they do not fit it is necessary to hunt further and reassess in greater detail.

> Making features fit is an important aspect of the assessment. If features do not fit, further assessment is usually needed

In general terms, it means making sense out of what the patient is able to say and demonstrate about the disorder. This applies to:

1. The history: making the onset of the disorder fit, or be acceptable or reasonable, when related both to the ways the disorder affects the patient, and to the physical examination findings.
2. The examination: making all of the findings compatible with each other and also with the patient's disabilities.
3. The changes that take place during treatment: working out why treatment predictions are sometimes not achieved, and why a movement or symptom does not improve when it should have in relation to other movements or symptoms which *have* improved.

4. Other treatments that might be used: deciding that because such-and-such is happening with treatment, an intra-articular injection, for example, might serve the patient better.

5. The end-result of treatment: making sense out of a compromise end-result, deciding whether maintenance treatment is indicated, deciding whether the symptoms and signs match with each other and with the whole story of the complaint, etc.

The mental processes involved in 'analytical assessment' are simply thinking *logically*, though they involve vertical thinking and lateral thinking (DeBono, 1980), inductive thinking and deductive thinking. It is in this area that the 'specialist' manipulative physiotherapist shines. As was stated by Hunkin (unpublished observations), 'Your achievements are limited by the extent of your lateral and logical thinking'.

## TWO INHERENT CAPABILITIES OF THE BODY

### The body's capacity to adapt

It is astonishing to realize the body's capacity to 'adapt to changes' forced on it by congenital abnormalities, trauma and lifelong heavy work. Knowing this to be a fact helps us to put our examination findings into a more precise context while making assessments. In other words, if a patient has had an accident or disease earlier in life, the body's **capability to compensate** for the damage can be so complete that the abnormal findings may have little or no bearing on the presenting disorder.

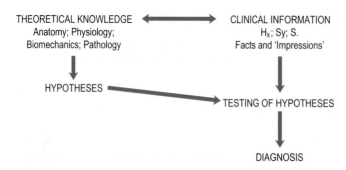

THEORETICAL KNOWLEDGE ⟷ CLINICAL INFORMATION
Anatomy; Physiology;              $H_x$; Sy; S.
Biomechanics; Pathology        Facts and 'Impressions'

HYPOTHESES

TESTING OF HYPOTHESES

DIAGNOSIS

**Figure 1.7** Flowchart demonstrating relationships and contexts for theoretical and clinical knowledge with related hypotheses. H, history; Sy, symptoms; S, signs (from *Physical Therapy of the Low Back* (1988). Twomey and Taylor, eds, p. 140. Churchill Livingstone). Reproduced with permission of the publisher

## The body's capacity to inform

Secondly, patients' *bodies* can tell them things related to their disorder that we can never detect even by the most thorough physical examination. These are frequently subtle messages that patients may comment on, and they can be priceless. The only way the manipulative physiotherapist can elicit these subtleties is by *listening to patients*, and by encouraging them to mention anything that might be relevant, irrespective of how trivial or unimportant it may seem.

Patients who are 'tuned in' to their body will be more aware of these subtleties. This is a process of educating patients to notice and report trivia. For example, in response to the question, 'What effect did the last treatment have?', a patient may say, 'I don't know – I can't explain it – it just feels different'. Such a statement demands an 'immediate-response question' (*see* pp. 35–36) – 'Is it a favourable difference or an unfavourable difference?'

Thus we reach an understanding of what the disorder is and what it is doing to the patient (*see Figure 1.7*).

## SUMMARY: THE 'CONCEPT'

The essential sections that make up this concept of treatment are founded on an understanding of the following 10 points. Naturally, many of them are included in the methods that others use, both during treatment and when teaching manipulation, but the emphases will vary from person to person. The fundamental ideas that have particular importance in this concept are identified by **bold print**.

1. *Diagnosis*: The realization that, although there is much in medicine that is still unknown, and although precise diagnosis is not always possible, **these need be no bar to precise, effective and informative manipulative treatment** provided the two-compartment ('brick wall') method of thinking is adopted.

2. *The relationships between techniques and assessment*: Keeping the theoretical area and the clinical area in their correct inter-relationships by visualizing the 'symbolic semi-permeable **brick wall**'.

3. *Theory*: **Not allowing theoretical knowledge** (which in fact may be false), or the lack of it, to obstruct seeing or finding clinical facts.

4. *Assessment and analytical assessment*: **Validation, proving each step** in the clinical situation. **Flawless analytical assessment** is the keystone to this concept of manipulative physiotherapy.

5. *Examination*: There are a number of characteristics of physical examination vital to the use of the concept:
   a) Making use of the patients' **functional** movements, with which they can demonstrate their disability or disorder.
   b) The importance given to *any* **combinations** of movements that produce **appropriate symptomatic responses**.
   c) Knowing the principles of **differentiation tests**, and the methods of performing them.
   d) Having a full appreciation that patients can have **different KINDS of pain** within one disorder. Appreciating the implications of '**pain-through-range**' '**end-of-range-pain**', '**latent pains**', '**pain inhibition**': and understanding the '**irritability**' of a disorder with its implications for guiding treatment.
   e) Making use of testing movements while **compressing** the joint surfaces, to compare that pain response with that found when compression is not applied during the same test movements.
   f) The depth of the detail of **palpation** *examination* of soft tissues and accessory movements.
   g) The use of '**movement diagrams**' in analysing physical examination findings.

6. *Appropriate wording*: Because there are many unknown aspects of theory, answers to questions

asked by professional people regarding the effects of manipulative treatment must **always be flexible, never dogmatic** and need to be protected by the use and explanation of the symbolic semipermeable 'brick wall'.

7. *Listening*: **Listening attentively** to the patients' every word in an **open-minded and non-judgemental manner**. **Believe** patients, yet question them. This is a very demanding skill, requiring a high level of **self-criticism**.

8. *Techniques*:
   a) An open-minded attitude to treatment techniques is essential, thus being able to **innovate freely, unhindered by theory**; but **relating** the techniques to **functional disturbances** and **presenting signs**.
   b) **Recording** the techniques by using grades of movement, rhythms of movement and the symptomatic response during the technique, so as to qualify the mode of the technique for accurate communication.
   c) A clear understanding of how to **treat** *pain* by using oscillatory techniques, which are **totally painless** and **do not include any** *stretching* whatsoever. Such treatment is not used in other concepts.
   d) A similar understanding of the application of a **compression force** of the joint surfaces while performing oscillatory movement techniques. Such treatment is also peculiar to the concept.
   e) A similar understanding of how to adapt techniques for treating stiffness, and the modifying of these techniques when muscle spasm limits movement.
   f) Relating the 'grades' and 'rhythms' of techniques to the clinical findings and any concurrent pathology.
   g) Using asterisks to highlight the recording of major information from the subjective and physical examinations.

9. *Relating treatment to the history, symptoms and signs*: Although the heading states the basis of the treatment concept, the treatment is also influenced by what is known as the diagnosis of the patient's disorder (*see* p. 87). Treatment also involves recording the fine details of the **effects of techniques both during and following** their performance. This is an essential involvement of treatment.

10. *The body's inherent capabilities*:
   a) **Believing** that the patient's body has an **enormous capacity to adapt and accommodate** to disorders without causing symptoms.
   b) **Believing** that the **patient's body can tell the patient** – and therefore, through the patient, the manipulative physiotherapist – subtle, but vital information, about the disorder, which is very important to assessment, treatment and prognosis.

**IT IS OPEN-MINDEDNESS, MENTAL AGILITY AND MENTAL DISCIPLINE, LINKED WITH A LOGICAL AND METHODICAL PROCESS OF ASSESSING CAUSE AND EFFECT, THAT ARE THE DEMANDS OF THE CONCEPT.**

# Chapter 2

# The doctor's role in diagnosis and referral for manipulative physiotherapy

## Adapted from the original text by Professor D. A. Brewerton, MD, FRCP

Every patient who is to undergo spinal mobilization or manipulation by a physiotherapist should have consulted or have access to a doctor, who has the dual responsibility of determining the diagnosis and deciding the best treatment. Therefore, the first purpose of this chapter is to guide doctors as to the types of patient who should or should not be referred to a physiotherapist for manipulation, mobilization or traction of the spine. The main emphasis is on the contraindications to such treatment. Unfortunately, any guide to doctors cannot yet be based entirely on an analysis of proven facts. However, there have been detailed studies of the results of treatment or controlled trials. At present it is still essential to draw on the experience and impressions of many doctors and therapists as well as contemporary evidence.

The physiotherapist must assess and examine the patient before treatment is begun, and repeatedly during a course of treatment. Without the ability to do this no physiotherapist should undertake the forms of treatment Mr Maitland describes. This type of examination is detailed and expert, but largely confined to the musculoskeletal system. Consequently, the second purpose of this chapter is to outline for physiotherapists some of the broader issues that a doctor must consider in the assessment.

Success depends largely on collaboration between doctor and physiotherapist and vice versa. The doctor's role is to make a broad diagnosis or classification of the disorder, and to discuss changes in the clinical situation that may develop during the course of treatment.

## ORGANIC DISORDERS NOT INVOLVING THE VERTEBRAE

The clinical history and examination by the doctor are essential in excluding a wide variety of disorders that may simulate spinal pain (*Table 2.1*). Special attention is always given to the patient who can move the relevant part of the spine freely without discomfort.

Most of the more serious diseases that are commonly quoted in textbooks cause diagnostic difficulties. More

**Table 2.1**    Disorders that may simulate spinal pain

| Cervical pain | Lumbar pain |
|---|---|
| Malignant lymphadenopathy | Peptic ulcer |
| Pancoast's tumour | Renal disease |
| Vertebral artery syndrome | Pancreatic carcinoma |
| Subarachnoid haemorrhage | Obstruction of aorta or |
| Coronary artery disease | iliac arteries |
| Polymyalgia rheumatica | Carcinoma of colon or |
| | rectum |
| Thoracic pain | Other pelvic carcinomas |
| Bronchogenic carcinoma | Endometriosis |
| Other lung disease | Pregnancy |
| Coronary artery disease | Disseminated sclerosis |
| Aortic aneurysm | Spinal cord tumour |
| Massive cardiac enlargement | Hip disease |
| Hiatus hernia | Short leg |
| Gall bladder disease | |
| Herpes zoster | |

problems are caused by gall disease, hiatus hernia or angina presenting with dorsal pain, or relatively minor peptic ulceration causing lumbar backache. Occlusion of the aorta or iliac arteries may present with lumbar pain on walking. No patient with dorsal pain should be treated without having had a chest radiograph.

There is no indication for manipulation if the cause of pain is not within the spine.

## PREGNANCY

Pregnancy, in the last months, is regarded by some authorities as a contraindication to manipulation. It is true that the pregnancy presents mechanical and technical problems, but if marked pain is clearly originating within the spine there is no absolute bar to manipulation provided sensible precautions are taken.

## DISEASE OF THE SPINAL CORD OR CAUDA EQUINA

Disease of the spinal cord or cauda equina, or any evidence of pressure on them, is an absolute contraindication to any form of mobilization or manipulation. This applies even to the slightest symptoms, such as mild bilateral paraesthesiae in the feet. The term 'spinal stenosis' describes a clinical syndrome that is usually produced by a massive disc protrusion compressing the cauda equina. This results in pain in both legs, with progressive pain, numbness and weakness on walking,

and is easily mistaken for intermittent claudication due to peripheral arterial disease.

## THE VERTEBRAL CAROTID ARTERIES

The vertebral carotid arteries may be occluded by atherosclerosis, or by disease or deformity of the spine. Some of the very rare tragedies following manipulation have been due to occlusion of, or injury to the vertebral carotid arteries, particularly on rotation or extension of the neck. Before performing any mobilization or manipulation of the neck, it is essential to ask specifically for any symptoms suggesting vertebral carotid artery disease, particularly any giddiness or disturbance of vision related to neck posture. The physiotherapist should gently rotate the neck fully in both directions and hold each position for a few seconds to be certain that this does not produce symptoms before attempting even gentle mobilization. Examination for vertebrobasilar insufficiency is discussed on pages 242–246.

## VERTEBRAL DISEASE

A classification of the vertebral causes of spinal pain includes many well-known pathological disorders (*Table 2.2*). In practice most patients have changes that are difficult to classify, and it is usually impossible to make a precise anatomical diagnosis. There is often a basis of underlying degenerative change, and this is sometimes aggravated by strains and minor trauma.

General medical assessment and radiographs of the spine are essential before advising manipulation of the spine at any level.

## SPONDYLOLISTHESIS

Spondylolisthesis is a contraindication to forceful manipulation at that level, but treatment is often successful when directed to the relief of a pain originating higher in the spine.

## OSTEOPOROSIS

Osteoporosis is an absolute contraindication to manipulation, and this restriction applies also to conditions likely to cause osteoporosis, including treatment with steroids. Age in itself is not a contraindication to manipulation, and some of the most worthwhile results are obtained in older patients.

Table 2.2    Vertebral causes of spinal pain

| Developmental | Tumour |
|---|---|
| Spondylolisthesis | Secondary carcinoma |
| Scoliosis | Myelomatosis |
| Hypermobility | |
| Various uncommon | Infection |
|   disorders | Staphylococcal |
| | Tuberculous |
| Degenerative | E. coli |
| Disc lesions without | Brucella melitensis |
|   root compression | |
| Disc lesions with root | Inflammatory |
|   compression | arthropathy |
| Disc lesions with compression | Ankylosing spondylitis |
|   of spinal cord or cauda | Rheumatoid arthritis |
|   equina | Reiter's disease |
| Osteoarthrosis of | Ulcerative colitis |
|   apophyseal joints | Crohn's disease |
| Hyperostosis | Psoriasis |
| Instability | |
| | Metabolic |
| Trauma | Osteoporosis |
| Fracture | Osteomalacia |
| Stress fracture | |
| Subluxation | Unknown |
| Ligamentous injury | Paget's disease |

## ANKYLOSING SPONDYLITIS AND RHEUMATOID ARTHRITIS

Ankylosing spondylitis and rheumatoid arthritis both commonly affect the spinal ligaments, which occasionally may lead to subluxation within the cervical spine and rarely to sudden death. Evidence of any inflammatory arthropathy of the spine is an absolute contraindication to neck manipulation, even if there is no clinical or radiological evidence that the involvement includes the cervical spine.

## NERVE ROOT PAIN

Root pain due to a disc protrusion or any local degenerative disorder may dominate the clinical picture, producing much more pain and restriction of spinal movement than its underlying cause. It is one of the first essentials to decide whether there is an element of root pain before choosing the best treatment for a patient. This is easy if there is a full root distribution of pain accompanied by paraesthesiae, but very difficult when the involvement is partial. The extent of the radiation

of pain may help; if it is beyond the elbow or knee, root involvement is probable. It is also more likely if the pain includes paraesthesiae or other qualities suggesting nerve irritation. With root involvement, a gentle spinal movement may readily produce radiation of pain to a greater distance than would otherwise be expected; and maintenance of a spinal posture, such as rotation of the neck towards the pain, may reproduce the root symptoms if the position is held for 10–20 seconds.

## NERVE ROOT PAIN AND MANIPULATION

Experts do not all agree whether patients with root symptoms should be subjected to forceful manipulation. Some claim that it is justified if there are no neurological signs; others advocate manipulation provided the symptoms do not extend beyond the elbow or the knee, using the argument that reference of pain that far need not imply root involvement. My own practice is to avoid forceful manipulation for all patients with any evidence of nerve root involvement, but this is a controversial issue that will not be settled until there have been detailed studies of patients with root symptoms to determine more accurately which do well and which do badly. While this knowledge is awaited, it is probably wise to exclude from forceful manipulation all patients whose symptoms appear to arise from root compression, however mild; but to permit manipulation of patients with pain of a similar distribution, provided that it is confidently diagnosed as being due to spinal derangement without root involvement. Nevertheless, it must be admitted that physiotherapists who are expert at passive mobilization and manipulation sometimes produce dramatic relief of symptoms from arm pain or sciatica, even when there are neurological signs. Also, it is probably right to make an exception when a patient has root symptoms of very long standing and then appears to get a stiff neck or back due to a mechanical derangement of the spine unrelated to the chronic nerve root pain.

## NERVE ROOT PAIN AND TRACTION

Traction can be applied constantly to a patient confined to bed with severe root pain arising in the cervical or the lumbar spine, or intermittently on an outpatient basis. Traction in bed is used mostly for patients with particularly painful sciatica that has not settled after treatment by bed rest alone. The traction undoubtedly immobilizes the lumbar spine more effectively, and probably the distraction aids in pain relief.

## Intermittent traction

Intermittent traction on an outpatient basis is preferably given daily, and can be applied to the cervical or lumbar spine. Cervical traction for patients with arm pain thought to be due to root compression has been the subject of a thorough study (*British Medical Journal*, 1966). This showed that virtually every patient had marked relief of pain during the application of the traction, which was usually applied with the head in a flexed position. Often the pain relief lasted for a matter of hours, but the treatment did not influence the natural history of the condition or the long-term results. Three-quarters of the patients improved substantially within a month whether traction was used or not. This means that intermittent traction for outpatients should probably be reserved for patients with severe pain, who will be grateful for the temporary relief of pain even if the overall rate of recovery is not improved. Lumbar traction is commonly applied to patients with sciatic pain, although there has not yet been adequate statistical evaluation of the results.

## IMPENDING NERVE ROOT COMPRESSION

Patients between the ages of 15 and 35 years who develop acute lumbar or cervical pain are more likely to have true disc protrusions than older patients. Lumbar pain in the younger age group frequently presents in a way that suggests the likelihood of sciatica in the near future, and this is a contraindication to manipulation.

## THE REMAINDER

Although the great majority of patients who complain of spinal pain cannot be classified or diagnosed, this mixed and complicated group contains the patients who are most suitable for treatment by spinal mobilization or manipulation. The essence of selection is to choose patients whose pain originates in the spine, and then exclude all those in whom there is any evidence of involvement of the spinal cord, cauda equina, nerve roots or vertebral arteries, and those with any evidence of disease affecting their vertebrae or spinal ligaments.

In the management of this large remainder there are virtually no absolute contraindications to treatment, provided the correct techniques, as outlined by Mr Maitland, are chosen. The main objects of treatment are to use the gentlest techniques that will produce the desired result, and to modify the treatment on the basis of the patient's progress and repeated reassessments by the physiotherapist. Treatment starting with gentle mobilization and a small amplitude of movement should be perfectly safe for all patients in this mixed group. Everything depends on the techniques used; no one would recommend the use of traction for a patient with acute lumbar back pain or forceful manipulation for a patient with sciatica or brachial neuropathy accompanied by neurological signs.

Some authorities advocate more clear-cut indications for treatment based on more accurate diagnosis, but it is doubtful whether such accuracy is really feasible. Although the origin of the pain may be located at the correct level within the spine, in the absence of root symptoms it is often only possible to make intelligent guesses as to whether the cause is a degenerative or protruded disc, vertebral instability, degenerative changes in an apophyseal joint, a torn interspinous ligament or some other precise diagnosis. Furthermore, it is impossible to give definite indications and contraindications for treatment within this ill-defined group of patients. Nor is it wise to say categorically which techniques are most likely to be effective; different manipulators get their best results with different techniques. At present all that can be said is that when these patients are treated by experienced physiotherapists many of them do well, and they appear to recover more rapidly than with other methods. Regrettably, we must await more detailed investigations and assessments before anything is more definite.

## POSTURE AND WORK

Any physiotherapist treating a patient with spinal pain should automatically review with the patient the use of the spine for all everyday activities, emphasizing any posture or movement that aggravates the pain. It is wrong to concentrate on spinal mobilization while the patient is regularly making the pain worse by some unwise posture or by a repeated activity at work.

## PSYCHOLOGICAL FACTORS

Pure psychogenic pain in the neck or back is not common, but virtually all chronic spinal pains are influenced by social and psychological circumstances, and the doctor's assessment is never complete if based on physical grounds alone. Given a chance to talk, many patients with these symptoms pour out their problems and make it obvious that they are suffering from depression, anxiety, marital or social problems or something else that demands help in its own right. Sometimes the patient has been told that the problem is 'arthritis of the spine', and wishes to be protected from the ravages of a widespread, crippling disease.

While it is true that patients whose symptoms are predominantly psychological in origin may benefit considerably from manipulation and the general support given by the physiotherapist, this approach to treatment can never be an adequate substitute for psychological help, and better long-term results are usually obtained by doctor and patient facing up to the real problems. Furthermore, prolonged physical treatment with indifferent results may confirm the patient's suspicions that the problem is an organic disease that is too difficult to treat. This description applies to many patients who go from therapist to therapist receiving years of unsuccessful treatment.

Among patients with chronic spinal pain there are many with moderate or severe depression. They reject immediately any suggestion that their problems are psychological, and usually they will not talk about their problems until they have received a course of anti-depressive drugs or other treatment. This is a much better approach for most of them than to retreat into physical treatment.

A chronic anxiety state may be a form of depression, to be treated accordingly, or it may be based on a personality disorder. Obviously the personality cannot readily be changed, but these patients often have insight and recognize that they have had other symptoms due to tension. They may be surprisingly willing to discuss their pain in psychological terms. An explanation that 'some tense people get peptic ulcers, while others have tense neck muscles and a painful neck' may be understood and accepted, with obvious relief that the cause is nothing more serious.

Sometimes a double approach is required. When patients cannot accept at once that the pain is psychological in origin, they may tolerate the suggestion that psychological factors predominate provided they are also told that they have a minor organic condition that will probably respond to physical treatment.

# Chapter 3

# Communication

## (with a contribution by J. Graham, MB, BS, FRACP)

One of the most important aspects of this concept of manipulative physiotherapy, as stated in Chapter 1, is assessment, and this has been further emphasized by extending the subject into analytical assessment (*see* pp. 12–13). It is, as has been said, the keystone of the concept, and if the keystone needs further refining, this lies in the skill of retrospective assessment. In retrospective

assessment, it is the assessment of the patients' awareness of changes to their symptoms that is the most important element. The only method of getting this information is via skill in communication. If it requires stating, the most important part of this sixth edition is without doubt understanding the skills of communication with the patient in retrospective assessments throughout treatment. It is for this reason that this chapter has been written in such detail.

> Skills of communication with retrospective assessment are keystones of the concept, as this contributes to patients' awareness of the changes in their symptoms

Dr John Graham has put force into projecting the importance of this chapter by writing an introduction. Dr Graham is the Visiting Specialist Physician at the Flinders Medical Centre, with important roles in the Pain Clinic and the Coronary Hypertension Unit, and his knowledge of communication, with all its ramifications, goes far beyond the scope of this text. Because of his skill and knowledge, I am pleased to begin the chapter with his introduction, which is quoted in full.

The health professional who has the good fortune to possess or read this book on manipulative physiotherapy will be exposed to the thinking of an unusually clear and perceptive mind.

As one who has had the opportunity of watching Mr Maitland assess patients both directly and on video-tape, I was on the one hand excited and on the other intrigued to see over and over again the techniques of a highly skilled communicator.

It is this communication skill which you have an opportunity to learn as you read this book. Just as you may wish to read over and over again a particular assessment method, so I recommend that you read and re-read this immensely valuable chapter on communication.

Mr Maitland speaks about 'how I think', about 'analytical assessment' and about 'flexibility'.

He understands that flexibility in thinking involves 'inventiveness', 'creativity' and 'trying a new way', but always evaluating the new way against old ways.

He is ever prepared to try a new sequence. Thus flexibility is 'not being rigid'. He understands that 'the map is not the territory'. A map is a representation of territory. Names are representations of things.

He has developed his solid metaphor of 'the semi-permeable brick wall'. Brick walls are opaque, and hard to get through.

On this side of the brick wall are the history, symptoms and signs (HSS). This side is open to the clarification of more elegant and precise history taking, correct checking of what the symptoms are and careful eliciting of physical signs. The other side is 'the pathology', and that is mostly inferred.

The chapter on communication is about this side of the brick wall. Clarifying HSS is checking to see that the message sent is the message received.

New information to any person makes sense to that person by their comparing it to what is already in their minds (*memory, maps*).

Mr Maitland is prepared to visit carefully and thoughtfully that subjective world of his patients to ensure that he really does approximate his way of thinking to that of the patient.

His approach conveys very clearly that he cares about his patients, that he understands that they have resources which will help them to achieve specific successful outcomes.

He enters a close, point-to-point, moment-to-moment feedback loop with his patients. They can perceive this, and co-operate the more because of it. His eye contact, ready-to-respond smile, sense of humour, touching the patient in appropriate ways and at appropriate times, allow his verbal message to match his non-verbal communication.

If he encounters difficulties, he is prepared to ask questions which clarify or specify, or make it easier for the patient to find an answer.

In his language of communication, he frequently reveals to the patient that he has more than one technique available to himself and to them. For example: 'One of the things I could do is . . .', implying that there are other things.

He also frames his questions in such a way as to allow patients to find small changes both during the session and in between sessions. They know, therefore, where to look for success.

By making his own hypotheses explicit to himself he is free to confirm or reject what he discovered. (Some people really never do know what they are trying to achieve with a technique, so they don't know they have already disproved a hypothesis which wasn't explicit to themselves.)

So Mr Maitland says 'using a technique . . .', knowing what you want it to do, while performing it.

Consider this masterly piece of reframing: 'the patient has been a problem to get better . . . there is a wealth of information in that.' Rather than falling into a pessimistic or negative way of thinking, he decides to find out why a patient could be a problem, knowing that this very matter suggests that some special extra information is 'embedded' in the problem.

He is prepared to seek 'all evidence', think of 'any method' and pioneer the extension of concepts (consider the 'slump' test).

The question for the teacher becomes 'how would you pass on to the student the information that she needs about that technique and what it can do? Or for the student, 'What exactly is Mr Maitland doing here?' 'How can I do it as well?.

This book goes a long way towards achieving these goals. You can build your experience from your own knowledge, and from the wealth of Mr Maitland's learnings and experience expressed in these pages.

Most people consider that communication between two people who speak the same language is simple, routine, automatic and uncomplicated. However, even in normal household conversations there are many instances every day when misunderstandings occur. Each of us has been involved, at one time or another, in a conversation when he or she fails to impart a point of view, finding it difficult to put thoughts into words. This lack of success can be very frustrating, particularly if the other person has a different point of view and wishes to put it to you. Within a group of people, the theme of a conversation often changes rapidly as each person leads the conversation off at a particular tangent. This can occur just as easily in communication between only two people. Normal conversation, therefore, is not as simple and straightforward as might be thought.

There are two interviewing skills of which therapists must be aware; these are hearing/listening, and seeing/looking. Therapists may well hear what they expect to hear rather than listening to the words the patient uses. The following quotation is worthy of recording.

> Listening is itself, of course, an art: that is where it differs from merely hearing. Hearing is passive; listening is active. Hearing is voluntary; listening demands attention. Hearing is natural; listening is an acquired discipline. (The Age, 21 August 1982)

Similarly, therapists may see patients without looking at their nuances of expression and body language.

Looking (observing) is itself a skill; that is where it differs from merely seeing. Seeing is passive, looking is active. Seeing is natural; looking is an acquired discipline.

> Listening and observing are essential skills in communication

Doctors, counsellors, physiotherapists and people of many other professions who are required to understand the problems of their patients need to appreciate the complexities surrounding communication. Clear, successful communication may be difficult to achieve. It is not so difficult, however, when we develop ways of thinking about words and behaviours that help each word, word group and behaviour to be decoded.

Attention to one level of communication (for example content, meaning of words) can be practised until, step by step, we can develop a high level of skill in uncovering meanings. When we learned language originally, we did in fact build it word by word, gradually increasing our understanding of the special meaning of any word, and the context in which it was used. Any other level of communication can be studied in the same step-by-step manner. When we have skills at two levels, we can much more comfortably use the skills at the same time or in sequences to serve our goals of skilful and comfortable communication.

Experts in communication, such as Virginia Satir and Milton Erickson, have spent thousands of hours learning by observation and by practice, choosing words thoughtfully, and making many mistakes (Zeig, 1980). Their success depended greatly on their willingness to learn, and to learn by trial and error, checking out the responses of their patients and clients as well as their friends and relatives.

A good way to discover more about our own style of interviewing is to record it on video-tape or audio-tape and play it back to ourselves and to constructive peers or supervisors. Such a practice can give a great opportunity for us to notice the possibilities for understanding and for misunderstanding our own words and intonation. The skill must be developed to a high level if a patient's problem is to be understood without any detail being missed. Skill in communication is necessary if instructions need to be given to a patient, so that any possibility of being misunderstood is avoided. The learning of this art or skill requires patience, humility, clarity and self-criticism. Without them, good rapport with patients will not be achieved. Words, phrases and intonation need to be chosen carefully when asking questions to avoid being misunderstood, and patients must be listened to carefully so that the meanings of the words they use are not misunderstood. When communication mistakes do occur during this learning process, the physiotherapist should look at herself for the mistake and not blame the patient (for the purposes of clarity throughout this book, the physiotherapist will be referred to as 'she' and the patient as 'he').

Over the years, many cartoons have appeared that depict the problems of communication. Figure 3.1 is an excellent and rather clever example.

It is the last three lines that bear greatest significance:

> what you heard
> is not
> what I meant!

This could be saying, 'what I said was so badly worded that it didn't express the thought that was in my mind', or it is possible that the receiver tuned in, or listened closely, only to those parts of the message that fitted their own way of thinking, and ignored other parts that did not. It is also

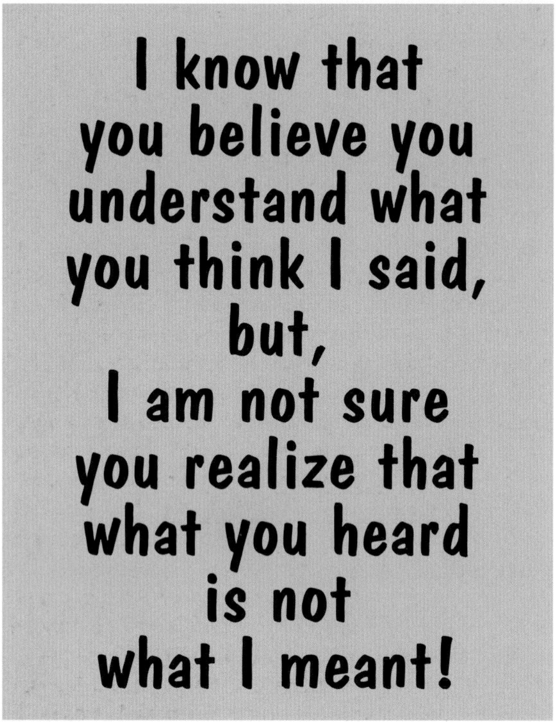

# I know that you believe you understand what you think I said, but, I am not sure you realize that what you heard is not what I meant!

**Figure 3.1**    One of the problems of communication

*possible that the hearer's attention was altered by his or her expectation or frame of mind.*

It is equally important to 'read, mark, learn and inwardly digest' the first lines also:

*I know that*
*you believe you*
*understand what*
*you think I said*

These words put before us two other facts. The first is that the person listening to what is being said frequently does NOT accurately hear what is being said, even though he thinks he does. Secondly, it is often NOT understood nor interpreted correctly (*see* Figure 3.2, 1st process).

*Regarding the words*:

understand what
you think I said

*two facts are put forward. The first is that in fact we do not always*

understand

*what is said; the second is that what the listener thinks is said may, in fact, be slightly different from what has been said, and therefore the listener will get the wrong message.*

Communication consists of both non-verbal and verbal components with the latter including aspects such as tone of voice.

> Both verbal and non-verbal components are essential elements of communication processes

The non-verbal component consists of the nuances of behaviour that must be observed and interpreted by the physiotherapist and used by her when she speaks to the patient.

The verbal component requires skill in the choosing of both words and phrases to formulate questions.

In summary:

*the choice and arrangement of words in such a way as to get an idea as exactly as possible out of one mind and into another.*    (Sir Ernest Gowers, 1979)

*Listening is itself, of course an art: that is where it differs from merely hearing. Hearing is passive; listening demands attention. Hearing is natural; listening is an acquired discipline.*
(*The Age*, 21 August 1982)

*Looking (observing) is itself a skill: that is where is differs from merely seeing. Seeing is passive; looking is active. Seeing is natural; looking is an acquired discipline.*    (G. Maitland, 1990)

## NON–VERBAL COMMUNICATION

The first aspect of communication that must be stressed is the non-verbal or 'body language' aspect. It is the *sine qua non* of communication. The impact of non-verbal signals is usually stronger, quicker and more direct than the impact of words. The signals are frequently more informative than words, and have the advantage of transmitting messages as a subconscious reflex action before sufficient time has elapsed to choose the best words. Because non-verbal communication is reflex in type and therefore less easily controlled, it can be expected to be more genuine. It also has the advantage of expressing more subtle messages more precisely and distinctively than can words.

There are of course many non-verbal signals that are consciously used by the patient and which do not always agree with their verbal messages. It is very important to notice the verbal and non-verbal messages together and to be aware of when they match (congruency) and when they don't match (incongruency).

In any event it is important to respond to (and respect) BOTH communications.

To make the best use of the patient's non-verbal communication, the physiotherapist needs to be very observant, alert and receptive. She should consciously look at the patient from the beginning, so that a basis of trust can be established within the first few minutes of being with the patient. Nevertheless, it would be unreasonable for all people to develop such a trust within a short time. It could be appropriate for some person, having received unsatisfactory treatment elsewhere, to be suspicious of the new therapist. A way of handling this might be as follows.

'It seems that previous treatments haven't been successful. Knowing that, I would like you to know that I need your help, for you to look closely at what I do and for you to tell me anything that raises any queries you may have. I need to know all you can tell me, even things that you may feel are trivial or unimportant. Also don't expect a cure, or you will be disappointed if I join the line of failures.'

What you are then asking is the reasonable request of 'look before you leap', and raising the idea of 'how would you know when you can trust the helping person?'. The patient's nuances of behaviour can be extremely informative, and so can those of the physiotherapist. If she reads his nuances of behaviour well and handles her own nuances well, she can gain the patient's confidence quickly and help him to recognize her concern for him. The tone of voice, the intonation and associated facial expression are also components of non-verbal communication that can be used to great effect.

People have different personalities, different characteristics, different levels of intelligence, and so on. During an interview with every patient, the manipulative physiotherapist can adapt her mannerisms to fit his. She should follow his patterns; she should not try to change him so that he responds to her patterns. Another way of expressing this aspect is to say that the patient's peculiarities should form the 'common denominator', not the physiotherapist's peculiarities. It is interesting to discover how we came to our own pattern of peculiarities in a unique way, with many learnings from mother and father as well as from other people with whom we have lived, played and worked. So too, the patient, by a different life journey, came to his or her own peculiarities. When we now meet, it becomes a task of some importance to move into an adaptable position that fits comfortably with the patient's position. Bandler and Grinder (1975a) call this process 'watching and pacing'.

It could include such things as sitting with our head at the same angle as the patient's head (though not to mimic them if they have an acute 'wry neck'), to have our hands in the same sort of position as theirs, and even to include breathing at the same rate and speaking with about the same loudness, tone and tempo. All of this would need to be done in a natural and comfortable way. It is important for this matching to be done gracefully or artfully, and not to be forced or unnatural.

As with verbal communication, the physiotherapist should not assume she is interpreting the patient's nuances correctly, because his frame of reference is probably quite different from hers. Also she should be aware of her own state of mental and physical well being, because it affects how she interprets the patient's non-verbal signals. When necessary, any possible assumptions she may make, related to his nuances, should be clarified so that misinterpretation is avoided. Likewise, if there is a disparity between the verbal and non-verbal messages, the correct interpretation needs to be sought.

The patient's facial expression and eye movements as well as leg, foot, arm and hand movements are extremely informative in providing spontaneous information, and the physiotherapist should be alert and equipped to interpret these messages. It was interesting to read a novelist using the words, 'His mouth was wreathed with unspoken language' (Macdonald, 1970).

There is much to be learned and appreciated in the area of non-verbal communication, and the reader is recommended to read a text such as *Bodily Communication* (Argyle, 1975) and to follow up the relevant references listed in its bibliography.

In the paragraphs above, non-verbal communication has been discussed as it relates to the question–answer situation during the subjective examination of a patient. The following is a common example of how the non-verbal nuances of behaviour can be used when examining a patient's joint movements.

During the physical examination of a patient's movements, the physiotherapist may say to a patient, 'I want you to bend forwards until you feel discomfort in your back. As soon as you do feel anything, STOP, and immediately stand up straight again'. Despite the precision of the instruction, it is common for a patient to bend further and further, feeling more and more discomfort. During the bending forward the patient may, quite unconsciously, display a non-verbal message such as beginning to purse his lips. If this is seen by the physiotherapist, it will enable her to stop him bending further, return him to the upright position and ask him if he felt any discomfort. She is then able to reinstruct him on the necessity to 'STOP', thus making the test precise and safe.

## VERBAL COMMUNICATION

The process of obtaining a clear picture of a patient's symptoms, either at an initial consultation or during the course of treatment, depends very much upon successful verbal communication. For some people expressing their thoughts comes easily, while others have difficulty. However, communication skills can be learned. Later in this chapter, examples of conversations between a patient and a physiotherapist are given for the purpose of helping the physiotherapist to learn the special communication skills required for accurate assessment.

In summary, it is important to realize that the patient's responses to questions will be modified by his lifelong background of experiences – that is, his 'frame of reference' will be different from the physiotherapist's. Of equal importance is the fact that the physiotherapist's interpretation of the patient's statements will be influenced by her own 'frame of reference'. These components should be borne in mind throughout every treatment session.

## INTERVIEWING SKILLS

Probably the first requirement during interviews with patients is that the physiotherapist should retain control of the interview at all times. This is difficult with the garrulous patient. However, the garrulous patient readily reveals all of his problems, whereas it can be extremely difficult to draw out from the reticent patient all the information that may be required.

Retaining control of the interview with the garrulous patient is fundamental. In the interview, it is useful to be able to stop a garrulous patient as soon as the information from him either:

- exceeds your own ability to assimilate it, or
- changes to a subject that you are not finding relevant.

The stop could be called a 'disruption', and this can be achieved by saying 'I'm sorry, but what I need to know is . . .', naming the last subject you were following, or 'I was interested to hear about X, could you tell me more about that point?', or 'I'd like you to remember this matter Y, but may I come back to it after I make myself clearer about X in more detail?.

A versatile physiotherapist has many ways of stopping or changing the conversation, as well as an ability to recall the subject that the patient may like to return to in due course.

Another approach is to allow the patient to say some of what he wishes to say while the physiotherapist continues to show an interest, but when it is obvious that helpful spontaneous information is not forthcoming, she may interpose a question at a volume slightly greater than his, while also involving non-verbal techniques such as raising a hand, or touching his arm just before starting to ask her question. This tends to interrupt his train of thought, and means the question can be asked without the need for a calculated increase in volume. The manipulative physiotherapist, in particular, repeatedly uses the strongest form of non-verbal communication, which is 'touch'.

The reticent patient needs to be kindly told that it seems he finds it hard to talk about his complaints but it is necessary for him to do so. He should be reassured that he is not complaining but rather that he is informing, and that what he does not tell her, she will never know.

To gain the most out of an interview with a patient, the physiotherapist should try to 'feel' the kind of problem the patient has; she should put herself 'in his shoes', so to speak, and let it be seen that she understands his plight. She should show that she takes him at his word, even if she has doubts. Her facial expression and the quality of her voice should engender confidence and show empathy.

There are many ways in which the physiotherapist can modify the questions she needs to ask to make them easier for the patient to understand, thus making it easier for him to respond more accurately. As an example, during an interview it is important to *use the patient's language* whenever possible, even pronouncing words as he does whether it is correct pronunciation or not, as this makes things that are said or asked much clearer, easier and quicker for him to understand. No question therefore should contain technical terms, and we need to watch for a puzzled look, slightly dilating pupils, roving eyes or altered facial expression, as indications of the patient's searching for a meaning.

It is important to remember to use the following four strategies:

1. Speak slowly.
2. Speak deliberately.
3. Keep questions short.
4. Ask only one question at a time.

Each of these aspects makes it easier for the patient to answer questions accurately. It is important always to bear in mind that the patient is in unfamiliar surroundings, and that his complaint is his all-pervading thought. If questions are long and awkward, the words may just encroach on his mind rather than make an impact. This may lead to the import of the question being lost.

At an initial interview, it is natural for a patient to have a strong desire to explain all aspects of his problem that HE believes are important. Therefore, he should be given a reasonably free hand to express these aspects. However, at no stage should the interview be allowed to get out of hand. By allowing the patient a degree of controlled latitude, the physiotherapist can learn much about the patient as a person as well as his problem. For example, the manner in which the patient makes his initial spontaneous comments about his problem tells the examiner the relative importance he places on each of the facets of his problem. For example, if two patients are talking about their shoulder problems, one patient may say that his arm is too stiff to tuck the back of his shirt into his trousers, while the other may say he has so much pain he is unable to put his hand behind his back to tuck his shirt in. On these two statements alone, it is likely that each of these two patients will require different treatment. Such initial spontaneous comments will show the patient's attitude towards his problem, and may also indicate his 'pain threshold' and pain acceptance.

When a patient is responding to a question, he may include in his reply a comment outside the scope of the question. For example, he may have been asked 'When did the symptoms begin?', and in his reply he may have included the comment that he had changed jobs. He must have had some reason for saying this. Perhaps the 'changing of jobs' is related in some way to a change in his symptoms. The physiotherapist should therefore interpose the question, **'Do you relate that to the onset of your symptoms?'** and then follow with 'When was that?'. At that moment in the dialogue, the patient's thought processes centre on the change in jobs. If the above question is interposed at this stage, the answer will be more accurate and will be made more quickly than if the patient is allowed to continue talking, changing his train of thought. Conversely, if the question is left until a later stage the patient will have to start afresh to re-orientate his thinking before he can reply. This takes extra time, and thoughts that might have been 'on the tip of his tongue' to mention may unfortunately be lost. The skill of making use of the patient's line of thought is immensely valuable. The only danger with the technique lies in losing one's own train of thought. This *paralleling* of questions with the patient's mental processes is an important skill to develop.

When a question is apparently misunderstood, *the physiotherapist should blame herself*, not the patient, for the communication error; she should note the misunderstanding and track it (e.g. by rephrasing the question, if necessary in several different ways). For example, the physiotherapist could say, 'I'm sorry, what I really meant was, did so and so . . . etc.?'. It is this process of self-criticism that is our best teacher.

One very important element of the initial interview is the insight it provides into the kind of person the patient is, for this guides the physiotherapist as to how to conduct the remainder of the interview. By the end of the interview, the physiotherapist should be able to make a reasonable judgement as to the patient's sensibility and credibility.

## WORDING SKILLS

### PARALLELING

This has been touched upon on page 28, and it is only learnt by experience. What is meant is this. When a patient is talking about an aspect of his problem, his mind is running along a specific line of thought. It is likely that, along this specific line of thought, he could have more than one point he wishes to express – in fact, there could be three or four points. To interrupt him may make him lose his place in his story. Therefore, unless you, the therapist, are in danger of losing your place, do not stop him (unless he is just rambling on), because if you do interrupt he is likely to lose his place and you may well lose important points that he may fail to retrieve at any later stage of the questioning.

### BIAS

While the method described here may sometimes be appropriate, it is important for the therapist to be aware that:

1. Some people are very open to suggestion.
2. Some people are very opposed to suggestion.

There is a skill in learning when to use any particular style of question – 'A time to use it and a time not to use it'.

There are skills in the wording of questions that the physiotherapist should learn if 'assessment' is to be used to its maximum effect. The first of these is that, unless care is taken to prevent it, the physiotherapist's questions will probably have a bias. It is most important that questions should not be biased in any way towards the answer hoped for. In fact, this statement can be carried one stage further – if the physiotherapist is hoping for a 'yes' answer to a particular question, assessment is better served if the question is worded so that it is biased towards a 'no' answer. For example, when a patient attends for the third treatment and the physiotherapist is hoping that he will have shown some subjective improvement, she could ask him, 'Did my last treatment make you worse in any way?'. This will influence the patient to say something like, 'No, well not much anyway'. To ask, 'Are you feeling any better from the last treatment?' will influence him (especially if the changes are minimal) towards saying, 'Yes, thank you, I think I am', rather than giving her the most important information contained in the first response, 'No, well not much anyway'.

## BREVITY

When asking questions and responding to a patient's answers, the number of individual words used by the manipulative physiotherapist should be kept to an absolute minimum. This avoids confusion in the mind of the patient and misunderstanding, and it also conserves time. However, when using conversation to establish rapport with a patient any number of words can be used, and they should be accompanied by plenty of pleasing non-verbal signs.

Often a single word can ask a question adequately, and that one word will not only save time in asking the question, but will also hasten the answer because the patient's thinking processes are thrust into the quick answer situation. For example, if a patient has said that the pain spreads across both sides of his back, the question, 'Equally?', calls for a much more rapid and positive response than does, 'Do you get more pain on one side than the other?'. Another good word is 'because'. For example, 'I couldn't walk for half an hour'. This is a statement of fact, not a comparison; convert it to a comparison by asking 'because?'. 'I couldn't walk for half an hour.' 'Because . . . (pause)?' 'Because the pain in my back was killing me.' This is still not a comparison, so ask 'Is that the same as usual or worse than usual?'.

## SPONTANEOUS INFORMATION

Another important skill is that of asking questions in such a way as to provide opportunities for spontaneous comments in the patient's reply. Any spontaneous comment is far more valuable than a direct answer to a direct question. This is because it provides quality to the answer given. The quality is of the kind that provides an insight into the patient's personality, his ability to accept (or not accept) his symptoms, while also putting his symptoms in a context that is correct for him (*see* pp. 28 and 36).

## KEYWORDS

Finally, a patient's answer to a question often includes a phrase that requires an *immediate follow-up question*, or he uses a word, such as 'Saturday', which must have been stated for a reason. The reason should be sought while it is still fresh in the patient's mind. To follow the patient's line of thought is a far better policy than following one's own line of thought.

---

Summary of interviewing skills:

- Retain control of the interview
- Reassure the patient that the information given is important to the physiotherapist
- Use the patient's language and words whenever possible
- Speak slowly
- Speak deliberately
- Keep questions short
- Ask only one question at a time
- Allow spontaneous information, as this may reveal much about the illness experience of the patient
- Use paralleling skills
- Be aware at all times of possible errors in the communication process
- Use feedback loops for clarification and deeper understanding

---

## ERRORS IN VERBAL COMMUNICATION

That people run into difficulties of misunderstanding is indisputable, but the whole subject is really much easier to understand when we examine the following idea:

*The map is not the territory and the name is not the thing named.* (Bateson, 1980)

What this really means is that a thought is a representation of some external thing (visual, auditory or kinaesthetic). A map of Adelaide is a representation of Adelaide – it is not actually Adelaide, but merely a coding of some data about Adelaide. The information in a human mind is such a map (or model, or representation) and is used to make sense of new or old information.

There is a transformation (or a coding) when a thing becomes a perception. Naming is always classifying, and mapping is essentially the same as naming. The next vital point is that people operate out of their internal maps (models) *not* out of direct sensory experience. They can only make sense of new information by comparing it with what they already have coded.

Since people code their information at different times and in different ways, they tend to have ideas linked together in their own individual ways.

People (unconsciously) retrieve information from their minds when they hear words, and communicators need to check what the receiver accesses (retrieves). The retrieving is called 'a transderivational search' by Bandler and Grinder (1975b), i.e. the person makes a derivation through a searching process. Let us look at this in the context of a physiotherapist carrying out an interview. The words that she uses are a way of representing what she is thinking. By understanding the possibility of using 'unspecified search language' or 'increasingly specified search language', the physiotherapist gains great power in choosing words well and developing modifier questions as she enquires further in the search for meaning.

Following general introductory remarks would come the presenting complaint, which allows the physiotherapist to hear an 'unedited' expression of the problem. It is here that the physiotherapist can greatly increase her own skill to obtain an accurate transfer of information from the patient to herself.

The process could be called interpretation, but it always depends upon accurate checking with the patient to confirm that she has the right meaning. This is a feedback loop. *Without feedback loops, communication between people would be at grave risk of being very inaccurate.* This also means that the hearer is really aware of the danger of making assumptions.

There are many identifiable areas where mistakes in verbal communication can and do occur. They occur in the physiotherapist's thinking surrounding the asking of the question, in the words used when asking the question, and then in the way in which the patient hears and interprets what is said. The errors are further multiplied by the patient's thinking processes in preparing his response, and in the words he then uses. Finally, mistakes occur in the physiotherapist's thought processes in interpreting the patient's answer to her question. *Figure 3.2* shows these areas for mistakes in an example where one question is asked by the physiotherapist, answered by the patient and then interpreted by the physiotherapist.

There are three main areas where physiotherapists make mistakes during an interview. The first is not expressing their thoughts clearly, as in the ditty 'what you heard is not what I meant' (*see* pp. 25–26). The second is misinterpreting the patient's answer to the question, and the third lies in the area of ASSUMING a meaning of the patient's answer. The words chosen by the patient and the intonation used may be quite misleading. These factors, therefore, are areas with which the examiner has to take the greatest care. It is wiser to confirm the meaning with a patient than to let it pass. This 'confirming' is a frequent requirement, not a rarity.

There are very many influences that lie behind the way a patient expresses himself and, although it is impossible to identify all of them here, some common ones need to be mentioned.

## MISINTERPRETING

First, if a patient has a high pain tolerance he will use weak words when expressing the level or grade of his disorder. The examiner will make an error of judgement if she has not picked up during the interview that his pain tolerance is high. This patient is usually reticent in talking about his aches and pains. The opposite may also be the case; that is, the examiner may wrongly judge the severity of a patient's problem when the patient has a low pain tolerance and uses extravagant language such as 'excruciating', 'agony', etc., to describe his pain.

*High pain tolerance* involves multiple factors, e.g. culture, peer group expectations, and the reason for playing a symptom or point of the problem up or down.

*Low pain tolerance* is again multifactorial, and the patient may use extravagant language such as 'excruciating' and 'agonizing'.

The words may convey the psychological impact of injury upon the patient, or his need to impress others with the 'seriousness' and change in his lifestyle consequent upon the injury. Alternatively, the patient may be wanting to be sure that the physiotherapist will be gentle in the examination, assessment and treatment.

Some outside issues such as an insurance claim may alter the degree to which the symptom is presented either psychologically or somatically, consciously or unconsciously. The physiotherapist needs to recognize and understand that people always have reasons, conscious or unconscious, physical or psychological, for their exact mode of presentation, and that it expresses a certain need.

The physiotherapist should therefore never be critical of the way a patient presents. The very presentation *itself* is a message, needing to be decoded just as much as the other findings that the history and examination reveal.

Secondly, a patient may be reticent in talking about his symptoms, even though they are sufficiently restricting for him to be seeking treatment. It is extremely easy to misinterpret the severity of the disorder if this aspect of the patient's character is not perceived. When it is perceived the physiotherapist should guide him to talk about his symptoms, explaining that without his co-operation errors of interpretation will occur and important information may be missed.

Thirdly, when a patient is not fluent in the language of the physiotherapist, his only means of expressing

**Therapist**

Error

**1st process**
THE REASONING BEHIND THE QUESTION WHICH IS TO BE ASKED
The fundamental error that lies behind much poor questioning is having insufficient theoretical and clinical knowledge to guide the precise information required from a patient

**Patient**

**2nd process**
WORDING THE QUESTION
The error occurs when the question asked does not clearly ask what the physiotherapist needs to know

Error

**3rd process**
HEARING AND UNDERSTANDING THE QUESTIONS
Two errors can occur at this stage:
1. A word or words may be used which the patient does not understand

2. What the patient hears may be biased away from what he should have heard

Error

**4th process**
CONSIDERING THE REPLY
Because the patient has particular thoughts about his complaint, he may assume different reasons for the question from those of the physiotherapist. Also his memory of facts which are involved in answering the question may be incomplete or inaccurate

Error

**6th process**
HEARING AND UNDERSTANDING THE WORDS USED IN THE PATIENTS ANSWER
Patients may use descriptive words which are difficult to understand, particularly when describing bizarre symptoms. The error lies in assuming the meaning of them rather than asking questions to be certain of the meaning

Error

**5th process**
PUTTING THE ANSWER INTO WORDS
To translate thoughts related to answering the question into words is even more difficult for the patient than for the physiotherapist because of the comparative lack of experience

Error

**7th process**
INTERPRETING THE ANSWER
Because of the physiotherapist does not have the patient's symptoms herself, she has to interpret the answer in the light of her own experiences (including her experiences with other patients). The interpretation may be wrong if the answer is not clarified

Error

**8th process**
RELATING THE ANSWER TO THE QUESTION
If the physiotherapist accepts the patient's answer as providing all the information when in fact it does not, the subsequent examination will be open to major errors

Error

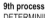

Error

**9th process**
DETERMINING THE NEXT QUESTION
If the was insufficient knowledge on which to base the first question, irrespective of the accuracy of the patient's answer, the basis for the second question must also be in the error

If there has been no error in any of the proceeding eight processes there should be no error in this 9th process

Error

Figure 3.2   The area for mistakes in verbal communication

how bad his symptoms are may be to gesticulate in an exaggerated manner. It is essential to recognize that such nuances of behaviour are simply methods of non-verbal communication, which are exaggerated when verbal communication is difficult. *Because it is so easy to misjudge the patient's disability, the physiotherapist's manner has to be tempered with understanding.*

Fourthly, a patient's ethnic background influences the mannerisms he adopts in expressing his problem. People from some countries are hardy and tough, while in other countries they are expected to groan and 'carry on' while the whole family flocks around to help with dressing, walking, etc. The physiotherapist needs to be very aware of these ethnic characteristics to avoid misinterpreting the verbal and non-verbal messages.

Fifthly, it is easy to misjudge (or interpret wrongly) the expression of a patient's disability when factors such as litigation, family or social situations, or financial problems are involved. It is equally easy to misjudge the influence of a patient's psyche. To avoid such communication mistakes the examiner should give the patient the benefit of any doubt, at least until it is proven that, for example, the emotional element is a major factor in the persistence of his symptoms. Frequently such judgements can only be made (and perhaps *should* only be made) in retrospect. It is interesting that Miller (1978) makes the statement that the patient (his illness) 'is innocent until proved guilty'.

Sixthly, some patients will only comment on the symptoms that remain and do not comment on other aspects of the symptoms that may have improved. If subjective asterisks (*see* pp. 60–61) are utilized, the skilled physiotherapist can seek the positive side of the symptomatic changes rather than accepting the patient's negative approach. The opposite situation may be equally misleading.

Finally, a mistaken interpretation can occur when a patient's present symptoms are an exacerbation of symptoms that are always present but at a lower intensity. Such a patient has come to accept a certain amount of discomfort as being normal and thus, when describing his present problem, he is likely to express a lower degree of severity (or disability) than would be expressed by a patient with the same pain but who is normally symptom-free.

---

Misinterpretation of the information is possible due to:

- Differences in individual pain acceptance, which may lead to different verbal and non-verbal presentations of the pain
- A reticent patient, i.e. the patient who is unwilling to reveal all relevant information due to stoicism, fear of finding out something is seriously wrong, or a dislike for the medical and associated professions
- Exaggerated non-verbal communication, because of difficult verbal communication
- Cultural differences
- Known social or psychological problems
- One-sided focus on the remaining symptoms or on the improvement of symptoms
- The individual illness experience

---

## THE REASON BEHIND THE QUESTION

During the learning stages of asking patients questions and interpreting their answers, it is difficult to know where to start. There are certain questions that have to be asked to avoid 'the finger of negligence' being pointed at the therapist; questions about dizziness in patients with cervical disorders, for example, or the possibility of cauda equina involvement in lumbar disorders. It is necessary to ask about the effect of rest and activities, of sitting, of getting up from a chair after sitting for half an hour, or the effects of coughing, sneezing and deep inspiration, etc. BUT do the therapists always know the reasons behind these questions? And do they know what to do with an answer when they get one? In other words, they have to learn the reasons behind the questions. Certainly they can be taught some of the reasons, under some circumstances, but not every circumstance can be covered. This element of communication (*see* Figure 3.2, 1st process) is probably the key to most of the problems a beginner has. Putting this into one clinical example may make it easier to understand.

One specific question asked of patients with low lumbar problems is, 'How does it feel when you first waken in the morning before you get out of bed?', followed by, 'And how does it feel when you first get out of bed in the morning?'. The reason for asking the first question is that the therapist needs to know whether prolonged rest lessens the symptoms compared with short-term rest, and also to know whether the patient is wakened by the symptoms, or whether he wakens and then becomes aware of the symptoms. The two common answers by the patient are that:

1. When he changes position in bed (such as turning from lying on one side to the other) he feels a sharp twinge of pain:
   a) Where does he feel it?
   b) Does he need to have been in bed for a substantial period of time before this occurs, or does it

occur if he changes position almost as soon as he lies down?

c) Does the twinge disappear quickly without getting any worse throughout the night? This latter response indicates that the physical examination should be able to determine the provoking position and movement. In treatment it will be this position of the patient and this movement by the therapist which will probably be used as the treatment technique.

2. He may be wakened by an increased intensity of the aching, sufficiently for him to have to get out of bed and walk around until the increased aching subsides.

If the therapist DOES know the reason behind the question, has she got the answer? No! So, not having the answer based on her reasoning, what should she do? The thing she should NOT do is believe that she does have the answer and move onto the next question (this happens far too easily, and destroys the validity of the subjective examination). The next question could be, 'Does the same thing happen if you lie on the other side?'. If the answer is 'NO', that is, he can lie on the other side without any problems, then it is likely to be a positional factor. If it is the position that is the cause, then the physical examination will reveal the movements in certain positions that provoke and ease the symptoms. For treatment, whether the symptoms need provoking or not is a separate decision that is made at the conclusion of both the subjective and the physical examinations. However, if the answer is that it makes no difference how he lies – he is still wakened by increased aching, which forces him to get out of bed – then the problem may be an inflammatory disorder, or at least have a large inflammatory component. Therefore, *question*! What other subjective question should be asked? 'What happens when you get out of bed'? *Answer*: his back should be notably stiff, not necessarily painful, it should take in excess of 1 hour after rising before it wears off, and it may not always completely loosen. She now has the answer to the original question: he has either ankylosing spondylosis, an intradiscal disorder or perhaps a locked joint.

## ASSUMING

If a patient says his pain is 'constant', it is wrong to assume that he means constant throughout the day and night. He may mean that when he has pain it is a constant pain, but it isn't present all day long. It is important to check the more exact meaning – constant meaning 'steady' or 'unchanging in degree', constant in location, or constant over time?

Although the following catchphrase takes an extreme view of the problem, it is one well worth remembering:

NEVER ASSUME ANYTHING

If we add to the possible mistakes explained above the communication problems created by language differences, personality, distress, etc., it is easy to understand how physiotherapists can both misunderstand and be misunderstood.

## VERBATIM EXAMPLES

It was very gratifying to read that Macnab (1977), in his book *Backache*, considered the dialogue of history taking sufficiently important to portray it in verbatim question and answer form. This, from a man of Macnab's stature, gives the inclusion of literal quotations in a book the element of acceptability. Taking an accurate history is no less important than making an accurate assessment of the subjective and objective changes that take place during treatment. For this reason verbatim text is used here to provide guidelines which will, it is hoped, help the physiotherapist to achieve the depth of accuracy and refinement required for good assessment.

The process of learning how to word questions, and what automatic follow-up questions should be asked when certain answers are given, can be hastened by understanding the guidelines that are presented in the following dialogues. The guidelines should not be interpreted as preaching to the ignorant, or treating readers as schoolchildren; they are given to show the extent to which the rule 'never assume anything' should be taken. Similarly, they also show the process of confirming messages so as to avoid mistaken interpretations. It is more realistic to understand that we cannot avoid making assumptions or hypotheses – but if we make any assumptions explicit to ourselves, we are in a good position to know that they are assumptions, and to know when they are wrong or confirmed or in need of changing. They will also show how accuracy can be achieved without the patient being made to feel he is being treated as an imbecile, and without irritating him by excessive repetition of questions. In fact people have enormous amounts of information stored in the computer that we call the mind, and it is a genuine respect for this matter and a care for the quality of our communication that gives us the potential to create a good relationship environment.

Before asking a question, it is vital for the physiotherapist to be clear about four things:

1. What it is she wishes to know and why.
2. What is the best possible way to word it.
3. What different answers might she get.

4. How the possible reply to her questions might influence her planning ahead for the next question.

It is probably the last of these that picks out the good physiotherapists from the less good.

A mistake that occurs with trainee manipulative physiotherapists is the accepting of an answer as being adequate when in fact it is only vaguely informative, is incomplete, or is in insufficient depth. The reason for the physiotherapist accepting the inadequate answer is usually that she does not clearly understand why she is asking the question, and therefore does not know the number of separate answers she must hear to meet the requirements of the questions. The same reason can lead to another error; that of allowing her line of thought to be diverted by the patient, usually without her realizing it.

To enable most value to be gained from the following verbatim text in terms of learning how to avoid communication errors, the physiotherapist's questions will be identified by the letter 'Q' (question); her thought processes will be identified as 'ET' (examiner's thoughts); and the patient's verbal responses will be identified as 'A' (answer).

In the verbatim texts that follow, the communication skills exemplify certain aspects:

- Awareness of the body's capacity to inform.
- Not irritating the patient.
- Keeping questions brief.
- Making features fit.
- Assuming nothing.
- Controlling the interview.
- Paralleling questions.
- Asking leading questions.
- Using spontaneous answers.
- Knowing the question's purpose.
- Emphasizing/using key words.
- Immediate-response questions.

When the patient's problem is pain, with or without limited movement, guidelines for particular questions can be discussed in the following groups:

1. Immediate-response questions – immediate questions in response to certain of the patient's statements.
2. Keywords – words that indicate a patient's line of thought.
3. Specificity – assisting the patient to make meaningful assessment.
4. At initial consultations, questions about:
   a) The history
   b) The behaviour of the symptoms.
   Questions about pain responses during test movements.

5. At subsequent treatment sessions, questions about changes in the symptoms.
6. During a treatment session, questions about:
   a) Changes in pain response during reassessment of test movements
   b) Pain response while a technique is performed
   c) Changes in pain response after a treatment technique is performed.
7. At review sessions, questions:
   a) During a retrospective assessment
   b) After each three to five treatments
   c) When progress has slowed or stopped
   d) Following a break from treatment.

The greatest percentage of a physiotherapist's patients seek treatment just because of their pain, while all other aspects of their problem, as far as they are concerned, pale into insignificance. Only a very small percentage of patients seek treatment because of either painless stiffness resulting in loss of function, or muscle weakness. The treatment concept which this book outlines is clearly not one that takes into account pain to the exclusion of all else, but it does recognize that MOST patients are patients because of pain; without pain they would not be patients. The purpose in raising this point is that in the verbatim texts used, nearly all refer to a patient's symptoms of pain.

If pain were the only consideration, the first question asked of a patient at an initial consultation would always be, 'Where is your pain?'. However, a patient may reply bluntly, 'I don't have any pain', whereupon a trainee manipulative physiotherapist might feel lost and wonder, 'Where do I go now?'. Therefore, the opening question should be, 'As far as you are concerned . . . (pause) . . . at this stage . . . (pause) . . . what do you feel . . . (pause) . . . is your . . . main . . . problem?'.

## IMMEDIATE–RESPONSE QUESTIONS

Many questions have to be asked of a patient during a first consultation, and the patient's answers to these questions are normally statements of fact. However, during subsequent treatment sessions, because it is the effect of treatment that is to be assessed, answers to these questions have to be changed from *statements of fact* to *comparisons*. For example, a patient may answer a question by saying, 'I had pins and needles in my hands when I hemmed a skirt'. This is a statement of fact and is of no value as an assessment unless it is known what would have happened with 'hemming a skirt' before treatment. From a communication point of view, the aspect to be emphasized is that the statement, 'I had pins and needles in my hands when I hemmed a skirt', demands the immediate-response question, 'How does that compare with what would have happened if you had hemmed a skirt before we began treatment?'. Much time is wasted and valuable information lost if the method is not continually followed.

---

### CONVERT STATEMENTS OF FACT INTO COMPARISONS

There are many responses to therapist's questions that are statements of fact and which, if accepted at face value, can give false impressions. For example, following the question, 'How have you been?' the patient may say, 'Better, thank you'. Rather than assuming that this means he has improved as a result of treatment, the statement 'better' must be followed by 'Better than *when*?', 'Better than *what*?', or 'Better in *what way*?'. In actual fact, 'Better, thank you' may be meaning better than the 24-hour exacerbation he had following the treatment (of which he had been warned).

The following examples should clarify when immediate-response questions must be used automatically. They are presented in groups, to illustrate the different kinds of answers that may be given by patients. The groups are:

1. At initial consultations.
2. Clarifying subjective assessments.
3. Subjective differences.
4. At subsequent treatments.
5. Non-verbal responses.

### 1. AT INITIAL CONSULTATION

At the first consultation a patient may have symptoms that could be arising from a cervical disorder or a glenohumeral disorder. During the subjective examination, the patient may make the comment, 'I feel it mostly with quick movements'. The immediate-response question, which the physiotherapist *must* ask, is:

Q   'Quick movements of what?'

and then, following the patient's answer, ask

Q   'In what direction?', or

Q   'Are you able to show me that quick movement now?'

A patient may have a definite opinion about what he has wrong with him. Any expression of this kind requires immediate follow-up so that the point he makes is neither misunderstood nor ignored. For example, he may say, 'When I get the pain, it feels like a pinched nerve'. Such a statement is also an example of a 'keyword'.

The immediate-response questions are:

Q   'What is it about the pain that makes you feel it is like a pinched nerve?', and

Q   'Where do you feel the nerve is pinched?'

The patient who made this statement had a sharp intermittent pain deep in one spot in his buttock. His history of episodic back and buttock pain would have led the examiner to ASSUME that he was describing a pinched nerve in his back, whereas his symptoms were relieved by treating his hip.

### 2. CLARIFYING SUBJECTIVE ASSESSMENTS

When determining the effect of the last treatment, there may be particular aspects learned at the first and second consultations which should be followed up, such as the patient having pain putting his shoes and socks on first thing in the morning, or pain provoked by walking.

Q   'How was your leg with walking this morning?'

A   'Oh, VERY GOOD.'

Because it is important to know how the leg symptoms are changing in response to treatment, the statement 'very good' must be fully clarified. Four immediate-response questions are given as examples of what might be asked:

Q   'How does that compare with yesterday or other mornings?'

Q   'Do you mean 100 per cent?'

Q   'Is there any difference between the feeling in your right and left legs now?'

Q   'Same as the other leg – nothing at all – 100 per cent?'

### 3. SUBJECTIVE DIFFERENCES

In response to the question 'How have you been?', a patient will often respond in a way that indicates that he feels there is a difference yet he is unable to explain it clearly. As a comparison is being sought, the immediate-response question can always be asked in the terms of the example given. It is a valuable way of converting the uninformative *statement* into a useful *comparison*.

Q   'How have you been?'

A   'I feel that something in my back has shifted.'

The immediate-response question is:

Q   'Is it a favourable "shift", or unfavourable?'

Patients are able to feel things that the physiotherapist is unable to assess by any physical examination. She is then reliant upon the patient's statement. It is very important that a physiotherapist should accept what the patient says and put it to good use by well-chosen questions. The answers will reveal the value of his statement.

Q    'How have you been?'

A    'It feels different.'

Time can be saved by asking simply, 'Is it a good difference or a bad difference?', instead of spending time offering suggestions as to the ways in which it might be different. In fact, the patient's answer to the 'good or bad difference' question may give more answers than expected.

## 4. AT SUBSEQUENT TREATMENTS

All the following examples are responses to the first question asked at the beginning of each treatment session – 'How have you been?', 'How has it been?', or 'How are you? Any different?.

There is a necessity for the patient to understand that he has a very important role to play in the assessment of changes (for good or ill) that are taking place at the treatment session and from session to session. The fact should be explained to him at the first session that it is comparisons the therapist needs, NOT just 'statements of fact'. This subject is discussed more fully in Chapter 4. Nevertheless, if the following dialogue is looked at in depth, it is possible to see that there are many examples where the patient can understand the need for comparisons – he is, in fact, being educated as to how he needs to think.

(1)  A    'Not too bad', or 'Good thank you'.

Q    The immediate-response question is 'Any different from usual?' or 'What does that mean?'.

(2)  When a patient attends the second session and says he's 'just the same', it is a necessary part of the education process to confirm his statement strongly.

Q    'Do you mean you're neither better nor worse?'

A    'That's right.'

Q    'With all I did last time, did I stir it up at all?'

A    'That's right.'

Q    'How did you feel when you walked out of here compared with when you came in?'

A    'Just the same.'

Q    'And you had no reactions later?'

A    'No.'

This depth of questioning *is* necessary at the first assessment so that the patient learns the precision in answering that is being sought. All four questions are necessary immediate-response questions.

(3)  Q    'How has it been?'

A    'The first burst of incredible pain was at 3 am'

ET    *This response is a statement of fact: the rule is to make it a comparison. I wonder if this is unusual and if it is related to my treatment? My immediate-response question must be something akin to the following.*

Q    'How does that compare with your usual pattern of pain?'

(4)  Q    'How has it been?'

A    'Saturday was a much better day.'

The kind of immediate-response question required here is:

Q    'Is that unusual?', or 'Before beginning treatment, could you have had days which were much better, as you say Saturday was?'

(5)  Q    'How has it been?'

A    'A lot, lot better; it's incredible.'

ET    *It would seem reasonable to assume he has made substantial improvement, and that it is probably related to treatment. However, I wonder if he considers he is cured and does not require any further treatment? Therefore the immediate-response question should be along the following lines.*

Q    'Do you mean you are 100 per cent and we can stop treatment?', or 'Do you not have anything left in the way of symptoms?'.

(6)  Q    'How has it been?'

A    'A bit stiff.'

ET    *This is informative in that his main feelings relate to stiffness. However, it does not qualify the stiffness in any way other than to say that it is mild rather than a rigid stiffness. The immediate-response question is:*

Q    'Do you mean stiffer than usual?'

(7)  Q    'How has it been?'

A    'I was not wakened last night by the pins and needles.'

The immediate-response question is:

Q    'Is that unusual?'

(8)  Q    'How has it been?'

A    'Worse.'

'Worse' is a statement that must ALWAYS be clarified in depth. Many times a patient will make this response when, on more detailed investigation, the worsening may be treatment soreness rather than the disorder itself having been made worse.

Q    'In what way has it been worse?', and so on.

(9)  Q    'How has it been?'

A    'More sore.'

Q    'And do you think that is from the treatment?'

A    'Yes.'

Q    'When were you first aware of it being more sore?'

ET    *It is better for me to ask the question this way to elicit a more spontaneous response rather than asking if it was sore when he finished treatment.*

A    'Fairly soon after I left here.'

Q    'Do you mean 2 minutes, or an hour or so?'

A    'I would say it started to become sore within a quarter of an hour.'

ET    *What needs to be determined is, is the soreness a 'treatment soreness' or 'disorder soreness', that is, has the treatment technique irritated the disorder and made it more sore, or is it a soreness that has resulted from the pressure of the thumbs (for example) used as the treatment technique.*

Q    'Are you able to tell whether it is just soreness from my thumbs, or is it the problem we are treating which is more sore?'

ET    *Patients are not always able to differentiate the soreness in this way but at least two-thirds of the patients are, so it should always be sought.*

A    'I'd say it was your thumbs.'

Q    'Good – thank you. That's most helpful.'

(10)  Q    'How have you been?'

The garrulous patient will take a long time to answer, and may not give much information that is comparative. He may give an item-by-item description of the symptoms he felt from the time immediately following the last treatment until the moment the question 'How have you been?' is asked. The patient must be permitted to say what he feels is necessary, provided the physiotherapist *does not lose control of the interview*. The immediate-response question, which should be asked as quickly as appropriate, is:

Q    'Overall, what effect do you think the last treatment had?' or 'Do you feel the last treatment has made you any worse?'.

## 5. NON-VERBAL RESPONSES

### Example A

All of the above examples of immediate-response questions have been related to verbal communication, but there are many examples when the examiner must recognize a non-verbal response either to a question or to an examination test movement. The physiotherapist *must* qualify such expressions. For example, in response to the question, 'How has it been?', the patient may respond simply by wrinkling his nose. The immediate-response question is:

Q    'That doesn't look too good. Do you mean it has been worse?', etc.

### Example B

During the physical examination, when the patient's movements are being tested, the patient may screw up his eyes or make an appropriate cringing movement. When such nuances of behaviour occur, the physiotherapist must return the patient's joint to a pain-free position and immediately ask:

Q    'What exactly did you feel and where did you feel it?' '. . . was there anything else?'

It is also necessary to follow up then with questions to determine whether the pain was an increase in intensity, or an increase in the distribution of the symptoms.

Other common nuances that require an immediate-response question are: the first movements of squeezing the eyelids or wrinkling the nose; altering the position of the head; clenching the teeth or fist; and pursing the lips. There are many more to add to the list.

## KEYWORDS

Frequently during questioning a patient will use a word or phrase that has a special significance. Failure to recognize this means that an opportunity to improve the standard of the assessment is lost, and the assessment made may then be incorrect.

The following dialogue is a true record of the questioning of a particular patient who was not a good witness. Her main symptom was an aching shoulder.

Q    'How have you been?'

A    'Quite well thank you.'

Q    'How has your shoulder been?'

A    'Just the same – sore since Monday.'

ET    *There are two things to latch on to and use here, one is 'sore' and the other is 'Monday'.*

Q  'Do you mean the soreness has been just the same?'

A  'Yes.'

Q  'So the last treatment didn't do anything either to help the shoulder or to make it worse?'

A  'No, it's just the same.'

Q  'You have referred to the shoulder as *aching* previously, and today you are talking about soreness; are these different or are they the same feeling and you are just using different words?'

A  'Oh, I don't know. It's just that it has been sore.'

Q  'Was it sore before?'

A  'I suppose so, it's just the same.'

This discussion regarding soreness may seem too trivial to justify pressuring the patient for clarification. However, it is very important for the manipulative physiotherapist to be accurate, because it is the subjective assessment that frequently provides finer and more accurate information than does the physical assessment.

*The conversation quoted so far is neither satisfactory nor complete; a patient does not change her description from 'aching' to 'soreness' without reason. From some things the patient has said it would seem that there has been a change of some kind in her symptoms, despite the fact that she insists that she is 'the same'. The probing enquiry must therefore continue.*

The patient used the word 'soreness' rather than 'aching', which should alert the physiotherapist to the fact that there *has* been a change in the symptoms. This one word, the keyword in this example, demands that the physiotherapist recognizes the implication of the word and therefore knows that she must question the patient until the significance and meaning of the word are clarified.

The patient in her original statement said that her shoulder had been sore 'since *Monday*'. Irrespective of how poor a witness the patient is, there must be a reason why she chose spontaneously to mention Monday. The conversation should therefore continue, and the following is the actual verbatim record.

Q  'Back at the beginning you made the comment that your shoulder had been sore since Monday. What is it that makes you relate the soreness to Monday?'

A  'Well, because that's when it became sore.'

Q  'Was it sore on Sunday?'

A  'No, it was Monday.'

Q  'When on the Monday were you aware of the soreness?'

A  'It was sore while you were treating it.'

Q  'Is this the first time that it has been sore during treatment?'

A  'Yes.'

Q  'Is it still sore?'

A  'Yes.'

Q  'Is it just as sore as it was on Monday?'

A  'Yes.'

Q  'If it is *now* sore, why do you feel it is "just the same" as it was before Monday?'

A  'Well, because it is aching just the same as it was when I first began treatment.'

The list could go on, but all that is necessary is to know:

1.  How to spot the language limitations.
2.  How to get the patient to search for helpful answers by specific questions.

It is necessary to have only a little understanding to realize how somebody who has pain can insist that it is the same, because the original pain has not changed, even though there is soreness superimposed.

The value of having carried this analytical assessment of the subjective changes through to a conclusion lies in the fact that, now, the physiotherapist knows two things:

1.  Her technique did not improve the patient's symptoms.
2.  Her technique did produce soreness, which has not yet subsided.

Therefore, she must change her treatment technique to avoid that soreness. Without the information being clarified, a wrong technique might well be used.

There are many instances of keywords, such as 'no, not much', or 'no, not really', which indicate there is something, and so should be followed through. If a patient says 'today it's all right', this indicates that yesterday it wasn't – follow it up. 'Nothing really' means there is something. The list could go on for ever; the important things are: don't miss the key words; and don't fail in following them through to obtain the complete answer.

## SPECIFICITY

The use of extreme alternatives can assist the patient to make an answer easier and more accurate. Numerical scales may also be helpful. For example, the patient may report being 'somewhat better'. The physiotherapist can make this specific by providing the patient with a 0–10 scale on which the patient must place his own assessment of progress. Percentages likewise may be useful. Verbal extremes may jog the patient into being more specific. For example, during a retrospective assessment the patient may report being 'better'. This is a vague statement (note, a statement, not a comparison), and the physiotherapist will make the patient be more specific by replying, 'Do you mean cured?', to which the patient's response may be, 'Oh no, not that much better'.

Similarly, when taking a patient's history the physiotherapist may enquire as to how long ago some incident occurred. The vague patient may say, 'Oh, ages ago', while the garrulous patient may reply, 'Well, I think it was when I was in India, or maybe it was Burma'. To make either reply more specific, the physiotherapist could follow up or intervene with '2 years or 20?'.

## AT INITIAL CONSULTATIONS

It is impossible to cover every possible 'question–answer–question' situation that might occur during initial consultations. However, once the introductions and learning to pronounce the patient's name (as he pronounces it and perhaps recording it phonetically) have been completed, the opening question can be made succinct if the following guidelines are utilized:

1. If the patient has recently had a manipulation under anaesthesia or has recently discarded a support, the opening question might be, 'Do you have anything in the way of symptoms now?'.

2. If you know that the patient has had some form of treatment which has been of benefit and that he may be at a stage of being able to return to work, the opening question might be, 'What are you still unable to do?'.

3. When you know that the patient has a chronic disorder, or has a disorder which has involved multiple areas, the opening question might be 'What are your problems at this stage?', or, 'What is your MAIN problem now?'.

The response to the examiner's first question will guide the next question into one of two directions:

1. The history of the complaint.
2. The behaviour of the symptoms.

Each will be discussed separately.

## HISTORY (INITIAL CONSULTATION)

History taking will be discussed in much more detail later (Chapter 6); here the discussion relates to

communication guidelines. Nevertheless, it is necessary to divide the patients into two types: the first is the group whose recent history involves trauma; the second is the group where no injury can be recalled or, if an injury can be recalled, it is a trivial one, such as a slight twinge felt during lifting. This second type is very common, and it is very important to determine the factors that contribute to the onset of the pain to enable the state of the abnormality to be understood and treated objectively.

Communication problems are greatest in the history taking of the second group of patients because, as there is no obvious injury that has caused the disorder, much probing is needed to determine the predisposing factors involved in the onset. In this situation, the patient does not appreciate the fine quality of detail that the physiotherapist requires. The following text is but one example of the probing necessary in the history taking of the second group of patients.

ET  *If I ask a vaguely directed question, he may, by his spontaneous answer, help me considerably to understand those parts of his history which he feels are most important. The points that are important to me I can seek later, if they do not unfold spontaneously.*

Q  'How did it begin?'

ET  *This may save my having to ask when it began.*

A  'I don't know. It just started aching about 3 weeks ago and it isn't getting any better.'

ET  *It is necessary to know what precipitated the pain, whether it was mechanical or not. If there was an incident that precipitated the episode, it was either so trivial he doesn't remember it, or he doesn't associate it with his symptoms. Before sorting this out, it may save time for me to know if he has had previous episodes. If he has, they may provide the key to recognizing the historical pattern of a particular disorder, and they may even provide the key to this kind of precipitating onset for the present symptoms.*

Q  'Have you ever had this, or anything like it, before?'

ET  *I have to be alert here because he may say, 'no' on the basis that previous episodes have been called 'fibrositis' and he therefore does not associate them with his present problem, which has been called 'arthritis' or 'disc lesion'.*

A  'No.'

ET  *I can now direct my questions in several ways, but probably the most informative, because his present thoughts are directed along 'past history' lines, is to spend a little time verifying his 'no' answer.*

Q    'Do you mean you've never had a day's back-ache in your life?'

A    'No, not really.'

ET    Ah . . . 'Not really' means to me that he has had something; so I must clarify it.

Q    'When you say, "Not really", it sounds as though you may have had something.'

A    'Well, my back gets a bit stiff if I do a lot of gardening, but then everyone has that, don't they?'

ET    Now it's coming out. What I need to know is the degree of stiffness related to the degree of gardening.

Q    'How long does it take to recover from a certain amount of gardening?'

A    'It might take 2 or 3 days to get back to normal after a whole weekend in the garden.'

ET    That's very useful information. It helps me to know what his back can tolerate. I realize I don't yet know whether his back is deteriorating or remaining static, but to save time I'll leave that determination until later – provided I don't forget to find out. I will need to know this factor, because it will guide the vigour of treatment required and guide prognosis requirements. The answer may come during other parts of the examination. What I really need to know now is how this episode began. His initial vagueness indicates I am going to have to ask searching questions to find the answer.

There are many ways the questions can be tackled, and the answer for each will take about the same length of time to determine. The following is the line taken.

Q    'You said it came on 3 weeks ago. Did it come on SUDDENLY?'

A    'Yes, fairly quickly.'

ET    Fairly quickly means 'suddenly' to him, but it's not precise enough for me; so I'll need to probe deeper.

Q    'What were you FIRST aware of?'

A    'It just started aching.'

Q    'During the morning or the afternoon?'

A    'I don't remember.'

Q    'Do you remember if it came on, on one day? In other words, did you not have any aching one day and have an ache the next day?'

After a delay, while he ponders the question, the answer comes.

A    'Yes, I think so.'

Q    'What day was that, can you remember?'

ET    To pursue this line of thinking I will guide his memory, which may help him to remember something that might otherwise be lost.

A    'It was on the Thursday.'

Q    'Was it aching when you wakened that day, or did it come on later in the day?'

A    'I think I wakened with it. Yes, I'm sure I did because I can remember saying to my wife during breakfast that my back was aching.'

Q    'And when you went to bed the night before you did not have backache? Is that what you mean?'

A    'Yes, that's right?'

He might well have said, 'No, I don't think it started like that'. The next question would then need to be, 'Before the aching began, did you have any other feeling in your back such as tiredness or stiffness, or even just being aware of your back? In other words, did it just sneak up on you gradually without your realizing it initially?'. He may reply, 'Yes, now that I look back at it, I think it was like that'.

ET    That's that part of the question solved, or at least as much as I need at the moment. Now to find out what provoked it. The first thing is to make him think about whether there was any trivial incident which occurred during the day before the backache started. If this proves negative, then I'll ask about 'predisposing factors'.

Q    'Did you do anything at all on the WEDNESDAY that hurt your back, even in a minor way, or made you AWARE of your back in any way?'

A    'No, I've been trying to remember if I did anything, but I can't remember any time I could have hurt it.'

ET    So now I have to resort to the 'predisposing factors' referred to above. While his mind is orientated towards physical activities, if I continue with questions associated with activities, he will probably be able to answer more quickly and the answer will be more reliable. To ask him about the non-physical-activity 'predisposing factors' (fatigue, sickness, etc.) will force him to change his train of thought.

The next question probes for this. To do this first and then return to the predisposing physical activities later will result in delays in his mental re-orientation. It may also result in missing out on a relevant piece of information, which might have been on the 'tip of his tongue', so to speak.

*This technique of paralleling questions with a patient's line of thought is an important communication technique to follow at all times, unless there is a very strong reason for departing from it.*

Q  'Had you been doing any UNUSUAL work on that Wednesday or about that time?'

A  'No.'

Q  'Had you been doing any HEAVIER work than usual?'

A  'No.'

Q  'Had you been doing any particular work for LONGER than usual?'

A  'No.'

ET  *So there isn't any OBVIOUS physical activity which has provoked this ache. The next step is to investigate the other 'predisposing factors' – there MUST be a reason for the onset of aching on the Thursday morning.*

Q  'At that time, were you unwell, or overtired, or under any stress?'

A  'Well yes, I was pretty tired. I'm overdue for holidays and we have had two men off work sick – and now you mention it, we had been working longer hours than usual to meet a deadline – I'd forgotten that; and I was involved in a lot of lifting and carrying that day.'

ET  *It often takes quite a long time (which is quite reasonable) for a person to retrieve pieces of information, so, rather than thinking 'Why didn't you say that when I asked you earlier', I should think, 'Well, at least I didn't miss out on that bit of information'.*

Q  'And that is unusual for you, is it?'

A  'Well, yes, it is. I do have to do quite a bit of lifting, but the pressure was really on at that particular time.'

ET  *Thank you very much, that's just what I was looking for. Now it makes sense, the history and the symptoms are compatible.*

The above is not the end of the 'history' questioning, but sufficient dialogue has been presented to show a communication pattern which can be adopted. As well as the unanswered *'So long as I don't forget'* question mentioned earlier, the physiotherapist needs to know if there has been any spontaneous recovery or worsening of the symptoms over the 3-week period. Also, there are many facets of the patient's past history which need to be sought, and any question you think of later may still be valuable. These will be discussed in Chapter 9, as this chapter is concerned only with communication.

Another communication guideline – which applies particularly when a patient's response to the opening question, 'When did this begin?', is 'Oh, ages ago' – is as follows:

ET  *His response infers that it didn't start last week, but that's all. The method that will most quickly bring out the answer is to provide him with two clear reference points and thus force him to be more specific.*

Q  'Do you mean 6 months ago, or 6 years ago?'

A  'Oh no – no, only about 2 or 3 months ago.'

As already mentioned, when interviewing garrulous patients, trying to keep control of the interview is extremely difficult. During history taking, these patients tend to go off at tangents and give a lot of irrelevant detail. For example, the opening question and answer might be as follows:

Q  'When did it start?'

A  'Well, I was on my way to visit an old aunt of mine, and as I was getting onto . . .'

Whether the physiotherapist allows him to continue as he chooses, or either brings him back to answer her question or gently coaxes him to answer some of her other questions, will depend on two things. The first is, how much of his talk is likely to be talk for talking's sake? The second relates to the amount of spontaneous information of good quality she might learn if she allows him to continue. If it is the former, she intervenes. Some examples of intervening questions that will enable the physiotherapist to keep control of the interview are as follows:

Q1  'What happened?'

Q2  'Did you fall?'

Q3  'How long ago was this?'

Such questions should be skilfully interposed by gently increasing the volume of the words used in the question so that the patient's thoughts are pulled away from his current line and subtly directed to that of the interposed question. The important thing is that the examiner can retain control of the interview without insulting or upsetting the patient.

Nevertheless, it is important that every effort should be made to make patients feel that they are not complaining; rather, they should be told that they are *informing* – 'What you don't tell me, I don't know'.

One of the best ways of enhancing the intervention is to touch the patient (their knee, arm, hand etc.) and to say simultaneously 'Did you fall?'. The 'touch' has the effect of immediately changing the direction of their thinking. Some people dislike being touched, so for them still use 'touch' but do it through their sleeve (thereby lessening the skin-on-skin situation); make it both brief and light.

## BEHAVIOUR OF SYMPTOMS (INITIAL CONSULTATION)

Without experience in the choice of words or the phrasing of questions, an enormous amount of time can be taken in determining the behaviour of a patient's symptoms. Unfortunately, time has to be spent if the skill is to be learned, for nothing teaches as well as experience. The information required, relative to the behaviour of a patient's symptoms, is:

1. The relationship symptoms bear to rest, activities and positions.
2. The constancy, frequency and duration of the intermittent pain and remissions, and any fluctuations of intensity.
3. The stage of stability of the disorder.

The following is one example that provides a guide as to the choice of words and phrases that will save time and help the therapist to avoid making mistaken interpretations and incorrect assumptions. The conversation that follows is between the examiner and the same man interviewed above, who has had 3 weeks of backache. The text relates only to the behaviour of the backache.

ET  *Earlier in the interview he said his backache was 'constant'. 'Constant' can mean 'constant for 24 hours of the day' or 'constant when it is present' as compared with the momentary sharp pain. This is borne out by the fact that a surprising number of patients say their pain is constant, yet when you ask them, immediately prior to testing the first movement, 'Do you feel any symptoms in your back at this moment?', they will answer, 'No'. The 'constant ache' and 'no symptoms' are incompatible. To avoid misinterpreting his use of 'constant', it is essential that it be clarified. It may be possible to gain a more positive answer by tackling the question from the opposite direction.*

Q  'At this stage, you don't have any period when you are without some degree of backache?'

A  'No, it's there all the time.'

ET  *The next question is to ask him if he has any ache if he wakens during the night, because this is the most likely time for him to be symptom-free.*

Q  'How does your back feel if you waken during the night?'

A  'All right.'

Q  'Do you mean it is not aching then?'

A  'That's right.'

Q  'So you do have SOME stages when it isn't aching?'

A  'Only at night. It aches ALL day.'

*The word 'CONSTANT' when used by patients is one of the words that always require clarifying.*

ET  *That's now clear. His thinking processes at the moment relate to 'no symptoms in bed' and 'it aches all day'. Two associated aspects of the daytime to which I need to know the answers are:*

1. *Does the ache vary during the day? (and if so, how much, why, and how long does it take to subside?)*

2. *Does he have any lumbar stiffness and/or pain on getting out of bed first thing in the morning?*

*To make use of his current train of thought, the following is the question asked, and it should quickly follow his answer '. . . it aches ALL day'.*

Q  'Does the ache vary at all during the day?'

A  'Yes.'

ET  *Well, that doesn't help me much, but it does provide a point from which to work. There are many ways I can tackle the next few questions. Basically, what I want to know is, does it increase as the day progresses or does it depend on PARTICULAR activities or POSITIONS he may adopt? How can I get the answer most quickly? I'll try this first.*

Q  'What makes it worse?'

A  'It just gets worse as the day goes on.'

Q  'Do you mean there is nothing you know of which makes it worse – it just gets worse for no obvious reason?'

A  'Yes, that's right.'

ET  *Because assessment is easier if there is something he can do that increases his ache, a more leading question needs to be asked.*

Q  'Is there anything you can do, here and now, which you know will hurt your back?'

A  'Well I know that while I've been sitting here my back has ached more.'

ET  *Because he may have been performing some activity before he arrived which has caused the increased ache, rather, or as well as, the sitting waiting for me, the following question must be asked:*

Q  'Do you mean sitting normally makes you ache?'

A  'Yes, if I sit and watch television it aches.'

ET   *I still wonder if there is not an activity which will cause aching. I also wish to know how long it takes for the ache with sitting to increase, and whether he has any difficulty getting out of a chair. The answers to these questions provide useful information regarding the severity of his problem. As he is thinking about aching while watching television, it is wiser to follow his current thoughts and ask an associated question rather than to search for an activity which causes the symptoms; that can be left until later.*

Q   'After watching television, do you have any problem getting out of the chair or can you immediately stand up straight and walk away normally?'

A   'No, it takes me a while to straighten up.'

ET   *This information is very valuable, because it is one fact that fits a recognizable pattern of low back pain disorder and it is one that responds to mobilization. For the pattern to be correct, his answers to certain other questions should match established expectations (making features fit). One such expectation is that his lumbar spine should be stiff on first getting out of bed in the morning. He may have difficulty with putting socks on or leaning over the handbasin to wash or to clean his teeth. The stiffness may be mild and last for only 10–15 minutes. However, if his activities were restricted by his ache (he has already indicated that they are not), the stiffness would be greater and would last for longer. I must ask the question in such a way as to receive a spontaneous answer, because it provides a much clearer indication of the quality and degree of his stiffness. Therefore, I should not ask, 'Is your back stiff when you get out of bed in the morning?'. The reason is worth a moment's thought. If I were to ask this, he need only answer 'yes', which gives no indication of its relative importance to him in the context of his total problem. Therefore I should ask the question more vaguely.*

Q   'When you first get out of bed in the morning, how does it feel?'

A   'I suppose it's a bit stiff, because I have some difficulty putting my socks on.'

The greater value of this answer is that *he* has used the word 'stiff' without being guided to it, and because he has talked of stiffness, not pain. Also, because he has spontaneously reported stiffness, which fits a recognizable pattern, he has shown that his disorder is genuine. The spontaneous answer to the unbiased question provides the exact quality and degree of the stiffness being sought. The questioning in this way has another facet; we decided between choosing a more specific question which needs only a 'yes' or 'no' (or 'I

don't know') answer or a more open-ended, less specific question.

Q   'How long does the stiffness last?'

A   'Only a few minutes. I'm still aware of it when I lean over the handbasin to wash my face, but by breakfast time it has gone.'

ET   *Now I'll return to the question about activities, but make it double-barrelled by seeing if different activities make any difference to the ache or the stiffness on getting out of bed the next morning.*

Q   'Do you have more trouble getting out of bed in the morning following a very active day? For example, if you garden at the weekend, do you have more trouble with aching or stiffness than during the week?'

A   'Yes, I do. It takes me a lot longer to get to sleep and I'm quite a bit stiffer the next morning.'

ET   *Good – this fits the pattern referred to earlier and strengthens the judgement about the diagnosis.*

Some readers may consider the above answers are too good to be true. However, as the physiotherapist learns how to ask key questions to elicit spontaneous answers, so the answers become more informative and helpful in understanding both the person and his problem. At the same time, the patient quickly gains confidence in the physiotherapist. Also, because the 'spontaneous' answers enable more accurate judgements to be made, the assessments are of greater value for reporting progress to the referring doctor.

The behaviour of the patient's symptom of stiffness may also be significant when there is some pathology involved. For example, during the early part of an initial consultation the examiner may feel that the patient has an early ankylosing spondylitis; the conversation and thoughts may be something like this:

ET   *I want to know if his back feels stiff on getting out of bed in the morning. If he does have ankylosing spondylitis, his back should be quite stiff and probably painful. Even if it is not very painful, the stiffness should take more than 2 hours to improve to his normal degree of limited mobility. To gain the maximum value from his answer I must not ask a leading question.*

Q   'How does your back feel when you first get out of bed in the morning?'

A   'Not so good.'

ET   *If he does have ankylosing spondylitis he should say his back is stiff, so, still avoiding a leading question, I ask:*

Q   'In what way isn't it good?'

A      'It's stiff.'

ET    *This is a statement, and all statements need to be made factual if they are to be used for prognosis assessment purposes.*

Q     'How stiff?'

A      'Very stiff.'

Q     'How long does it take for this stiffness to wear off?'

A      'Oh, it's fairly good by about midday.'

ET    *His job may involve shift work, so I must not assume the stiffness lasts for approximately 5 hours.*

Q     'What time do you get up in the morning?'

A      'About seven o'clock.'

ET    *That means he's stiff for at least 4 hours. That's too long for any ordinary mechanical back problem.*

## PAIN RESPONSES DURING TEST MOVEMENTS (INITIAL CONSULTATION)

To assess the behaviour of the patient's symptoms during the physical examination, some questions require much repetition. Because of this, care must be taken to avoid irritating a patient by repeatedly asking the same question with the same words. If a patient has both local spinal pain and referred pain, it is essential to know how each is affected by movement. It is dangerous to assume that the behaviour of the referred pain parallels the behaviour of the spinal pain. The wording of the questions should therefore be well planned, because it is essential to retain the patient's confidence. It is hoped that his confidence will be enhanced by the thoroughness of the examination.

For the purpose of the verbatim text, the patient has constant pain extending from his right sacroiliac area through the buttock and the right posterior thigh to the calf. The buttock and calf are the areas of greatest pain. It is assumed that there is no contraindication to examination of all movements through a full range. Before testing movements, it is essential to know the state of the symptoms.

Q     'While standing there now, what do you feel in your back and leg?'

A      'The whole lot.'

Q     'Equally throughout?'

A      'No, the thigh isn't too bad.'

Q     Your buttock and calf are more painful, are they?'

A      'Yes.'

Q     'Which is the worst?'

A      'They're about the same.'

ET    *Right, that's clear. Now to test forward flexion.*

Detailed description of how movements should be examined is provided in Chapter 6. The following text, while it exemplifies the depth of questioning required of the physiotherapist to know clearly the behaviour of the symptoms, also shows the words that can be chosen to speed up the process.

The patient is asked to bend forward and then return to the upright position.

Q     'Did the pain change?'

A      'Yes.'

Q     'What happened?'

A      'The buttock pain increased.'

Q     'Did the calf change?'

A      'No.'

Q     'And nothing else changed either?'

A      'No.'

Q     'Good. And now, has the buttock pain subsided back to what it was before?'

A      'Yes.'

Q     'Did that happen immediately you started to come up, or did it take a while to subside?'

A      'It only hurt more while I was fully bent forwards.'

ET    *That's ideal answering. I now have a very complete picture of how the symptoms behave with forward flexion. Now let's see what happens with other movements.*

Q     'Now arch backwards', which he does, while I watch his movement and his nuances, 'and up again: any pain that time?'.

A      'Yes.'

ET    *The movement will probably have hurt in the buttock and/or the calf. Accuracy and time are the essential factors that influence the words used in questioning him about the pain.*

Q     'Where?'

A      'In my buttock.'

Q     'Can you show me the part which is affected?' (which he does).

Q     'No calf?'

A      'No.'

ET    *Now I need to know two things: one, did he have more pain bending forwards or more on bending backwards; and two, has the pain subsided following arching backwards as it did after forward flexion? Because the 'lingering' aspect (see pp. 63–64, 188–189) may require more careful thought for the patient to answer, I will ask it first.*

Q  'Has the buttock pain subsided again?'

A  'Yes.'

Q  'In the same way as it did when you bent forward?'

A  'No, it's only just subsided now.'

ET  *That's useful information. I must record it and mark it with an asterisk before I forget it.*

Q  'Did your buttock hurt more when you bent backwards or forwards?'

A  'Backwards, I think.'

ET  *As the answer is, 'I think', then the difference can't be great. It may be that the delay taken for the symptoms to subside influenced his answer. It is this delay associated with bending backwards that I am going to assess most closely during treatment.*

This example demonstrates how much close attention the pain responses to the joint movement deserve. To omit precision in this area would be a grave mistake. Conversely, once the behaviour of the pain is established, the treatment techniques can be suitably modified and the appropriate care given to treatment and assessment.

The intonation of the patient's speech can also express much to the physiotherapist, provided she listens with her mind as well as her ears. During the consultation, every possible advantage should be taken of all avenues of both verbal and non-verbal communication. The more patients one sees, the quicker and the more accurate the assessment becomes.

Q  'Now let me see you bend to your left side.'

And so the examination continues.

The examples given should show how it is possible to determine very fine, accurate information about the pain responses to movement without great expenditure of time. Obviously it is not always as straightforward as the example given, but it is nearly always possible to achieve the precision.

Some patients become quickly irritated by being asked the same questions in the same detail. The physiotherapist who is tuned in to the patient's non-verbal communication will very quickly get this message. One way around this, without losing precision, is to vary the question. On testing the fourth movement, when asking about the pain response, just say:

Q  'Buttock again?'

A  'Yes.'

On testing the fifth movement:

Q  'Only buttock?'

A  'Yes.'

On testing the sixth movement:

Q  'Same?'

A  'Yes.'

This mode of questioning respects not only the patient's temperament, but also his intelligence. And at the same time, he will come to respect your perceptiveness and consideration for his feelings.

It is to be hoped that he is learning his role in making judgements about his disorder.

Non-verbal communication was discussed in detail earlier in this chapter. The quality, speed and precision provided by body language is invaluable, but the examiner must be alert and perceptive if it is to be fully utilized. Perhaps the following example helps show its value in modifying the verbal communication. Let us assume that we are still looking at the movements of the man who has pain extending from the sacroiliac area to the right calf, the buttock and calf being the areas of greatest pain.

Following the subjective examination and testing forward flexion, the expression on the patient's face may mean, 'How much longer is this going on?', or 'If she says, "Did that hurt?" and "Where did it hurt?" once more, I'll scream'. The physiotherapist should be alert to these expressions and, more importantly, should respect them and act upon them. Sometimes it is even necessary to balance the importance of the need to determine the information against that of not upsetting the patient. On determining that the latter is the more important, she could temporarily assume some of the answers and, if it is quite safe to do so, defer some of the examination to a later session. She could ask the patient 'Can you, and your back, cope with just three more movements?', implying that this is the last.

ET  *I can see he's getting irritated so I must be careful how I handle him.*

Q  'Just bend backwards.'

ET  *I'm going to watch his face like a hawk and, at the slightest sign of change in expression, I'll stand him up.*

Let us assume that after bending backwards 20° he starts to wrinkle the muscles around his left eye; the immediate response must be:

Q  'Up you come' (at the same time encouraging the return by assisting it).

ET  *I should be careful how I ask where it hurt. Although to make assumptions is wrong in principle, this is a time when, as mentioned above, an exception must be made. Under these circumstances, if I assume correctly that it was his buttock that hurt, it will be good policy to say this and then all he has to do is say 'yes' or even just nod his head.*

Q  'I assume that was hurting in your buttock and not your calf?'

A  Affirmative nod.

Q  'Just two more movements, then I'd like you to lie down. Bend over to your left side . . . now to your right' (using the same observations and questioning as above).

## AT SUBSEQUENT TREATMENT SESSIONS

### CHANGES IN SYMPTOMS (SUBSEQUENT SESSIONS)

Let us assume that the patient is a good witness with right-sided buttock and calf pain, and that he has lost all antagonism he may have had to the questioning of the initial interview. The last treatment was 2 days ago.

ET  *I want to determine the effect of the last treatment in the most informative way possible. My first questions should seek out spontaneous replies because they provide quality to the statements of fact.*

Q  'Well now, how have you been?', or 'How do you feel now compared with when you came in last time?'.

A  'Not too bad.'

ET  *That tells me nothing, so . . .*

Q  'Any different?'

A  'I don't know whether this is usual, but I've been terribly tired.'

ET  *At least this tells me that his symptoms have not been significantly worse. If they had been, he would have said so straight away. Because the tiredness can be related, and because it can be a favourable sign, the response to his answer should be as follows:*

Q  'Yes, it is quite common and it can be a good indicator. How have your back and leg been?'

A  'A bit worse.'

ET  *Most responses need qualifying, but for 'worse', clarifying is mandatory. I need to know:*

- In what way?
- Which part?
- When?
- Why?

Spontaneous answers are still important; so I'll keep my questions as non-directive as possible.

1.  In what way?

    Q  'In what way is it worse?'

    A  'My buttock has been more painful.'

    Q  'Sharper, or more achey?'

    A  'It's more difficult to get comfortable in bed.'

    ET  *That's not really answering my question, but it is telling me something positive, which for the moment I'm going to accept as being enough answer.*

2.  Which part?

    ET  *Because he may have a nerve root problem I should determine if his calf pain has changed, and it would be better to do this before finding out the 'when' and 'why' of his increased buttock pain. Because I hope his calf pain hasn't worsened too, I am going to ask the question in a way that will influence him to say 'yes, the calf has been worse too'.*

    Q  'Do you mean your calf?'

    A  'No, that's about the same.'

    ET  *That makes the answer to what I wanted to know very positive. I know there are three particular times when changes in symptoms are most likely to have been due to treatment and thus more informative for me (see pp. 71–72), but I don't want to question him regarding these three times unless I cannot get the answers spontaneously.*

3.  When?

    Q  'When did you notice the buttock worsening?'

    A  'Last night.'

    Q  'How about the night before?'

    A  'No different from usual.'

    Q  'So there was no change from the time you left here after treatment until last night?'

    A  'That's right.'

4.  Why?

    ET  *It is essential that I must make the patient feel able to say that he feels his increase in pain was caused by the treatment.*

Some patients are quite prepared to say angrily, 'You made it worse', but many more are not aggressive and do not like to say that it was the treatment that made them worse, even when they feel it was. They are sufficiently thoughtful to avoid making the statement, if they possibly can.

No one likes the feeling associated with having made a patient worse and being told so. However, these feelings must be overcome; the information being sought is more important than the physiotherapist's emotions, and it is essential to know what has made the symptoms worse. The best way to ask the question, which helps to overcome one's inhibitions and to make it easy for the patient to answer is to say straight out:

Q    'Do you think it was what I did to you last time which made it worse?'

A    'Not really, because the night before last was all right. And, actually, when I left here I felt better, and I think I even had a better night than usual.'

ET    *That is a good answer – it's surprising how helpful a 'good witness' can be. I now know treatment didn't make him worse last night, but something must have.*

Q    'Do you know of any reason why last night should have been worse?'

A    'It may be because I had to sit in an uncomfortable chair for two and a half hours at a meeting that evening – my buttock was quite sore during the last hour.'

ET    *Thank you – most helpful.*

Q    'And how did you feel this morning compared with other mornings?'

A    'Back to what it has been all along.'

ET    *That's excellent. This is useful information to help my judgement of the present stability of the disorder. I also have a guide as to how much vigour I can use, and may need to use, in treatment.*

The following is an example of a patient not answering the question. It is important to remember the information you are seeking; this is the only way to avoid being led away from the point, quite unintentionally, by the patient's answer. The question is asked:

Q    'How does IT feel' (be non-specific, therefore use 'IT') 'compared with before Friday's treatment?'

A    'It's terribly sore, right in the centre.'

This is not an answer to the question, and the physiotherapist could be led off the track. The follow-up question should be:

Q    'Yes that's how it is now, but how does it COMPARE with when you came in for treatment on Friday?'

A    'It's about the same.'

## DURING A TREATMENT SESSION

### CHANGES IN PAIN RESPONSE DURING REASSESSMENT OF TEST MOVEMENTS (SUBSEQUENT SESSIONS)

The test movements in reassessment follow the same lines as described for the initial interview, but with two exceptions. The first is, the only movements that have to be tested are those that were abnormal. However, having said this, sometimes it is necessary to confirm that particular movements, such as lumbar flexion and straight leg raising, are still normal. The second exception is that, when one is checking a test movement, it is often helpful to know the patient's opinion of the test movement compared with when the physiotherapist last tested it by asking:

Q    'How does that feel to you compared with when you *came in* for treatment last time?'

A    'Different – easier.'

ET    *I could not detect any difference in range or quality of movement; so his comment is of value to me.*

### PAIN RESPONSE WHILE ONE IS PERFORMING A TECHNIQUE (SUBSEQUENT TREATMENT SESSION)

It is important to know when performing a technique on a patient what pain response may be taking place during the performing of the technique. There may be no pain; or no pain to start with but soreness may occur as the technique is continued; or while performing the technique there may be soreness or reproduction of the patient's symptoms, which may behave in one of three ways:

1.  The symptoms decrease and disappear (they may increase during the first 10–20 seconds and then decrease).
2.  The symptoms may come and go in rhythm with the rhythm of the technique.
3.  An ache may build up, which is not in rhythm with the technique.

The communication issues associated with determining the behaviour of the symptoms during the performance of the technique are related to trying to help the patient understand what the differences might be, so that he can give a useful answer.

ET    *Now that I have started performing the technique I must know straight away what is happening to the patient's symptoms.*

Q  'Do you feel any discomfort at all while I am doing this?'

A  'No, I can't feel anything other than the stretching.'

ET  *This state of affairs may change fairly quickly, so in about 10 seconds I will ask again.*

Q  'Still nothing?'

A  'No, I can feel a little in my left buttock now.'

Q  'And that wasn't there when I started?'

A  'Yes it was there, it's always there.'

Q  'Has it changed since I started?'

A  'Yes, it's slightly worse.'

ET  *What I need to know now is whether this is a grad-ual build-up into an ache, or whether it is going to 'come and go' in rhythm with the technique. To make it easier for him, the question is better asked in such a way that he can choose one of two statements:*

Q  'Does it come and go in rhythm with the movement, or is it a steady ache?'

A  'It's just a slight ache.'

ET  *What I need to determine as quickly as I can is whether it is going to increase with further use of the technique, whether it will remain the same, or whether it will decrease and go.*

After a further 10 seconds, the question is asked:

Q  'Is it just the same or is it increasing?'

ET  *The question is asked this way, because it is hoped that the symptoms will be decreasing and therefore it is better to influence the answer towards what is not wanted rather than to get a false answer by influencing it towards what is wanted.*

A  'It's about the same.'

Ten seconds later:

Q  'How is it now?'

A  'It's less, I think.'

In another 10 seconds:

Q  'And now?'

A  'It's gone.'

ET  *That is an ideal response.*

To know what is happening in such depth while one is performing a technique is vital to proving the value of the technique.

This next patient (a man with a cervical problem) was not a good witness. On performing the technique, he responded to a question by saying:

A  'Yes, I can feel something while you're doing that.'

Q  'Is it like the pain you can get?'

A  'It's hard to tell.'

Q  'Is it a nice feeling or a nasty feeling?'

A  'I don't know.'

Q  'Does your neck like it or dislike it?'

A  'I don't know.'

Q  'Does it feel as though what I'm doing is getting at the thing that is wrong with your neck?'

A  'Oh yes, it certainly is.'

Only the last answer provides the information needed, and questioning has to continue until this is achieved.

When you are performing a technique using your hand on a painful area and the patient responds with 'under your hand' when you ask if he is feeling any-thing, the immediate-response question should be:

Q  'Is it the pressure of my hand, or is it the move-ment reproducing your pain?'

A  'I don't know.'

Q  'Is it on the surface or deep inside?'

A  'Oh, definitely not surface.'

Of course, if the answer is not as decisive, you can change your contact as well to see if the pain changes.

## PAIN RESPONSE AFTER A TECHNIQUE IS PERFORMED (DURING A TREATMENT SESSION)

To determine the effect of a technique, both the subjec-tive and physical aspects must be assessed. The patient is asked to stand so that the physiotherapist can reassess his movements. Before testing the movements, the patient is asked whether he feels any different as a result of the technique. The following conversation shows how this can be done quickly, without sacrificing the depth of information required.

Q  'How do you feel now compared with when I last had you standing?'

A  'About the same.'

ET  *So subjectively he is unchanged – now to check the movements.*

Q  'Now bend forwards – come up again. How was your buttock that time?'

ET  *I've noted that the range was 5 centimetres further, and the quality of his movement looked better.*

A    'It didn't make my buttock any worse that time.'

Q    'And now that you're upright, is it any worse as a result of having bent forwards?'

A    'No.'

Q    'Before you had any trouble with your back, how far could you bend forwards?'

A    'I think that's as far as I could ever bend.'

ET    *Well, at least it seems forward flexion is much better, because pain is no longer provoked by that movement. Now let us see what has happened to the other movements.'*

And so the routine continues.

It may be useful, especially if the patient feels that his symptoms have not changed, to ask if he feels that the quantity or quality of his movement has changed. There are sometimes situations where the patient starts to move more freely and with more quantity but the pain is still the same, so the patient experiences it as being the same, although parts of his movements are changing already. By asking the patient about other aspects of the movement that is being tested, he may learn about this and concentrate more on these aspects of the test-movement as well.

## AT REVIEW SESSIONS

### QUESTIONS DURING A RETROSPECTIVE ASSESSMENT (AFTER EACH THREE TO FIVE TREATMENTS)

It is frequently necessary at the third, fourth or fifth treatment sessions to make an assessment of the progress in the patient's symptoms and signs compared with those at his first visit.

Q    'How do you feel compared with before we began?'

This question is extremely valuable, because the answer enables the physiotherapist to see the progress in its proper perspective. It is not uncommon for a patient to report at each successive treatment that he is feeling better, 'Yes, I am sure I'm a bit better', yet at the fourth treatment session, if he is asked how he is compared with the first day, he will 'um' and 'ah' and hesitate and finish up by saying:

A    'Well . . . I'm not any worse.'

It is for reasons such as this that the retrospective assessment must be made a routine part of treatment.

If, however, there has been progress, the assessment may be made in the following manner:

Q    'What do you feel the percentage of improvement has been compared with when we began?'

Because some patients are unable to think in these terms, it is necessary to add to the question. In doing so, it is better to bias the question towards an unfavourable answer:

Q    'Well, are you less than halfway to being completely better?'

A    'Oh no, I'm more than half better thank you.'

## WHEN PROGRESS HAS SLOWED OR STOPPED

Making a reappraisal of the effect of treatment at a stage when progress is not continuing as it should is as difficult as, or more difficult than, a first consultation. The communication aspect is much the same as has already been discussed. The problems, from a teaching point of view, are setting down what it is you wish to find out. For this reason, discussion is dealt with separately (*see* pp. 78–79).

## CHANGES IN SYMPTOMS AT REVIEW SESSIONS FOLLOWING A BREAK FROM TREATMENT

Review consultations are conducted to assess the changes that have taken place during an interval following cessation of treatment. It is only the communication aspect as it relates to assessing changes in the patient's symptoms that will be discussed here.

The patient to be reviewed is the same male patient who was a good witness and who had right buttock pain greater than calf pain. He last received treatment 10 days ago. Following the introductory pleasantries, the questions and answers take on the more serious vein.

Q    'Well now, how have you been?'

ET    *To seek spontaneous statements the opening questions should be vague, so as to encourage him to describe aspects as they come to his mind. In this way they will come in the order of importance in which he sees them.*

A    'Better, I'm pleased to say.'

ET    *Well that's a happy start; but what I need to determine is what is better, in what way is it better, how much is due to treatment alone and how much* is spontaneous recovery. To make these determinations I need first to know in what way he has improved and when the improvement occurred. The how much better question can come later if it isn't mentioned spontaneously. I do have particular questions related to his symptoms that I can ask, having recorded them and marked main points with asterisks at his last treatment. However, it is the spontaneous responses that take precedence.

Q    'That sounds good. Tell me, in what way are you better?'

A    'The aching doesn't bother me during the day now, and when I get out of bed in the morning I don't have any difficulty putting on my socks and shoes.'

ET   He hasn't mentioned sitting, but I must first clarify what he means by, 'doesn't bother me during the day'. He has said it 'doesn't bother' him, so it sounds as though there are still some symptoms persisting. I wonder in which area?

Q    'I presume you mean you still have some symptoms during the day but that they are less than they were. What is it that you do feel?'

A    'My buttock aches after I've been sitting for a long time.'

Q    'Sitting for how long?'

A    '2–3 hours.'

Q    'Do you still have difficulty getting out of the chair?'

A    'No, not now.'

Q    'And is that all?'

A    'Yes.'

ET   Well, that's answered sitting, at least in part, without my having to ask, but I may need to qualify it more, later. Now I want to learn the answers to two separate questions: one relates to calf pain; the other relates to when he gained the improvement and whether he is continuing to improve. The latter could prove to be lengthy, so we'll clear up the calf first.

Q    'How is the calf?'

A    'Oh, that's all gone.'

ET   That answer may make asking about spontaneous recovery easy, especially if the buttock and calf symptoms are directly linked.

A    'When did that go?'

A    'I haven't had any calf symptoms for the last 4 days.'

ET   And I haven't seen him for 10 days. So without asking him, it appears that there has been continuing improvement throughout the 10-day interval. As I must not assume this, I'll ask about changes in buttock symptoms.

Q    'And what has happened to the buttock aching and sitting over the last 4 days?'

A    'I think it's lessening.'

Q    'You think?'

A    'Well, I don't sit a lot every day, but I have the impression it's improving.'

ET   This reinforces the estimate that he is continuing to improve even though he is not having treatment, but I'll give him the option to disagree with this.

Q    'Do you feel you have improved evenly over the 10 days, or do you think that most of the improvement came in the first few days and that you've been static since?'

ET   By putting this question in the particular sequence chosen, I am deliberately influencing him away from the answer I am expecting.

A    'Oh no, I'm sure it's still improving.'

ET   I needn't chase this any further. It seems certain he is still improving, and at a rate which appears satisfactory to him. I'll probably suggest reviewing him again in approximately 3 weeks' time, with the options that he can telephone and cancel the appointment if he is free of symptoms or that he may come in sooner if he stops improving or worsens. However, we'll see whether the progress of his test movements matches the subjective progress. If it does, it will strengthen this plan for review.

## CONCLUSION

Although this discussion about communication and its problems may seem lengthy, it merely touches the surface of the subject – and it must be recognized that this is all it does. Nevertheless, all of the main issues have been included. From the author's point of view, the primacy of the subject will show on reading the section on 'retrospective assessments'. It is hoped that, if the foregoing has been understood and absorbed, it will make retrospective assessments a powerful tool for the manipulative physiotherapist, equipping her to be an essential consultant in assessing the patients' neuromusculoskeletal disorders.

# Chapter 4

# Assessment

Over the years, various diagnoses have been put forward by manipulators to explain what they are doing with the many spinal pain syndromes they treat successfully. Many of the suggested causes of the patient's problems are not wholly accepted by the medical profession, and consequently treatment by passive movement is not used to its fullest advantage. How much better off we and our patients would be if passive movement treatment were used and controlled by proper assessment so that its role in the overall management of neuromusculoskeletal problems could be learned.

During the last few years, passive movement has gained greater recognition as an effective mode of treatment. Furthermore, its use as a source of information regarding the behaviour of joint disorders has been realized by some doctors to be of great value if the joint movements are assessed accurately throughout treatment. Without assessment, treatment is merely an application of techniques lacking guidelines. Assessment within the concept has been referred to in Chapter 1 (pp. 4, 12–13). Its real identity may more readily be seen by reference to *Figure 4.1*.

Examination is described in Chapter 6. However, for the purpose of this chapter on assessment it is necessary to elaborate on certain points, because without accuracy and detail in examination the proper assessments cannot be made.

Medical diagnosis only discloses that mobilization or manipulation could be a treatment of choice. Further detailed examination of movements is essential to determine the exact choice of treatment

There are two thinking processes on examination. The first is seeking the *source* of the disorder, and the second is the *cause* of the *source*.

*PART ONE*

**A. The *SOURCE*(s) of the symptoms**
1. Name as the *possible* sources of *any part* of the patient's symptoms that *must* be examined.
   Joints underlying symptomatic area(s)   Joints that refer into the symptomatic area(s)
   Neural/supportive elements that refer into the symptomatic area(s)   Muscles underlying symptomatic area(s)
2. List joints above and below the lesion that should be checked (when appropriate):
   ...............................................................................................
3. Are there any special tests indicated?
   a. Neurological examination ......................................................................
   b. Other – specify ..............................................................................

**B. Influence of symptoms and pathology on examination and first treatment**
1. Is the pain severe? (*Yes/No*) or latent? (*Yes/No*)
   *Give the example on which the answers are based.*
   a. *Local symptoms*
      i. Repeated MOVEMENT causing pain – or go just beyond P1 ...............................
      ii. Severity of pain so caused ...............................................
      iii. Duration before pain subsides ...........................................
   b. *Referred/other symptoms*
      i. Repeated MOVEMENT causing pain – or go just beyond referral of pain ...............
      ii. Severity of pain so caused ...............................................
      iii. Duration before pain subsides .........................................
2. Does the nature of the disorder indicate caution? (*Yes/No*)
      i. Pathology/injury – specify .............................................
      ii. Easy to provoke exacerbation or acute episode .........................................
3. Are there any contraindications? (*Yes/No*) Specify ...........................................

**C. The kind of examination**
1. Do you think you will need to be gentle or moderately firm with your examination of the movements?
2. Do you expect a comparable sign to be easy or to be hard to find? Why?

*PART TWO*

**D. The CAUSE of the SOURCE of the symptoms: Associated examination**
1. Provocative neuro/musculo/skeletal/medical factors leading to the cause of the symptoms.
   What associated factors must be examined:
   a. As reasons why the joint, muscle or other structure have become symptomatic and/or
   b. Why the joint or muscle disorder may recur? (e.g. posture, muscle imbalance, muscle power, obesity, stiffness, hypermobility, instability, deformity in proximal or distal joint, etc.) ....................................
2. The effect of the disorder on joint stability ...........................................

**E. Treatment**
1. Which short-term or long-term goals of treatment are pursued?
2. Do you expect to be treating pain, resistance, weakness or instability?
3. Are there any precautions or contraindications which need to be respected?
4. In planning the TREATMENT (after the examination), what advice should be included to prevent or lessen recurrences?

Adapted from *Neuromusculoskeletal Examination and Recording Guide* (1998), with kind permission of Lauderdale Press, Adelaide.

**Figure 4.1** Assessment at an initial stage of treatment: two compartment thinking processes, seeking the *source* of the movement disorder as well as seeking the *cause* of the source will guide treatment procedures

In Chapter 2 Professor Brewerton has given information regarding the diagnosis, indications and contraindications for manipulative therapy, and it is obvious that diagnosis is vital before manipulative treatment is undertaken. This diagnosis may only disclose that the patient has a neuromusculoskeletal disorder, signifying that mobilization or manipulation could be a treatment of choice. If a physiotherapist is asked to treat by passive movement, it is then necessary for her to examine individual movements in detail.

First, and most importantly, examination of the patient should reveal which particular intervertebral level or which neural component is responsible for his symptoms, and what effect the disorder has on his movements. It is by restoring these movements to normal that his symptoms will be relieved.

Secondly, abnormality of the movement of the faulty component should be determined by passive movement tests, testing each intervertebral joint separately, and the examination must divulge:

1. The presence and behaviour of pain through the available range.
2. The movements that are restricted or hypermobile.
3. The extent, quality and behaviour of stiffness (including the relevant symptomatic response) during movement or at the limit of range.
4. The extent and behaviour of muscle spasm during movement or at the limit of range.

Behaviour of the symptoms is the most important aspect.

The 'behaviour' of the aspects listed above relates to movements of the faulty intervertebral joint and the concurrent symptomatic response at the time *and after* treatment. In relation to the pain-sensitive structures in the vertebral canal and the intervertebral foramen (i.e. the dura, the nerve-root sleeves and the nerve roots), their movements must also be examined for range and the behaviour of any resulting pain. The same movement assessment needs to be made of the neural structures. Also, in the daily management of the vertebral disorders, it is essential to know the state of conduction of the nerves in those patients whose symptoms indicate involvement of the nerve root.

Many tests can be used to assess the joint movements mentioned above; among the principal ones are the

movement tests produced by pressures on the palpable parts of the vertebrae. These are described in detail in Chapter 6 (pp. 150–162).

## LISTEN AND BELIEVE

The physiotherapist must be prepared to listen to the patient attentively and believingly. It is extraordinary how often doctors and physiotherapists do not listen or do not listen carefully enough, and certainly do not listen at sufficient depth, to their patients. It is wrong to make academic judgements on what should be done to help a patient in preference to making a clinical judgement based on information the patient can give, tempered by what is known academically. A 74-year-old healthy woman who had been unable to comb her hair or do up her brassiere for 6 weeks because of shoulder weakness and discomfort was told that the only options open to her were 'major surgery' or to 'put up with it'. This was based on gross arthritic changes shown on the X-rays. She refused surgery, preferring to put up with it. Because her sister, who 'had had exactly the same problem' was 'cured by physiotherapy', she pressed for the same treatment. The diagnosis was 'osteoarthritis' and certainly she had gross joint changes, which were obvious both clinically and radiologically. Physically, she had a 35 per cent reduction in range, pain on stretching, and considerable dry crepitus during active movements. When the shoulder was moved passively with the glenohumeral joint surfaces compressed, crepitus was increased and discomfort (not pain) was provoked. Prior to the onset of symptoms 6 weeks previously, although she knew she had an arthritic shoulder, she did not have the disability. The 'major surgery' was based on the radiological findings interpreted academically. Seven weeks previously her radiological findings, one would expect, would have been much the same. Clinically her problem was an 'end-of-range' problem rather than a 'through-range' (gross osteoarthritis) problem. Her shoulder responded quite satisfactorily.

In assessment, listening and perceptive questioning are essential to gain information that cannot be revealed by any other form of examination

*A person's body, with all the parts that combine to form it, can tell the person things that we are often unable to find out by any form of examination other than (1) listening and (2) asking perceptive questions that assist him to say the things he feels because his shoulder (or whatever part it is) is telling him. For example, the person's body (with its disorder) is able to differentiate between different kinds of soreness,*

Assessment is the keystone of effective, informative treatment, without which treatment successes and treatment failures lose all value as learning experiences. Like the keystone, assessment is at the summit of treatment, locking the whole together

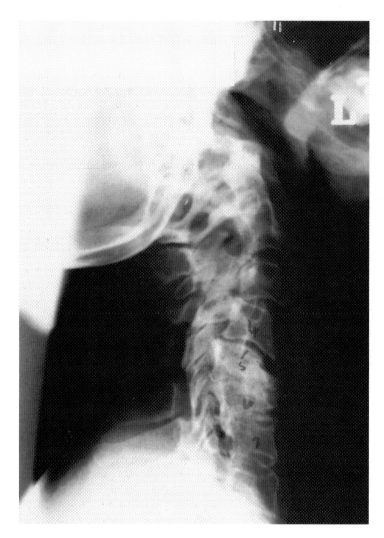

**Figure 4.2** Radiograph of the cervical spine of a 73-year-old woman. *Cervical spine:* The cervical spine is curved convex to the right. There is quite marked anterior angulation at C4–5 with slight anterior subluxation of C4 on 5. With flexion there is also anterior subluxation of C3 on 4. There is narrowing of all the inter-vertebral disc spaces below C2 but this is most pronounced at C5–6 and C6–7. Osteoarthritic changes are evident in the uncovertebral joints below the level of C2 bilaterally. There is encroachment on the intervertebral foramina on the left side at C2–3, C3–4 and C4–5, C5–6. There is some asymmetry of the superior facet of C2; this is partially accounted for by rotation and the curvature of the cervical spine. *Impression:* Severe degenerative changes in the cervical spine as described. Was there any previous injury?

*and it is good assessment to ask the question, 'Is it the thing that is wrong which is sore, or is it just bruising soreness from treatment?'.*

*Another example where a patient needs help to be able to explain what his body is telling him is, 'We both agree that your movements look better, but you obviously feel that your symptoms aren't any better; are you able to explain what it is that doesn't feel better?'. Information revealed by such believing questioning can reveal invaluable information. We must listen, and we must search.*

The manipulative physiotherapist must be fully educated in the theoretical aspect of diagnosis and treatment, but she must be even more educated in the clinical possibilities. The human body has an enormous capacity to adapt and accommodate to the insults and disease inflicted upon it, and the above lady is a perfect example of this. So also is the lady whose radiograph

of the cervical spine is shown in *Figure 4.2*. She is 73 years old, and for more than 72 years of her life she has not had any sign of any symptoms, not even one day of neck stiffness. By the appearance of her X-rays this hardly seems possible, yet it is so. One must be careful about what one does with theoretical knowledge.

Assessments are made both from subjective and from physical examination; they require the patient's co-operation and the examiner's skill in interpreting the patient's verbal and non-verbal signals, of which there are always many.

> Interestingly, as treatment reaches say the third session, the patient realizes that he is being educated as to how to think and of what to take notice

The patient is then able to make very pertinent answers to questions, and the assessment process becomes quicker and more accurate.

It is important for the physiotherapist to realize that the patient is able to 'feel' far more that the manipulative physiotherapist can ever determine by examination – his body can inform him of very fine changes, and it is her responsibility to listen and acknowledge. Therefore, it is important to say the following at the time of the first consultation:

1. 'What you don't tell me, I don't know.' 'Your body can tell you things which I cannot determine by examining you, so if you don't tell me, I don't find out about it – and that might mean I miss out on relevant information.' 'So you can see, you can't tell me too much, but you can tell me too little.'
2. 'There is a big difference between "not much" (when referring to symptoms) and "nothing at all".'
3. 'You must not feel you are complaining when you tell me about the symptoms or what causes them. You must feel that you are *informing*, not complaining.'
4. 'You may think of things that you don't feel are related to your problem, or are unimportant. You must tell me about them; let me be the judge.'
5. 'Can you see what an important role you have in the treatment of your disorder?'

In manipulative physiotherapy, assessment has many facets, all of which will be discussed. However, there are two different kinds of assessment that should be defined first:

1. During the initial examination of a patient, an assessment is made of:
   a) The diagnosis, including its history in terms of the stage of the disorder and its present stability
   b) The ways in which it affects the patient
   c) The symptomatic response to test movements, as being the pertinent part of a total examination.

2. Throughout treatment, assessments are made of the changes that occur, and judgements are made as to their degree, their relevance, and the influence they have on modifying treatment and modifying judgements of diagnosis and prognosis. On rechecking (i.e. assessing) the patient's original abnormal movements, it should also be possible to interpret the value of that technique as applied to that particular joint at that particular state of the disorder. This is the whole purpose of assessment: EVALUATING THE EFFECTS OF EACH TREATMENT TECHNIQUE.

There are two different kinds of assessment:

1. At initial examination of a patient
2. Throughout the treatment series: at the beginning of each session, during the performance of a technique, after a technique has been performed, at completion of a treatment session, over a 24-hour period immediately following the last treatment session, retrospectively, every third/fourth session, after a break from treatment, at the completion of treatment – analytical assessment

## ASSESSMENT AT INITIAL EXAMINATION

The first of these two applications is discussed elsewhere in this book (Chapter 6), but in relation to this chapter there is one important aspect, which is:

*MAKING FEATURES FIT.*

This concept, 'making features fit', comes into every aspect of examination and treatment, and into every aspect of assessment.

Making features fit is one of the most essential aspects of assessment. The manipulative physiotherapist will tell the patient that his problem is like a jigsaw puzzle, and it is her job to make 'all the pieces fit'. She needs his help to do this, and it is her ability to communicate that makes the difference between her being successful in helping him with his problem or not

In making a diagnosis the history of the onset is important, and to make an accurate diagnosis the onset must 'FIT'; that is, be compatible with the objective determinations found during examination. An example is given in the section on history taking, where a man was severely disabled by a sudden onset of severe pain when all he did was to reach to take a cup of tea from his wife. The disability doesn't 'FIT' the story of the onset. Therefore, there HAS to be one of two kinds of reason behind the minor 'incident' and the major disability. Either there were predisposing factors of a physical nature or there must be some disease-type process as the underlying diagnosis. The ability to seek out the answers is the basis of successful assessment in this area.

There are other problems associated with diagnosis. For example, an initial diagnosis may need to be changed in retrospect when it is seen how the patient's symptoms and signs alter with passive movement treatment. An example will clarify this.

A woman was referred from an orthopaedic surgeon, who requested manipulative treatment for 'disc prolapse causing C7 nerve-root symptoms and compressive signs'. On examination, the three cervical movements of extension, lateral flexion to the left and rotation to the left were all markedly restricted and all reproduced tingling in the patient's forearm and hand. She had diminished sensation in the pad of the terminal phalanx of the index finger, marked weakness of the triceps, and a diminished triceps reflex. She was in considerable pain. Traction was the treatment chosen, and by continual assessment over the first 4 days noticeable improvement was apparent in pain, cervical movements and neurological changes. She only required 10 treatments, with mobilization and gentle manipulation being added for the last sessions. At the conclusion of treatment, there was complete recovery of cervical movements and all neurological changes had returned to normal.

After re-examining the patient, the orthopaedist appreciated that the patient could not have responded so quickly if the original diagnosis of disc prolapse had been correct. In retrospect, he considered that the symptoms were caused by synovitis or inflammation of the synovial joint reducing the diameter of the intervertebral foramen and thus compressing the nerve.

> Clinical note: a patient's symptoms may arise from more than one source (e.g. a shoulder and a cervical component), which have both to be addressed in treatment

A further problem related to making a diagnosis is the fact that some doctors consider that a patient can have one diagnosis only. There are instances, however, where careful assessment and skilful planning of passive movement treatment will show that a patient having pain (say) arising at the base of the neck and radiating to the shoulder and mid-upper arm may have a shoulder disorder causing the shoulder and arm pain, coupled with a cervical joint disorder causing the neck and scapular pain. Examination of the joint signs for both the cervical spine and the glenohumeral joint should be accurately assessed at the initial examination. If joint signs are found both in the shoulder and in the appropriate intervertebral joint, then ideally treatment should be applied only to the cervical spine at first. The joint signs in the spine may improve, resulting in the patient losing his neck and scapular pain but retaining the shoulder and arm pain. Re-examination of the glenohumeral joint may reveal that the glenohumeral joint's

signs have remained unchanged. Under these circumstances treatment should then be applied to the glenohumeral joint in an effort to clear its joint signs, so gaining an improvement in the shoulder and arm pain. There are many such examples of combined joint involvement to explain the different pain patterns and syndromes that occur from patient to patient.

Another example of multiple causes for a patient's pain is seen frequently with patients having pain in their back that radiates down the full length of the leg. In relation to this area of pain, physiotherapy students may find themselves in a dilemma when learning dermatomes. Confusion is understandable when one diagram may show the L4 dermatome as starting in the low back area and spreading throughout the buttock and leg to the top of the foot (see Figure 6.4), while another may show the L4 dermatome starting below the knee and radiating down the shin into the foot. There is good reason for each of these presentations. There are various causes of referred pain from pressure or irritation of a nerve root – for example, there may be a prolapse of the nucleus pulposus, or the prolapsed material may be in direct contact with the nerve root (and not the dura or nerve-root sleeve). Under these circumstances the pain will only be felt below the knee. An important point is that if the pain is felt only from the knee downwards, and if it can be shown that this pain is arising from the back, then the pain must be due to irritation or compression of the nerve root alone.

Another example, which is far more common, is the patient who has a diagnosis of L4 referred pain extending from the centre back area through the buttock and leg to the top of the foot. The reason for this *may* be that the extruded disc material is irritating other pain-sensitive structures in the vertebral canal, such as the posterior longitudinal ligament, the dura and the nerve-root sleeve, as well as the nerve root. Under these circumstances, we may have four contributory causes for the patient's pain.

If a patient has pain radiating from the buttock down the leg to the top of the foot and he complains that the worst part of the pain is in the lower leg, then one can confidently assume that the nerve root is involved, particularly if spinal movements reproduce all of this pain (and in particular the distal pain). When pain is felt from the lower spine to the foot, the disc and adjacent posterior longitudinal ligament may be causing some of the proximal pain and the nerve root and its sleeve may be the source of the distal symptoms. Therefore, more than one factor is causing the patient's pain. From the foregoing it is easy to see that there are many problems associated with diagnosis, and there is still much more that medicine has yet to unravel. However, the problem must be tackled, and

**Table 4.1**    Taking the history

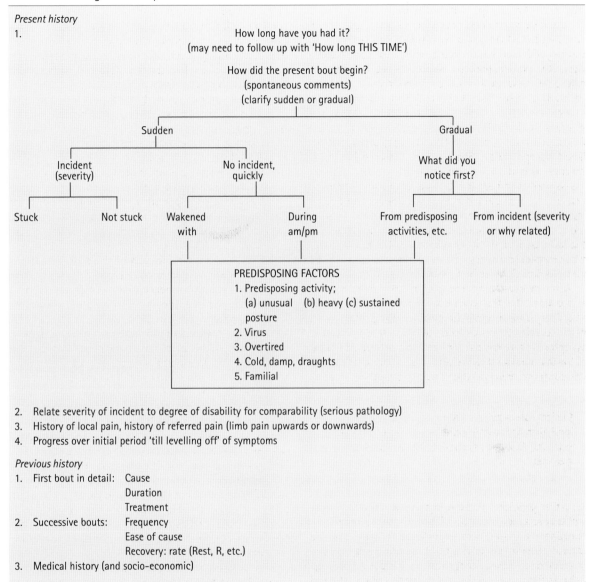

*Present history*

1.
How long have you had it?
(may need to follow up with 'How long THIS TIME')

How did the present bout begin?
(spontaneous comments)
(clarify sudden or gradual)

Sudden — Gradual

Incident (severity) — No incident, quickly — What did you notice first?

Stuck — Not stuck — Wakened with — During am/pm — From predisposing activities, etc. — From incident (severity or why related)

PREDISPOSING FACTORS
1. Predisposing activity;
   (a) unusual    (b) heavy (c) sustained
   posture
2. Virus
3. Overtired
4. Cold, damp, draughts
5. Familial

2.    Relate severity of incident to degree of disability for comparability (serious pathology)
3.    History of local pain, history of referred pain (limb pain upwards or downwards)
4.    Progress over initial period 'till levelling off' of symptoms

*Previous history*
1.    First bout in detail:    Cause
                               Duration
                               Treatment
2.    Successive bouts:        Frequency
                               Ease of cause
                               Recovery: rate (Rest, R, etc.)
3.    Medical history (and socio-economic)

in the meantime when a diagnosis is incomplete the ability to make the proper use of 'two-compartment' thinking makes it possible to use manipulation within routine medical care, and the treatment is made safe and informative by virtue of good assessment.

## ASSESSMENT THROUGHOUT TREATMENT

This is an area of multiple complexity, especially in interpreting the findings. It is one of the areas of the greatest development in manipulative physiotherapy in recent years, and has become the one area that picks 'the wood from the trees' among manipulative physiotherapists. The aspects of assessment which have shone through as being the ones providing finest value lie in the areas of:

1.    Communication.
2.    Behaviour of pain, stiffness and muscle spasm.
3.    The comparisons between normal and abnormal examination findings.

Each of these needs to be discussed in detail, but before this is done an outline of 'assessment throughout treatment' will be explained.

An important part of assessment is the ability to recognize patterns of syndromes. Also, it is necessary to be aware of the extent of improvement that may be achieved with treatment. The only way to gain this proficiency is by clinical experience based on accurate critical assessment. Armed with this competency, and as a member of a team, the physiotherapist can offer constructive suggestions to the referring doctor regarding the physical side of the management of the patient. Achieving this competency is a slow process and is not to be rushed. Miss Jennifer Hickling, a physiotherapist of note in this field in England, once said to me:

Manipulation depends upon clarity of thought and critical thought. People have to be trained at it in a most detailed way. It is easier to achieve this with undergraduate students than with postgraduate people because the latter have got into the habit of thinking in other ways, and it is difficult to undo these habits.

This business of methodical, critical thinking resulting in adding brick to brick is terribly important. Novices must expect to get fewer results more slowly than the experienced person, and they must resist the temptation to try short-cuts.

Novices need to clearly understand that every little bit of clinical knowledge they get out of a patient, provided they are certain about what it is and what the results are, adds up to a brick which is clear-cut; a fact that is not only useful for that patient but also for other patients they must meet.

For example, an experienced person who is prepared to take a calculated chance, not in an unscrupulous or unprofessional way but mentally, may go straight for a particular technique and say, do rotation to the left as a V, right at the beginning of treatment, and she may get a quick result. Others who feel their way into it might finally come to the conclusion that this V is necessary, but it might take them six or seven treatments to get there.

It is much better to have taken six or seven treatments to get there and to have justified all the way along the line that rotation is the right choice, and that the dosage is the right one. To arrive at the result by guesswork does nothing for the novice's future good management of manipulation generally, whereas arriving at the right result more slowly, having proved to her satisfaction the correctness of every step along the way, will pay hands down in the future.

Unless novices are prepared to sort out their knowledge as far as possible into these clear-cut

> Assessment of changes in the patient's symptoms occurs throughout the treatment process
>
> 1. Initial examination
> 2. At the beginning of each treatment session
> 3. During performance of a technique
> 4. After performance of a technique
> 5. After completion of treatment session
> 6. Retrospective assessment at each 4th/5th treatment session
> 7. At completion of treatment

proven facts they will end up with a welter of rather wishy-washy knowledge which is of little use in the different situations which come along.

Assessment of changes in the patient's symptoms and signs throughout treatment is made at the following times:

1. At the beginning of each treatment session (so that a judgement can be made as to what should be done today).

2. During the performing of each treatment technique (to be aware of changes the technique is having on the patient's symptoms while it is being performed).

3. After the technique has been performed (to determine the immediate effect of a technique and make a judgement about what should be done now).

4. At the completion of the treatment session (so that the present effect of the whole treatment session is known, as distinct from what may appear to have changed with each technique).

5. Over the 24-hour period immediately following the last treatment session (because this is often the most important informative period).

6. As a retrospective assessment:
   a) At the beginning of each fourth or fifth treatment session (often out of interest done to confirm the day-to-day assessment)
   b) When the amount or rate of progress has slowed or stopped (to determine the reasons and plan the action required)
   c) Following an assessment break from treatment (to establish the place of further treatment).

7. At the completion of treatment (to make judgements on prognosis and prophylaxis).

## ASTERISKS

Before discussing assessment under these headings, the use and value of asterisks (*) in the recording of examination and treatment needs explaining and putting into the proper context. In order to précis (successfully) and commit to paper both examination and treatment findings, one is forced to be clearer than would be the case if recording were not done. The asterisking must be carried out at the time of recording each piece of information *during* the consultation, and not left until the end of the consultation. Having been thus enforced, the next step is to select out of the recording those subjective and physical findings that must improve if the patient is to be made well again. This asterisking must be carried out at the time of recording each piece of information thought to be worthy of an asterisk, throughout and during the consultation (not at the end of the consultation). Identifying these main assessment markers with a large, obvious asterisk not only enforces a commitment, but also makes retrospective assessments quicker, easier, more complete and therefore more valuable.

---

Asterisks are an invaluable aid in assessment. Use an asterisk to highlight the following in the recording:

- Primary symptoms or disabilities/activity limitations
- Signs that reproduce a patient's symptoms
- Other information that is important
- Key issues that need to be followed up

---

There are three levels of distinguishing markers:

1. Asterisking items that the patient identifies as being primary symptoms or disabilities.

2. Asterisking information that the clinician considers to be aspects of major importance, even if the patient does NOT see them as being major (e.g. tingling pins and needles felt intermittently along the lateral border of the foot).

3. Key issues that must be followed up because of doubtful diagnosis and the possibility of evolving disease. These can be marked with an asterisk and by also 'highlighting' the appropriate written section.

Asterisks are a means to an end, not an end in themselves; they are not jargon, neither necessary to nor peculiar to manipulative physiotherapy; they are, nevertheless, an invaluable aid in assessment. The asterisks must be written into the record as the information is recorded. By doing it this way, the therapist recognizes what is worthy of an asterisk more quickly.

## COMPONENTS – 1

For each patient, asterisks should be used to identify the ways in which he knows he is affected by his spinal disorder ('subjective asterisks'). From among the points he mentions, asterisks should be applied to the following:

- Any functions he is unable to perform normally and which relate to different components of his diagnosis. For example, he may not be able to walk as briskly because the increased stride length required is limited by a 'canal' component (*see* p. **000**), i.e. limited straight leg raising; he may not be able to stand erect because of a discogenic component, which may be totally unrelated to the canal component. To just mark one of these two with an asterisk could result in not appreciating that, although one component of his disorder (as he sees it) is improving, the other is not.

- If he has a 'positional' component (that is, he is unable to lie on his right side) and a 'movement' component (he has sharp stabbing pain when climbing a ladder), each must be identified with an asterisk for the same reasons given in (1).

- When a patient has more than one pain, at least one 'subjective asterisk' should be used for each pain.

Some patients' symptoms are only of an intermittent nuisance quality. It may be difficult for them, on first being questioned, to provide a reliable subjective asterisk by which progress may be assessed. Under such circumstances the point must be pursued:

Q 'How will you be able to tell if your neck is improving?'

A 'I don't really know.'

Q 'How can you find out' – 'What provokes the uncomfortable feeling?'

A 'It just seems to come of its own accord.'

Q 'How often does this happen?'

A 'Oh, it's not regular.'

Q 'How long can you be without it?'

A 'Oh I have something every day.'

Q 'Is it really early in the day or at the end of the day?'

A 'It's usually there when I first get up in the morning and then perhaps at the end of the day.'

Q 'Is this a fairly regular pattern?'

A 'Well, yes, I suppose it is now that you put it that way.'

This is an example of the mental discipline the manipulative physiotherapist must exercise to arrive at the vital issue – the point cannot be glossed over.

## COMPONENTS – 2

In the physical examination, some relevant tests relate to one component of the patient's disorder and other tests relate to other components. Just as asterisks are needed for different components of the subjective findings, so are they equally necessary for the different components of the physical examination findings. This is most clearly seen in the example of a patient who has pain radiating from his back down to his foot, where there is diminished sensation along its lateral border. All of the following should have an asterisk:

1. A movement that provokes sback pain alone.
2. A movement that reproduces the referred pain.
3. A movement (such as straight leg raising) that indicates restricted canal/foramina movement as compared with intervertebral joint movement.
4. A pain-through-range movement as compared with an end-of-range pain (that is, a movement that is only felt to be painful at the end of range).

There are many other kinds of components and, when more than one can be identified in a patient's disorder, each should be marked by an asterisk.

Following the physical examination of the patient's movements, the main findings should be identified by asterisks. However, it is important that these should be selected findings; not every item is worthy of an asterisk. To use asterisks indiscriminately destroys clarity and indicates lack of thinking. Asterisks should be used to identify and highlight the different components of a patient's symptoms. The following are examples of different components, some or all of which may exist concurrently in a patient:

1. A canal sign from a joint sign.
2. A 'stretch-pain' sign from a 'compress-pain' sign (see p. 188).
3. An 'irregular-pattern' movement sign to identify it from among a collection of 'regular-pattern' movement signs (see p. 136).
4. A pain-through-range movement sign to identify it from an 'end-of-range-pain' movement sign when both are found on examination (see p. 188).
5. When a patient has more than one component to his pain, a movement that produces each component should be identified with an asterisk. An example of this is when cervical rotation to the right produces only scapular pain, and lateral flexion to the right produces only tingling in the index finger.

As treatment progresses, the asterisked symptoms and signs will change; some may go, some may change in character and new ones may be revealed. Nevertheless, throughout treatment the subjective asterisks must match the physical asterisks; this is another example of MAKING FEATURES FIT.

Although it is not without value to go through the process of assessment as a mechanical process, it lacks quality; it is non-discriminatory and leads almost nowhere. However, if the findings are related to the expectations of the treatment technique, the diagnosis history and prognosis, and the possibilities in the availability of selection of techniques, the assessment becomes very discriminatory, mature and valuable. The paths for learning that such a process of assessing and 'making features fit' are infinite. And if the process is carried into the realms of speculation (see pp. 7–8), the mental processes have no boundaries. It is in this area that assessment changes to analytical assessment.

Earlier in this chapter, the following areas were stated as being the areas of greatest growth in assessment:

1. Communication.
2. Behaviour of pain, resistance and muscle spasm.
3. Identifying normal and abnormal findings.

## COMMUNICATION

This subject has been dealt with in detail in Chapter 3.

## BEHAVIOUR OF PAIN, RESISTANCE AND MUSCLE SPASM

### BEHAVIOUR OF PAIN

> Pain can behave in a variety of ways in relationship to movement, including recovery pain, release pain, latent pain and after pain. Different pains can occur in different movements with the same patient

Pain is a subjective experience, it is influenced by an enormous variety of factors, and it presents in many different ways. It is the most common reason for a person seeking, or being referred for, manipulative physiotherapy. Rote learning can teach much about pain, but to experience pain oneself, or 'feel' it vicariously with empathy, is far more valuable. *Table 6.1* mentions the influences of psychosocio-economic factors – such influences as patients wishing to please, the variations in patients' psychological and physiological pain thresholds and pain-acceptance levels – all of which vary from person to person. Assessing a patient's threshold of pain may be assisted by firmly stretching one or two of the patient's *normal* joints and noting their response. Keele (1967) stated that 23 per cent of people have a physiological low pain threshold, 17 per cent have a high pain threshold, and 60 per cent have an average, normal pain threshold. For the clinician, the basic requirement is to listen, to believe and be seen to be understanding what the patient is trying to express. If the manipulative physiotherapist cannot learn to do this, she should give up before she starts. If the patient says, 'My arm feels heavy' or, 'My back feels as if it's in a vice', accept the statement, treat him with selected techniques and then, on standing him up to assess the effect of the technique, ask, 'How is that heaviness now?' or, 'How is that "vice" feeling now?'. If we use their words, they readily recognize the questions and can answer them valuably and we can make a more foolproof assessment. If the patient's terminology (and pronunciation) are used, the assessment is quicker, more accurately translated and gives the patient a feeling of being understood. A patient does not have to be stupid to have bizarre symptoms, and it is iniquitous to label his disorder as psychosomatic unless it is proven to be so. To repeat a previous statement, the patient's psyche is innocent until proven guilty, not the reverse.

The presentations of local and referred pain are discussed in detail in Chapter 8 (pp. 183–212), but there are other equally important facets of pain which require separate mention here.

## Recovery pain

In this category, the patient feels pain as he brings his body back to the upright starting position following test movements. For example, during examination of the trunk movements of a patient with central low back pain his trunk flexion is tested. The range may be full and painless, yet as he returns to the upright position from the fully flexed position he experiences low back pain during an arc of the return movement. From an assessment point of view, if, following treatment, the pain felt on the return movement to the upright position after flexion is less severe, or if the arc becomes smaller, this indicates improvement.

## Release pain

This phenomenon is common in the cervical spine (and sometimes the thoracic spine) with rotation, and in the lumbar spine with lateral flexion. It occurs almost exclusively with elderly patients. When the spine is taken to the limit of any of the movements suggested above and over-pressure is applied, the movement may be quite pain free; however, the instant the patient starts the return movement sharp severe momentary pain is experienced. Such a response should be classed as being abnormal, and treatment should be aimed at eliminating it.

## Latent pain

Because most types of latent symptoms arise from disorders which are difficult to help, assessment needs to be precise to detect small (e.g. 1 per cent) changes. There are many varieties of latent pain:

1. Pain occurring when a test movement is sustained. For example, a patient presents with pain in his scapula and triceps areas. On examination, the routine cervical test movements are found to be full range and painless. However, if cervical extension is sustained (for say 10 seconds) while some over-pressure is also maintained at the limit of its range, the pain may be reproduced only at the end of 10 seconds. Also, when the patient's head is returned to the upright position it may take some seconds for that pain to subside. This kind of behaviour is a very accurate measuring stick. If treatment is successful, the sustaining time required to reproduce the pain will increase, or the time taken for the symptoms to subside will decrease. The goal of treatment is to achieve symptom-free movement no matter how long the extension position is sustained, even if it is sustained while applying very strong over-pressure.

2. Pain occurring some seconds after a sustained test movement is released.

3. Summation of pain either as test movements are continued or as a test position is sustained. It can also occur with repetitive oscillatory movement.

4. A surge of pain occurring after a group of test movements have been performed. This surge of pain is a reasonably frequent finding, and an example will help to explain it. A patient may have pain in his left scapula radiating into the back of the upper arm. During the examination of his cervical movements, all are full range and painless. However, immediately following the examination of his movements, the patient may have a surge of pain into the scapula and arm. When this occurs the first time, it will not be possible to know which of the test movements has stimulated this latent pain. The examiner should see this phenomenon as a

warning to be gentle with examination movements and do fewer of them. If the patient sits quietly without moving his head, this latent surge of pain will subside. The length of time taken for the exacerbation to settle will vary from patient to patient, but will be consistent with any one patient. (This is another example when the time taken for the symptoms to subside is a valuable measuring stick.) When these test movements are repeated, they should be examined in a slightly different manner to elicit the exact behaviour of the pain with each direction of movement. Let us take examination of cervical lateral flexion first. This movement should be tested towards the side of pain, and if no pain is found at the limit of the range, over-pressure should be applied. If the movement is still painless, the position should be sustained for a short time (say 10 seconds). The patient's head should then be returned to the upright position. The patient is then asked to remain sitting for 10 or more seconds to determine whether there is any resulting surge of pain (i.e. latent pain) from that movement. If there is no pain from this test, then rotation towards the side of pain should be tested in the same manner, with care being taken to allow enough time for latent pain to show up. If these test movements prove negative, all other movements should be tested (a) in a calculated sequence and (b) with sufficient time for accurate assessment between each test movement. When the particular movement producing the latent pain is determined, the next step is to discover how much movement is needed to produce how much latent pain, i.e. the intensity and area of pain. The time taken for the latent pain to subside should also be noted. These fine assessments of the behaviour of pain on movement may seem tedious and time consuming. They are important, however, and familiarity with the different ways pain can behave with movement makes the examiner dextrous in carrying them out. Assessment is made of the time taken for the surge of pain to occur, its intensity at its peak and the time taken for it to recover.

5. Lingering pain, which may take from 30 seconds to 5 minutes to subside after being produced by movements or sustained positions.

6. Latent exacerbation – pain that appears in an increased form between 30 minutes and 5 hours after treatment.

Assessing changes in the first five types of latent pain described above requires three judgements to be made each time. The first is timing the onset of symptoms and the diminishing of symptoms in seconds; the second is assessing the severity of the symptoms at their peak; and the third is assessing quality of the symptoms caused. These last two are personal judgements, requiring maximum appreciation of the patient's non-verbal communication. These three judgements must be intimately linked with the causing test movement or position – that is, with its strength, amplitude, sustained time and duration, and any pain response occurring during the test.

## 'After' pain

Because this pain response occurs 'after' the cause, some readers may link it with latent pain – and according to the dictionary definition of 'latent', the word can be used to describe this 'after' pain. However, because it does not occur at any stage during the treatment session and (more importantly) because it is a definite entity that can occur in response to treatment, the entity is more readily remembered and identified if given a separate title.

'After' pain is a pain response that may not occur until waking on the morning following the day of treatment, or within the first hour or so of getting out of bed. Pain that comes on 2–4 hours or more after treatment is a pain response of the same kind, but at that time interval it is easier and clearer to assess as being a result of treatment. When it occurs the following morning, it is less easy to understand it and to be prepared to relate it to one's own treatment. However, it is not an uncommon happening. Among many different onsets of spinal pain that patients have, there is one particular history finding that occurs quite commonly and provides proof that the 'after' response is a reality. A patient may, towards the end of a day's physical work, feel a slight twinge of pain or just a slight ache, but the symptom goes quickly. The next morning, however, the patient is unable to get out of bed because movement causes severe pain. Relating this to assessment, it is important to point out that treatment as advocated in this text will not provoke the above degree of response. Nevertheless, the 'after' response is a reality and must be remembered when one is planning and carrying out treatment, and in assessing the effect of the last treatment.

During any test movement that causes pain, the movement and its pain responses should be assessed fully and with care to allow assessment by re-examination to show if there has been improvement following a treatment technique, even if this improvement is only in the order of 1 per cent. An example of the depth of detail required is exemplified in a patient who feels pain on the left side of his neck at the mid-cervical level. During the examination he is asked to turn his head to the left until the symptoms are first felt. This range is estimated and recorded (for example, 70°). The physiotherapist then guides the movement through a further 5°, and judges how the pain behaves with this further movement. If the patient reports that the pain has not changed, the movement is taken further, even to the extent of over-pressure at the end of the available range of movement. This further movement may result in a marked increase in the left neck pain. Some readers may doubt that such detail in examination is necessary. The answer to these doubts is that the findings give the physiotherapist a guide as to the treatment technique to use, while providing a very fine measure by which the effectiveness of the chosen treatment techniques can be assessed. For example, having made the initial assessment of rotation as detailed above, the physiotherapist carries out a selected treatment technique, then sits the patient to reassess the rotation, taking note of the three facets of the rotation test. Favourable changes of the above example would be indicated by any of the following findings:

1.  As the patient turns his head to the left he feels the same pain as he did at the initial test. Over-pressure is applied, with the result that the movement can be pushed further without increasing the pain.

2.  If the patient's active *range* of rotation to the left is unchanged although it becomes symptom free, and the response to over-pressure is as it was at the initial examination, the fact that he can turn actively without pain indicates improvement.

3.  When the patient turns his head to the left he feels no pain, nor does the first gentle over-pressure provoke any pain. With firmer over-pressure, however, pain increases as it did in the initial test. These findings indicate greater improvement than (2) above, even though the patient still feels the same degree of neck pain with the stronger over-pressure.

4.  If the patient can turn his head without pain and the over-pressure also does not cause any pain, the patient's disorder is obviously improving favourably.

If the treatment technique is of no help, the signs found on re-examination will not have altered.

Should the treatment technique have made the condition worse, then either:

1.  The patient's cervical rotation to the left will be slightly more limited and pain will start earlier in the range, OR

2.  The active range of rotation and its associated pain may be unchanged, but with even the slightest over-pressure applied to the movement his pain will increase more than at the initial test.

As the first use of the technique is very gentle, any worsening of the signs will be minimal and not harmful, and the changes will be informative.

## Two or more pains

There is yet another problem associated with careful assessment of a patient's movement and his pain. A patient may have two or more pains. One movement (or a group of combined movements) may be found to reproduce one particular part of the patient's symptoms, while a different movement reproduces a second and different part of the patient's pain. This is particularly important if we can accept that it is *not uncommon* for a patient to have more than one kind of pain, either in the same area or in a closely linked area. It is important for the physiotherapist to be fully aware of these possibilities lest differences be missed during examination. For example, it is common for a patient to complain of two distinctly different kinds of headache. The patient must be adequately questioned to determine the differences, and each pain should be examined, treated and assessed independently.

Patients have many descriptions for pains, yet it is surprising how often they use similar terms, most of which are readily recognizable. This is so even with patients in different countries and with different cultures. It is probably stating the obvious to say that, if a pain changes to an ache, the change is favourable. 'I feel I'm standing straighter', or 'I feel more secure', are favourable comments, whereas 'It feels delicate', 'It feels precious' or 'It feels unsafe' are unfavourable comments. A patient saying, 'It recovered more quickly after tennis than I would have expected', is another kind of favourable change. However, a patient is often able to answer the question, 'How does it feel now?', only by saying, 'I don't know, I find it hard to explain, it's . . . it's just different'. The question, 'Is it a favourable difference or an unfavourable difference?' should follow automatically, and the patient can nearly always make a clear distinction.

When assessing progress, the physiotherapist should be alert to situations where improvement in symptoms and signs do not occur synchronously. There are times, particularly if the patient has severe pain, when the signs may show improvement without the patient being able to appreciate any change in symptoms. Severe nerve-root pain fits into this category. In these situations the slight improvements in the movement signs indicate that the same treatment should be repeated; improvement in the symptoms will soon be noticeable. Conversely, circumstances may arise where the symptoms improve quite dramatically but progress in the joint signs is not so rapid. The adolescent disc lesion is a good example of this phenomenon. If either the subjective or the physical assessment shows improvement, then it can be considered, with one very important exception, that the disorder is improving.

The important exception to this rule concerns patients who have severe nerve-root pain and neurological changes. These patients should be examined neurologically daily by the physiotherapist, and any worsening of neurological changes, or the appearance of neurological changes that were not apparent before, should be reported immediately to the doctor. It is common for such patients to report dramatic improvement in symptoms over a period of 1 or 2 days, even to the extent of becoming symptom free or almost symptom free. In these cases pain does markedly and rapidly lessen, while the neurological changes either appear or worsen considerably. As has already been stated, the referring doctor should be notified at once because the patient may require immediate surgery.

When a patient has restricting local pain arising from the vertebral column, he may say that his pain has not changed when he is still unable to swing a golf club. The physiotherapist should then check other asterisked signs. It may be that this patient can now turn in bed without pain whereas it was impossible before. In other words, the greater demand (the golf swing) has not improved, but the disorder is in fact improving because the lesser demand (turning in bed) has improved. Minor aspects of a patient's complaint usually improve before the major complaint.

## Assessing changes in pain

Reference has been made to assessing changes of latent pain and 'kinds of pains', but there are two other situations that bear recording.

The first is that a patient may report, at the beginning of a treatment session, that his symptoms are unchanged; however, when his movements are assessed, the quality of a particular movement may appear freer. In fact the patient feels unchanged because after, say, turning his head 45° to the left, he can go no further because of pain, the intensity of which (and the position at which it occurs in the range) is the same as at his last treatment. On more detailed examination, it may be that pain felt between 20° and 35° is much less than it was at his last treatment. Ordinary local pains are able to change in many favourable ways, such as the above, without the patient necessarily being aware of them. Relating the above example to movement

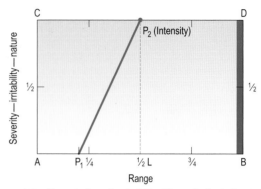

**Figure 4.3**  Presentation of pain felt with cervical rotation to the left on Monday

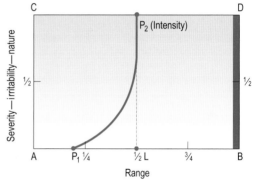

**Figure 4.4**  Presentation of pain – reported as 'unchanged' – felt with cervical rotation to the left on Wednesday

diagrams, *Figure 4.3* would be the presentation of pain felt with cervical rotation to the left on Monday and *Figure 4.4* would be the representation on Wednesday when he reports it being 'unchanged'.

The second is that, at the beginning of a treatment session, the patient may say that his symptoms have not changed because movements or a movement may be just as painful as when he began treatment, or as they were when he had his last treatment. However, on examination of the painful movement, improvement may be indicated by the fact that the unchanged pain is in fact experienced later in the range than at his last visit (*Figure 4.5*), or that his FIRST awareness of pain with the test movement is later in the range (*Figure 4.6*). Even when both positions have improved and the pattern of pain during the movement has also improved (*Figure 4.7*), the patient may still say that his symptoms have not changed because the intensity of the pain IS unchanged. His statement is correct and should not be argued against, but at the same time examination must be accurate enough for the assessment to reveal the favourable change.

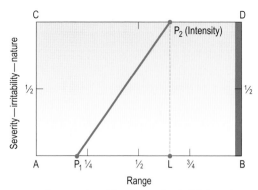

Figure 4.5    Presentation of 'unchanged' pain felt later in range with cervical rotation to the left on Wednesday

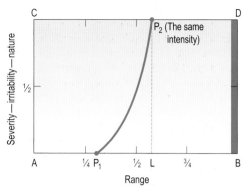

Figure 4.7    Presentation after improvement of pain felt with cervical rotation to the left on Wednesday

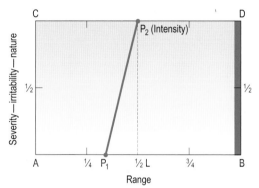

Figure 4.6    Presentation of pain first felt later in range with cervical rotation to the left on Wednesday

> Minor changes in a movement diagram may be examples of improvement of which the patient may be unaware

> In assessing a change in symptoms, it is also of relevance to assess changes in disability and in quality and quantity of movement

Relating the movement diagram to the three situations given above, and using *Figure 4.4* as the original presentation, the movement is still limited by the intensity of the local pain but the positions of $P_1$ and $P_2(L)$ have changed, as also has the behaviour of pain between $P_1$ and $P_2$.

*Figures 4.4–4.7* are all examples of improvement of which the patient may be totally unaware. Even when he is aware of the changes, their significance will be interpreted differently by the patient and the manipulative physiotherapist. If the manipulative physiotherapist realizes that the improvement is of greater significance to her assessment than does the patient, it will help her in her attitude towards him.

## Getting used to pain

On assessing changes in symptoms, patients quite frequently say, 'I think it's just the same – I think I'm just getting used to it'. During the comparatively short time patients have treatment, they DO NOT 'get used to' pain; the response therefore can be accepted as an indication of slight improvement.

## Weather changes

Patients who have 'joint' disorders often consider themselves good barometers because their symptoms change with changes in the weather, and this is fact, *not* fantasy. The fact that some people's symptoms increase just before the weather changes, while others change as the weather changes or immediately following the change, makes assessment difficult. However, the helpful feature for assessment is that, although the person's joint symptoms increase, the associated movement signs do NOT exhibit any proportional change.

## Treatment soreness and disorder soreness

Patients often report soreness following a previous treatment session. This must *always* be clarified. Is it the disorder that has become sore, or is it just soreness from the manual handling of the treatment technique? 'Is it a surface bruised feeling from my hand, or is it "the thing" that you have got wrong with you which is sore?' (this is another example of an 'immediate automatic follow-up' question).

## Wrong technique

On the occasions when it is determined that a patient's symptoms have been aggravated by the previous treatment, it is not always that the wrong technique was used – it may be that it was performed too strongly, with too much movement, for too long, or in the wrong position. Therefore, an effort must be made to see if the patient is aware of what it was about the technique that was the cause. This is particularly relevant if previous use of the technique had been producing ideal progress.

## BEHAVIOUR OF RESISTANCE

> Resistance to movement may manifest as a loss of the friction-free feeling through the range of stiffness, increasing as the movement is carried further into range

Consider now the differences in the behaviour of joint stiffness. In the normal person, the movement of one joint surface on its companion is a completely friction-free movement. However, examination of a patient's joint may show that while the range is full, yet on oscillatory movements through range it lacks this feel of friction-free movement. With experience it is possible to feel a slight resistance to movement as described above, even though the range is full. This resistance may be accompanied by crepitus, although this is by no means always the case. It is important that physiotherapists develop the skill of feeling this lack of friction-free smoothness.

When a joint is limited by stiffness, there are two common ways in which this resistance may behave:

1. In the first part of the joint's movement slight restriction to the friction-free movement may be felt through a large part of the range, and it only increases markedly in strength at the limit of the range (*Figure 4.8*).

2. Resistance may be felt early in the range and the further the movement is carried into the range the stronger the resistance becomes, until a point is reached where the physiotherapist is not prepared to stretch the joint further. In other words, the rate of increase of strength of the resistance is proportional to the movement through range (*Figure 4.9*).

The physiotherapist must be aware that these variations in joint stiffness can and do exist; proficiency in assessment of their differences will come only with clinical experience.

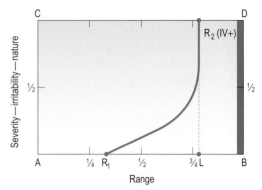

**Figure 4.8** Increase in stiffness of joint chiefly at limit of range

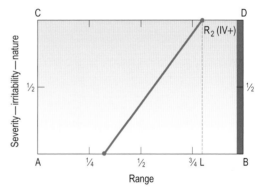

**Figure 4.9** Increase in stiffness of joint proportional to movement through range

## BEHAVIOUR OF MUSCLE SPASM

> Muscle spasm may be felt as a quick reflex response to pain or as a strong involuntary protective contraction

There are two basic categories of muscle spasm that can be found on examination of joint movement, and these are described in detail in Appendix 1.

The first of these is a muscle contraction that comes into effect as a reflex response to pain provoked by movement. The pain may be provoked because the movement is jerkily performed or because the joint is poorly supported. However, if the joint is handled well, this spasm does not make itself obvious. Nevertheless, when it does occur, it is an indicator of the intensity of the pain. It can be differentiated from a voluntary muscle contraction by virtue of the speed with which it is invoked by the provoking movement; the reflex spasm contracts much more rapidly than the voluntary spasm.

The second category of muscle spasm is related more to what is wrong with the joint rather than being directly related to a pain response. It is always a strong contraction of the muscle fibres, and most commonly is the limiting factor in a particular direction of movement of a joint.

For those interested in the movement diagram representation of these two spasms, they are described in Appendix 1.

There is another type of muscle response that is sometimes found when one is examining joint movement, and this is a 'holding' rather than a spasm. Although a small minority of patients will voluntarily contract the muscles that support the joint to prevent its being moved, this can very clearly be seen as a voluntary muscular contraction. As compared with this, the 'holding' is different. It is not a sudden muscular action, but rather an inability on the patient's part to be able to let the muscles relax. Patients exhibiting this 'holding' are usually totally unaware of their unrelaxed state.

Both the muscle spasm that limits range and the 'holding' muscle response reveal improvement changes by showing a decrease in intensity and an increase in the range found on examination. Also, in relation to 'holding', improvement on re-examination is demonstrated by an improvement in the quality of the movement through which the muscle holds.

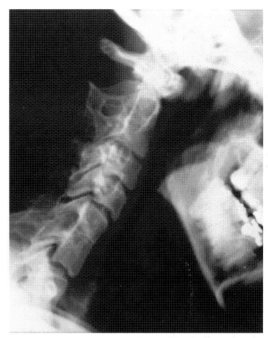

**Figure 4.10**  Radiograph of cervical spine of a 76-year-old woman, showing congenital fusion between second and third cervical vertebra. *Cervical spine:* There is a congenital fusion of C2 and 3, C6 and 7 and T1 and 2. Flexion is grossly limited. Both C3–4 intervertebral foramina appear a little narrowed. There is congenital cleft in the fused right laminae of C6–7

## IDENTIFYING NORMAL AND ABNORMAL FINDINGS – WHAT IS NORMAL? WHAT IS ABNORMAL? HOW CAN THEY BE DEFINED?

Useful hypothetical categories are to think of the spine as being:

- ideal – normal in every respect
- average – disadvantaged but not overtly symptomatic (i.e. clinically silent)
- abnormal – disadvantaged and symptomatic

It is accepted as being normal to have one leg or one arm slightly shorter than the other, yet this is in fact abnormal because they are asymmetrical. In a slightly different vein, a person may have an idiopathic scoliosis, which is obviously abnormal, yet he may not have any pain arising from the spine. Also, a person may have marked spondylitic or arthritic changes in the spinal joints yet have no pain. *Figure 4.10* is the radiograph of the cervical spine of a woman aged 76 who had never had any symptoms, not even a day of mild stiffness or soreness arising from her neck, up to the week prior to the film being taken. Differentiating the relevant from the irrelevant findings is therefore very difficult.

The following define the 'ideal' spine, the 'average' spine and the 'abnormal' spine.

### IDEAL SPINE

The 'ideal' spine refers to a series of intervertebral motion segments (i.e. interbody and zygapophyseal joints with all their supporting ligamentous and motor structures) which are normal in every respect; that is, none is disadvantaged in any way by injury, wear and tear, structural anomaly or disease – each motor segment is perfect.

### AVERAGE SPINE

The 'average' spine is not 'ideal'. It does not consist of a series of perfect motor segments. One or more of them is abnormal in some way, even if they are not causing any symptoms of major consequence.

Although the 'average' spine has been defined as having no symptoms of major consequence, this needs qualification. Some people have no symptoms whatsoever, while others have minor symptoms of a kind which they accept as being 'normal'. The three kinds of imperfection in the average spine are explained as follows:

1. Congenital or acquired structural anomalies.
2. Degenerative changes.
3. Disease processes or changes resulting from trauma.

## Congenital or acquired structural anomalies

There are people whose spine is disadvantaged by a congenital or acquired structural anomaly. Examples include a bifid spinous process that lacks one of its processes, a spinous process that inclines towards the left or the right, or congenital fusion between the second and third vertebrae, which is not uncommon (*Figure 4.10*). Such anomalies are of themselves painless, but they do indicate either asymmetry, or that more stress is placed on adjacent intervertebral segments.

Anomalies of neural elements must also be considered. There are many references in medical literature giving evidence of differences of nerve-root origins from the spinal cord and their exits from the vertebral canal. Such anomalies must be taken into consideration when assessing the origins of a patient's referred pain. *Figure 8.2* is a good example.

Prefixed and post-fixed plexuses also form part of the anomalies that exist. According to Brain and Wilkinson (1967), 12.1 per cent of people have a prefixed brachial plexus and 10.7 per cent of people have a post-fixed plexus.

There are other examination findings that should be considered as being normal or common, or even abnormal, yet do not require treatment:

1. Many people are unable to touch their toes, and this applies even to children.
2. Different body types have different normal ranges of movement.
3. On examining the range of movement available in the vertebral canal structures (the slump test described on p. 144), some people, even the young, have a marked restriction without it necessarily causing pain.

## Degenerative changes

The first of the three subdivisions (i.e. congenital or acquired structural anomalies) is quite different in kind to the other two, and should be thought of and

seen to be so. The spines of people in the first subdivision are only 'disadvantaged', because in all other regards the individual segments fit the 'ideal' group.

Elderly people commonly have a reduction in range of movement (most noticeable with the movements of cervical rotation and extension) without requiring treatment. This statement needs some qualification and expansion because it applies to many patients.

The elderly person who has no cervical symptoms yet has restricted rotation will feel discomfort if the movement is on the side to which it is stretched. This is perfectly normal provided that, when the stretch is applied in the opposite direction, the discomfort is again felt on the side to which the head is turned. However, it may be that when the rotation is stretched to one side the discomfort is felt on the opposite side. This is equally normal, provided that when the stretch is applied in the opposite direction it too causes discomfort on the opposite side. The examination finding that is not accepted as being normal is when the discomfort is felt only on one side whether the rotation is stretched towards it or away from it. Another abnormal pain response is the 'release pain', which is felt when 'over-pressure' to a movement is released.

The quality of the sensation created by stretching the cervical rotation as discussed in the preceding paragraph should also be stated so that it may assist in assessing the differentiation of normal from abnormal. When the movement is stretched, discomfort is normal and 'hurt' may be normal or abnormal (depending on the person's pain threshold, pain acceptance, personality, etc.), but when the person experiences a sharp 'bite' of pain, this is not normal.

## Disease processes or changes resulting from trauma

This group includes people whose spines show evidence of joint changes due to disease or trauma and who have symptoms for which they may or may not have had adequate treatment, yet who accept these symptoms as being their normal despite the fact that they interfere with their normal life. On examination, their joint movement are painful when stretched and palpation findings are obvious.

## ABNORMAL SPINE

The 'abnormal' spine is a symptomatic spine for which the person seeks treatment. On examination, significant comparable signs will be palpable at the appropriate intervertebral level. The title 'abnormal' is used to signify an abnormal degree of symptoms rather than abnormal joints, which, as has been stated, may be totally painless.

This labelling into groups is not a facetious act; it is a realistic situation and highlights important clinical connections between symptoms and examination findings that can be assessed. The value of the different groupings lies in our ability to recognize the differences between findings that relate to a patient's symptoms and those that are not necessarily related. Such differentiations can then also be related to treatment expectations. For example, it is possible to recognize, through the interpretation of the findings, that the realistic goal of treatment may be a minimally symptomatic 'average' state or a pain-free 'average' state rather than an 'ideal' state.

Unfortunately, very few people over the age of 40 have a total complement of 'ideal' intervertebral joints. Most people, for one reason or another, fit into one of the 'average' groups. If a group of 40-year-old people who have no pain or discomfort and consider their necks to be normal were examined by palpation, abnormalities would be found in nearly all of them. The question is, when such a person has a spontaneous onset of neck pain and seeks treatment for it, how does the examiner differentiate between the findings that relate to the present problem and the findings that were present before the spontaneous onset of the neck pain? A similar difficulty arises when attempting to determine the degree of disability that can be attributed to a recent injury and the degree that is attributable to pre-existing yet painless 'average' joint findings.

## NEW/OLD TISSUE CHANGES

Obviously if an intervertebral joint suddenly starts to cause pain for no obvious reason something must have happened to it, and therefore tissue changes of some kind will be present.

If these recent tissue changes have occurred in an 'ideal' joint, the only findings that will be detected by palpation examination will be of the 'new' or 'recent' kind, as with, for example, a sprained ankle.

If these recent tissue changes have occurred in an asymptomatic 'average' cervical joint, then on examination by palpation there will be new tissue changes superimposed on the older 'average' tissue changes.

Success in differentiating between the new and old changes makes prognosis, related both to the success of present treatment and to the likelihood of future recurrences, easier to assess.

If these recent tissue changes have occurred in a symptomatic 'average' segment, there will be 'recent' tissue changes superimposed on the changes that were already painful when stretched or palpated. Because the patient had symptoms before the exacerbation, the palpable tissue changes would not have been as 'old' as those in the pain-free 'average' group. Differentiation between the 'new' and 'old' changes under these circumstances is much more difficult.

The abnormalities sought by palpation are of the following kinds:

1. Soft-tissue changes.
2. Bony anomalies.
3. Movement abnormalities.

### Soft-tissue changes

These changes are to be found in the ligamentous, capsular, muscular and connective tissues as thickening or muscle spasm. Palpation of them will reveal tenderness.

The abnormalities of 'feel' in ligamentous, capsular and connective tissues are that the older they are the harder they feel, and the more recent they are the softer they feel. For example, palpating old capsular thickening around the zygapophyseal joint will be like pressing against leather; there are even variations in the hardness of the leathery feel. Thickening from more recent stresses will give a softer or spongier feel, which may overlie an older leathery feel.

Thickening within the muscular tissue is usually more diffuse and never feels like hard leather. Nevertheless, when thickening is present it has a stringy feel if it is 'old' and a smoother feel if it is 'new'.

### Bony anomalies

Under this heading the features that can be determined by palpation are: abnormal deviation of a spinous process from the central line without or with vertebral rotation; absence of one process of the bifid spinous process; abnormal position of one cervical vertebra relative to its neighbour; and the osteoarthritic osteophyte formation of the margins of the zygapophyseal joints.

The abnormalities of deviation of spinous process and positions of vertebrae can be confirmed by X-rays. If a positional finding is long standing, the shape of the associated vertebrae will have changed from their symmetrical appearance to accommodate the changed positions.

The articular pillar abnormalities that indicate osteoarthritic (or osteoarthrotic) findings are readily determined by palpation, and can also be confirmed by X-rays. If the changes are 'old' and totally inactive, the bony margins of the exostoses will be hard and clean without any sign of soft or leathery covering.

### Movement abnormalities

These abnormalities consist of the following: hyper- or hypomobility; abnormal quality of movement through range; and stiffness and spasm. Such abnormalities can be determined by palpation being applied in a manner that produces intervertebral movement. Abnormalities of movement should be qualified in terms not only of the available range of movement, but also of any change in the normal free-running movement through the range up to the end of the available range. This may be disturbed by such factors as arthritic change, stiffness in supportive capsular and ligamentous structures, or protective muscle spasm.

An 'old' hypomobility has a hard end-feel at the limit of the range, with movement before the limit of the range being a smooth, friction-free movement. A 'new' hypomobility, on the other hand, has stiffness occurring earlier in the range, building up in strength of resistance until the end of range is reached; that is, there is 'resistance through range'.

When crepitus is present during movement, it will be painless if it is unassociated with presenting symptoms and painful if it is associated.

In 'ideal' joints, when the synovial joint surfaces are strongly compressed and move, the movement will be painless (Maitland, 1980a). There are circumstances when pain is experienced during a large amplitude of the range, and it is sometimes possible to heighten this pain by holding the joint surfaces firmly compressed while moving the joint through the same amplitude of the range.

### Pain response

The pain response felt by the patient during the palpation examination of tissues and movement is most important. The pain or discomfort may be felt either through range or at the end of range; it may be felt deeply, or it may reproduce the patient's symptoms.

Superficial and deep local pain can occur in both 'new' and 'old' situations. Severe pain felt by the patient when only moderate pressure is applied to a soft tissue, or applied to produce movement, is always 'new'. When a patient has referred pain that can be reproduced by palpation examination, the indication is that it is associated with a 'new' disorder.

## ASSESSMENT

### AT THE BEGINNING OF EACH TREATMENT SESSION

Assessment of changes in symptoms and signs at each treatment session needs to be carried out in a particular manner. There are three times when the patient's

interpretation of the effect of treatment (i.e. the symptoms he feels) are most valuable:

1. Immediately following treatment.
2. During the evening of the day of treatment and that night.
3. On first getting out of bed the following morning.

It is important not to ask the patient initially for this information, because to do so may block the flow of spontaneous comments from the patient; questioning should be so planned that the physiotherapist can evoke spontaneous remarks, which then prove to be very informative.

When assessing at the beginning of a treatment session, the first question should be, 'How have you been?'. The answer will be valueless if the patient takes it as a general remark and answers, 'Fine thanks, how are you?'. However, if the patient says, 'Much better, thank you', then useful information has been expressed.

If the first question produced a valueless answer, the next question should be, 'What do you feel was the effect of the last treatment?'. The reply, 'Better' or 'Worse', needs further clarification. For example a patient may, in wishing to emphasize the degree of his present pain, give the impression that he is worse, whereas on closer questioning it may be proved that he was better after his treatment until he performed some activity which aggravated his pain. Under these circumstances, treatment helped rather than made him worse. This kind of information may be gained through the following questions:

'In what way is the pain worse' (is it more severe, sharper, changed to a throbbing pain, or has it increased in area, etc.?)

'When did it start to become worse?'

'What do you think made it worse?'

'Was it related to treatment or did you do something which may have aggravated it?'

The physiotherapist must be prepared to accept the possibility that she has performed a technique too strongly. If a patient comes in feeling cross, saying 'What you did to me yesterday made me a lot worse', the beginner is going to feel disconcerted and disheartened. She will find it easier to accept the blame if she can reply, 'Good – not that I wanted to make you worse, but it shows me exactly what to do and how to do it'; or she may say, 'If I can make you worse by too much or too heavy mobilizing of your spine then I should stand a good chance of being able to improve it'.

The sequence of questioning to determine *when* and *why* a patient's symptoms were worse is important.

The first questions can be, 'When did you notice it starting to worsen?', and, 'Do you know what made it become worse?'.

Assuming the answers being sought are not elucidated by the above questions, the next step, relative to *when*, is, 'Did you waken with it being worse or did it come on later in the day?'. Patients can usually answer this. If the answer is, 'It was worse when I first got out of bed', and if it refers to the morning following treatment, the possibility then exists that the worsening was due to the treatment. The second step, relative to *why*, should be tackled only after the answer to *when* is known. The purpose of the assessment is to determine whether the worsening was due to treatment (which is a known quantity) or to other factors. If it is due to other factors, the degree of the cause must be determined so that it can be related to the degree of worsening; by this the degree of stability of the disorder being treated may be learnt. If the patient's answer to 'when' is, 'When I got out of bed next morning', the automatic immediate-response is, 'Does it sometimes fluctuate like this, being bad one morning for no known reason, or is this unusual?'. If the answer is, 'No, this is unusual', the question has to be pursued; 'Did you do anything yesterday which might have aggravated it?', 'Were you more tired than usual yesterday evening?', 'Do you think it could be due to yesterday's treatment?'.

Only after all of this questioning has proved fruitless can the following be asked: 'How did you feel when you left here yesterday after treatment compared with when you came in for that treatment?'. Then can follow, 'How did you feel later in the day after the treatment?'. And lastly, 'What did it feel like when you went to bed?'.

The following is an example presented to show how carefully the questions have to be asked to gain the information being sought, and to show the care necessary in interpreting the patient's responses. The patient, a young man, had severe low back pain with a vague referral into the right buttock and right posterolateral thigh.

At his first visit last Friday, following a limited examination he was treated using a grade of lumbar rotation for sufficient time to produce a change in the symptoms or signs if it were the right technique to use. There was a small but definite improvement, showing that it could be the right technique.

The second treatment was on Monday, and the following is the conversation that was required to determine the effect of the treatment.

Q   'How have you been?'

A   'It was terrible on Saturday but it's better now.'

ET   *That is an unqualified statement and must be converted to an informative comparison.*

Q   'Better than when?'

A   'Better than Saturday, but then I haven't been doing anything.'

ET   *I still don't know whether he's better than before treatment on Friday.*

Q   'How do you feel now compared with when you were in here before treatment on Friday?'

A   'Oh, I don't know … about the same … or … it might be a bit better.'

ET   *That isn't really the clear-cut kind of response I'm looking for and the line of questioning is not getting me very far. I still don't know the effect of the treatment. I think I shall chase the 'bad on Saturday' part and see if that gives me any information.*

Q   'You said that you were bad on Saturday – when on Saturday?'

A   'I don't know.'

Q   'Did you waken feeling bad on the Saturday morning or was it later in the day?'

A   'I don't know, I think I was all right in the morning; I think it was later in the day.'

Q   'Did you do anything that could have made it bad?'

A   'No, I've only been resting.'

ET   *He is not very decisive with his answers; this really is hard work.*

Q   'What were you doing during the afternoon?'

A   'Oh, resting.'

Q   'Did you get up at all?'

A   'Well, now you come to mention it, my wife did go out about midday and I was at home on my own. The phone rang four times and I had to answer it. That meant bending down to reach the telephone because it was on the floor.'

While saying this he demonstrated how he bent down to the telephone, and the action certainly looked awkward.

Q   'Thank you.'

ET   *At last I've got the answer, but I should take it a little further to be sure.*

Q 'Was it before that, or after, that your back worsened?'

A 'Yes, it was after the phone calls.'

Q 'How did you feel on Sunday?'

A 'Oh, I was a bit sore Sunday morning, but it got better as the day went on.'

Q 'And now you're about the same as before treatment on Friday, is that right?'

A 'Yes I think so.'

ET *Having got that clear I must move on to my next part of assessing.*

Q 'How did you feel after treatment on Friday compared with before the treatment?'

A 'I certainly knew I'd been moved round a fair bit.'

Q 'Do you mean that you had more pain than when you came in?'

A 'I don't think so, I was about the same.'

Q 'Well, what were you aware of, when you refer to knowing you had been "moved around a fair bit"?'

A 'It just felt different.'

Q 'What felt different?'

A 'My back.'

Q 'In what way was it different?'

A 'It felt a bit sore.'

Q 'How long did it last?'

A 'Only for about 5 minutes.'

Q 'And then how did you feel?'

A 'Back to the usual.'

ET *This is hard work and I'm not getting very far.*

Q 'Do you remember that during treatment on Friday you were lying on your side and I was twisting your back?'

A 'Yes, I certainly do.'

Q 'At the time, I thought you said that you felt better.'

A 'Yes, that's right.'

Q 'Despite the 5 minutes of soreness?'

A 'Yes.'

Q 'How long did it remain better?'

A 'Well, I don't really know, because my wife drove me home while I lay on the back seat and that wasn't very comfortable.'

ET *At last I know, as precisely as is possible, where my treatment stands in relation to his symptoms, and I know that, unless I find that his test movements on examination are worse, I must continue with the rotation for at least one more treatment if I am going to learn its value. To change techniques would be a wrong decision, because a stage has not been reached when the value of rotation has been proved.*

The extent and depth of the subjective questioning may seem to some people to be tedious, unnecessary and a waste of time. Tedious it might seem, unnecessary and a waste of time it is not. It is vital to the interpretation of the effect of treatment to be able to understand the effect of the treatment in the patient's terms. It is not tedious, it is challenging and stimulating.

If the vital spontaneous information sought is not forthcoming, it may be necessary to ask the direct questions:

'How did you feel when you got up first thing the next morning compared with how you felt when you came in for the last treatment?'

'How did you feel for the rest of the day and that night?'

'How did you feel when you got up first thing the next morning?'

Should the answers still not give a clear assessment, the physiotherapist may need to ask, 'Has your pain altered at all as a result of treatment?'. If the patient has to hesitate before answering, then it is fairly clear that the symptoms could not have changed much, if at all.

If the patient reports feeling better from the treatment, it is equally important to clarify what it is that has improved and in what way it has improved. This is particularly relevant when a patient has referred pain.

At each treatment session, when making the initial assessment of the subjective changes, the manipulative physiotherapist must be able to understand clearly the effect of the previous treatments. If the patient gives garbled or conflicting information, she may need to ask the patient, '*Thinking overall*, what effect do YOU think the last treatment had?'. It may be necessary to ask, 'How did you feel when you left here after the last treatment in comparison with when you came in for that treatment?' – in other words, 'What do you think was the immediate effect of the treatment?'. Such a commitment frequently gives a better balanced assessment of the overall effect of treatment than is determined by asking specific questions about specific stages during the interval between the two sessions.

## Written records by the patient

There are times when it is necessary for a patient to *write* a running commentary of the behaviour of his symptoms. For example, a patient may be a very poor historian, in which case he may be asked to write down how he feels immediately following treatment, how he feels that night, and how he feels on first getting out of bed the next morning. There are also times when it is critical to know precisely what happens to a patient's symptoms for the first 4 hours immediately following a particular treatment.

When a patient is having to interrupt a sequence of treatment for business or other reasons, it is useful to ask him to write down the behaviour of his symptoms over the first 48 hours from the time of the last treatment. Some readers may feel this is encouraging a patient to become a hypochondriac, but this is not so, and even if it were the advantages of the written record far outweigh any supposed disadvantages.

When a written record is used, it should be handled by the manipulative physiotherapist in a particular sequence:

1. On receiving it from the patient, it should be placed face down.
2. The patient should be asked to give a general impression of the effect of the last treatment.
3. The subjective assessment of the effect of the last treatment should be taken through to its conclusion.
4. The written record can then be assessed and any discrepancies clarified.

It is not uncommon for a written record to give a wrong impression because it is read out of context with all other elements of the assessment. It may read as though the patient is worse, whereas, because he has not recorded some important facts (not asked for), he has in fact improved.

So this is where the manipulative physiotherapist must become skilled at interpretation and use her asterisks from the initial consultation chart.

## Patient records

After completion of the subjective assessment questioning, it must be recorded on the case notes.

The FIRST entry at every treatment session is always the assessment of the subjective changes, including in particular the patient's opinion of the changes effected. It is therefore mandatory for the manipulative physiotherapist to develop the habit of beginning the written record with words that the patient uses (abbreviated if necessary) to express HIS opinion of the effect. This must be recorded in quotation marks so as to indicate clearly that this is the patient's opinion. It may not be the manipulative physiotherapist's opinion, but it certainly is the patient's. If there is a variance of opinion, which cannot be resolved, both opinions must be recorded.

Occasionally a patient will comment that following the last treatment he felt extremely tired, and in fact many have slept for as long as 3 hours. This effect usually occurs following the initial treatments, and can be considered to be a favourable response to the treatment.

The above is the *subjective* assessment of the effect of the previous day's treatment. This is followed by re-testing the previously abnormal movements and assessing the quality of any change resulting from treatment. Changes in these signs will hopefully agree with the findings of the subjective assessment, so reinforcing each other. This will then make the total assessment more reliable.

## ASSESSMENT DURING THE PERFORMANCE OF A TREATMENT TECHNIQUE

Two points are important here; one is the intention of the technique, and the other is the kind of change it may be effecting.

> Assessment during a technique:
>
> • Are goals achieved?
> • Does no undesirable side effect occur?

## Intention of technique

Following the examination and assessment of the patient's disorder it may be the intention to select the position and treatment technique that provokes a controlled degree of his symptoms, i.e. point (2) below, or the opposite may be the intention. (This intention must also be remembered when making the assessments following the use of the technique.)

## Kind of change

Two pain responses can occur while performing a technique: first, is that pain may be felt in rhythm with the oscillations of the technique; and second, an ache may develop during the performing of the technique.

Pain felt in rhythm with the technique, i.e. point (3), may change in the following ways:

1. From a pain-free start, the disorder may begin to hurt in rhythm with the technique. The technique should be continued without any change whatsoever being allowed to take place in its:
   a) Speed
   b) Rhythm
   c) Amplitude
   d) Position in range.
   To achieve this perfection requires total concentration. After 10 seconds, while the technique is still continued, a comparison is made of the rhythmic pain. If it is increasing, the technique may be continued provided a careful watch is kept so that it does not continue to worsen the symptoms. If it does, the technique must be stopped.

2. A rhythmic pain may decrease as the technique is continued with the constant speed, rhythm, amplitude and position in range. A judgement is made of the amount and rate of change related to the amount and kind of technique required to effect the change. This gives an idea of the likely prognosis, particularly when the percentage of improvement retained over 24 hours is related to the kind of treatment and the amount of treatment.

3. The rhythmic pain may increase for the first 10–30 seconds before then starting to decrease. The pain may continue to decrease and even disappear. If the initially increasing pain is calf pain of recent origin, the technique is not continued for the 30 seconds. However, if it is local spinal pain or nearby referred pain (particularly if it is chronic in nature), the constant speed, rhythm, amplitude and position in range are continued for the 30 seconds, provided of course it is not steadily worsening as each second goes by. If the patient is unable to tolerate the intensity of pain before the peak is reached (and the manipulative physiotherapist must communicate to know this), it may be necessary to move to an adjoining more comfortable joint temporarily. When she returns to the offending joint it will often be less hurtful. Assessing such changes requires not only verbal communication but also awareness of the non-verbal nuances of behaviour, the patient's ability to relax more and the technique being easier to produce – all play their part. The degree of concentration and skill required under these circumstances is demanding, and the extent of (a) talking to the joint and (b) feeling for

the joint resembles that of the pianist playing a concerto in conjunction with an orchestra and, at the same time, being aware of the composer's emotions.

4. The last rhythmic pain response is when the pain worsens as the technique progresses and continues to progress. Just as much care is required under these circumstances as in (3) above, because it is necessary to assess whether the disorder is telling the manipulative physiotherapist, 'I don't want to be moved like this, please stop – you're making me worse', or saying, 'You're moving me too quickly', 'You're pushing me too far into the painful range' or 'You're moving me jerkily'. These comments are not facetious, they are very real and this depth of information *can* be assessed by listening and by responding with careful modifications in handling the technique. If the pain still continues to worsen, then it is really saying, 'Hands off, you're making me worse'.

When the physiotherapist is carrying out a passive movement technique on a patient, she should first ascertain whether the patient has any pain while positioned for the treatment technique to be carried out. Before testing the patient's movements to assess the objective changes, the question must be put to the patient, 'What symptoms do you feel at the moment, while you are standing there, before I test your movements?'. This same question must be asked when the patient is asked to stand (for assessment purposes) after a treatment technique has just been completed: 'How does it feel now compared with before I did that technique?'. Then test the required movements for the physical assessment.

Special care is required when the patient has latent or lingering pain. The technique is then performed at a chosen grade, and the patient is asked whether the technique is causing any alteration to the symptoms. This information is necessary from three points of view:

1. The patient may have referred pain while positioned for treatment. As the treatment technique is carried out, this pain may gradually lessen and go, it may remain at the same level throughout, or it may worsen. Assessment during the technique will guide the decision as to whether to continue with the technique or perform it more gently, or whether a change of technique is indicated.
   a) For example, in the early stages of treatment of a patient who has pain radiating throughout his leg, if treatment initially causes slight calf pain (and especially if this calf pain increases as the technique is continued), then the physiotherapist

should discontinue that technique. She should stand the patient and reassess the other movement signs before going on to the next technique.

b) On the other hand, if the condition is more chronic in nature, it may be necessary to provoke this calf pain with the treatment technique to gain improvement. On reassessment, it would be hoped that the provocation had brought about a definite improvement in pain-free range of active movement.

c) While performing the treatment technique, only the back pain (and not the referred pain) may be reproduced. If this occurs, the technique should be continued. Whether it should be repeated depends on the assessment of its effect.

2. The patient may have no pain while positioned prior to performing the technique, but during the performance of a technique he may feel centre back pain. It should be determined whether it is the symptoms being reproduced, whether what is being felt bears any resemblance (in kind or site) to the patient's symptoms, and it should also be determined whether the pain is due to the pressure being used or the movements being created. The physiotherapist may choose to continue with the same technique at the same grade, and ask the patient several times during the performance whether the centre back pain remains the same, improves, or worsens. If pain increases, she may lessen the grade of the technique or she may stop. If there is no change in the symptoms or they improve, she may need to do the technique more firmly.

3. There is one other response that can be determined during treatment. It is a difficult assessment to make, because misunderstandings between physiotherapist and patient occur easily. It is useful to know when performing a technique whether pain is provoked at the limit of the oscillation only, and the easiest way for the physiotherapist to make this assessment is to say to the patient, while performing the technique, '*Does – it – hurt – each – time – I – push?*'. Another way to ask is 'Is it in rhythm with what I'm doing or is it a constant feeling that is increasing as I continue?'. The words in italics are said in rhythm with the strongest part of the treatment technique. The patient then easily understands this question and has no hesitation in answering clearly.

These assessments of what is happening while every technique is being performed must mandatorily be recorded on the treatment record (pp. 75, 108–109, 225).

## AFTER THE TECHNIQUE HAS BEEN PERFORMED (TO DETERMINE THE IMMEDIATE EFFECT OF A TECHNIQUE AND MAKE A JUDGEMENT ABOUT WHAT SHOULD BE DONE NOW)

The main points to be considered under this heading have already been covered in the section on assessment at the beginning of each treatment session (*see* p. 72). Care must be taken; first in the manner of questioning, and secondly in the accuracy of testing movements, which form the basis of comparison.

Having carried out a treatment technique at a chosen grade long enough to achieve the expectation from the technique chosen, the physiotherapist asks the patient to sit up (or stand up) for the assessment.

The first mandatory question is, 'How does that feel now?'. If there is no immediate spontaneous response, she asks, 'Does it feel any different?'. Again, accuracy in questioning and interpretation are important to subjective assessment. It must be remembered that any statement made in response to these questions must be converted to a comparison and clarified.

The patient's movements are then re-tested, and a comparison made with those present before the treatment technique was used.

When reassessing the movement signs, the same sequence of test movements must be used each time. The reason for this is that one movement that provokes pain may alter the signs for the next movement tested. Similarly, if cervical movements were tested in standing at the beginning, they should be reassessed in standing. It is inconsistent to test movements one time in standing, another while sitting in a chair, and a third time with the patient sitting on the treatment couch without foot support.

It is hoped that the subjective and physical assessments will agree.

In principle, when a physiotherapist is in the learning stages of treatment by passive movement, this assessment should be made following each use of every technique. As experience is gained, she learns to expect a certain improvement when particular techniques are applied to particular disorders. For example, if she is treating an elderly patient with general neck pain that can be reproduced at the limit of all movements, all of which are stiff, she can assume that there will not be much change during one treatment session although there may be considerable improvement over two treatment sessions. In these circumstances it would not be necessary to assess after each technique, but assessment should be made by comparing the symptoms and signs at the end of the second treatment session with those at the beginning of the first treatment session.

If the physiotherapist is able to judge that changes in symptoms and signs may be expected to take place quickly, she should assess them after each application of a technique; if the *rate* of change is not as much as desired, then a change in technique should be made. This procedure should be continued throughout the treatment, changing from technique to technique to find the one that produces the quickest and best improvement.

## ASSESSMENT AT THE COMPLETION OF THE TREATMENT SESSION (SO THAT THE PRESENT EFFECT OF THE WHOLE TREATMENT SESSION IS KNOWN, AS DISTINCT FROM WHAT MAY APPEAR TO HAVE CHANGED WITH EACH TECHNIQUE)

The amount of treatment that can be undertaken at any one session depends upon:

1.  The severity of the patient's pain.
2.  The nature and stability of the patient's disorder causing the pain.
3.  The 'irritability of the painful disorder.

The more care required in treatment, because of the foregoing factors, the less can be done at one session. If the amount of treatment is limited, then so also is the number of changes in technique that can be attempted. Under these circumstances the 24-hour assessment is critical, because these are the patients who are likely to suffer exacerbation of their symptoms following too much treatment. Signs of exacerbation may not be apparent at the time of treatment.

With a patient fitting the above category, not only should an assessment be made of the effectiveness of a *technique*, but also at the end of the treatment *session* a comparison of the subjective and physical findings should be made with those that were present at the beginning of the treatment session. In this context it is helpful if the patient can summarize his subjective changes (throughout the treatment session), giving an indication of whether he felt a particular technique was helpful or whether he might expect some reaction later.

Patients who fit into the group where one movement provokes only a local pain, which goes immediately on releasing the movement, do not need the same assessment of the effectiveness of the total treatment as do patients in the foregoing category. However, it is often useful to know if the patient thinks any one particular technique helped more than another. It may be that he can also state whether one particular technique 'gets at' the disorder more than another.

## ASSESSMENT OVER A 24-HOUR PERIOD IMMEDIATELY FOLLOWING THE LAST TREATMENT SESSION (BECAUSE THIS IS OFTEN THE MOST IMPORTANT INFORMATION PERIOD) AND SUBSEQUENT 24-HOUR PERIODS UP TO THE NEXT TREATMENT SESSION

When a patient's pain is localized to the nearby spinal area, only reproduced at the limit of one movement (or perhaps two), and immediately relieved on releasing the movement, then it is likely that two uses (or even one) of a technique may be enough to assess its effectiveness.

If the patient has no signs of any aching whatsoever, no symptoms at night, a totally stable disorder, and no increase in the symptoms with repetitive painful movement, then many changes in technique can be made at one treatment session, and the 24-hour assessment is less important.

With all patients who do not fit into the above category, assessing the effect of the treatment over an interval of 24 hours following the treatment is essential. The fact that the patient can feel worse on getting out of bed the morning following treatment, as a result of that treatment, demands that this 24-hour assessment be made before a final judgement as to the effect of a treatment session can be made.

All of the details regarding any analytical assessment of the subjective changes over this interval have already been described (p. 72). The analytical assessment of the physical findings, particularly as they relate to different components of the patient's disorder, have also been described (asterisks, pp. 60–61).

## AS A RETROSPECTIVE ASSESSMENT (SO THAT AN OVERALL ASSESSMENT CAN BE MADE OVER THREE OR FOUR TREATMENT SESSIONS)

Even when it is possible confidently to make a physical assessment that progress has been made, it is still of value to know how the patient feels he is progressing.

> In reassessing the effect of a treatment, it is essential to evaluate progress from the perspective of the patient as well as from physical examination findings

When questioned regarding his symptoms, a patient's answer may well be influenced by factors related to his work, his home problems, compensation, his ethnic group, his desire to please the physiotherapist, etc. Therefore the physiotherapist must be sure the patient is giving accurate answers to her questions and that she interprets them as he means them. In the context of 'question and answer', she must *never assume anything*. At the beginning of treatment it is not uncommon for a patient to reply day after day that he is feeling much better. Then, when asked after, say, four treatments, 'How do you feel now compared with before we started treatment?', he may say cautiously, and after a long period of thought, 'I'm sure it's a little better; at least it certainly isn't any worse'. Such a retrospective answer makes the physiotherapist realize that she is not making as much daily progress as she thought she was.

It can be of help to ask the patient, 'What percentage of progress do you think you have made compared with when we began treatment?'. Often the patient finds it difficult to use percentages, but he may answer by some other equally useful comparison – e.g. 'On a scale of 0–10, if 0 was where you were when I first saw you on Monday the 23rd of September and 10 was no pain at all, where would you put yourself on that scale now?'.

The physiotherapist should make her own percentage assessment before putting the question to him. If there is agreement in judgement, then obviously communication and assessment are good.

Sometimes the subjective and physical assessments do not agree. For example, a patient's pleasure at improvement in his symptoms may not be equally reflected by improvement in his signs. The converse may also occur. However, these are exceptions to the general rule, and usually at a slightly later stage of treatment they will agree.

Even when a patient has clear objective signs on which assessments can be made, it is still important to find out how he considers he is progressing. It is poor policy to just continue treatment time after time without making this 'retrospective assessment'. It is very easy to continue treatment unnecessarily, leading to perpetuation of the joint disorder.

To avoid this situation, a gap of twice as long as usual between treatments can clarify the symptomatic response and clear the manipulative physiotherapist's thinking process.

### When the amount or rate of progress has slowed or stopped (to determine the reasons and plan the action required)

This is the most important assessment skill and the one in which the specialist manipulative physiotherapist, particularly if her goal is to be a consultant, must be perfect. It is the assessment that requires the greatest mental agility, alertness and discipline in the whole field of manipulative physiotherapy.

> In retrospective assessment, communication has to be at its most successful level in order to determine changes from the perspective of the patient and to (re) determine further treatment goals

In this retrospective assessment, it is the subjective assessment that plays the greatest role. It is the area where communication must be at its most successful level, and it is an area where experience makes judgement easier and more reliable. The technique of asking the questions, and knowing the reasons why the questions need to be asked, can be learned by anyone who has seen or witnessed its importance and is willing to be patient with patients.

In the relevant section of Chapter 3 (p. 50) the dialogue used for retrospective assessment was omitted, because it was considered more important to be able to include in the text at this stage the kind of information being sought. The information being sought is:

1. When does the patient consider he stopped improving?
2. Why does he consider the improvement stopped?
3. Did he consider he had made progress with earlier treatment?
4. Did he consider progress was brought about by the treatment?
5. At what stage of treatment did the improvement take place?
6. Was the improvement progressive?
7. If treatment helped him, were there any particular techniques or times that helped him more than others?
8. Was it a technique done in a *particular manner* that helped him?
9. Was there any particular technique, or technique done in a particular manner, that aggravated his symptoms at any stage?
10. How is he now compared with before treatment began?
11. How does he compare now with how he was before the onset of this episode?
12. Does he consider he is back to *his* normal?
13. What treatment goals need to be achieved from this session onwards (especially improving certain impairments and disabilities).

Once you have determined his opinions in relation to all of the above questions, it is the right stage to start a full re-examination, both subjective and physical, as though he were a new patient. The questions would then be:

'What is your problem at this stage?'

'When does it bother you most?'

'Is there anything you can do here and now to demonstrate to me a way in which you can provoke the symptoms?'

'Are there any other aspects of your symptoms, or the ways in which they affect you, that you think might be helpful to my understanding of your problem?'

**A retrospective assessment as outlined above can take as long as, if not longer than, any initial examination.** The searching for detail is much more important at this point, because the future management of the patient's disorder may be a big and important decision to make. On it hang factors that may make all the difference to his future life. This may seem a very dramatic statement to make, and it is a major decision only with a small percentage of patients. Nevertheless the decision, when it has to be taken, is a very important one both to the patient and to the physiotherapist, because her reputation on the one hand and her skill as a practitioner on the other depend upon it.

### Following a planned assessment–break from treatment (to establish the place of further treatment)

Many patients have a disorder that the manipulative physiotherapist realizes cannot be made normal in every regard. Under such circumstances, the end-result of treatment will be a 'compromise result'. It is not easy to know when that compromise result has been reached, and there is only one way to determine it. First, a time will be reached when the patient's symptoms and signs do not continue to improve, and in fact there is a possibility that the treatment perpetuates the symptoms. The second stage is for the patient to be given a break from treatment of approximately 2 weeks, after which an assessment of the symptoms and signs can be made. The third stage is to determine whether another three or four treatments should be given to see if further progress can be made, or whether it would be better for the patient to have another 2-week break from treatment followed by reassessment. The following is an example of such a process.

### EXAMPLE

This relates to a patient who presents with symptoms arising from a low-grade active arthritis, where it is known that to regain a full painless range of joint movement is impossible. The question is, when does one discontinue treatment?

In the early stages of passive movement treatment for such patients, a gratifying improvement in movement

and pain can be expected. Later during treatment, a point will be reached when the patient's symptoms remain static and it is difficult to be sure whether the range of movement is improving very slightly or not at all. The physiotherapist should know that a stage can be reached when, in fact, the mobilizing is perpetuating the complaint. At this point the patient can be asked the direct question, 'Do you feel you have continued to improve over the last three or four treatments?'. If the answer is 'NO', then the treatment should be discontinued for a period of approximately 2 weeks, after which the patient's signs and symptoms should be reassessed and the following actions taken:

1.  If the symptoms have improved, the patient should be left for a further 2–3 weeks and then reassessed. If there is then additional improvement, the patient can be discharged on the assumption that the symptoms will continue to improve without treatment.

2.  If the symptoms and signs have remained the same, the patient should be given four or five more treatments and then taken off treatment again for 2 weeks. At the end of this period it will be possible to determine whether the extra treatment produced any improvement, and whether a further few treatments should be administered.

This pattern of management must be very accurately assessed if it is to be used constructively. It may be of interest to mention here that when these patients have recurrences (and they always do have recurrences), usually:

1.  They seek treatment at an earlier stage of the exacerbation.
2.  They respond more readily to treatment.
3.  They have progressively longer periods between exacerbations.
4.  Many of their exacerbations recover quite quickly without treatment.

### AT THE COMPLETION OF TREATMENT (TO MAKE JUDGEMENTS ON PROGNOSIS AND PROPHYLAXIS)

A point to be considered in relation to assessment at the end of treatment is, 'What is normal in the way of pain and movement for this patient?'.

People have widely differing norms. For example, forward flexion of the trunk in standing can vary from one person being able only to reach just beyond the knees, to someone else being able to put hands flat on the floor. Such variations also occur in other movements.

It is necessary to bear in mind these ordinary variations if an accurate assessment is to be achieved.

*Example 1.* Consider a patient who presents for treatment of low back pain. On examining forward flexion it is found that he can only reach his knees, and at this point his back pain is reproduced. On first seeing this it might be considered that flexion is markedly limited and painful, and therefore the patient's condition is assessed as being quite bad. However, if this patient had been asked, 'How far could you bend before the onset of your pain?', he might have replied, 'I've never been able to bend much further than my knees'. This information puts the interpretation of the flexion disability into a different perspective.

*Example 2.* An elderly patient with neck pain also shows radiological evidence of gross degenerative change. Passive movement treatment is very helpful for a patient such as this, but the assessment must take into consideration the fact that rotation to either side will never reach 90°. The same will apply to all his other cervical movements. Therefore the assessment must take into account the range of movement that is likely to be normal for this patient. The role of treatment will be to eliminate the painful aspect of joint movement. The end-result will be slightly improved movement, although movements will remain stiff in all directions. Importantly, the neck pain will have gone.

The next point to be made under this heading is that the effect of treatment cannot be clearly known until an interval of 2–3 weeks has passed following the last treatment session. If a patient has retained full-range pain-free movements and has continued to be symptom free over this interval, the effect of treatment is clear-cut.

There are occasions when a patient with chronic symptoms yet little to find on examination of movements may not show any signs of symptomatic improvement throughout treatment. However, this same patient may find that the symptoms disappear after a 2-week break from treatment. This is not uncommon.

At the time of the last treatment and assessment, the manipulative physiotherapist must know the degree of improvement she has been able to effect, and how close this result is to an ideal result. She should also know how easy it might be for the symptoms to recur. Part of the judgement in this regard would be based on the history and diagnosis of the disorder as well as the stability of the disorder at the time of treatment. Based on these judgements, she should be able to predict how careful the patient may need to be in looking after his spinal problem. It is in this area that prophylactic treatment, in terms of re-education, stabilizing or mobilizing exercises, is considered.

Although it is outside the scope of this book to discuss prophylaxis, there is one facet that does not seem to be widely appreciated. Among the many people who have frequent episodes of mechanical spinal pain, there is a significant percentage who have episodes because their joint movements have never been made as good as they could be in their pain-free periods. Despite the fact that it only requires two or three treatments to make them symptomatically well, they are left with a residue of joint signs which, although they are not causing any symptoms, leave the patient's spine in a state such that a combination of factors may cause a recurrence of the symptoms. However, if these movements were made symptom and sign free, any factors that might influence the onset of another episode would need to be more vigorous because of the better state of the joint. This is a very common finding among patients who have had episodes of pain for which they have gained relief with a few treatments from lay manipulators. If the manipulative physiotherapist is able to continue treatment beyond the symptom-free stage to reach the point when the movements are also sign free, then the frequency of episodes is markedly altered.

## ASSESSMENT ASSISTING IN DIFFERENTIAL DIAGNOSIS

At the initial examination of a patient, the doctor may not be able to make a definitive diagnosis. If the problem is a musculoskeletal disorder, then under some circumstances passive movement treatment can be applied in such a way as to assist in making the diagnosis.

For example, a patient may have pain in the region of his shoulder and the referring doctor may not be certain whether the pain is emanating from the patient's shoulder or from his neck. The patient can be referred to a manipulative physiotherapist with a request that he be treated in such a manner as to assist in forming the diagnosis.

To do this successfully the physiotherapist needs to examine both the neck and the shoulder in the kind of detail mentioned earlier in this chapter so that all joint signs, both cervical and glenohumeral, are revealed in detail. She should then treat the cervical area first and assess the effect of this treatment both on the cervical and on the shoulder signs. If treatment to the cervical spine produces favourable changes in both cervical and shoulder signs, then the cervical treatment should be continued. However, if there is no improvement in the shoulder signs within three treatment sessions, despite trying all techniques applicable to the cervical spine, treatment to this area should be discontinued. The shoulder should then be treated and its response assessed. In this way the response to treatment will give the answer as to whether the cervical spine is involved, thus assisting the diagnosis.

## ANALYTICAL ASSESSMENT

Assessment is the keystone of effective, informative treatment, without which treatment successes and failures are not learning experiences. Assessment can be performed as a mechanical process, and is used to prove the value of a technique. Analytical assessment goes a stage further. It literally implies analysing one's thoughts about all aspects of a patient's disorder and treatment to arrive at clearly defined answers. As well as enforced discipline, it requires an agile, sceptical and methodical mind, a mind with the ability to be open-ended and accept 'cause and effect' in opposition (if need be) to accepted principles, a reproachful-of-self attitude and an attitude of 'well – if you think so – *prove it*'. It involves the process of: THINK, PLAN and EXECUTE (to) PROVE.

This does not always mean performing a technique to prove its value at a particular stage of a patient's disorder; it may mean any of the following:

1. Proving a negative by, for example, treating a structure vigorously in a particular manner to prove that there is nothing wrong with it.

2. Sending a patient home without treating him to prove that the progress, which seems to have been achieved, has in fact been as a result of the treatment and has not been spontaneous recovery.

3. Forcing oneself not to give way to the temptation of trying a second technique, so that the interpretation of the next assessment cannot be confused or be ambiguous.

This last point is critically important in the planning of a treatment session. The most important goal (other than relieving the patient of his symptoms) is to execute a plan of treatment so that there is no possibility of being confused by the patient's answer to the initial question 'How have you been?' when a mixture of techniques has been used. Although a patient may be able to say, 'I'm pretty sure the traction helped me but when you did that twisting of my back I don't think that did it any good', the statement cannot be relied upon to be exactly right. Whereas if, in assessing the effect of the traction, it did not seem to have made much immediate change either subjectively or physically, the analytical mind has to think and decide the relative values between:

1. Shall I try rotation as a treatment technique to see if it will effect any immediate change? Favourable

change may result but it may not; it may leave me in exactly the same position as after the traction. Then, do I ask myself, 'Well, shall I try such and such a technique, or is this just getting me deeper into confusion'

OR

2. Would I be better off to leave treatment at this point and assess the effect of the traction over the 24-hour assessment period? I might find, if I try rotation, that this produces a marked change. The one thing I do know for certain is that, if I leave treatment at traction only for today, *I cannot possibly be confused when I see him tomorrow.*

One of the important mental processes in analytical assessment is to plan today's treatment with thoughts of tomorrow's assessment in mind. In other words:

DON'T CONFUSE TOMORROW'S ASSESSMENT.

The following is an example of deciding to send a patient home without treatment to achieve these very ends. This man had right buttock pain. Forward flexion showed a slight list to the left, which, if countered, reproduced the pain. The slump test was positive when the right foot was dorsiflexed, reproducing the buttock pain. The pain was markedly reproduced when, while in full lateral flexion to the right, he was flexed.

On reassessing him at the third visit, he said he was 70 per cent better. He did not have as much reaction after the second treatment as that following the same treatment on the first day. Following the second treatment, he said he felt uncomfortable for half an hour and then the pain cleared and had not returned since.

It *could*, but may not, be assumed that the improvement was from the treatment.

NEVER ASSUME ANYTHING.

The following immediate-response question was asked: 'When you left here, did you do anything different or unusual which could have been responsible for the improvement in your symptoms?'. After a long deliberation he responded, 'Not that I can think of'. On asking him if he had periods of freedom like this at other times he said, 'Yes'. The next immediate-response question was, 'Do you feel the improvement has been as a result of treatment?'. The answer was, 'I'm not sure'. This was a surprise because it seemed to conflict with several things: his elation at saying he was 70 per cent better, the timing of the improvement, and the lessened reaction from the second treatment. It seemed the improvement should have been from the treatment; he should have been able to say quite spontaneously,

'Oh yes'. On examination it was found that there was slight improvement with the slump dorsiflexion test and also a slight change in the quality of the pain when flexing from the lateral flexion right position. Further questions about other symptoms such as stiffness on getting out of bed in the mornings indicated improvement, but again these were variable symptoms.

Thinking of 'don't confuse tomorrow' and knowing that if he were treated today and he then reported tomorrow being not as good, the current uncertainty of 'cause and effect' would be further confused:

Would the 'not as good' be due to treatment?

Was the last improvement a 'flash-in-the-pan?'

Would the 'not as good' have been just the same if he had not had treatment?

To make the best use of assessment, it was decided to give no treatment and to review in 4 days' time. Execution of the plan would mean that an unconfused assessment of the symptoms could be clearly associated or disassociated with treatment.

In fact the patient rang on the third day saying he wasn't as good as when last seen. The answer was then clear and treatment was continued.

The THINKING and PLANNING processes require a full appreciation of:

1. The patient's disorder (its pathology, if it is pathological, and its present stage).
2. The effects that particular techniques can be expected to have, both in terms of the amount of change that can be expected and retained, and the rate of change.
3. The patient as a person, and all that that implies.

Critical analysis of self and continuous seeking for certainties, if applied conscientiously to the treatment of every patient, leads to an invaluable accumulation of experience and reliability as a consultant. This goal is a responsibility we have to our patients and to the medical profession.

## CONCLUSION

Just as there are communication difficulties in normal conversation, arising out of misinterpretation of the meanings of things said or not said, so there are difficulties in assessing the patient's subjective response to treatment. Because of these difficulties, the physiotherapist should be most careful in questioning to assess any variations in the patient's symptoms.

None of the patient's feelings about his pain should ever be assumed. For example, if a patient is asked to bend forward, and he does so and says 'Ouch!', the physiotherapist should immediately follow up with 'Did that hurt?' – 'Yes' – 'Where did you feel it?'. As the examination continues and the patient repeatedly feels pain with each movement, it can be irritating to him to be continually asked 'Where did it hurt?'. Under such circumstances, when the patient cringes while testing movements, the physiotherapist can ask, 'In the same spot?'. This avoids reiteration while still getting the correct message. Assume nothing. If the pain alters in its area he will say where it is, even if only asked, 'In the same spot?'. It is this close communication between physiotherapist and patient that makes assessment so informative and valuable, and thereby makes treatment more specific and effective.

Although some will say this is too time consuming to be of value, successful treatment compels this degree of accuracy; it is essential if the physiotherapist is to remain in control of the treatment situation. Given practice and experience, it is not a lengthy procedure.

# Chapter 5

# Prognosis

This chapter is written for manipulative physiotherapists by a manipulative physiotherapist. It neither takes the place of medical prognosis, nor does it provide answers regarding percentages of disability, nor define the relative psychological/medical components of a disorder.

*Prognosis is the forecast of the probable course of a case of disease or injury, or it is the art of making such a forecast.*    (Shorter Oxford Dictionary, 1980)

Writing about prognosis is a daunting task for a manipulative physiotherapist, and some readers may consider prognosis as being outside the role or responsibility of the profession. However, the manipulative physiotherapist has more contact with the patient than the referring medical specialist, and often sees the patient in the presence of other members of the family. These visits can reveal much valuable information that can contribute to the medical specialist's final prognosis. The contribution that the manipulative physiotherapist is able to make depends upon her ability to communicate, empathize with and 'feel' what the patient feels, and to maintain an enthusiastic and positive attitude as well as on her skill to make a prognosis.

Throughout this book, persuasive and, I hope, convincing emphasis is placed on the importance of repetitive ASSESSMENT of changes in the patient's symptoms and physical examination findings. The aim is for the features of the symptomatic behaviour and history to make medical sense such that the physical findings can be added to make features fit (*see* pp. 57–58) and then, by showing what effect each single modality of treatment (or passive movement treatment technique) has on the patient and his disorder, the picture is made more complete.

The manipulative physiotherapist must always keep her mind open to ALL the incoming information and remain empathetic to 'feel' the patient's symptoms so she can 'walk their walk', but maintain an enthusiastic and positive attitude. Although it is tempting to start formulating a prognosis at the initial examination, this is still too early for forecasting. At the retrospective assessment, after three or four treatment sessions, the manipulative physiotherapist has enough information to begin forecasting.

However, as treatment continues further, the manipulative physiotherapist can refine the information to make her forecast more accurate and meaningful. The assessing process and resultant prognosis will also give her the information with which she can empower the patient to manage his disorder.

If this assessing process is implemented by the manipulative physiotherapist, she should reach a stage when her years of self-critical appraisal and clinical experience enable her to compile a valuable legal type of report within her field. This could contribute to a physical prognosis of the patient's future and enrich the medical specialist's final prognosis. The accuracy of a manipulative physiotherapist's judgement in a final analytical assessment depends upon her skills in examination and treatment, plus her years of self-analysis and clinical experience.

An excellent text, which should be read in conjunction with this chapter, is Eurig Jeffreys' book *Prognosis in Musculoskeletal Injury* (Jeffreys, 1991). The book is written for specialist doctors and lawyers and deals mainly with injuries, but any manipulative physiotherapist involved in providing reports, opinions or suggestions should be familiar with it. Jeffreys writes that prognosis:

> is an art, or skill, not a science. IT CONCERNS PROBABILITIES, NOT CERTAINTIES and it refers to INDIVIDUAL, not the general . . . Fortunately, although individuals differ in their response to insult, their ailments follow recognized patterns and it is possible to form GENERAL PREDICTIONS of the natural history of disorders

At the final analytical assessment stage the manipulative physiotherapist, through careful repetitive assessment, has collected information that can help her answer the following questions regarding prognosis.

## QUESTIONS REGARDING PROGNOSIS

### WHAT IS THE DIAGNOSIS?

Diagnosis is a critical issue when making a prognosis, but it is necessary to state that frequently it is not possible to make an 'accurate diagnosis' of a patient's disorder (Grieve, 1988b). For example, although it may be possible to state that a patient has been diagnosed as having rheumatoid arthritis, some of the symptoms may be coming from an osteoarthritic component. Treatment to relieve pain due to the osteoarthritis might provide more relief than relieving the rheumatoid pain. Another example of diagnostic difficulty could be a patient with symptoms in the regions of the shoulder, upper arm, scapula and neck, with contributing sources from the cervical spine, neural tissues and

glenohumeral components. It may be impossible to isolate one structure or even a group (e.g. a joint complex) of structures as the cause of symptoms and signs. This is where the manipulative physiotherapist can assist medical practitioners, by her manual skills and knowledge, and can add to the doctor's knowledge in formulating a prognosis. It is easy to understand the difficulties most readers would experience in having to give a diagnosis for patients with low back pain, unless of course they fit a clear routine presentation of patients they see often.

Grieve (1997) wrote most aptly to the editor of *Manual Therapy* about 'Diagnosis of spinal neuromusculoskeletal conditions'. For my part the word DIAGNOSIS means ascertaining the *locality* and the *nature*, in patho-anatomical terms, of the morbid changes that have occurred, in which tissue, together with the consequent disordered function. That is, not only WHERE it is, but also WHAT it is. Having read recent observations on the subject (Twomey and Taylor, 1987; Jull *et al.*, 1988; Durrell, 1996; Phillips and Twomey, 1996) there is a need for comment, since in my opinion many of these authors are not writing about diagnosis at all but only about localization – which, while highly desirable, does not amount to diagnosis. Simple localization is not diagnosis. Brewerton (1986), a consultant rheumatologist with much experience of working with manipulative physiotherapists, and with perception of their special clinical problems, remarks:

> the great majority of patients ... [with] spinal pain cannot be classified or diagnosed – using the word in the proper sense as is classically understood by clinicians world wide.

To make a diagnosis in terms that are meaningful to the manipulative physiotherapist we must remember the brick wall, analogy (*see* p. 6), and relate the clinical examination findings and assessment in its entirety to the areas of known medical knowledge.

The manipulative physiotherapist needs to attempt to decide:

1. What structure(s) does she think is at fault?
2. What is the stage of the disorder?
3. What is the stability of the disorder?
4. What factors are affecting the behaviour of the disorder?
5. What is the 'cause of the source'?

### What structure(s) does she think is at fault?

From the initial examination, she will determine:

1. The joints that lie under the area of pain.
2. The joints that do not lie under the area of pain but can refer pain into the area.

**Table 5.1**    Differentiation of structures

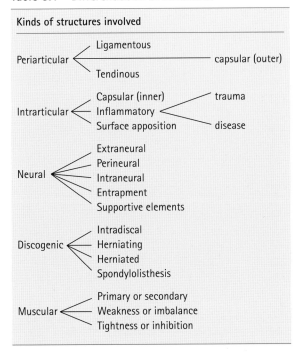

Kinds of structures involved

analyse the rate of progression of the disorder. This will assist in making a prognosis.

A detailed history will inform us if the symptoms are spreading or worsening in intensity. Consider the following:

- Are the attacks more frequent or disabling?
- Is there a familial history, and did the symptoms worsen or dissipate with or without treatment? If treatment was used, what method was it?
- Does our 'medical knowledge' help us to understand the patient's story?
- Is it subjective or structural impairment?

The natural history of an episode of non-traumatic onset is of resolution. Our aim is to speed up the process, ideally by provoking the body's own healing powers, and restore movement so it is full and pain free.

> The manipulative physiotherapist who is skilled in 'the concept' will learn to understand the path of progression of the disorder

Repeated episodes cause impairment, which will further guide the forecast.

## What is the stability of the disorder?

A detailed history of the current episode will inform the therapist how easily the problem is provoked and relieved. For example, did it take a long weekend (3 days) of digging up a lawn and replanting it to provoke symptoms such that the patient couldn't get out of bed on Tuesday morning? Or did he bend over to pick something off the floor and feel his back 'go'? (*see* Chapter 6, p. 118).

The past history will also help enormously:

- On previous episodes, did the back take more activity to provoke pain?
- Are predisposing factors implicated?
- Is the site or intensity of pain increasing?
- Is there altered sensation peripherally?
- By the third treatment, are the symptoms lessening or retracting centrally, or the opposite?
- Are the symptoms now more or less easily provoked?
- Is the backache worse but the leg symptoms have gone?

With a low lumbar disorder, the spine's ability to move freely during a repeated movement from full flexion to full extension will indicate its stability. Once a full range has been achieved, the movement of the spine is observed during the movement of full flexion through to full extension.

3. The neural sources that will be implicated in pain referral.
4. The muscles that lie under the area of pain.

See Table 5.1 for the differentiation of structures.

After three of four treatments, and analytical assessment, it may be possible to reduce these four possibilities to one or maybe two.

The thinking process is then related to:

- With what movement and how is the pain reproduced?
- Does the movement involve stretching or compressing?
- Are the joint surfaces opposed or distracted?
- With differentiation tests (*see* Chapter 6, p. 162), are the neural or muscular elements involved, and if so to what extent?
- Is there more than one structure implicated?

By careful assessment these questions can be answered. Note that in the vertebral column, and in particular in the lumbar spine, the disc is commonly a source of pain (the common features of its presentation are discussed later in this chapter).

## What is the stage of the disorder?

If it is possible to localize the structure, then we must think in terms of stage of the disorder, and specifically

Begin by stopping the movement at the upright stage so the disorder is not aggravated. This can be progressed by not stopping the movement in the middle and by increasing the speed of the movement. Lastly, by sustaining the full flexion for longer (e.g. 20 seconds) the effect is amplified.

**CAUTION**: This is not a test movement to be done in the initial assessment stages.

### What factors are affecting the behaviour of the disorder?

*The onset of the disorder*

If the onset is caused by a specific injury, the behaviour of the disorder is less predictable than if it is of spontaneous onset.

When the onset is spontaneous, two patterns emerge. The first group of patients is of those whose symptoms begin gradually, without there being any known remembered reason. By delving into their history it is revealed that they suffered an injury (sprain, strain) many years previously. Despite having had a good response to treatment at the time, this has laid down the foundation for gradually developing degenerative arthritic changes. The present episode may have begun very insidiously, such that they are unable precisely to remember its onset. This pattern can commonly occur in patients between 45 and 55 years of age, although similar radiological changes may be seen in a 74-year-old who has been symptom free for 74 years (*Figure 5.1*)!

> Some people have never experienced what they would call symptoms, yet the gross radiological osteoarthritic degenerative changes are obviously well established

The second group of patients consists of those who have symptoms as a result of repetitive functions, at work or in sport, which are in excess of what their bodies can accommodate. Examples include overuse, new use, disuse and abuse. If this is superimposed upon degenerative changes from a previous injury (possibly from childhood), the prognosis may involve more treatment sessions with a long-term (several years) maintenance programme involving exercises and/or stretches.

Finally, there are those patients who are recovering from trauma, surgery or other medical management for reasons other than an injury (e.g. nerve root compression with neurological changes). This latter group is discussed superbly by Jeffreys (1991).

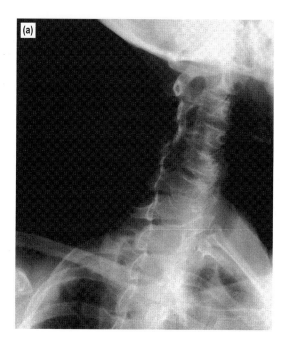

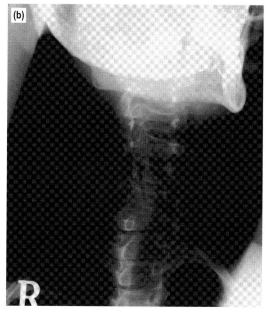

**Figure 5.1** (*a*) and (*b*) X-rays of a 74-year-old patient who is symptom free

*The nature of the injury*

The nature of the injury is significant in terms of how much violence or force is transferred. The type of injury itself is a factor. For example, in a car accident, the position of the cars at impact, the speed and direction of movement of both cars, the person's position in the car and his posture are all factors affecting the behaviour of the disorder. In another example, the injuring movement may have been a repetitive movement sustained by an assembly-line worker. These two examples will lead the therapist's thinking in two different directions regarding prognosis.

### Pre-existing signs and/or symptoms

Pre-existing signs and/or symptoms may indicate a 'weak link', which gives out when trauma (albeit minor) is forced upon the chain.

In the non-traumatic category, repeated past bouts may have an increasing frequency and/or severity, causing the current disorder to be particularly disabling. An inflammatory component may be emerging with successive bouts, or a previously dormant subclinical inflammatory component may emerge following a traumatic episode. Assessment of the treatment response and the method of treatment used (amplitude and depth of movement) help to clarify the prognosis.

### Age

If a boy aged 18 years can't swing a golf club without back pain, the prognosis will be very different to that if the same problem affects a man aged 60 years.

### General health

A person suffering from other disorders (not musculoskeletal) may be below average in their general fitness level, which may increase their vulnerability to problems.

### Gender

A man's physique is usually different to a woman's of similar age, and they will deal with physical stress differently.

### Occupation

The patient's occupation must be considered if it is proved to be a reason that the disorder is persisting.

With careful assessment the manipulative physiotherapist has a thorough understanding of the person's physical ability, and she can relate this to his work environment. For example, it may be that the patient is unable to turn his head further than 70° to the left without causing pain, although he can turn 90° to the right without discomfort. In his office the computer is placed to the left of his keyboard and he has a chair placed on his left where clients sit when he interviews them, which happens several times a day. Although he made good progress after two treatments, he was unable to retain

**Table 5.2**  Recognizable features of the presenting disorder

| Hypothesizing conjecturing |
| --- |
| Is it a: |
|     recognizable pathology? |
|     typical or atypical pattern? |
|     trauma situation (strain/sprain)? |
| DO FEATURES FIT? |
| DO THEY MAKE SENSE? |
| Is it: |
|     overuse |
|     misuse? |
|     new use? |
|     abuse? |
|     disuse? |
| Has it more than one component? |

more than 25 per cent of the improved movement gained at each session. By changing the placement of the computer and the chair used for interviews, he was free of signs and symptoms when assessed before the fifth treatment. In many cases, astute minor changes can improve the situation by altering the irritating repetitive movement.

Once the irritating posture or movement is eliminated the injured structure(s) can heal.

> A physiotherapy-specific diagnosis is concerned with movement disorders; therefore it is important to document the injuring movement directions and the direction of functional limitation

### Family history

A family history of similar disorders, inflammatory conditions or poor healing must influence prognosis.

Other questions that must be considered (*Table 5.2*) include:

- What is recognizable about the patient's condition?
- What does not seem to fit into the factors that guide the diagnosis?

## What is the 'cause' of the source?

To reach the stage of being able to complete treatment and arrive at a prognosis is to understand the possible underlying reasons why the structure has become the source of the symptoms; in other words, what is the 'cause of the source' (*Table 6.3*, Part Two). As well as trauma, it is necessary to consider items such as posture, muscle weakness or tightness, hypermobility of one side of an inter-vertebral segment making the other side of the segment work harder, or the segments above and below being similarly affected. Some aspects to be considered relate to the structures that are the source (or the cause of the source) of the symptoms (*Table 5.1*).

The examination emphasis is on the determination of the range of movements and their symptom responses, with:

1. Physiological movement tests.
2. Functional movement tests.
3. Combined movement tests.
4. Passive accessory movement tests.

> In the vertebral column, it is PALPATION that is the most important and the most difficult skill to learn. To achieve this skill it is necessary to be able to FEEL, by palpation, the difference in the spinal segments – normal or abnormal; old or new; hypomobile or hypermobile – and then be able to *relate the response, site, depth and relevance to a patient's symptoms (structures, source and causes)*. This requires an honest, self-critical attitude, and also applies to the testing of functional movements and combined physiological test movements.
> IT TAKES AT LEAST 10 YEARS FOR ANY CLINICIAN (even one who has an inborn ability) TO LEARN THE RELATIONSHIP BETWEEN HER HANDS, THE PAIN RESPONSES AND HER MIND

Comments by many manipulative physiotherapists make it necessary to emphasize again that:

> a stiff joint is not necessarily a painful joint

In other words, if a structure is limited in range it does not have to be the *source* of symptoms. On the other hand, it may well be the *cause* of related overworked structures becoming the *source* of symptoms.

Relating this fact to prognosis, it may be necessary to take the stiffness into account when grading the patient's likely future lifestyle (e.g. recurrence of episodes; *Table 5.2*).

## HOW DOES THE EFFECT OF TREATMENT INFLUENCE THE PROGNOSIS?

Although it is tempting to predict the outcome of certain treatment techniques, it is important to retain an open mind to the treatment response. This ensures the accuracy of the assessment, which is essential to proving the value of each treatment technique. The assessment process is explained in detail in Chapter 4.

The ideal response to treatment is gradual improvement to full pain-free movement in three to four treatments spread over 3–4 weeks. If there is a quick response, e.g. full recovery after one treatment, then either the joint signs have not been 'cleared' or the disorder may recur with very little provocation. If the response is slow, the manipulative physiotherapist must constantly be asking herself if the technique is the wrong choice, if its method of application (strength and her technique) is wrong, if it is her poor communication/assessment skills at fault, or is the disorder beyond her area of expertise?

Just as treatment techniques involve the assessment process to prove their worth, so do exercises. Before giving any person stretches or exercises, their effectiveness must be assessed. In many cases this process should continue until the usefulness of the exercises or stretches is proven. The manipulative physiotherapist must prove their value, and the patient will arrive at their own conviction. This is important so that they will 'own' the problem and take the necessary action. This is particularly relevant when we think in terms of prognosis, as both exercises (specific or general) and stretches become part of the necessary lifestyle changes. If the response to treatment is favourable and the joints are 'cleared', the forecast is good and the patient can feel in control. The patient must understand what provokes the disorder and therefore what to avoid (*see* predisposing factors, below). It may be possible to provide the patient with knowledge of what to do in terms of easing the pain (movement, heat, rest, etc.), should there be a recurrence.

## HOW DO PREDISPOSING FACTORS INFLUENCE THE PROGNOSIS?

When a trivial incident causes quite disabling pain, there may be factors that predispose the spine to 'giving way'. In taking the history these factors must be identified so that the manipulative physiotherapist and the patient are aware of them – the patient can then avoid them in the lifestyle changes he makes, and the manipulative physiotherapist can understand more fully the disorder she is discovering, and 'make features fit'. The presence of these factors therefore influence the forecast.

## WHAT DO WE UNDERSTAND ABOUT THE PATIENT AND HIS RESPONSE TO INJURY?

The manipulative physiotherapist is not qualified to give a psychological/medical opinion of the patient. However, with experience, and often after three to four treatment sessions, she may have evidence of the patient's response and his ability to communicate, and an understanding of the language he uses to communicate. This certainly has value as a medical opinion. We have no control over the other person's attitude and behaviour, but we have 100 per cent control over our own. Therefore to gain the best outcome possible for the situation we must be vigilant in keeping ourselves focused on:

1. *Understanding* the situation from the patient's perspective.
2. Making sure we are making our questions *clear*.
3. *Believing* the patient's story.
4. Using wise *non-verbal* signals.
5. Taking the blame if there is *miscommunication*.

It is too easy to place the blame for a poor outcome on factors other than our own lack of skill, and therefore to cast a poor prognosis.

With this understanding, the manipulative physiotherapist must consider expectations at the conclusion of treatment of the patient's disorder in relation to:

1. The likely restraints on lifestyle.
2. The likelihood of recurrences of episodes of the disorder, and the possible early warning signs the patient must heed to minimize the severity of the recurrence; and the steps the patient then needs to take.
3. The need for specific ongoing exercises, intermittent maintenance treatment or follow-up assessment.

As Jeffreys (1991) so delightfully puts it, 'In few disorders can prognosis be REVERSED (I dressed him, God cured him – Ambroise Pare)'.

The information thus gathered enables the manipulative physiotherapist to make a forecast of the probable course of the individual case she is treating. However, while 'no two backs are the same' it is, as Jeffreys states, 'possible to form general predictions of the natural history of disorders'. In a very broad sense it is possible to look for guidelines to direct one's thinking.

## THE CLINICAL APPLICATION OF PROGNOSIS MAKING

### CERVICAL SPINE

### Headaches and the upper cervical spine

For a complete discussion of cervical headaches (and dizziness), the reader is referred to Lance (1993) and Bogduk (1994a).

Many cervical headaches arise from the upper cervical spine, and the most common intervertebral segment involved is C2/3. However, this level needs to be clearly differentiated from C1/2 during the physical examination. When C2/3 is the source, C3/4 becomes involved, but only as a secondary component.

In the subjective examination, the area of symptoms may not include the neck.

> Palpation is an important part of examination and is enormously informative

The main findings by palpation are the following:

- Thickening of tissues around the articular pillar, frequently unilaterally.
- Thickening of the tissues in the interlaminar trough. This interlaminar area is normally a shallow bony dip; abnormally there is no dip but rather a prominence, which may be thick and hard (indicating its age), soft and spongy, or cystic.
- Prominence of the spinous process of C3.
- Limitation of C2/C3 intersegmental movement, especially with a unilateral PA technique directed 30–40° medially on the ipsilateral side.
- Reproduction of at least part of the area of the cervical headache symptoms, or local DEEP pain, can always be found with at least one of the many such palpation examination procedures.

> DEEP pain response is not accepted as being normal

Cervical spine headaches can arise also from the occiput/C2 (O/C2) articulations, which require another important physical examination technique (compression) that will provoke appropriate 'high' cervical (O/C2) symptoms and reveal limitations of range or quality of movement. It also assists in differentiating O/C1 involvement from C2/3.

If the compression is performed expertly (that is, with little or no movement occurring below C2), the therapist will be able to feel if there is limitation to the free movement in the lateral flexion direction. From the same compression position, lateral flexion is an easier restriction to assess than is rotation, flexion/extension or protraction/retraction. Any one of these test movements will provoke symptoms of which the patient is readily aware, and he will probably report them spontaneously.

The history may or may not involve trauma. If trauma has been a factor and the joint signs (primarily palpation) can be 'cleared', the likelihood of recurrences is diminished. However, once the patient has suffered headaches he has a propensity to suffer recurrences, although treatment can lessen their severity and frequency. It is important to determine the cause of the source.

If the symptoms include visual disturbances and/or dizziness, the prognosis is less clear. Objectively, while other routine tests may be useful, compression is likely to be the most informative.

The description of the many types of headache (Lance, 1998) helps us to put the cervical headache into perspective. Many headache sufferers will have a component of cervical source of symptoms, but they cannot be diagnostically called 'cervical headache', and this we must accept as fact.

## Headaches with a neural component

People who have headaches will seek treatment because of their severity, their constancy (even if mild, if they last too long), if they are not relieved with drugs, or because they are disturbing and involve other areas such as the face, eyes and tongue, or concentration, mood, dizziness, etc. Neural symptoms are different in their quality from musculoskeletal symptoms and the other symptoms that variously accompany pain/discomfort.

The cause of these headaches can be vertebral canal pain-sensitive structures. They can be differentiated by examining and comparing cervical movements in various positions (sitting, cervical flexion supine, prone and side lying left and right) and by adding different components of the slump test in the 'long sitting' position and noting the symptom response differences and different ranges available in the different positions (Breig, 1978).

The accuracy of prognosis as a final analytical assessment depends on the manipulative physiotherapist's skills in examination and treatment, plus her years of critical experience.

The ideal goals of treatment are to improve the headache symptoms and to restore to normal, as far as possible, the physical signs (especially the neural signs) that were found to be abnormal at the outset. The history of these cervical headaches is usually long, and the end result will probably be a compromise. This can be an impairment.

## International classification of impairments, disabilities and handicaps (ICIDH)

The World Health Organization established the ICIDH in 1980 as the following (WHO, 1980):

- An *impairment* is any loss of normality of psychological or anatomical structure or function.
- A *disability* is any restriction, or lack of ability, to perform activity in the manner of, or within the range considered normal for, a human being.
- A *handicap* is a disadvantage for a given individual, resulting from an impairment or disability, that limits or prevents the fulfilment of a role, depending on age, sex, social and cultural factors for that individual.

In 2001 a revised edition of the ICIDH (ICF) was published (WHO, 2000) in which the term 'impairment' was defined as an impairment of function and the terms 'disability' and 'handicap' replaced by 'activity' (level of personal activities) and 'participation' (concerns with social roles), in order to focus more on resources rather than on deficits. The ICF endeavours to describe levels of 'disablement' from the viewpoint of the different dimensions of health at both biological and social levels. In 2000 ICIDH-2 became ICF, International Classificaiton of Functioning.

Many manipulative physiotherapists will be mainly concerned with the evaluation of impairments (Van Baar *et al.*, 1998), however a change in focus towards restoration of full function currently appears to take place.

The term impairment is viewed slightly different by Jeffreys (Jeffreys, 1991). Impairment can be subdivided into *structural impairment* and *subjective impairment*, and both forms of impairment may singly or together contribute to disability.

- If the end result is an *improvement* in the headaches and the physical signs, the patient is left with an '*impairment*', both subjective and structural.
- If the symptoms are not provoked by the abnormal movement signs yet these are still neural signs at the appropriate level, the patient is left with a 'structural impairment'.

If there are no other complications or components, the non-traumatic history is not longer than, say, 2 years, and the patient is younger than about 30 years, it should be possible to make him symptom free. However, if there are appropriate changes present, such as indications of hypermobility, instability or a history of repeated bad episodes, then the final prognosis might be:

- An improved subjective impairment plus structural impairment, but not a disability or activity limitation.

- Structural impairment, but with a possible (or probable) likelihood of recurrences of subjective impairment.
- If restricted in his ability to do a normal day's work because of increasing headache and restriction of neck movements, the patient will have a handicap or participation restriction.

As to his future, only the manipulative physiotherapist's experience and the knowledge of others can give the possibilities. For example, if the prognosis is made at the end of treatment, it can only be recorded that there is a possibility that time alone *may* produce further improvement and that the subjective impairment may subside. The structural impairment may improve because the patient's body may accommodate for the restricted movement as it becomes less painful.

Periodic assessment of the disorder's components is required (one consultation in 3–6 months). If an even more reliable qualification of the prognosis is required, the periodic assessments may need to be extended and varied over a period of 2 years. This may show a disability status changing to an impairment status.

If there is no improvement in the symptoms although the movement signs have significantly improved, then the headaches must have a significant cervical component.

## THORACIC SPINE

### Scapular symptoms

When scapular symptoms are of cervical origin, they will spread over the scapula:

- To the middle, lower scapular and upper scapular (possibly C7)
- To the upper scapular (C4) or
- If there is some middle and lower scapular connection, a milder component of overflow from C5–C7.

As to the origin of the scapular symptoms, if there is no obvious cervical component then the source is more likely thoracic in origin. On thoracic examination, the manipulative physiotherapist is usually able to reproduce the symptoms. It may be necessary for the palpation techniques to be used in combined directions to achieve the reproduction.

> If the source is in the thoracic spine, the prognosis is better than if the source is in the cervical spine

The reason behind this statement is that the thoracic origin is more likely to be periarticular, whereas the cervical source *may* in part be intradiscal. The periarticular disorder is more likely to have a final prognosis of subjective impairment, whereas the cervical intradiscal would be a subjective impairment with the likelihood of exacerbations. The intervertebral disc does not repair as completely or as quickly as periarticular tissues, and therefore the cervical discogenic source is likely to have a compromise result from treatment and the likelihood of recurrences.

Two examination techniques provide valuable information towards making a favourable prognosis:

1. First, if the examination technique of caudal grade IV++ compression applied with the cervical spine in the position of the appropriate degree of ipsilateral flexion and rotation becomes pain-free, the likelihood of recurrences is significantly reduced. Recurrences would require a stronger cause, be less severe, and respond more readily to treatment.

2. Secondly, the prognosis is favourable when the patient has a *full painless* range of cervical extension with over-pressure. To test this properly, the patient moves to the limit of cervical extension and is encouraged to gain further extension by the manipulative physiotherapist stroking his forehead repeatedly to gain even further active extension, and finally by adding quite firm over-pressure (even controlled staccato nudges) at the limit of the range. If this can be achieved without causing flinching by the patient, the interpretation could be considered to be ideal.

Because a recurrence is still possible if the patient's activities in daily living require new use, overuse or abuse, the prognosis may need to be considered a disability.

### Upper limb and cervical symptoms

These symptoms are much more complex, because the symptoms may have their origin in:

1. The cervical spine, discogenic or posterior joints
2. The neural tissues, intra- or extraneural, with radiological or entrapment components
3. Irritative or compressive nerve-root sources, overuse, new use or abuse.
4. Thoracic outlet problems, etc.

When pain is referred distally from the spine, careful differentiation of the possible sources is important (*see* pp. 253–254).

If the source of the pain is the posterior joints, with no contribution from the disc and pain-sensitive structures of the neural canal, the prognosis is easier to forecast. Movement and postural correction may be used to ease the symptoms, but it will be unlikely to eliminate them completely. The pain is less debilitating and restricting of activity than discogenic or neural referral. If the cause of the source can be determined and changed favourably, prognosis is good. Lifestyle changes may be appropriate to prevent recurrences.

If the source of the arm pain is clearly only discogenic, with a spontaneous onset such as having painted the ceilings over a weekend and being woken during Sunday night with neck and arm pain, then the prognosis is initially unreliable. To clarify the prognosis it is necessary to determine the stage and stability of the disorder. This may be helped with knowledge of any past history. The result of treatment and assessment is critical to the forecast. If it is impossible to find a position or movement that relieves the distal symptoms, then the prognosis is poor. More often rotation, which opens the joint of the affected side, and/or traction are useful. If the pain is controllable this way and responds favourably to treatment such that by the third treatment the distal symptoms are minimal and very occasional, the prognosis is good. Extension (the injuring movement) may be the last movement to 'clear'. To provide a good prognosis, clearing the extension movement is paramount. The technique is explained in this chapter.

When the neural tissues and the thoracic outlet are involved, the prognosis is poorer and less predictable. If the treatment progresses favourably such that in the latter stages of treatment the patient can be instructed successfully to do his own stretches daily, causing the improved signs and symptoms to be retained for more than 24 hours, then the prognosis is improved.

## LUMBAR SPINE

### Low lumbar pain

It is common knowledge that episodes of lumbar pain among the general population are very common. Attempting prognosis for a high proportion of these, even those where injury is not involved, is not reliable. Even with all the aids at our disposal, imaging and injections, etc., we do not seem to be getting much closer to achieving accurate prognoses.

Making a prognosis is easier when it can be determined if the disc is involved.

To begin with, a detailed history of the patient's low lumbar disorder is essential in formulating a possible prognosis. It is not uncommon for a person to be unaware of the severity of the pain until the morning after unusual, heavy or sustained work in lumbar flexion. It is fairly safe ground to believe this is the case with a discogenic disorder.

Discogenic disorders have many reasonably clear characteristics (e.g. difficulty in putting stockings and shoes on when first getting out of bed, the longer response to treatment, back pain with coughing or sneezing), and the more of these that are present, the more likely the disorder is to be discogenic. Also, the more of these present, the more chance there is of progressing to a radicular problem with neurological changes requiring surgery and causing a degree of disability.

From the prognosis point of view, the clinician needs to know:

1. The vigour of the previous days' work.
2. The degree of disability so caused.
3. The patient's general state of health and well being.
4. A detailed history of previous episodes.
5. If there is a family history of similar back problems.
6. The age of the patient.
7. The behaviour of the signs and symptoms in terms of severity and site of referral. The more distal and severe, and the poorer the response to treatment, the poorer the prognosis.
8. Any pyschosocial factors ('yellow flags') hindering the recovery to full function.

Therefore low lumbar pain that can reliably be diagnosed as being discogenic without any other associated source of symptoms is quite a different problem – it is clear-cut from a diagnostic point of view, but *not* from a prognostic point of view. The prognostician needs to find answers to the following questions:

1. Will it be possible to make the patient symptomatic and disability free?
2. Will it be possible to make the patient asymptomatic, leaving the disc structurally healed and stable?
3. Will the problem worsen, with symptoms beginning to refer into the buttock or even into the posterior thigh?
4. Will symptoms spread to the toes?
5. Might neurological *CHANGES* occur?

If the intervertebral disc can be excluded, decisions regarding the prognosis are simpler.

Elderly patients who have extensive radiological changes and suffer an episode that starts from a trivial incident are very difficult to treat successfully. They require a few widely-spaced gentle treatments. Usually at the end of the treatment the result is one of an ongoing disability.

Other low lumbar pains can arise from the zygapophyseal joints, the ligamentous, capsular and muscular tissue, and other constructional impairments (including those affecting the pain-sensitive structures in the vertebral canal).

Competitive élite sports participants who have a genetic tendency to weakness in some area of their bodily system are likely to have problems achieving a lasting good result from treatment. Their age and the cause of the signs (misuse, new use, overuse, abuse) is also an indication of their problem and its prognosis. Depending on the history of the changes over the next 18 months, the prognosis becomes clearer.

An extreme example of the variation concerns two patients who started with the same onset of low lumbar pain on the same Wednesday. By Friday one of them was symptom free, and the other had pain referred into the big toe, weakness of the extensor hallucis longus and 50 per cent loss of sensation on the dorsum of the big toe. Eighteen months later the patient with low lumbar symptoms only had not had any episodes; the other required surgery and had a good result.

> BY ACCURATE ASSESSMENT THROUGHOUT
> TREATMENT WE CAN PROVIDE THE OPPORTUNITY
> FOR CLARIFYING THE PROGNOSIS

# Chapter 6

# Examination

(with a contribution by **B. C. Edwards,** OAM, BSc(Anat), BAppSci(Physio), Grad Dip Manip Th, MMPAA FACP Hon DSc (Curtin) (Specialist Manipulative Physiotherapist))

Intelligent manipulative treatment is based on the appreciation of the history of the patient's complaint and interpretation of the examination findings. It is taken for granted that all patients having contraindications to passive mobilization treatment are excluded by the referring doctor. Nevertheless, it is the responsibility of the therapists to recognize all danger signals. In mechanical problems of spinal joints, the examination is concentrated on finding which vertebral level(s) is responsible for the symptoms, and assessing how movement of the joint has been affected.

A plan that encourages a clear and methodical examination progresses through the subjective section of the examination to the physical section, with a 'planning' stage interposed between the two. The planning stage forces the inexperienced person to relate mentally the many facts of the patient's story to the parts that will require examination. These procedures are carried out automatically by the experienced physiotherapist, but do require adherence to such a flexible plan. The inexperienced person, however, must have a

starting point to encourage clarity and a systematic approach.

> After the subjective examination, a plan of the procedures of the physical examination needs to be made before it is performed

Although throughout this book most diagrams show both the patient and the operator as males, it would complicate the descriptive text if both patient and operator were referred to as 'he'. Some readers and reviewers have commented on this discrepancy, although all of them point out that it is of minor consequence. The word 'she' is deliberately chosen in referring to the operator in an attempt to emphasize the fact that passive movement treatment techniques can be very gentle procedures and that the additional strength a male manipulator may have is not necessary for the stronger manipulative techniques. One of the writer's aims is to present the subject of manipulation as one requiring skill rather than strength.

## SUBJECTIVE EXAMINATION

The subjective examination relates to the patient's account of his complaint and its past history. Methods of questioning will vary from patient to patient because although some patients are excellent witnesses, others frequently appear unable to understand some questions or are unable to answer them simply. Skill in extracting the appropriate information requires care, patience and a critical attitude. If the technique is good, much can be gained in addition to the answers to the questions. The patient gains confidence in the physiotherapist, who in turn is able to understand the patient's plight. The influences of social and environmental factors must be appreciated, and it is necessary to remember that this colours the examiner's thinking as well as the patient's.

> If the interviewing technique is good, much can be gained in addition to the answers to the questions. The patient gains confidence in the physiotherapist, who in turn is able to understand the patient's plight

Communication is difficult and full of pitfalls. The physiotherapist may not word the question in a way that clearly expresses what she means to ask, and the words used in the question may not mean the same to the patient as they do to the therapist, or the patient may misunderstand what is being asked. He may have problems that are important to him, and incorrectly assume that the question is directed at these (*see Figure 3.2*). Hence there are all manner of difficulties to spoil what is often assumed wrongly to be a simple process of discussion.

To make it easier for the patient, only one question should be asked at a time, and it should be persisted with, within reason, until the answer is obtained. The question can be directed in different ways if it is not clearly understood by the patient, and it should be carefully worded to avoid influencing the answer. If the patient gives what seems to be an incongruous answer to the question, then the fault may lie in the way the question was put. It is kinder to rephrase or explain the question than to restate it, even if it was so simply put that the error must have been the patient's. It is essential to approach each interview with a degree of humility and charity.

> To make it easier for the patient, only one question should be asked at a time and it should be persisted with, within reason, until the answer is obtained

The subjective examination can be divided into five parts:

1. 'Kind' of disorder.
2. Site of symptoms.
3. Behaviour of symptoms.
4. Special questions.
5. History.

The specific subject matter of these, for each section of the spine, is listed in the Tables and discussed in the text given in the relevant chapters on each section of the spine; the general subject matter is given below.

From the very first question asked, regarding what the patient FEELS is his main problem, the examiner begins thinking about possible hypotheses for the disorder, limited though they may be. The subjective examination questions that follow will be related to the hypotheses and have three main areas of thought:

1. The kinds of *structures* involved.
2. Clarifying the hypothesis about the disorder.
3. The disorder's *stage*, current *stability* and *irritability* or *severity* (*Table 6.1*).

## 'KIND' OF DISORDER

### First question

The aim of the first question (Q1) (*Table 6.1*) is to determine what the patient's main problem is in his own terms. It is important that he should be given every opportunity to express his reasons for seeking treatment. For example, with the first question being:

'As far as *YOU* are concerned' ... pause ... (this pause allows him time to realize that the therapist is specifically interested in the patient's OWN OPINION) ... 'what do *YOU* feel' ... pause ... 'is *YOUR MAIN* problem?'

The therapist may choose to include in the question, 'at this stage?'. If the patient is excessively talkative, this pre-empts him and he has to limit his answer to both the present tense and to expressing his own opinion – NOBODY else's.

Wording the question in a manner to encourage spontaneous comments will indicate the patient's priorities in relation to why he is seeking treatment. 'Is there anything it prevents you from doing?' is a useful

Table 6.1  Stages of generating and testing hypotheses during the procedure of the subjective examination

| Hypothesizing conjecturing | | Kinds of structures involved |
|---|---|---|
| IS IT A: | C/O SUBJECTIVE EXAMINATION (interrogation with empathy) | |
| Typical pattern? | OBSERVATION/INTRODUCTION/CLIN. CLUES (asterisk* as you go along) | intraarticular → capsular (inner); inflammatory → disease, trauma; surface apposition |
| Recognisable syndrome? | | |
| Trauma situation? | THE 'PERSON' Q1 | periarticular → ligamentous, tendinous, capsular |
| Recognisable pathology? | KIND OF DISORDER (e.g. trauma, #, chronic gradual) | |
| ATYPICAL? | Follow-up Qs (clarifying & hypothesising) | neural → extraneural, perineural, intraneural, entrapment, supportive elements |
| DO FEATURES FIT? | Symptoms behaviour (demo) HISTORY, Irritability | |
| Has it more than one component? | AIMED Qs (prove/disprove) | |
| | Special Qs, Routine Qs, Danger Qs | discogenic → intradiscal, herniating, herniated, spondylolisthesis |
| | STAGE of DISORDER STABILITY of DISORDER NOW IRRITABILITY of DISORDER | |
| | 'DISORDER' (Physical Diagnosis) | muscular → primary or secondary, weakness or imbalance, tightness or inhibition |
| | THEIR demonstration movements OUR DIFFERENTIATION OF THOSE MOVEMENTS | |
| | Thoughts on treatment PLAN and prognosis | |

early question. If the answer is 'Yes', the following bracket of questions will need to be asked:

'*What* does it prevent?'

'*What prevents* it?'

'Do you have any *reaction* from having tried to do it?'

When a patient does not put an emphasis on pain as his *main* problem and clearly indicates that it is his activities that are restricted, the next question is: 'Do you get much in the way of pain or discomfort?'.

There are many 'kinds of disorder' (*see* below), but the reply to the initial question is most commonly 'I get a pain across here', indicating the area. When this is the reply, it is usually best to clarify the area of the symptoms before asking questions about the history of the disorder.

Establish the 'kind' of disorder: why has the patient sought treatment or been referred for treatment? It will only be necessary to use direct or leading questions to establish the 'kind' of disorder if it is not revealed spontaneously during the initial open-ended questions.

In answer to the first question, the patient may respond with the following 'kind' of disorders:

1. Pain.
2. Stiffness.
3. Giving way.
4. Instability.
5. Weakness.
6. Loss of function.
7. Post-trauma:
   a) Surgery.
   b) Manipulation under anaesthesia.
   c) Hospitalized traction.

The pattern of thinking during the subjective examination (*Table 6.1*) depicts the questioning as an interrogation, but it differs from that held in a court of law because it is an **interrogation with empathy**. Being an 'interrogation' indicates the depth of questioning required to gain the detailed information related to both forming an hypothesis and knowing the kind of structures involved. 'With empathy' indicates the depth of questioning required to understand how the disorder feels to the patient in his terms.

> The subjective examination is an 'interrogation with empathy'. It indicates the depth of questioning and enables the therapist to get an impression of the patient's personal experience's of their disorder and the impact it has on their life

Committing the essence of the subjective examination to paper is a valuable learning experience in itself. It forces one to identify the things that are essential, and record them, and leave out the less valuable information given by the patient.

> Systematic recording of the information obtained is a valuable learning experience, as it helps to identify the essential elements, for further examination and treatment

The therapist should reassure the patient by saying, 'Don't feel that some things are too silly to mention. Your body can tell you things about its reaction to the disorder that I can't find out unless you tell me. You can't tell me too much, but you can tell me too little. Let me be the judge of what I need to know and what I don't'.

The relevance of using asterisks (*) or highlighting may be appropriately introduced here, as they form an important component of the written record of both the subjective and physical examinations. The asterisks serve two functions. First, they identify the points to which the therapist can refer back when making assessments for changes to the patient's symptoms and the clinical findings. This speeds up the assessment process and also makes it more precise. Secondly, it is a good teaching process, keeping the therapist 'on her toes', so to speak, to latch onto highly informative and significant words, phrases or functions that arise in the subjective examination. Similarly, it teaches the therapist the significant features during the physical examination. It is important that the asterisks be used at the instant of recording the feature, not on completion of the examination as a retrospective exercise. This is why *Table 6.1* states 'asterisk as you go along'.

> Using asterisks in the recording of information is essential. This serves two functions:
>
> - It identifies those points which can be used in the re-assessment of the patient's progress
> - It serves as a teaching process, to latch onto informative and significant words

It is important that the asterisk be used at the instant of recording the information, not on completion of the examination as a retrospective exercise. This is what is meant by 'asterisk as you go along'.

## Making features fit

As can be seen in *Table 6.1*, questions need to be asked to assess if the features of the history fit with the behaviour of the symptoms; and also to assess whether the behaviour of the symptoms fits with a recognizable syndrome or pathology.

> Making features fit:
> - Do the features of the history fit with the current behaviour of the symptoms?
> - Does the behaviour of the symptoms fit with a recognizable syndrome or pathology?

## Stage, stability and irritability of the disorder

From the moment of first seeing the patient, the therapist takes note of any nuances that may give the first clues as to what the patient is suffering from, anything that may help in knowing the patient's characteristics, etc. The second part of the meeting relates to anything in the introductory remarks and settling the patient in comfort and easing his mental state before the consultation begins. During this phase the therapist may notice some clinical clues to assist her to make judgements during the consultation.

'Asterisk as you go along' has been discussed (above), and is really a way of saying that the examiner should be able to pick up major issues to be used for assessment of changes of treatment and for highlighting key issues from the patient's or examiner's point of view; they must not be left until the end of the consultation.

> 'Asterisk as you go along' is an essential element of hypothesis generation, and it should not be left until the end of the consultation

Questions oriented to the history of the disorder should be asked so as to determine the **source** and the **stage** of the disorder (especially if information gained relates to the recognizable pathology development). When the stage of the disorder has been established, the current stability of the disorder should be determined. If there are wide variations in the severity of the symptoms, or if the site of the symptoms varies widely from one day to the next, this will indicate that the disorder is considered to be unstable, and therefore the physical examination will need to be modified to avoid exacerbation.

> Goals of questions relevant to the history of the disorder:
> - What may be the source of the disorder?
> - What is the stage of the disorder?
> - What is the stability of the disorder?
>
> If a disorder is considered 'unstable', then the physical examination has to be modified to avoid exacerbation

If the behaviour of the symptoms, when related to activities, indicates that exacerbations are both easily provoked and take a long time to subside, the **irritability** of the disorder is high. This indicates that the physical examination of test movements should only be taken to the point of onset of symptoms. Nevertheless, it may be wise to take the movement minimally beyond that point to know whether the further movement either heightens the severity of the symptoms or extends the spread of the symptoms.

The test movements also need to be taken only until the onset of symptoms if the activity that provokes the symptoms has to be interrupted because of the intensity of the pain. The disorder is not necessarily highly irritable if the symptoms subside immediately, but may still be sufficiently severe to require caution with test movements.

> If the patient's symptoms are considered irritable or severe, the physical examination or test movements should only be taken to the point of onset of the symptoms

## Hypotheses regarding structures involved

The right-hand side of *Table 6.1* lists the kinds of structures the examiner would have in mind.

Further the examiner should consider the ways in which the structures have been used and the different injuries which may have consequently occurred (*Table 6.2*).

Added to this list are many other elements (e.g. muscular, postural, biomechanical, ergonomic, positional, etc.). They are omitted from the present discussion, as they are considered to be mainly secondary or predisposing situations to the structures from which the symptoms are arising (*see* Part D of *Table 6.3*). Consideration must also be given to the structures that are the source (or the cause of the source) of the

**Table 6.2**  Types of 'use of structures' and the different injuries caused

| Method of injury | Type of injury |
| --- | --- |
| Misuse | Stress |
| New use | Strain |
| Overuse | Sprain |
| Abuse | |
| Disuse | |

**Table 6.3**    Planning the physical examination

There are two thinking processes on examination. The first is seeking the *source* of the disorder, and the second is the *cause* of the *source* (contributing factors).

*PART ONE*

**A.    The *SOURCE*(s) of the symptoms**

1.    Name as the *possible* sources of *any part* of the patient's symptoms that *must* be examined.
       Joints underlying symptomatic area(s)    Joints that refer into the symptomatic area(s)
       Neural/supportive elements that refer into the symptomatic area(s)    Muscles underlying symptomatic area(s)

2.    List joints above and below the lesion that should be checked (when appropriate):
       ..............................................................................................................................................................................

3.    Are there any special tests indicated?
       a.    Neurological examination ........................................................................................................................................
       b.    Other – specify ......................................................................................................................................................

**B.    Influence of symptoms and pathology on examination and first treatment**

1.    Is the pain severe? (*Yes/No*) or latent? (*Yes/No*)
       *Give the example on which the answers are based.*
       a.    *Local symptoms*
             i.     Repeated MOVEMENT causing pain – or go just beyond P1 .............................................................................
             ii.    Severity of pain so caused ...................................................................................................................................
             iii.   Duration before pain subsides .............................................................................................................................
       b.    *Referred/other symptoms*
             i.     Repeated MOVEMENT causing pain – or go just beyond referral of pain ......................................................
             ii.    Severity of pain so caused ...................................................................................................................................
             iii.   Duration before pain subsides .............................................................................................................................

2.    Does the nature of the disorder indicate caution? (*Yes/No*)
             i.     Pathology/injury – specify ...................................................................................................................................
             ii.    Easy to provoke exacerbation or acute episode ...............................................................................................

3.    Are there any contraindications? (*Yes/No*) Specify ......................................................................................................

**C.    The kind of examination (anticipation of findings)**

1.    Do you think you will need to be gentle or moderately firm with your examination of the movements?
2.    Do you expect a comparable sign to be easy or to be hard to find? Why?
3.    Which specific test procedures do you want to perform?
4.    When do you plan reassessment procedures?

*PART TWO*

**D.    The CAUSE of the SOURCE of the symptoms: Associated examination**

1.    Provocative neuro/musculo/skeletal/medical factors leading to the cause of the symptoms.
       What associated factors must be examined:
       a.    As reasons why the joint, muscle or other structure have become symptomatic and/or
       b.    Why the joint or muscle disorder may recur? (e.g. posture, muscle imbalance, muscle power, obesity, stiffness,
             hypermobility, instability, deformity in proximal or distal joint, etc.) ...............................................................

2.    The effect of the disorder on joint stability ...................................................................................................................

**E.    Treatment**

1.    Which short-term or long-term goals of treatment are pursued?
2.    Do you expect to be treating pain, resistance, weakness or instability?
3.    Are there any precautions or contraindications which need to be respected?
4.    In planning the TREATMENT (after the examination), what advice should be included to prevent or lessen recurrences?

Adapted from *Neuromusculoskeletal Examination and Recording Guide* (1998), with kind permission of Lauderdale Press, Adelaide.

symptoms – periarticular, intra-articular, neural and discogenic.

## Periarticular structures

These include the ligament, outer capsule and tendon.

Ligament disorders of relatively recent origin can be expected to be painful on stretching or squeezing them. They would be expected, therefore, to restrict the patient's functional movements, although on stopping the movement and thus releasing the stretch or squeeze the symptoms could be expected to cease. Also it should be possible to place the ligament in a position where it is painless. The history of the disorder would be expected to include sprains, strains or minor trauma, but abuse superimposed on fatigue or other predisposing circumstances may be the cause.

Ligamentous disorders of very recent origin (less than a week) would be expected to cause stronger symptoms, and would restrict functional activities greatly. There would also be other components contributing to the symptoms (e.g. inflammation, oedema). On the other hand, chronic ligamentous disorders will be painful on stretching and squeezing, but will withstand more tension than those of more recent origin. Finding painless positions for these structures is relatively easy: the more recent the onset of symptoms, the more the symptoms will be localized to the injured ligament; the more chronic the disorder, the greater the possibility of there being a degree of referred symptoms. With this thought in mind, it is necessary to state that it is not rare for a chronic ligamentous disorder to be the source of referred symptoms without there being any symptoms at the site of the ligament's disorder.

The outer layers of synovial joint capsules behave in much the same manner as described above. Tendons can be symptomatic and behave in much the same way as ligaments, but with one difference. If the disorder is at the tenomuscular or tenoperiosteal junctions, and there is no inflammatory component in the disorder, the stretch or squeeze situation will be the same as with ligaments. The differentiating test between tendon and ligament will be that an isometric tension applied through the tendon will be painful, compared with being painless for ligaments.

## Intra-articular

Most intra-articular capsular disorders have a different quality to their symptoms to that of periarticular structures. They are more constant than the end-of-range ligament disorders, and are usually more debilitating. Painless resting positions either do not exist, or the patient is only free of symptoms for an hour or so. A change of position is then needed, or a period of comforting movement is required. There are positions of resting which are more comfortable than others. The site of pain is always deep seated, and the patient is not able to actually touch it; however, if the therapist rocks the joint back and forth, the patient is able to identify it as the site. The disorder usually has a degree of inflammation, although this is not to say that it has a disease as its origin.

If the disorder is chronic, it is common for a movement in one direction to be freer than its opposite, and a movement in one direction can produce a sharp pain whilst a movement in the opposite direction, though hurtful, does not produce such a sharp pain or prevent further movement. However, none of the joint's movements are totally free of pain. Performing small range oscillatory movements (whether accessory or physiological) in a neutral mid-position will create an ache within the joint. If the movement is continued, the ache will increase proportionally to the duration of the oscillatory movements. The more severe the pain, the more restricted the movements. The history of the onset is gradual, and the patient is not aware of the cause.

Sustaining a squeezing of the joint surfaces together usually builds up an increase of symptoms; but only if there is a joint surface component to the disorder. However, if the disorder is chronic, both the duration and the strength of the compacting need to be increased. This differentiation test may need the addition of a tiny cardinal movement, or the comparison of pain provoked by the cardinal movement during sustained squeezing compared with the squeezing released (in part or wholly), to provide the answer. Symptoms (pain/discomfort) can be expected to be a 'through-range' probability. Anti-inflammatory medication can be expected to reduce the level of symptoms when the inflammatory component is an even more active disease process. This is not so if the inflammation is present only as a response to a mechanical process.

Inflammation can basically be one of two types. The first is as a result of previous injury (many years previously), which will have led to radiologically evident osteoarthritic changes. There can be long painless periods, unlike in active osteoarthritic disease or other forms of arthritis such as psoriatic or rheumatoid arthritis; these are rarely free of discomfort. The mechanical group of patients will have constant pain or discomfort, which has both a pain-through-range presentation as well as an end-of-range pain that provokes a marked increase in the intensity of the symptoms. It is this latter aspect that is the dominant clinical evidence differentiating it from the inflammation because of disease; the latter has a more gradual increase in intensity of pain as the joint is moved through its range. There is another differentiating aspect to this pain response to movement: the more active the pathology, the longer the exacerbation lasts following cessation of movement. There is an 'in between' classification of inflammation that occasionally confronts the clinician, known as 'subclinical arthritis'. The presentation is one of constant aching at the site of the joint involved, which increases in intensity with activity. The physical examination reveals through-range pain, yet there are positions where the symptoms subside considerably. None of the medical tests, such as blood tests or radiography, reveal the activity of disease or pathological changes. The response to passive movement treatment as outlined in this text is not the same as is the case with the mechanical variety of inflammation (or arthritis). Passive movement has no role to play other than to identify the situation as subclinical.

## Neural

One significant statement that can be made about neural symptoms is that they are different from musculoskeletal symptoms. The symptoms from routine uncomplicated musculoskeletal disorders are readily recognizable as such, and 'pain' or 'ache' are the predominant symptoms. Neural disorders, on the other hand, although they do have pain as a presenting factor, also have what are commonly considered to be bizarre or weird symptoms, and the patients frequently have difficulty describing them. When the neural system causes pain, it is almost certain to include some other symptoms of the bizarre variety – rarely, if ever, does it present as pain alone. Patients commonly wonder if they are being neurotic or hysterical, or if the problem is all in the mind. Even the pain can have a weird quality about it and is not like the usual pain most people talk about; it is ill defined in its area and often affects a whole hand, arm or leg. Other symptoms are whole-limb involvement, heaviness, a distal area of coldness, mental confusion and blurred vision. Frequently a patient will complain that all the symptoms are always on one side of the body.

Three extremely useful texts regarding this group of unusual complaints are those by Breig (1978), Grieve (1981) and Butler (1991), and further reading of the latter two texts is strongly recommended.

The responses to treatment of neural disorders by passive movement are often different from the responses of 'joint' disorders when the neural disorder is primary rather than secondary. When the joint structures are at fault and are irritating the neural structures, if the joint component can be cleared, the secondary neural irritation will improve in parallel with the primary joint component. However, should the source be nerve entrapment, it is often difficult to alter the entrapment by conservative management.

When intraneural disorders are caused by trauma, such as in a motor vehicle rear-end collision, they do respond to passive movement treatment, although the time taken to reach a satisfactory stage is markedly longer than when the 'joint' is causing an irritative state. The repetitive strain situation is much the same when it is a major contributor to the symptoms.

At this stage of our clinical and theoretical knowledge, it is probably advisable to think of the pain-sensitive structures in the vertebral canal, in particular the dura, as a subsection of the neural phenomena. Although many of the physical examination tests are the same for both, the structure and function of the dura are different. It is a very tough, strong, ligamentous-like tissue, and when the dura itself is the source of symptoms, it is a very difficult structure to restore to its full range of painless passive movement. However, it is far more common for it to be involved in a patient's symptoms on a secondary basis; that is, some *other* fault in the intersegmental movement results in irritation of the dura and causes it to contribute. Under these circumstances, restoring the intersegmental symptomatic state to normal will effect an elimination of the dural symptoms without having to treat the dura directly.

Referred pain from the dura is well documented as being non-segmental (Butler, 1991; Cyriax and Cyriax, 1993), and its physical examination (the 'slump' test) readily implicates its involvement.

## Discogenic

Discogenic disorders are less commonly the source of symptoms than was thought to be the case 15–20 years ago. However, they are still relatively common in the L4/5, L5/S1 and C5/6, C6/7 discs, with the lumbar discs being more prone to progress to the herniated (prolapsed) stage than the cervical discs.

Intradiscal disorders within an intact outer annulus in the lower two lumbar levels can usually be readily recognized by the history of the onset of the symptoms and by the behaviour of the symptoms. The history is usually one of lifting in a position of flexion plus rotation. The patient usually feels something happen in the lower back, but the pain need not be severe at that time. However, later the lower back may be uncomfortable and ache, and movements may be restricted by pain. It is quite common for the patient not to notice anything significant until the following morning when he first gets out of bed (or is unable to do so). Pain is considerable, but it is always felt in an area rather than a localized spot. The area is usually across the lower back, and it may be more painful on one side than the other. This may indicate that the disorder of the disc internally is more towards that side of the disc; if the damage is central, the area of pain will be felt more centrally. The site of the disc disorder may be in the nucleus or the inner annulus, or in both.

Certainly, if the current history is the third episode, both the nucleus and the annulus may be involved. It is not until the outer annulus is involved, resulting in a bulge of the disc, that there is any referral of symptoms to the gluteal area ('the weakened outer annulus' in *Table 6.1*). It is not until the symptoms extend into the thigh that the weakened outer annulus can be considered to be in a stage of progressing towards herniating. *Herniated*, *prolapsed* and *sequestrian* are the stages when the area of pain is likely to be radicular and include neurological changes.

The behavioural indicators of the intradiscal disorder will include one, some or all of the following:

1. Back pain when coughing and/or sneezing.
2. Difficulty in rising out of a slumped sitting position, and in being able to stand erect (or, if it is bad enough, the inability to stand straight at all).
3. Difficulty in getting out of bed in the mornings.
4. The inability to flex far enough to put on socks or stockings.
5. Difficulty in bending over the hand-basin to clean teeth, etc.
6. In order to sleep, the patient may need to lie supine with pillows under the knees to allow the lumbar spine to lower to a slightly flexed position or, when symptoms have a one-sided dominance, he may choose to lie on one side (usually the least painful side) with the top hip and knee flexed, or even in a foetal position.
7. A dislike of standing, or the half-flexed position adopted at the kitchen sink.
8. Evidence of a lumbar kyphosis in the standing position, or a list to one side (sciatic scoliosis; Maitland, 1961) on observation from behind. The list will often be contralateral in the case of an intradiscal disorder.

An *after effect* is quite common, and if present is indicative of a disc disorder. The 'after effect' means that, having performed activities in an unfavourable manner, the patient may not be aware of its having any effect, BUT will know all about it by the following morning.

In the cervical spine, the progress is not the same as described above for the lumbar spine. In fact, the cervical intervertebral discs are quite different to those in the lumbar spine (Twomey, 1992). A 'list' is not uncommon for the herniated intervertebral disc, but lists are nearly always contralateral.

The cervical intradiscal disorder may be more common than is generally thought, because the symptomatology seems to fit with Cloward's work (Cloward, 1959, 1960), especially with pain felt in the scapular area (*see Figures 6.1 and 6.2*). There is almost always muscle weakness of the triceps with C7 nerve root involvement (C6/7 disc), which is more common than C6 nerve root involvement (C5/6 disc). Recent investigations (Twomey and Taylor, 1992) show that the cervical discs are significantly damaged in whiplash injuries.

This section is an over-simplification, and is intended only as a guide for the more common presentations. The reader is referred to Bogduk (1987) for further details.

### Clarifying the hypotheses

This section follows the 'first question' in much the same way as does the section concerning structures

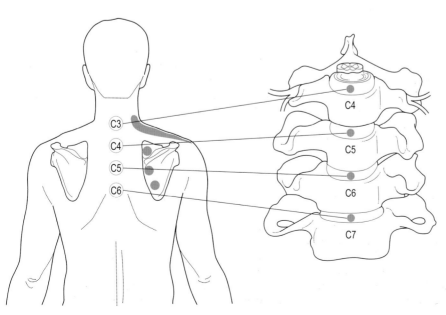

**Figure 6.1**  Discogenic pain, referred from anterior surface of lower cervical disc (Reproduced from Cloward, R. B. (1959) *Annals of Surgery*, **150**, 1052–64, with kind permission of author and publishers.)

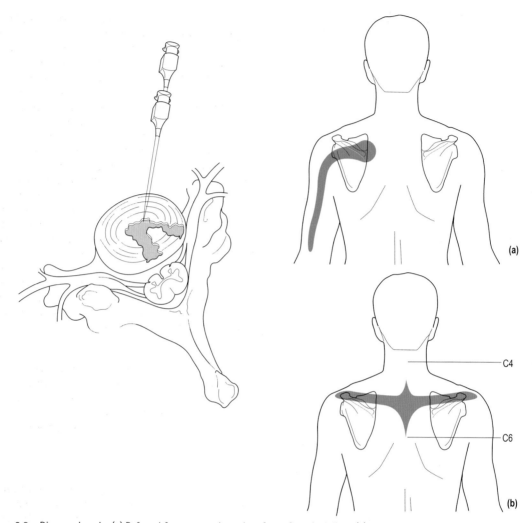

**Figure 6.2** Discogenic pain. (*a*) Referred from posterolateral surface of cervical discs. (*b*) Referred from central disc ruptures (Reproduced from Cloward, R. B. (1959) *Annals of Surgery*, **150**, 1052–64, with kind permission of author and publishers.)

involved. Here, use is made of experience gained from listening to the stories of other patients (*Table 6.4*).

The patient's disorders can be categorized into two groups:

1. Those whose symptoms have developed gradually without any significant trauma that they can recall.
2. Those whose symptoms have onset following trauma, whether a heavy fall, a motor vehicle accident or any other kind of severe injury, or surgery.

The first category of disorders, those of gradual onset, usually fit into a recognizable group of symptoms and examination findings. The patients may have a history which includes 'predisposing factors',

such as a familial (genetic propensity) background or an injury some years previously. It may therefore be that there is a pattern to the behaviour of the symptoms that the clinician recognizes. She is then in a position to direct her questions to certain other aspects of the behaviour of the symptoms not yet revealed. With this she can then confirm or deny the pattern.

> The clinician may recognize a pattern in the examination findings, which may be of help in determining the best treatment strategies. However, the examiner's mind needs to be sufficiently flexible to ask other questions that may fit any other typical patterns

**Table 6.4** Clarifying the hypotheses

| Hypothesizing conjecturing |
| --- |
| IS IT A: |
|     Recognizable pathology? |
|     Typical pattern? |
|     or |
|     Atypical pattern? |
|     Trauma situation? |
|     (Strain/sprain) |
|     DO FEATURES FIT? |
|     DO THEY MAKE SENSE? |
| IS IT: overuse? |
|     misuse? |
|     new use? |
|     abuse? |
|     disuse? |
| Has it more than one component? |

The 'recognizable pathology' referred to in *Table 6.4* is much the same as the 'typical pattern', except that its interpretation is wider in that it covers more than just the behaviour of the symptoms and examination findings. For example, it includes such things as the age of the patient, the history of the disorder, radiological anomalies, general health, etc. An example could be diagnosing ankylosing spondylosis in its early stages. 'Recognizable pathology' takes the questioning aspect further still, and demands knowledge of pathology and related clinical presentation. An example here would be the intervertebral discogenic disorders, which progress through the stages from low back pain at the beginning, to radicular pain with neurological signs and changes later. With this as an example, it is easy to see the importance of questions related directly to the 'stage of the disorder', plus the 'stability of the disorder' at the time when the patient is referred for treatment. If the symptoms and signs vary from one day to another, then it can be assumed that the disorder itself is varying, indicating that there is something unstable about it. Under such circumstances the treatment must be gentle, and the assessment skills must be of the very highest order during a treatment session and at each following session.

The 'trauma situation' is totally different, and must always be considered as having more than one component causing the presenting symptoms. It will therefore not present as a 'recognizable syndrome', and there will not be a 'typical pattern' to its presentation. However, it need not be classed as 'atypical'. The reasoning behind this statement is that even if the trauma renders the presentation being not fully compatible with the 'typical pattern' group, the 'recognizable syndrome' group or the 'pathology' groups, there may well be recognizable parts of the history, symptoms and signs. The therapist has to be alert, flexible and open-minded in her recognition of these possibilities, and extremely skilled in searching through her knowledge and experience as a 'critical-of-self' clinician to sort this out. The skill of 'making features fit' is important to this sorting out process. It may well take more than two or three sessions to enable the clinician to see where the features fit, just as it will take more than three or four sessions for the patient to understand what the clinician is endeavouring to find out and thence to contribute to the exercise.

> Problems that are traumatic in onset usually have more than one component involved and therefore it will be much more difficult to recognize patterns of clinical presentation. The skill of 'making features fit' is important to the process of sorting out different hypotheses

A patient's disorder may be totally 'atypical', and he may be referred to the therapist with the request to sort out any details that will help in making a differential diagnosis. This is making the best use of a manipulative physiotherapist at her highest level. The skills required in meeting this challenge are covered by all of the factors discussed above, in conjunction with two other elements:

1. The patient needs to understand his role in the management of his problem. This includes recording every change in the symptoms in a comparative way, plus what he feels may have contributed to the information in fine detail ('half of 1 per cent of zero'), and even including items that he might feel are irrelevant, thus leaving the therapist to be the judge. This is just as it should be.

2. The therapist must have good communication and assessment skills; she must also be very particular about details, open-minded, and honest in her own self-criticisms. She must base what she does in the techniques on sound reasons, and must prove their use in detail.

*The first question* regards the person. We remember and may even make written records of anything to be considered during the consultation that is going to be helpful for the patient. We recognize him as being a human being, a person who happens to have something wrong with him. The 'Q1' is discussed on page 98, starting with 'As far as YOU are concerned' … pause … etc.

*Follow-up Qs* (clarifying and hypothesizing) are of two kinds:

1. Those that are needed to achieve the amount of in-depth information required to answer the purpose of the question.
2. Those that may lead the examiner along a new path that is worth following while it is meaningfully in the patient's mind.

*History* is introduced at this stage, but can be determined at any stage (this is controlled mainly by the patient's line of thought). The subject is dealt with on pages 118–122.

*Behaviour* of symptoms is usually introduced early in the subjective examination, because the answer to Q1 makes it appropriate. The same applies to 'a demonstration', which may be spontaneously introduced by the patient as he explains his 'main problem'. If this does not happen, the procedure is to say to him 'Is there anything you can do, or any position you can put yourself into, that will bring on your symptoms?', or 'Can you do something here and now which will bring on your pain? (*assuming, of course, that pain is part of his main problem*).

*Aimed Qs* help to prove or disprove the hypothesis. Most of the time, questioning will be paralleling the person's line of thought. During this time, the examiner will be gaining information regarding the structures likely to be at fault and forming a hypothesis. However, the time comes when specific questions need to be asked that are directed at confirming the hypothesis (or proving the hypothesis wrong) and fitting with the structures thought to be causing factors.

## SITE OF SYMPTOMS

The first step is to clarify the area, depth, nature, behaviour and chronology of the symptoms, and to record them on a 'body chart'. Areas of sensory disturbance should also be included, as should brief comments regarding areas of maximum intensity and type of pain (*Figure 6.3*). Reference to such a body chart provides a quick and clear reminder of this patient's symptoms.

> The area, depth, nature, behaviour and chronology of symptoms, as well as the relationships between symptom areas, should be recorded on a 'body chart'

The area and depth of referred pain may sometimes be related to dermatomes, myotomes and sclerotomes, and areas of paraesthesia or anaesthesia can indicate a particular nerve-root involvement. Further information regarding referred pain is given on pages 188–189.

The patterns of pain distribution do not provide the answers as to the precise structure at fault, and nor is there total agreement on what kind or distribution of pain is produced by each pain-sensitive structure. There are also discrepancies between the academic findings on research on normal structures, and patients' descriptions of their symptoms. It is fair to say that no patients present with symptoms that can be identified as arising from a single structure; the symptoms always arise from a mixture of sources in combination. Realizing this to be so, the site and behaviour of symptoms can provide an indication as to the groups of pain-sensitive structures that are likely to be involved; and the physical examination can provide answers regarding the extent of the involvement. It is important to determine, in the lumbar and cervical spines (especially the lower segments of each), whether there is involvement of the pain-sensitive aspects of the intervertebral discs or the nerve-root sleeves. It is essential for the clinician to have in her personal library the books by Bogduk and Twomey (1991) and Twomey and Taylor (1994). Manipulative therapists (medical, paramedical or lay) cannot diagnose the source of pain by manual examination, but it is possible to have a good idea as to the intervertebral level of pain sensitive structures involved.

## Dermatomes

There are three kinds of dermatome charts:

1. Theoretical (embryological) representation, as can be seen in many anatomical texts (*Figure 6.4*).
2. Areas of pain when the nerve root is implicated in causing the pain (*Figure 6.5*).
3. The areas of referred pain found in most patients when they present with nerve-root involvement. Under these common circumstances, other pain-sensitive structures are involved in the pain mechanism (such as the nerve-root sleeve, dura and the posterior fibres of annulus fibrosis). These distributions are presented in *Figure 6.6*.

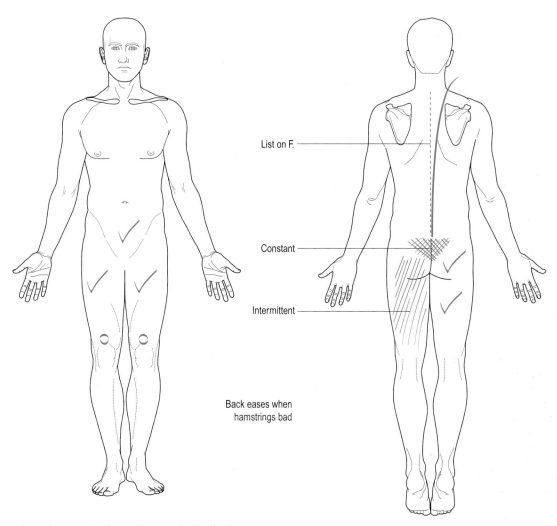

List on F.

Constant

Intermittent

Back eases when
hamstrings bad

**Figure 6.3**    An example of recording examination findings

The distribution of 'neural' symptoms or symptoms indicating altered neurodynamics is usually not dermatomal. These are not like point 3 above, and are discussed on pages 113–114.

Two nerve roots may be involved in musculoskeletal disorders of the lumbar spine. However, the possibilities of two adjacent posterolateral disc prolapses, or of two nerve-root anomalies, renders such a finding unlikely in musculoskeletal disorders of the cervical spine. When attempting to determine which intervertebral segment is involved when neurological changes can be attributed to a particular nerve root, the possibility of a prefixed or a postfixed plexus must be taken into account; it must also be remembered that, for example, the fifth lumbar nerve root may be implicated

by a disc prolapse at either the L4/5 or L5/S1 intervertebral spaces.

Some authors describe all deeply felt pain according to sclerotomes. However, patients are able to differentiate between pain felt deeply in the muscles and related tissues, and pain felt deeply in the bones, joints and ligaments.

## Myotomes

Many patients who have referred pain are unable to define the margins of their symptoms because they are deep and vague. Nevertheless, they are able to differentiate between superficial pain and deeper pain. Myotome charts, as used in this context, refer

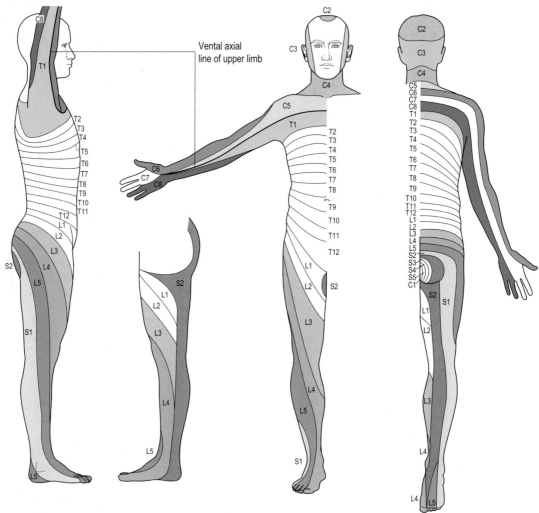

**Figure 6.4** Dermatome chart based on embryological segments

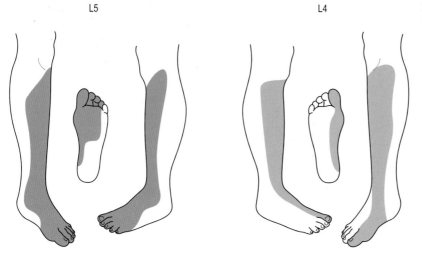

**Figure 6.5** Dermatome chart based on nerve root distribution

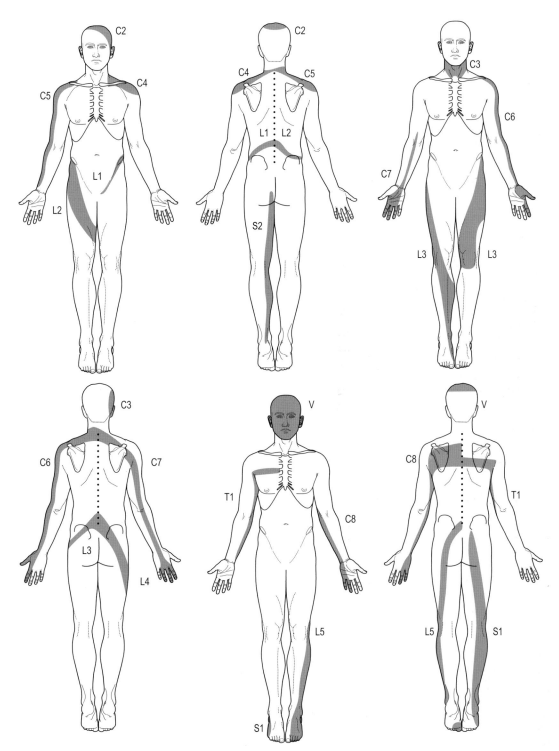

Figure 6.6   Dermatome chart based on areas of referred pain

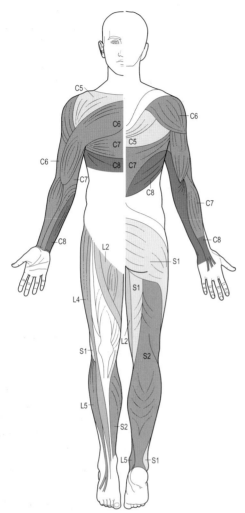

**Figure 6.7**  Myotome chart

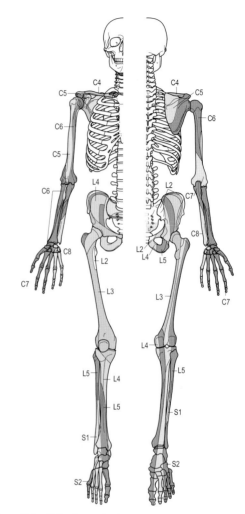

**Figure 6.8**  Sclerotome chart

to areas of pain (Paintal, 1960), not motor supply (*Figure 6.7*).

## Sclerotomes

A distinction should be recognized between two clinical presentations of pain felt deeply 'in the bone'; one is deep pain associated with the shaft of the bone, and the other is deep pain associated with peripheral joints (*Figure 6.8*).

## Cloward areas

Cloward, in the years since 1958, has contributed significantly to the recognition of specific areas of referred pain (Cloward, 1958, 1959, 1960). The significance of these areas lies in the fact that they complement the history of onset of many patients' symptoms,

thus indicating a possible diagnosis of discogenic disorder, even to the extent of indicating the stage of progression of the disorder. The two most commonly found areas of symptoms are shown in *Figure 6.9*. The symptoms usually have a vague distribution, and are felt as a deep gnawing ache or pain. There are variations of these two areas, and *Figure 6.10* provides a useful guide to the possible variations.

## Thoracic pains

Pain felt in the thoracic area is worthy of a body chart of its own, because it can occupy other areas than local spinal pain and referred nerve root pain. Of particular note in the posterior thoracic area are the sensory changes that can relate to the posterior primary ramus. They are always near the vertebral column. Nerve root pain spreads downwards from the spine in line with

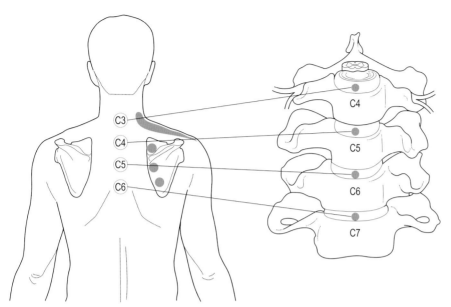

**Figure 6.9** Discogenic pain, referred from anterior surface of lower cervical disc (Reproduced from Cloward, R. B. (1959) *Annals of Surgery*, **150**, 1052–64, with kind permission of author and publishers.)

the ribs as it refers around the rib cage. Pain of spinal origin may spread horizontally across the back, and it may be felt to pass from the back *through* to the chest, in which case it *may* have an intradiscal origin. A further presentation is where an area or patch of pain may be felt anteriorly without any back pain (*Figure 6.11*). It should also be remembered that lower abdominal pain can be of two kinds; that arising from the low lumbar spine, and the groin pain referred from an L1 nerve-root disorder (*Figure 6.12*).

*Very few practitioners seem to realize the enormous importance which should be attached to establishing the precise site of the patient's symptoms.* Precision provides an invaluable foundation for the remainder of the examination:

1. The examiner must watch how the patient indicates the area of pain, and then she must use her own finger or hand to take over from his so as to identify the area exactly.

2. If a patient indicates an area across his back, the examiner should ask, 'Is it a line across your back, or an area across it?'. If the patient uses his hand or finger to demonstrate the area, he is in fact answering the question non-verbally – the use of hand indicating an area, and the finger indicating a line.

3. The matching of non-verbal messages both with verbal responses and with touching the area strengthens the exactness of the information.

4. One patient may be able to point to one precise spot of pain and another may use his whole hand, while yet another may only be able to indicate a large, vague area. Being able to point to a spot usually means that this is the exact site of the cause of the pain (however, see point 5 below).

5. The question should be asked, 'Are you able to touch the spot or is it deeper inside than that?'. The answer can differentiate between a deep myotome and a deep sclerotome. The large, vague areas indicate disorders of other structures (*see* p. 188).

6. Pain felt in the low lumbar spine may have its origin in the upper lumbar spine.

7. Patients can have musculoskeletal low abdominal pain arising from a low lumbar discogenic disorder rather than from a low thoracic nerve-root disorder.

> It is essential to establish the precise site of the patient's symptoms, as this influences the generation of multiple hypotheses and will be of paramount influence on the remainder of the examination

The many patterns of pain that are recognizable indicate not only the probable structure at fault, but also the intervertebral level that is at fault. Precision provides an invaluable foundation for the remainder of the examination.

Further reading of the texts of Cyriax and Cyriax (1993), Butler (1991) and Grieve (1988) will widen the clinician's mind to take in referred symptoms from entrapment neuropathies, peripheral joints, neural disorders, the autonomic nervous system and other sources.

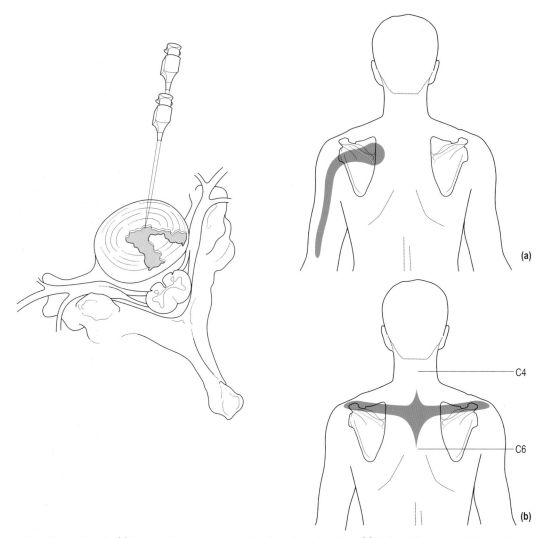

**Figure 6.10** Discogenic pain. (*a*) Referred from posterolateral surface of cervical discs. (*b*) Referred from central disc ruptures (Reproduced from Cloward, R. B. (1959) *Annals of Surgery*, **150**, 1052–64, with kind permission of author and publishers.)

There are many other areas and kinds of symptoms (not pain) that provide information as to their source. For example, patients may speak of numbness, yet on further questioning, it is a 'feeling of numbness' rather than an actual diminution of sensation. Under these circumstances, the area of that so-called numbness does not fit the pattern of a nerve root compressive loss of sensation; nor does it fit a pattern of peripheral nerve entrapment. A patient may comment that his whole arm feels heavy or cold, or there may be an area of hypersensitivity to light touch. All of these can have a spinal or neural source. The important things are to:

1. Listen to what the person says.
2. Believe him.
3. Record the information being provided.

4. Differentiate between the possible sources of the bizarre symptoms.
5. Know all there is to know about the neural and musculoskeletal anatomy, and the changes (not necessarily pathological changes) that cause symptoms.

David Butler has specialized within the field of musculoskeletal disorders to the extent that clinicians now have the opportunity to understand other sources of some of the previously unclear symptoms. We will have heard and believed them, noted and asterisked the appropriate places in recording them, and even recognized them within syndromes. The area considered must now include the nervous system, both in the title now being changed to 'the neuromusculoskeletal

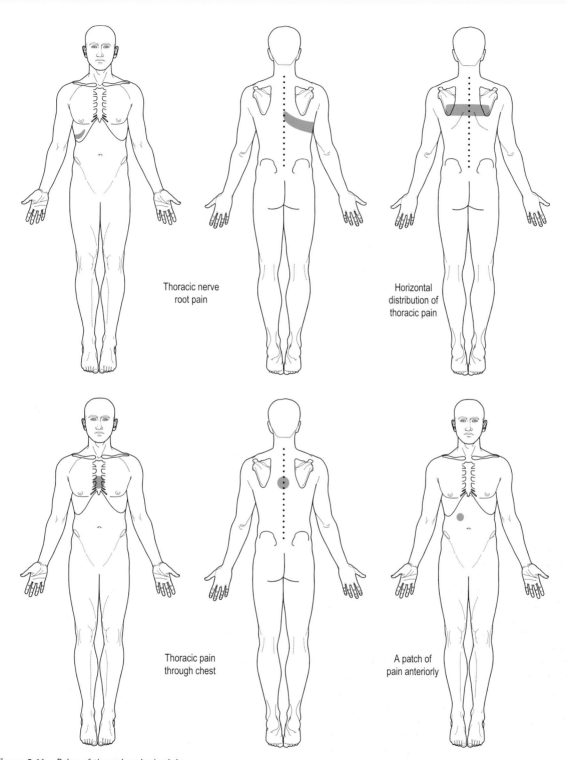

Thoracic nerve
root pain

Horizontal
distribution of
thoracic pain

Thoracic pain
through chest

A patch of
pain anteriorly

Figure 6.11  Pains of thoracic spinal origin

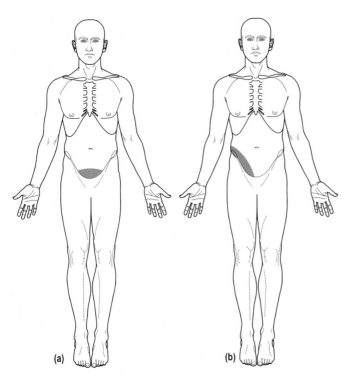

**Figure 6.12**   Lower abdominal pain referred from (*a*) the low lumbar spine or (*b*) an L1 nerve root disorder

system' and in the 'differentiation section' of the physical examination. As has been stated, patients may have unusual areas of symptoms that do not fit any of those mentioned on the preceding pages. They may have bizarre symptoms that they do not class as pain, and may not even mention them unless asked about them; or they may not recognize them as being related symptoms until they realize that the bizarre symptoms have disappeared in parallel with improvement of the primary symptoms for which they sought treatment. Examples common from the cervical/upper thoracic levels include heaviness of the whole arm, glove-stocking paraesthesia, blurred vision, head too heavy to hold up, etc. Butler (1991) refers to neuropathic pain, saying:

> *The clinical features … are not clear, and the suggestion to think of the nervous system when symptoms are a bit obscure is good … symptoms may jump from area to area, cervical one day, elbow another, glove-hand another.*

He also refers to 'lines' of pain and 'clumps' of pain. These features are very loosely grouped by therapists as being neural in origin, and include neuropathy. The two best texts on the subject are by Butler (1991) and Grieve (1988a), both of which are considered mandatory knowledge to the Maitland concept.

## BEHAVIOUR OF SYMPTOMS

Changes in the site and intensity of a patient's symptoms should be related to activities and positions, and to periods of short rest and long rest (the latter being throughout the night). During the questioning it is essential to differentiate the behaviour of the local pain from that which is referred; the two may be associated or they may behave in totally different patterns, the latter indicating different causes of the pains. *Figure 6.13* gives a clear indication of the general questions that should be asked.

The behaviour of the patient's pain with various activities will indicate how it affects him in and give an idea of its severity. Furthermore, it gives an indication of the level of disability, which can be expressed in terms of impairments, disabilities/activity limitation, and handicaps/participation restriction (ICIDH, WHO 1980, 1997). Questions should elicit facts against which subsequent progress can be evaluated. For example, a patient may say that he can walk as far as the front gate before his leg pain becomes severe. This fact is a basis for assessing progress if, during treatment, he reaches the stage of being able to walk further than the front gate. These subjective assessments then become objective facts.

An understanding of the causes and sources of a patient's referred symptoms can rarely be reached in a

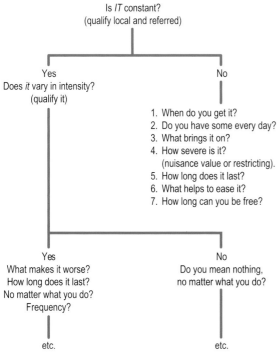

**Figure 6.13**   General questions for establishing behaviour of symptoms

single consultation: to reach it – ever – is difficult enough. There are so many influencing factors. The level of proven scientific factors is poor in itself. For further reading on the subject, Grieve's text (Grieve, 1988a) would be hard to better. One very real aspect that can be elicited from the patient is 'remembered pain' (or, in computer language, 'programmed pain'), and this needs to be determined. An example of this is that a patient may have buttock pain spreading along the lateral aspect of the thigh and calf, with the most severe part being at the lower third of the lower leg. Up to a certain stage of the subjective examination, this may be thought to be due to a nerve-root disorder. However, when it is discovered that the patient had a fracture 20 years ago at the lower third of the tibia and fibula, which caused considerable pain, the whole thinking must now include the possibility of programmed pain. The resulting effect may be that the examiner needs to rethink her priorities about the source of the symptoms.

## Irritability of the disorder

Questions should be asked to determine how easily the patient's symptoms are aggravated by his activities and how readily the symptoms subside, so that exacerbation of symptoms from excessive examination can

be avoided. This is later referred to as 'irritability', and is itemized in the 'planning sheet' (*see Table 6.3*).

To assess the irritability of a disorder, three aspects of the behaviour of a patient's symptoms must be related to a particular function or activity:

1. Determining the activity that provokes the patient's pain and knowing the vigour of that activity, particularly as it may relate to physical examination and treatment movements.
2. Knowing the degree and quality of the increased symptoms caused by that activity.
3. Knowing how long it takes for the increased symptoms to subside to their level prior to performing the provoking activity.

A comparatively minor activity, such as ironing for half an hour, that causes pain of a severity that forces the patient to stop ironing, but that subsides in half an hour such that another half hour of ironing can be carried out, indicates minor irritability of the disorder. This therefore permits a full examination plus some treatment on the first day without likelihood of exacerbation. If, however, the symptoms did not subside until the patient had had a full night's sleep, the disorder would be considered to be irritable and the examinations and treatment would have to be tailored, taking cognizance of the irritability, so as to avoid exacerbation.

No matter whether the patient's pain is constant or intermittent, present at rest or on activity, there will be movements, positions or activities that will aggravate or ease the pain. These positions or activities should be carefully noted, as they may well guide the choice of positions to be adopted or avoided during treatment.

Care is required when assessing the effect of rest on pain. Frequently the patient will say the pain is worse when in bed, when in fact the symptoms may only be worse for the first hour or so as a result of the day's activities. On further questioning, the pain is found to be considerably relieved by the following morning. However, pain that is worse at night and is severe enough to make the patient get out of bed requires careful investigation because of the possibility of more serious pathology than the mechanical problems usually referred for physiotherapy.

> Irritability can be defined as a little activity causing a lot of pain that takes a long time to settle. Sometimes it is useful to describe the symptoms of the patient as 'severe' if the activity that causes the symptoms has to be interrupted because of the intensity of the pain. All aspects of irritability and severity require care, both in the performance of examination tests and in the progression of treatment

Great difficulty can be encountered when endeavouring to assess the severity of the patient's pain. The whole subject of pain is enormously complex (Melzack and Wall, 1984), full of considerable known knowledge but also subject to many unknown and hypothesized features. Patients may describe symptoms in many different ways for widely differing reasons, but often there is a degree of uniformity, giving useful expressions for the clinician to recognize. Probably the most important fact always to have in mind is that symptoms can have a physiological basis (whether understood or not), and there can be psychological influencing aspects. The paper by Keele (1967) is still valuable in that it discusses the different physiological thresholds of pain determined by physical tests. Too often in the clinical situation, patients are not given the benefit of the doubt when they describe either unusual or bizarre symptoms for which there is no proven theoretical knowledge as yet. Treatment does not seem to have an effect on them, and unhappy patients become tagged with the label that their pain is purely psychological. Grieve (1981) and Butler (1991) provide much useful information about the possible reasons for the clinical types of symptoms encountered, and they certainly make sense to clinicians. The primary points at this stage of knowledge are that patients should be listened to and believed because (a) their descriptions help us to understand from what they are suffering, (b) they can show things about their personality, and (c) we stand a better chance of making an improvement by treatment.

Assessment of pain may be assisted by applying stretch to one or two of the patient's normal joints while watching his reaction. Weighing this information against both his history and his description of what he is unable to do because of his pain will all help in assessment.

The aim of the questioning is to know the patient's symptoms and problems so completely that the physiotherapist can 'live' them herself. It is then a natural step to ask about the onset and history of the present episode before asking about relevant previous history. Putting 'history' at the end of the sequence facilitates constructive questioning for the inexperienced physiotherapist.

## SPECIAL QUESTIONS

This section covers particular questions that *must* be asked so as to be aware of any inherent dangers for manipulative treatment or factors that may limit treatment (e.g. vertebrobasilar insufficiency, osteoporosis, etc.). The questions vary for each section of the spine, and are discussed in the relevant chapters.

Special Qs, routine Qs and danger Qs are set special questions that must be asked. Special questions include the effect of prolonged rest (a night's rest in bed as compared with a half hour's rest), the effect of activities, the degree of symptoms at the end of the day compared with on first getting out of bed in the morning and the middle of the day, etc.

Routine questions relate to general health, weight loss, fatigue levels, home and work relationships, previous operations and illnesses, medication, etc.

Danger questions relate to vertebrobasilar symptoms, cauda equina symptoms, osteoporosis, surgery, etc.

## HISTORY

As can be seen by reading the Tables for the *subjective* examination of the cervical, thoracic and lumbar spines (*see* pp. 230, 303 and 339), the history can be taken at any stage of the questioning and may be sought in segments during the remainder of the questioning whenever it seems most appropriate. When confronted with a chronic non-episodic disorder, the history is best left to the end because the area and the behaviour of the symptoms will guide the questioning, enabling the examiner to exclude irrelevant information from the patient's story. Because it is usually pain that causes most people to seek treatment, the example that follows will be presented in the sequence used if the patient's answer to the question is 'I get a pain across here'.

History taking is a skill that requires knowledge and practice. Macnab's chapter of history (Macnab, 1977) should be read, understood and applied by all. The finer details relating to the present episode of symptoms, together with those of any earlier history, can provide – even in the absence of being able to make a precise diagnosis – invaluable information about the state of the structures at fault.

It is not enough to know that a patient's symptoms came on 'gradually', as it may not be clear what this 'gradually' means. Ask, 'do you mean it insidiously, sneakily inveigled its way on you?'. If the answer is 'yes', the 'gradual' probably means that the patient would have gradually become aware of the symptoms over 1–4 weeks. Better information is gained by offering him two extremes – 'Was it gradually over a few days, or was it over a few weeks?'.

It is also necessary to separate this kind of 'gradual' from that which came on gradually over one day. Ask, 'Can you recall whether it began on ONE day, even if only very mildly, and that the day before you were perfectly normal?'. If the answer is 'yes', then it is necessary to know the following:

1. 'Did you waken with it?' – which would indicate that something had happened during the day(s) before. Questions should then be pressed to determine predisposing factors such an unusual activities or forgotten trivial incidents (*see Table 6.5* and relevant text).

2. 'Did it come on later during the day?' – which would indicate, in the absence of any trivial incident or unusually heavy or different work, that something had been gradually developing asymptomatically, and that the day when the symptoms began was just 'the last straw'.

**Table 6.5**    Taking the history

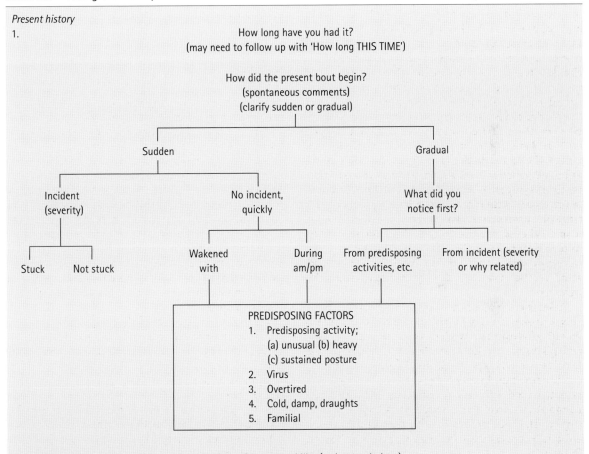

*Present history*

1.

How long have you had it?
(may need to follow up with 'How long THIS TIME')

How did the present bout begin?
(spontaneous comments)
(clarify sudden or gradual)

Sudden | Gradual

Incident (severity) | No incident, quickly | What did you notice first?

Stuck    Not stuck | Wakened with | During am/pm | From predisposing activities, etc. | From incident (severity or why related)

PREDISPOSING FACTORS
1. Predisposing activity;
   (a) unusual (b) heavy
   (c) sustained posture
2. Virus
3. Overtired
4. Cold, damp, draughts
5. Familial

2. Relate severity of incident to degree of disability for comparability (serious pathology)
3. History of local pain, history of referred pain (limb pain upwards or downwards)
4. Progress over initial period 'till levelling off' of symptoms

*Previous history*
1. First bout in detail: Cause
                        Duration
                        Treatment
2. Successive bouts: Frequency
                     Ease of cause
                     Recovery: rate (Rest, R, etc.)
3. Medical history (and socio-economic)

When a minor incident precipitates an onset of symptoms on the following day, the severity of symptoms, the degree of the incident and the patient's ability or inability to continue working provide invaluable information regarding the degree of the damage of the structure at fault. Similarly, the comparison of the symptoms on getting out of bed the morning following the incident, along with the state of the symptoms before going to bed, provides information relating to the underlying degree of disorder of the structure on which the minor incident has imposed its effect. Such disorders often progress from local pain to include referred pain. It is then necessary to know whether the pain has spread gradually, or whether it involved referred pain from the outset.

> Symptoms that have developed 'gradually' need further clarification

In questioning regarding the history of a patient's symptoms, it is necessary to recognize that the patient may have two disorders. A new problem may overlap with an older, longstanding one, and every effort must be made to differentiate between the contribution each is making to the patient's disability.

> A patient may present with symptoms that can come from two disorders. Every effort has to be made to differentiate between the contribution each is making to the patient's disability

Sometimes a patient presents with symptoms that fit the later stages of a recognizable disorder without realizing he has an associated history, and the manipulative physiotherapist may recognize that it is quite unusual for a patient to have these as his first presenting symptoms. In these circumstances, the patient must be pressed vigorously for previous symptoms that he may have had, yet considered to be normal (remember: 'You can't tell me too much, you can tell me too little; let me be the judge as to its relevance').

When trauma of a more major degree (such as that resulting from a car accident) causes symptoms, it is necessary to know the following:

1. The degree of the trauma – ascertain the extent of bruising, its colour and duration, the damage to the vehicle.
2. Whether the patient was aware that he or his car was going to be hit – that is, was he able to be prepared for the blow or was it an unguarded blow (the latter always imposing the greater danger)?

The main areas of history concern:

1. The onset and development of the present episode.
2. The present stage of the disorder.
3. The present stability of the disorder.
4. The previous history, including episodic development and the possibility of genetic components.

The most common spinal disorders treated by manipulative physiotherapists, where the disorder has a primarily spontaneous onset, are:

1. Ligamentous and capsular disorders due to accumulated stress from poor posture, overuse, misuse or abuse.
2. Ligamentous and capsular disorders from a minor sprain.
3. Locked or blocked joints.
4. Disorders of structures in the vertebral canal and intervertebral foramina.
5. Mechanically disturbed arthritic (-otic) disorders.
6. Discogenic disorders.

All of these have recognizable patterns of onset and development.

Ligamentous and arthritic (-otic, -osic) disorders of the spine have exactly the same history patterns as peripheral synovial joints with the same disorders. Examination of the history of patients with ligamentous disorders must be directed towards determining the parts played by:

- Stress
- Strain
- Sprain
- Overuse
- Misuse
- New use
- Abuse
- Disuse.

Arthritic disorders will have a prolonged history of constant awareness of discomfort studded with exacerbations. In some patients the disorder will be linked with previous trauma and in others there may be a familial link, but in all there will be through-range pain, and crepitus may be present. The history of discogenic disorders, which may or may not involve the nerve root and other structures, is detailed on pages 192–194. The history of a locked joint is very specific (see pp. 232–233). Referred pain has characteristics that can indicate the structure from which it is coming (see pp. 108–109).

Taking the history of the present episode first provides information that enables questions about the total history to be more positively directed. If the first question is, 'How long have you had it?' and the patient starts his answer by saying 'Twenty years ago, I ...', he should be gently interrupted by saying, 'No, I'm sorry, what I mean is how long have you had it this time?'. After you have determined when, the next questions determine how it began and what caused it. Patients will often say 'It began suddenly', which to the manipulative physiotherapist may mean at a particular instant, but to the patient may mean over a period of 2 or more days. A gradual onset usually means an insidious onset (discussed above), but whatever terms the patient uses, they must be clarified. If the onset was gradual, determine whether the patient knows any reason why it should have begun – what he first felt that made him aware something was wrong.

Each question that is asked must lead towards being able to make a diagnosis. Therefore, the clearer the picture the examiner has of the history patterns of the different disorders, the more information can be gained by asking the right questions to strengthen the judgement regarding the diagnosis.

Those patients who had an incident that caused the disorder will fit into one of three categories:

1. Those who had a fall or injury.
2. Those who had a minor or trivial incident but noticed little else until the next morning.
3. Those who merely twisted or bent, felt sudden pain, and were unable to return to the normal position.

It is very important to be able to MAKE FEATURES FIT.

For example, a very fit 45-year-old farmer, while sitting at the breakfast table, had a sudden onset of disabling pain when he reached across the table to take a cup of tea from his wife. Any movement provoked severe pain. He was carried to bed and the doctor was contacted. He had never had trouble with his back previously, despite a life of heavy work on his farm. A trivial yet disabling incident in isolation, such as that described, is totally unacceptable as it stands – there has to be a reason for the spine to react so violently to such a trivial event. The reason has to be either that there is a serious pathology present in the spine, or that there must have been factors present that predisposed to the spine 'giving way'.

Considering the predisposing factors, elements must be sought which, when added together, are compatible with his reaching for the cup of tea disabling him so. Interestingly, 2 weeks prior to the cup of tea incident, while out on the farm the farmer's small car had a puncture. Having no jack, the farmer lifted the corner of the car at the appropriate moment while his son changed the wheel. There was no sign of back trouble. One week later, he had to drag and lift a young calf into his stationwagon, again with no sign of back trouble. Then, a week later, he reached for the ruinous cup of tea. The incident of the cup of tea becomes much more acceptable when it is seen as 'the last straw'.

> Asking about 'predisposing factors' in the history of a patient's problem is essential, as it aids in understanding the features of a patient's problem, and guides in treatment progression and in the choice of prophylactic measures

In searching for the cause of a patient's episode, it is necessary to know how the symptoms first appeared and then to be able to find satisfactory reasons that are comparable. Such matching is equally important whether the patient has a postural backache, an incident of disc damage, or an exacerbation of an 'arthritic' disorder.

It is necessary sometimes to be prepared to probe extensively, even extending the probing over a period of the first two consultations, to make the features of the history fit the features of the patient's complaint. But 'fit', they must.

Delving into the past history is essential, particularly in relation to the original onset, if the progress of the disorder is to be understood. The garrulous patient can make this process irksome for the novice, who must learn what can be discarded or ignored from a 20-year history. However, after sorting out the original onset, the intervening years can be covered by such questions as:

'How long have your pain-free intervals been?'

'How many times have you had trouble?'

'Has the frequency of episodes changed over the last couple of years?'

'Have you been confined to bed because of it?'

'What has caused the episodes?'

'What kind of treatments have helped you best so far?'

With the present history it is essential to know the progress of the symptoms from the time of onset to the present moment, as well as knowing the effect of any treatment that may have been instituted. Questions regarding medical history and socio-economic history should also be asked. *Table 6.6* provides a quick reference for the general points mentioned; specific histories will be discussed later in the relevant chapters.

**Table 6.6** Planning the subjective examination

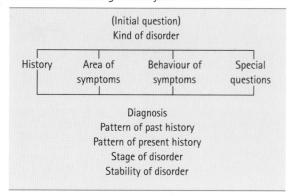

**PLANNING**

## PLANNING THE SUBJECTIVE EXAMINATION

The tables on pages 99, 119, 230 and 339 list all the subject matter related to the questions asked of the patient at an initial consultation. As mentioned earlier, the sequence of introducing the history can be varied to suit the circumstances. As one gains experience both by the process of examining every patient in detail and also in communication skills, the pattern of asking the individual questions to reach a diagnosis can be varied to a very wide degree. For the beginner, it is essential that variations in the sequence of asking questions should be made only as confidence in the skills makes it possible. It is vital that at no stage should the physiotherapist lose her train of thought, for once the train of thought is lost, essential questions can very easily be forgotten. *Table 6.6* shows the planning for the subjective examination. In planning the subjective examination, the first point to make use of is observation of all aspects of the patient's movements and attitudes as well as the small nuances of behaviour while being ushered into the place where the consultation will be carried out. The second stage consists of the introductory questions in the consultation. The first pointed question, directly associated with the examination, is 'At this particular stage, what do you consider is your main problem?'. Following on from the answer to this question, the plan is to establish the 'kind of disorder' of which the patient complains. (This is related to all of the items in *Table 6.6*).

During the questioning, it is very important to be sufficiently alert to pick up key words and statements that require 'automatic immediate-response follow-up questions', while endeavouring to parallel questions

with the patient's line of thought at any given moment. The goal is to make sense out of everything the patient says in an endeavour to 'make features fit'.

Having established the kind of disorder, the pattern of questioning can be directed along one of three paths. The three paths suggested above are:

1. History
2. Area of symptoms
3. Behaviour of symptoms.

If the patient has an acute onset, or is in severe pain, then the history probably comes first. However, if the disorder is chronic then it is possible that the behaviour of the symptoms, once the therapist has a general idea of the area of the problem, should be followed next. The third possibility is that the patient may have an area of referred pain into a limb, and because it may be necessary to decide whether this referral is radicular or not, it may be necessary to define clearly the area of symptoms before going into either the history or the behaviour of the symptoms.

Whichever area is chosen first, the final goal is to arrive at an informative diagnosis (*Table 6.7*). To plan the subjective examination the physiotherapist should be thinking along the following lines:

1. Thoughts should be aligned with the doctor's thoughts on the diagnosis.
2. Thoughts should be related to the observation of the patient when being ushered into the room.
3. Thoughts should also be related to the kind of disorder from which the patient may be suffering.

## PLANNING THE PHYSICAL EXAMINATION

After the subjective examination has been completed the manipulative physiotherapist should have a clear mind as to where to go in relation to (a) the diagnostic subjective findings, (b) the physical examination, and (c) making treatment prognoses, assessments and an estimation of end-results (*Table 6.8*).

When planning the *physical* examination the physiotherapist should have three distinct thoughts in mind:

1. What structures must be examined to determine the source, or sources, of the patient's symptoms? (*see Table 6.8*, part A).

2. Are there any limitations to the extent of the examination imposed by the pathology, irritability or severity of the disorder, other disorders such as structural damage or the behaviour of the symptoms? (*see Table 6.8*, part B).

Table 6.7  Chart demonstrating relationships and contexts for theoretical and clinical knowledge with related hypotheses (H$_X$ = history; Sy = symptoms; S = signs)

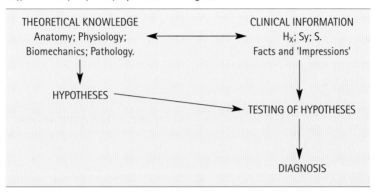

Before the physiotherapist starts the physical examination procedures, she needs to have a clear plan in mind of which structures she needs to examine and she needs to consider; whether there are limitations to the extent of the examination imposed by pathology, irritability or severity of the disorder, or other aspects such as structural damage. Furthermore, she needs to have hypotheses about the possible causes of the disorder and factors contributing to the development of the disorder

Having made decisions regarding these two aspects, the therapist should be able to commit her thoughts regarding the kind of examination procedures she should use (*see Table 6.8*, part C). The next step is to consider the remaining physical examination from a different point of view.

3.  What other aspects of physical examination, distinct from discerning the source of the symptoms, should be looked at as being the possible reason why the source of the symptoms became symptomatic? (*see Table 6.8*, part D).

Clinical evidence and experimental work have shown that pain from a muscle lesion is localized to the site of the lesion, although it spreads in area as the intensity increases. Lesions of synovial joints and the supporting inert structures, on the other hand, can also cause pain referred for some distance from the joint. Synovial joint lesions can sometimes be responsible for referred pain without any pain in the region of the joint. For example, it is well known that the osteoarthritic hip can cause knee pain, and lesions of the vertebral column frequently refer pain to the abdomen and thorax. Clinical investigation has shown that the intervertebral disc is capable of causing local and referred pain without any sign of herniation or nerve root compression (Cloward, 1959). It would seem that this pain is never more pronounced in the distal segment of a dermatome. However, when herniation of disc material compresses a nerve root the pain is commonly felt more severely in a distal area such as the calf or forearm. Symptoms can be referred into superficial areas, which may become hyperaesthetic (Glover, 1960); into the muscles, making them tender; or to joints, which may then themselves become painful on movement (Brain, 1957).

The plan can be considered in four sections, which are mentioned below, and they must be thought of as having two goals. *Table 6.8* shows that the physical examination has TWO distinct goals:

1.  PART ONE is entirely related to determining the structures that are the source(s) of the symptoms and to finding movement directions that are abnormal and need to be addressed in treatment.

2.  PART TWO is directed towards determining the factors that are the underlying causes of the structures becoming the source of the presenting disorder.

Parts one and two are not synonymous. Part two involves a different line of thinking to Part one – why should the particular structures have reached a stage of causing symptoms? Part one is a relentless examination to find the structures from which the symptoms are coming. They are quite different and *must* be clearly seen as separate parts of the examination. They must *NOT* be run together and thought to be the same.

**Table 6.8**    Planning the physical examination

**A.    The sources of the symptoms**

1.    Name as the possible sources of any part of the patient's symptoms every joint and muscle which must be examined

| Joints which lie under the symptomatic area | Joints which refer symptoms into the area | Muscles which lie under the symptomatic area |

2.    List joints above and below the lesion which should be checked.

    .............................................................................................

    .............................................................................................

3.    Are there any special tests indicated?

    (a)    neurological examination

    (b)    other – specify ....................................................................

    .............................................................................................

    .............................................................................................

4.    Are you going to test for vertebral artery insufficiency?    Yes/No

5.    Are you going to test for cord signs?    Yes/No

**B.    Influence of symptoms and pathology on examination and first treatment**

1.    Is pain 'severe'?    Yes/No    or 'latent'?    Yes/No

2.    Does the subjective examination suggest an easily irritable disorder?

    Local symptoms    Yes/No,    Referred/other symptoms    Yes/No

        Give the example on which the answers are based.

    (a)    Local symptoms

        Part (i)     Repeated movement causing pain ..........................

        Part (ii)    Severity of pain so caused .........................................

        Part (iii)   Duration before pain subsides ..................................

    (b)    Referred/other symptoms

        Part (i)     Repeated movement causing pain ..........................

        Part (ii)    Severity of pain so caused .........................................

        Part (iii)   Duration before pain subsides ..................................

3.    Does the 'nature' of the disorder indicate caution?    Yes/No

    (i)      pathology/injury – specify ...............................................

    (ii)     easy to provoke exacerbation or acute episode ......................

    (iii)    personality ......................................................................

4.    Are there any contraindications?    Yes/No

    Specify.............................................................................................

**C.    The kind of examination**

1.    Do you think you will need to be gentle or moderately firm with your examination of movements?

2.    Do you expect a 'comparable' sign {to be easy    or    to be hard} to find?

3.    What movements do you expect to be 'comparable'?

4.    Which test procedures will you carry out?

5.    When do you plan to perform reassesment procedures?

**D.    Associated examination**

1.    Provocative 'neuro/musculo/skeletal/medical' factors leading to the cause of the symptoms.

    What associated factors must be examined

    (a)    as reasons why the joint, muscle or other structure has become symptomatic    and/or

    (b)    Why the joint or muscle disorder may recur? (e.g. posture, muscle imbalance, muscle power, obesity, stiffness, hypermobility, instability, deformity in proximal or distal joint, etc.)

2.    The effect of the disorder on joint stability?

**E.    Treatment**

1.    Which short-term and long-term goals of treatment are pursued?

2.    Do you expect to be treating pain, resistance, weakness or instability?

3.    Are there any precautions or contraindications which need to be respected?

4.    In planning the TREATMENT (after the examination) what advice should be included and/or measures would you use to prevent or lessen recurrences.

There are four sections that need to be considered in the planning of the physical examination:

1. With the thorough knowledge of the patterns of pain from disorders affecting muscles, discs, synovial joints, 'neural' and nerve roots, it is possible to list the joints, nerves and muscles that must be examined as possible causes of pain:
   a) The joints that lie under the area of pain.
   b) The joints that do not lie under the area of pain but can refer pain into the area.
   c) The neural elements.
   d) The muscles that lie under the area of pain.

2. The second part to consider is the effect of the pain on the patient.

3. The third indicates the kind of examination (for example, the extent and strength of test movements) required.

4. The last aspect deals with examination of the underlying abnormalities to ascertain the reasons that may have been predisposing factors to the onset of the patient's pain, or that may, if uncorrected, lead to recurrences.

*Table 6.8* shows an example of a 'Planning the Examination' sheet.

In the discussion that follows, aspects of examination relating to general health, posture, muscle balance and other allied factors are omitted. Although they are of relevance in treatment, they have been omitted deliberately for the purpose of emphasizing the aspects that are so vital to the choice of the mobilizing and manipulating techniques to be used during treatment, and to the assessment of their effect.

An example will make the point of 'planning' clearer, and in this example the word 'joint' (as throughout this book) refers to the inert structures affected by passive movement.

A patient has pain spreading from C6 to T6 centrally and laterally across the right posterior thoracic wall from the top of the shoulder to the inferior angle of the scapula. The pain spreads into the right triceps area and down the posterior aspect of the forearm to the wrist (*Figure 6.14*). If the spread of pain from joints, muscles or nerve-root lesions is borne in mind, it will be necessary to examine the following structures as being the possible cause, in part or in full, of these symptoms:

1. *The joints that lie under the area of pain*:
   C6–T6
   a) Right costovertebral joints T1–T6
   b) Intercostal movement between the first and sixth ribs on the right
   c) Scapulothoracic movement on the right

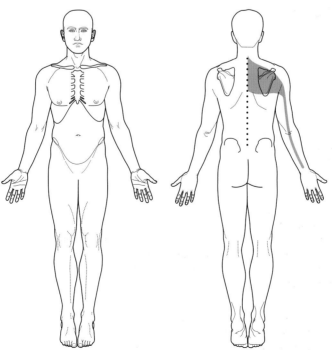

Figure 6.14   Distribution of pain

d) Right glenohumeral joint and rotator cuff
e) Right elbow
f) Right wrist.

2. *The joints that do not lie under the area of pain but can refer pain into the area* (other joints need to be included to allow for a pre- or post-fixed plexus and for errors of interpretation of pain areas):
   a) C4–C6
   b) T6–T8, including the costovertebral joints and intercostal movement.

3. *The neural/supportive elements that can refer into the symptomatic area(s)*:
   a) C3–C9 articulations
   b) The first and second ribs
   c) Entrapment and traction.

4. *The muscles that lie under the area of pain*:
   a) Elevators and retractors of scapula
   b) Extensors of elbow
   c) Extensors of wrist and fingers.

Experienced physiotherapists will examine some of the structures listed only briefly, because the history and behaviour of the pain make it clear that these structures are unlikely to be causing pain. However, such examination should never be completely omitted on the assumption that the structure is *not* contributing to the pain.

## PHYSICAL EXAMINATION

There are large differences in the background to the thinking of orthopaedic surgeons, orthopaedic physicians, manipulative therapists and the patient, and never the quartet shall meet. However, there is no reason why they can't work, think and discuss as a team. It is easy to see the orthopaedic surgeon and the physician being able to understand each other's thought processes; it is easy to see the manipulative therapist and the patient being able to see each other's thought processes. However, bringing the former two and the latter two thought processes together is not easy. It can be achieved, but it needs to be based on a personal understanding of each other rather than a professional one. Their frames of reference are greatly different. It is not reasonable for a member of an orchestra, or a soloist, to have the same thought processes as a conductor or the composer, but that does not prevent the team of all four working together to produce a good result. Their frames of reference are not the same. The humility and recognized acceptance that the one can establish with the other, again on a personal basis, is the key to opening the door to a wider understanding of each other's thoughts. Certainly the professional bodies can work towards such an understanding; their acceptance is on a consensus basis. However, the person-to-person basis is the key to the best and most successful result, and it is towards this end that each must work for the patient's sake. The manipulative physiotherapist can only provide a physical diagnosis (which naturally must be limited by training and experience) and a physical prognosis, which are more functional and movement-related compared with the other professionals; this must always be remembered.

The purposes of the physiotherapist's physical examination are first, to interpret the patient's concept of his disability into terms of muscles, joints and nerves causing their symptoms; and secondly to determine physical factors that may have predisposed the patient to the onset of the disorder. It is possible, by tests using isometric resisted contraction and passive movements, to differentiate between pain from muscles and pain from joints. It is also necessary to make an assessment of active movements to indicate the functional limits caused by the condition and to show the patient's willingness to move.

When the inert structures of a joint are painful, passive movement of that joint will be painful at some point in the range. To elicit the pain it may be necessary to move the joint while holding the joint surfaces compressed at one end of the possibilities, to test accessory movements at the other end. When a lesion occurs in a muscle, passive joint movement will not be painful unless it is a movement that stretches or pinches the muscle. However, pain will always be reproduced when fibres involved in the lesion are made to contract strongly. Joint problems are therefore determined by passive movement tests, and muscular lesions by isometric muscle contraction tests, which reduce joint movements to a minimum.

The isometric tests do not always provide clear answers, because an isometric test necessarily results in compression of the joint surfaces. Similarly, isometric tests in the lumbar and cervical areas always produce considerable intervertebral movement. Under these circumstances, the isometric test may cause pain because the joint is moving. Therefore, it may be necessary to test the muscle isometrically in different positions of the joint range, and to compare the degree of pain produced by a resisted active movement with that of a passive movement.

Examining a joint does not differentiate between pain caused by the intervertebral disc, the apophyseal joints, capsules or their ligaments. It does, however, reveal a disturbance of movement. It should be remembered that consideration of movement must not be limited to that of the disc and apophyseal joints. The spinal cord and its investments and the nerve roots with their sleeves must be able to move freely in the vertebral canal and intervertebral foramina. Tests for movement of these structures must also be part of the physiotherapist's physical examination.

The examination of the intervertebral segment can be divided into the following sequence:

1. Active tests
   a) Active movements – movements which the patient can perform to reproduce his pain (*see* pp. 127–133)
      – physiological movements
      – combined movements.
   b) Auxiliary tests associated with active movement tests, for example joint compression tests and tests for vertebrobasilar insufficiency.
   c) Neurological examination, which forms an essential part of the examination of the neural elements.

2. Passive tests
   a) Movement of the pain-sensitive structures in the vertebral canal and intervertebral foramen and neural linked movements.
   b) Physiological spinal movements.
   c) Palpation, including accessory movements.
   d) Passive range of physiological movement of single intervertebral joints.
   e) Differentiation tests.

## ACTIVE TESTS

Following the subjective examination and planning, a decision needs to be made as to whether the test movements of the physical examination should be taken to the limit of the available range (move to limit), or whether they should be taken only to that point in the range when pain commences or starts to increase (dominance of stiffness or pain respectively).

> Before starting the test, a decision needs to be made whether the test movements should be taken to the limit of available range or only to the beginning or increase of pain

Under the latter circumstances, some assessment should be made of the behaviour of the pain just beyond that point in the range where the pain commences or where the constant pain begins to increase.

When pain is the dominant factor in the patient's disorder, test movements are taken only to the point in the range where pain commences (and just beyond to assess the pattern of increase or spread). When

stiffness is more important than pain, the test movements should be taken to the limit of the available range and, if necessary, over-pressure (OP) applied.

*Move to limit* – gentle or firm over-pressure must be applied to all test movements in order to determine:

- The end-of-range 'feel' of the movement
- The symptom response to the OP.

*Move to pain* – when the patient has the severest of pains, the accessory movement tests should be performed in neutral physiological positions that are fully supported, as free of discomfort as possible and avoiding compression of joint surfaces. It also means that the accessory movement should only be taken to the point in the range when the pain is first felt (or where it is first felt to increase). When this assessment has been made, the movement should be taken fractionally beyond this point to assess how quickly the pain increases or how quickly it spreads.

A movement *cannot* be classed (or recorded) as normal unless the range is pain free both actively and passively; as well, over-pressure (OP) applied at the limit of range should not cause pain other than normal responses. Recording a range of flexion as being normal would be 'F✓✓' where the first tick (✓) refers to range, and the second tick refers to pain responses.

> A movement cannot be classed as normal unless the range is pain-free actively and passively, and with the addition of passive over-pressure at the limit of the active range. The recording of a normal movement in relation to its range, quality and symptom response is recommended as ✓✓

## Active movements

*Movements that the patient can perform to reproduce his symptoms – functional demonstration tests*

This is a fundamental, first line of approach to sorting out the source(s) of a patient's problem. It is basic and mandatory to the thinking process involved in the 'Maitland concept', and cannot be emphasized enough. It should become embedded in a therapist's mind and become a natural process (*see* pp. 86–87, 99, 236, 307 and 343–344).

The patient should be asked to demonstrate any activities that reproduce his symptoms. The physiotherapist should then analyse the movement component that is related to the symptoms.

An example may help in understanding the analysing process. A golfer is able to cause the pain by going through his golf swing. On asking him to repeat the swing, but to stop at the stage where he feels the pain, he may have to swing many times before he is clearly aware of the part that provokes his pain. In this example, the golfer is able to say that it is during his follow-through. The therapist then watches the patient's spine (at the site of his symptoms) while the swing is repeated, endeavouring to decide what the directions of movement are at the moment of pain. She decides it is a combination of thoracic rotation left, moving into extension and lateral flexion to the right. To test the validity of the thinking, the golfer puts himself into the position, whereupon she supports him and applies manual over-pressure in the directions she feels are at fault. An increase in the pain with one or more of the directions will prove or disprove her thinking. If there is no increase with any of the directions, she starts the whole process again until she finds what she is looking for and proves it.

> A demonstration of an activity that provokes the patient's symptoms is of help in analysing the components at fault and finding the abnormal movement directions, which will be addressed in treatment. Furthermore, this activity can be used as a control parameter in reassessments of treatment. The latter is especially important, as the movement demonstrated is a reflection of the patient's perception of his normal activities rather than the perception of the physiotherapist's, as is the case when she asks him to perform anatomically oriented tests like flexion or side flexion

### Physiological movements

When a joint is found to cause pain, a careful assessment of active and passive movements should be made. The active movements should be tested first because the patient will perform these within his own limits of pain, and therefore safely; the assessment of these movements will indicate the severity of the disability and guide the examiner in how much passive handling the joint will tolerate. Active movements of the thoracic and lumbar spine are tested while standing, except for rotation, which should sometimes also be tested while sitting. Sitting is also the position most suitable for testing cervical movements, because the trunk is more stable.

*Move to pain* – In the physical examination tables for each section of the spine, the statement is made 'Move to pain or move to limit'. This refers to the two methods that are used when examining the patient's active movements. If the severity or irritability of the patient's symptoms or the nature of the disorder causing them (*see* Planning Sheet, *Table 6.8*) are such that caution should be exercised when examining movements, the patient should, as a first step, be asked to move to the point where the symptoms commence, or commence to increase, then immediately stop and return to the upright position.

*Move to limit* – On the other hand, if the severity or irritability of the patient's symptoms or the nature of the disorder causing them indicates that movements can be taken to the limit of the range and stretched, then this is in fact what is done for each direction of movement. Whether movements are tested to pain or to the limit, they should both be taken, as a second measure, beyond the point so as to assess the behaviour of these symptoms with the further movement.

Before testing movement, the patient's present symptoms should be assessed. If he has no pain before moving, he should be asked to move in the direction being tested until pain is felt. If he has some pain present before moving, he should be asked to move until the pain begins to increase. Measurement of the range should be made, noting the area in which pain is caused by the movement. If the pain is not severe, nor of a kind that must not be aggravated, the patient should be asked to move further into the range, reporting any increase in the severity of pain or any alteration in its distribution, so that the severity and the behaviour of the pain with the further movement can be determined.

When no restrictions need to be placed on the examination of movements, the patient should be encouraged to move to the limit of the range and the physiotherapist should then apply controlled over-pressure to determine the 'end-feel' of the movement and any change in the quality of the symptoms. This over-pressure is essential if, on examination, a movement appears to be full range and painless. It is incorrect to record the movement as being normal unless firm pressure producing small oscillatory movements can be applied painlessly at the limit of the range. Care is required when applying this over-pressure to certain movements. With cervical extension, whether the pressure is applied by lifting under the chin or by pressing against the forehead, care should be exercised to prevent the movement being merely one of traction or compression.

There are three points to be mentioned in relation to testing active movements; points that apply when a movement reveals little in the way of pain:

1. Occasionally it is necessary for a patient to perform a test movement quickly if pain is not provoked by the full-range movement performed at the usual

speed. For example, a patient may say that turning his head is painful yet, on examination of movements at the usual speed, the movement is normal and over-pressure can be applied at the limit of the range without pain. However, if he is asked to turn his head sharply, the pain may be reproduced.

2.  If a patient says forward flexion of the lumbar spine is not very painful, yet the movement is limited, it is as well to find out how far he could bend before his symptoms began. There are some people who cannot reach their toes normally, including some who are unable to reach beyond their knees. Cervical rotation, in the presence of marked spondylitic change, is another movement of which prior knowledge of range is helpful. Stiffness under these circumstances may not be a primary physical sign in the patient's present condition.

3.  When flexion of the thoracic and lumbar spines appears to be normal, it is useful (particularly if on continued examination little is found) to tap sharply each spinous process in turn, either with the reflex hammer or with the fingertips. A joint causing pain is found to respond painfully to this tap-test.

Following the test for range and pain, the patient should (provided pain permits) move back and forth from the starting position while the physiotherapist watches for disturbances of the normal rhythm of intervertebral movement. Repeated movements should be avoided if a movement is very painful, as they unjustifiably provoke and increase the patient's discomfort. The experienced manipulative physiotherapist is able to assess the rhythm of movement during the assessment of movement for range and pain described in the preceding paragraphs. Initially, however, she may require the patient to make many movements.

Disturbances of the normal rhythm of intervertebral movement during flexion and lateral flexion of the lumbar and thoracic spines are readily seen from behind (*Figures 6.15* and *6.16*). Abnormalities in trunk rotation are much more difficult to notice. To watch

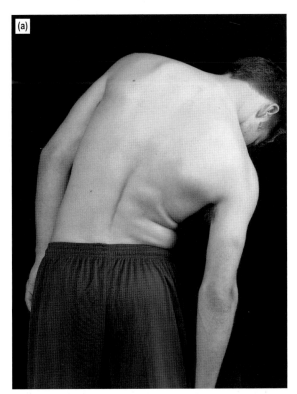 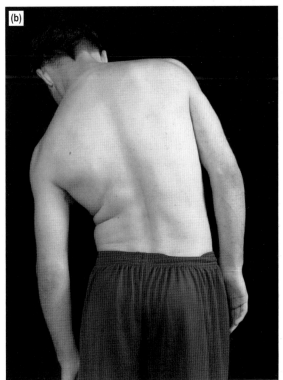

**Figure 6.15**   (*a*) and (*b*). The patient, when examined, appeared to bend equally to each side. In the two figures there is a difference in the appearance of the lumbar spine which looks like a limitation of movement when the spine is laterally flexed to the left. When the patient laterally flexed continuously from one side to the other it was easy to see that with movement to the left, the section of the spine between L1 and L3 remained straight. This stiffness had the same appearance as would be seen when bending a piece of hose that had an inch or two of cement somewhere within its length. There was no such stiffness with lateral flexion of the spine to the right

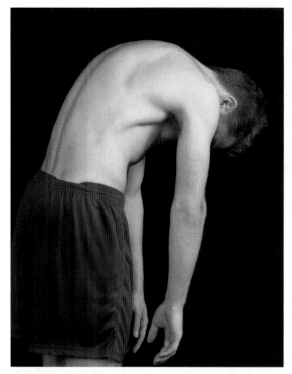

**Figure 6.16** This figure shows a limitation in the range of forward flexion at two levels of the thoracic spine. Between approximately T5 and T8 forward flexion is very limited, whereas between T10 and L1 the movement appears to a lesser degree. The movement above T5, below L1 and between T8 and T10 appears to be normal

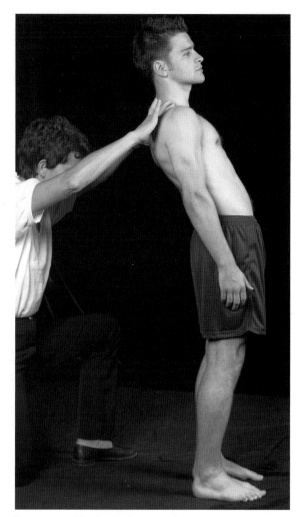

**Figure 6.17** Viewing lumbar extension

intervertebral movement during lumbar extension, the physiotherapist may need to kneel behind the patient while supporting his shoulders to prevent his overbalancing (*Figure 6.17*). If the position of testing lumbar extension is performed as shown in *Figure 6.18*, overpressure can be emphasized at single segments. The technique provides the examiner with any differences in 'end-feel' and symptom responses.

> Localized overpressure at a painful lumbar movement may provide the examiner with any differences in 'end-feel' and symptom responses

All spinal movements can be tested by moving either the upper spine on the lower spine, or the lower spine under the upper spine. In fact, these two modes can be combined; for example, the standing patient can be asked to rotate to the right as far as possible, and then, while his thorax is held in this position by the

physiotherapist, the patient can be asked to rotate his pelvis to the left. Moving joints in the same direction yet doing it in different ways can produce quite different pain responses, and should be investigated.

> Movements from the 'top down' may be compared with movements from the 'bottom up', as they can produce quite different pain responses

It should also be remembered that testing a movement in a weightbearing position may provoke a different pain response when comparing it with the same movement performed in the non-weightbearing position.

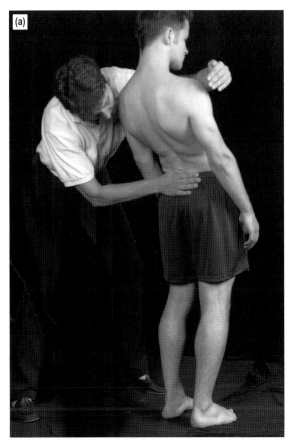
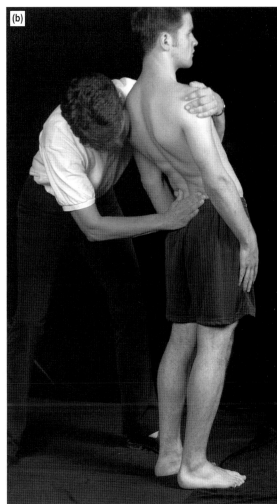

Figure 6.18   Assessing lumbar extension by over-pressure. (a) Preparatory positioning. (b) Over-pressure applied

---

Compare responses of test movements in weight bearing positions with non-weightbearing positions

---

All cervical movements should be watched carefully from the front because each can reveal useful information (*Figure 6.19*), but the contour of the neck when fully flexed is best seen from behind or above. The patient may rotate his neck with more flexion when turning to one side than to the other, possibly indicating a painful lesion in the middle or upper cervical area. Any abnormal movement found on examination must be present each time the movement is repeated for it to be judged significant.

The importance of watching the repeated movement lies in the fact that if a movement is tested only to note the range at which pain begins, only the gross movement of the vertebral column is assessed and insufficient account is taken of what is happening at the level of individual segments.

---

Do not only observe the gross movements of the spinal column and the beginning of the symptom response, but also the quality of the movements at the level of the individual vertebral segments

---

*Protective deformity.* An abnormal rhythm of movement may be present because of a painful lesion, or it may be due to an abnormality such as a joint stiffness, which is

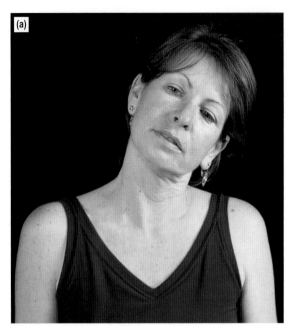
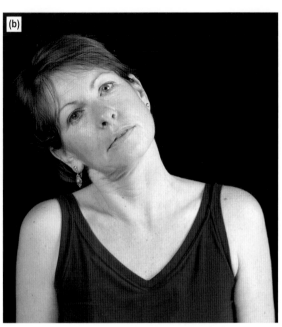

**Figure 6.19** (*a*) and (*b*). These two figures may appear, at first balance, to show a normal range of lateral flexion to each side. There is, however, a difference in the ranges of lateral flexion to each side taking place above the mid-cervical level. The restriction is shown by the lack of curve of the right neck contour above the mid-cervical level during lateral flexion to the left (*a*) when compared with the left neck contour during movement to the right (*b*). This limitation is easier to see when the patient repeatedly moves her neck in this plane. The therapist should observe the movement from ventral as from dorsal

painless. If it is caused by a painful lesion, pain will be provoked by preventing the abnormality occurring during the movement; if it is caused by joint stiffness, there will be no pain response. For example, if a patient who has a painful neck flexes his neck more when turning his head to the left than to the right, the physiotherapist should support his head and neck to prevent the flexion occurring during rotation to the left. If there is no pain response during this test, the abnormality is unrelated to the lesion causing the patient's pain. If the patient's pain is reproduced by this test, this is an example of a 'protective deformity'.

> Correct any deviation of a movement to determine if it indicates a protective deformity

Two common examples of static protective deformity are sciatic scoliosis and wry neck. Passive correction of these deformities will also cause pain. Most of the descriptive titles for these abnormalities are open to misinterpretation. For example, a so-called sciatic scoliosis commonly occurs when a patient has no sciatic pain but only back pain. Under these circumstances, it should not be called a 'sciatic' scoliosis. The clearest method is to name it as an ipsilateral or contralateral list, depending on the relationship of the list of the patient's thorax or head to the side of the pain. An ipsilateral list is a lateral displacement of the patient's thorax of head towards the painful side, and a contralateral list is when the displacement is away from the side of the pain. The relationship of the list to the side of the pain is important, but even more important is what happens to the list during movement; sometimes it will straighten out, and at other times it will increase and further movement will be impossible. A patient whose list increases with further movement will respond less easily to conservative treatment than will the patient whose list decreases or disappears.

Whenever a deformity of the section of spine under examination is evident, whether as a static protective type of deformity or as an abnormal movement, it may be tested by countering the abnormality so that its significance in relation to the patient's complaint can be determined. The degree of reproduction of the patient's pain caused by countering the deformity is the important assessment, but an attempt should be made to relate the deformity to previous history. The same protective deformity may have been present during previous episodes and may not have completely recovered; the significance of a current protective deformity would then be less. For example, if a patient on standing is seen to have a lumbar kyphosis, some of his deformity may be of a longstanding nature, particularly if previous episodes of back pain have been of similar severity. As such deformity does not usually completely disappear, at least 50 per cent of his present lumbar kyphosis is likely to be unrelated to his present pain. Another common example of 'old' mixed with 'new' is an arc of list that is visible during forward flexion of the lumbar spine. These are rarely if ever totally eliminated by treatment.

There is much yet to be explained about the protective lists, but there are more reasons than just for the protection of a painful root or its dural investment. There must also, on some occasions, be a mechanical disturbance, and this disturbance is sometimes irreversible (Maitland, 1961).

*Arm pain*. When the origin of a patient's arm pain is in doubt, it may be necessary to try to reproduce the pain by cervical movements. It is unwise and unnecessary to do this with severe nerve-root pain. If the normal tests of cervical movement do not reproduce the pain, rotation and lateral flexion (especially towards the painful side) and extension are three movements that should be tested in a special way. The head should be moved to the limit of the range or to the point where pain begins. If there is no pain or the pain is felt only in the neck, gentle pressure should be applied, increasing the movement and holding it for 10 seconds to see if pain spreads into the referred area. Occasionally referred pain may not be felt while the position is being held, but may occur when the movement is released. A similar test can be performed in the lumbar spine, using the movements of lateral flexion towards the side of the pain combined with extension. There is one further test that can be applied to the cervical spine to determine whether a referred pain is intervertebral in origin. It involves applying compression to the crown of the head while the cervical spine is slightly laterally flexed towards the painful side and minimally extended. The compression should be applied slowly and only increased to stronger pressure if the lesser pressure is not painful. Reproduction of the referred pain indicates that it is of cervical origin. Similar compression tests can be applied to the thoracic and lumbar spines, but they rarely reproduce referred pain.

## Combined movements

The combining of routine physiological movements to form test movements makes up a large part of the text of this book. In terms of examination, they are combined initially in directions that either open or close one side of the intervertebral segment. By performing them in this way, a *pattern* of painful movements may be found. Even if a pattern is not found, the movements should be combined in an effort to find a combination that relieves or increases the patient's symptoms. That is, if a patient flexes his trunk to the point where he feels pain in his lumbar sacral area, then the examiner should, in this position of flexion, assist the patient to flex laterally to the left and then to the right. On performing this movement, if pain is provoked with lateral flexion to the left, she should then add rotation of the trunk to the left and then to the right in this position of combined flexion with lateral flexion to the left. This is only one sequence of combining movements, but it does give an idea of how the movements can be combined to find the information being sought. Combining movements is discussed in each chapter of the different levels of the spine.

> Combinations of test movements are performed to find a combination that relieves or increases a patient's symptoms

## Movement patterns

by B. C. Edwards, OAM, BSc (Anat), BAppSci (Physio), Grad Dip Manip Th, MMPAA, FACP, Hon DSc (Curtin) (Specialist Manipulative Physiotherapist)

The movements of the vertebral column are complete and as yet not fully understood. The articulations are such that each vertebral segment, when moved, involves the movement of three different joints; two zygapophyseal joints and the disc. In the cervical spine the uncovertebral joints of Luschka also play a part, while in the thoracic spine the movements are complicated further by articulations of the ribs. As well as the shape of the articulations, the amount and type of movement that is possible at each level is affected by the soft tissue structures between the bony articulations and the structures within the neural foramina and vertebral canal.

Movements of the vertebral column do not occur in isolation, but rather in a combined manner. Some aspects of this have already been investigated (Farfan, 1975; Rolander, 1966; Troup *et al.*, 1968; Loebl, 1973). Gregerson and Lucas (1967) found that axial rotation in the lumbar spine was to the left when the subject bent to the left, and to the right when bending to the right. Interestingly, they found that in one subject the reverse was the case. Stoddard (1959) stated that the direction of rotation during lateral flexion in the lumbar and thoracic spine varies depending on whether the lateral flexion is performed with the whole spine in flexion or extension. He suggested that rotation is to the same side as lateral flexion when the movement of lateral flexion is performed in flexion, but to the opposite side when performed in extension. Kapandji (1974), however, stated that contralateral rotation occurs in conjunction with lateral flexion, but he did not mention any variation when the movement is performed in extension or flexion.

Personal laboratory observations on unpreserved lumbar spine specimens (which were removed within 24 hours of death and then frozen) would seem to indicate that the direction of rotation is in the opposite direction to that which the spine is laterally flexed regardless of whether the spine is in flexion, extension or neutral. There does appear to be some variation, however, depending on the presence or absence of degenerative changes within the zygapophyseal joint or disc.

There appears to be little dispute as to the direction of rotation in the cervical spine (C2–C7). This has been investigated by several authors (Lysell, 1969; Kapandji, 1974; Parke, 1975; Mesdagh, 1976; Penning, 1978). The direction of rotation appears to be the same regardless of whether the movement of lateral flexion is done in flexion or extension. Investigations so far appear to show that the combination of lateral flexion and rotation is always to the same side, and is related to the effect on the movement by the zygapophyseal joints. However, as mentioned previously, the involvement of the soft tissue, muscle, ligaments and structures within the canal and foramina all play a part in the type of movement possible at each level.

Because of the combination of movements that occurs in the vertebral column, the examination of the patient's movements can (and sometimes must) be expanded to incorporate these principles. In other words, there are times when to examine the basic movements of flexion, extension, lateral flexion and rotation is inadequate, and other movements combining these basic movements must be examined. Some aspects of this have already been described (Edwards, 1979, 1980). The symptoms and signs that are produced by examining rotary or lateral flexion movements performed while the spine is maintained in the neutral position in relation to other movements can be quite different from the signs and symptoms produced when the same movements are performed with the spine in flexion or extension. Testing movements while the spine is maintained in flexion or extension causes symptoms to be accentuated or reduced, and may change the symptoms from those of local spinal pain to those of referred pain.

> Examining rotary and lateral flexion movements in varying positions of flexion and extension helps to establish the type of movement pattern present

Combining movements gives an indication of the way signs and symptoms change when the same movement is done in flexion or extension. For example, the amount of rotation that is possible between C2 and C3 will vary depending on the amount of flexion or extension in which the movement is performed. Similarly, in the lumbar spine, the amount of lateral flexion may vary depending on the amount of flexion or extension in which the movement of lateral flexion is performed. Because of the above, the symptoms produced by testing movements with rotation in the cervical spine and lateral flexion in the lumbar spine may vary quite considerably, depending on whether the movement is done in the same degree of flexion or extension. Left rotation, say, of the cervical spine may produce left suprascapular fossa pain when the rotation is done in neutral. This pain may be accentuated, however, when the same movement is done in extension, and eased when done in flexion. In the lumbar spine, left lateral flexion may produce left buttock pain when the movement is done in neutral; however, the pain may be accentuated when the movement is done in extension and eased when done in flexion.

The movements described above involve the combining of two movements. However, the combining of three movements may also be performed. For example, lateral flexion and rotation can be done either in flexion or in extension. These movements can be performed in any section of the spine. *It is vital to realize that the sequence of performing the movements may also be varied and produce different symptomatic responses.* This is because whichever movement is performed first may reduce the available range of the second movement, and obviously the available range of the third movement. When using these combinations of movements as examining movements, care must be taken to ensure that each position is maintained while performing the next movement. It should also be understood that in the cervical spine, the flexion component of the movement, when performed in left rotation, requires the neck and head to be moved more in relation to the shoulder towards which the neck and head are turned, rather than approximating the chin towards the chest, as is the case in flexion of the cervical spine when performed in the anatomical position. An idea of the possible variations of sequence can be seen in the examples of lateral flexion and rotation to the left for the cervical spine:

1. Flexion first, lateral flexion to the left second, and rotation to the left third.
2. Flexion first, rotation to the left second, lateral flexion to the left third.
3. Lateral flexion to the left first, flexion second, and rotation to the left third.
4. Lateral flexion to the left first, rotation to the left second, and flexion third.
5. Rotation to the left first, flexion second, lateral flexion to the left third.
6. Rotation to the left first, lateral flexion second, and flexion third.

Different movements of the spine (i.e flexion, lateral flexion one way and rotation one way) can cause similar stretching or compressing movements on the side of the intervertebral joint. When flexion is performed in the sagittal plane, the articular surfaces of the zygapophyseal joint slide on one another, the inferior articular surface of the superior vertebrae sliding cephalad on the superior articular surface of the inferior vertebrae, while the interbody space is narrowed anteriorly and widened posteriorly. Rotation to the left can cause similar movement on the right zygapophyseal joint, as does left lateral flexion. This causes an opening movement, which is similar on the right of the intervertebral joint. The movement is similar in that it is an opening movement on the right, but it is *not* an identical movement.

The facts regarding a detailed analysis of combined movements can be related to the patients who have pain on movement. Some of the combinations of painful (or pain-free) movements follow recognizable patterns. Basically, there are two types of movement patterns that can be found on examining patients' movements that are mechanically disordered. They are regular and irregular; the regular patterns are stretching or compressing patterns.

> Regular patterns of movement combinations are stretching or compression patterns. They produce similar movements at the intervertebral joints, while producing similar symptoms

### Regular patterns

These are patterns in which movements produce similar movements at the intervertebral joints while producing the same symptoms, although these symptoms may differ in quality or severity. If the symptoms are on the same side to which the movement is directed, the pattern is a compressing pattern – that is, compressing

movements produce the symptoms. The reverse is the case if the symptoms are produced on movement to the opposite side, when the pattern is a stretching pattern.

Examples of compressing regular patterns:

1. Right cervical rotation produces right suprascapular pain, and this pain is made worse when the same movement is done in extension and eased when done in flexion.

2. Cervical extension produces right suprascapular pain, and this pain is made worse when right rotation is added to the extension and made worse still when right lateral flexion is added.

3. Right lateral flexion in the lumbar spine produces right buttock pain, which is made worse when this movement is done in extension and eased when done in flexion.

Examples of stretching regular patterns:

1. Right lateral flexion in the cervical spine produces left suprascapular pain; this pain is accentuated if the same movement is performed in flexion and eased when performed in extension.

2. Flexion of the cervical spine produces left suprascapular pain, and this pain is made worse when right lateral flexion is added and worse still when right rotation is added.

3. Right lateral flexion of the lumbar spine produces left buttock pain, and this pain is accentuated when the movement of right lateral flexion is performed in flexion and eased when right lateral flexion is performed in extension.

There are many patterns other than the simple stretching and compressing ones described above. These no doubt relate to biomechanical components, of which much still has to be understood. The influence of the changing instantaneous axis of rotation is one of the many confusing elements.

There is a further component to patterns of movement. So far, for the sake of making the subject simple to understand, only physiological movements have been mentioned. However, there are patterns of movements that include accessory movements with physiological movements. Two examples of regular patterns are:

1. Pain and restriction of movement on extension of the lower cervical spine matched by similar pain and restriction with postero-anterior pressure over the spinous process of C5.

2. Pain and restriction of movement on extension and on right lateral flexion of the lower cervical spine matched by comparable findings on postero-anterior pressure on the articular pillar of C5/6 at the intervertebral level.

> Other combined movements may include combining physiological with accessory movements

**Note**: The importance of palpation has been emphasized throughout this book. This being so, palpatory examination techniques must be included in every combined movement test that provokes or reproduces pain. It is best for the palpation to be added at the end-position of the combined physiological movements, rather than sandwiching it between physiological movements.

> Palpatory examination techniques must be included in every combined movement test

### Irregular patterns of movement

All patterns that are not regular fall into the category of irregular patterns. With irregular patterns, there is not the same conformity as described above. Stretching and compressing movements do not follow any recognizable pattern. There appears to be no correlation in the examination findings obtained when combining movements that either compress or stretch. There is a random reproduction of symptoms, despite the combining of movements that have similar mechanical effects.

> Irregular patterns of movement combinations do not follow any recognizable pattern of stretching or compression in the intervertebral joints

Examples of irregular patterns of movements:

1. Right rotation of the cervical spine (a compressing test movement) produces right suprascapular pain, and this pain is made worse when right rotation is performed in flexion (a stretching movement) and eased when the movement is performed in extension (another compressing movement).

2. Right lateral flexion of the lumbar spine (a compressing movement) produces right buttock pain, and this pain is accentuated when the same movement is done in flexion (a stretching, not a compressing movement) and eased when done in extension (a compressing movement).

3. Left lateral flexion in the lumbar spine (a stretching movement) produces a right buttock pain, and this pain is made worse when the same movement is done in extension (a compressing movement) and eased when the movement of lateral flexion is done in flexion (a stretching movement).

The many examples of irregular patterns, and combinations of painful movement, frequently indicate that there is more than one component to the disorder – for example, the zygapophyseal joint, the interbody joint and the canal and foraminal structures. Generally, traumatic injuries – e.g. whiplash – and other traumatic causes of pain do not have regular patterns of movement. Nontraumatized zygapophyseal and interbody joint disorders tend to have regular patterns of movement, because the movements of flexion, extension, lateral flexion and rotation have similar effects on the joints.

For a detailed description of Brian Edwards' original work (1992) in this area of combined movements, his book *Manual of Combined Movements* must be read. The book also contains details on the selection of techniques in treatment management.

## AUXILIARY TESTS ASSOCIATED WITH ACTIVE MOVEMENT TESTS

These tests are the performance of movements with the joint surfaces compressed together. Other tests such as those for vertebrobasilar insufficiency and neurological integrity come under this heading. These tests are described in the different spinal chapters as they occur.

### Neurological examination

There is a difference between neurological *signs* and neurological *changes*; 'changes' are objective physical deficiencies, whereas 'signs' are subjective abnormalities that can be determined on physical examination BUT are dependent upon the patient's statements and CAN be unreliable. A loss of sensation along the lateral border of the foot is a neurological change when, on examination, the patient does not flinch if the examiner gives a sharp jab with a pointed object (such as a pin or needle), especially if the jab produces detectable indentation. However, if the patient says he cannot feel a light wiping with a tissue on his symptomatic foot, as compared with the same degree of wiping on his sound foot, then it is a subjective finding; being dependent upon the patient's say-so, it is not an objective finding. Nevertheless, it can be acceptable to the examiner if the diminished sensation features fit with other clinical examination features.

The physiotherapist must report to the doctor any deterioration in neurological changes that may occur during treatment. This means that the physiotherapist must examine for and repeatedly assess possible neurological changes at the commencement of each treatment session.

## Referred pain

Referred pain having its origins in the nerve root or rootlets is called radicular pain; referred pain from other structures is simply referred pain and is not then a radicular pain.

It is a well-proven fact that referred pain can be caused by compression of the nerve root (Smyth and Wright, 1958) and by other sections of the intervertebral segment (Feinstein *et al.*, 1954). It may be difficult to describe precisely the difference between a nerve-root pain and a referred pain from other structures. Nerve-root pain can frequently be identified by its character; it is not just an ache, but a pain, often severe. The severity of the pain frequently shows in a patient's facial expression or in his description of the pain, or in the way he holds the limb. It is typically a very unpleasant sickening pain, and is most frequently greatest in the distal part of the dermatome. The pain is not necessarily reproduced by normal movement tests, but it frequently increases *after* a particular movement has been performed. The referred pain can, however, sometimes be reproduced if certain movements are held at the limit of the available range for some seconds (*see* p. 133). Referred pain from other sources does not behave in this way.

Not all nerve-root pain is severe, but when it is, the patients require especially careful neurological assessment and treatment must be gentle to avoid exacerbation if the best treatment results are to be gained.

To refer to the many diagrams of dermatomes is confusing unless it is understood how different structures refer pain. If the nerve root is the source of the patient's symptoms, they are frequently felt only in the distal part of the dermatome. This explains the type of charts supplied by Cyriax (1975). Clinical examples are patients whose pain starts distally, or patients whose back or neck pain disappears and is replaced by distal limb pain. However, it is common to have patients referred with pain in the spine continuous with the pain in the limb, which may or may not be worse distally. The reason for this may be that, while the nerve root causes some of the limb pain, other pain may be present as a result of disc pathology (Cloward, 1959). The disc may in turn be irritating other pain-sensitive structures in the vertebral canal, such as the nerve-root sleeve or dura (Cyriax and Cyriax, 1993). Supportive muscles and ligaments, with the apophyseal joints, disturbed by the disc damage, may also give rise to some of the local and referred pain. Referred pain of this kind indicates the need for charts showing pain locally and throughout the limb.

Muscle weakness resulting from nerve-root compression is best assessed by isometric (static) tests, and although each nerve root supplies more than one muscle, some muscles tend to be supplied by predominantly one root. The root or roots quoted are those found to have greatest clinical significance (*Figure 6.20*). While the patient lies supine, the power of the appropriate arm muscles can be assessed quickly in the order shown in *Table 6.9*. However, when assessing neurological muscle weakness, the tests may need to be extended considerably to ascertain the extent of weakness and nerve involvement. *Table 6.10* lists the muscles of the upper and lower limb, showing the nerve-root origin for the motor supply and the related peripheral nerve supply.

The relationship of sensory disturbance to nerve root involvement is simplified by remembering that the thumb and index finger are supplied by C6; the index, middle and ring fingers by C7; and the ring and little fingers by C8. Dermatomes of C5 and T1 reach to the wrist on the lateral and medial aspects respectively. In the foot, the dorsomedial aspect of the foot to the big toe is supplied by L4; the dorsum of the foot over the top of all the toes to the ball of the foot by L5; and the lateral aspect of the foot and the little toe by S1 (*see Figure 6.4*).

The biceps and triceps reflexes are the main reflexes in the arm, tested to elicit disturbances caused by nerve-root compression, although this test can be extended to the supinator, finger flexors and deltoid. To test the biceps reflex, the patient's slightly flexed arm muscle must be fully supported and completely relaxed. The thumb, placed firmly over the biceps tendon at the elbow, is then tapped with the percussion hammer. The triceps reflex is tested by tapping the triceps tendon behind the elbow while the patient's hand rests on his abdomen and his flexed elbow is supported in the physiotherapist's hand (*Figure 6.21*).

To test the knee jerk with the patient lying supine, the physiotherapist must slightly flex the patient's knee to approximately 30° and ensure that the quadriceps is relaxed before tapping the patellar tendon. When the response is weak, some reinforcement may be gained by asking the patient to grip his hands together in a monkey-grip and pull strongly.

If the ankle jerk is tested while the patient lies prone, the distal end of his tibia should be supported to flex his knee to approximately 30°. The tendo-Achilles is then tapped. This reflex activity is increased when the patient kneels erect on fully supported lower legs with his feet over the edge of the couch.

Normality of reflex activity is not complete without applying repeated tapping, at least six repetitions, to assess any degree of fatigue in the briskness of the

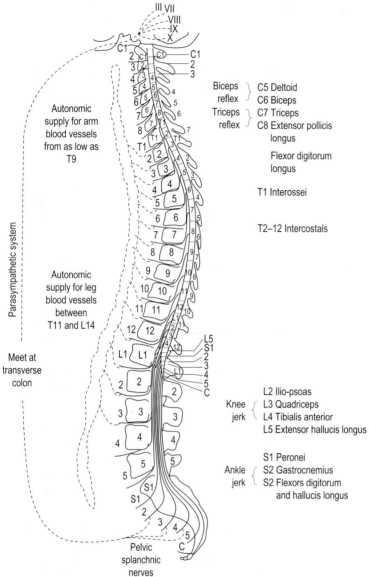

Figure 6.20   Nerve roots and the spine

response. Repetition is as important in the test of reflex activity as it is in the test of neurologically affected muscle power.

Finally, as a result of our interpretation of the neurological tests, we should realize that although nerve-root signs involving two roots can be due to benign pathology in the lumbar area, dual root signs are unlikely to have a benign origin in the cervical area.

> Dual root signs in the cervical spine are unlikely to have a benign origin

## PASSIVE TESTS

There are many passive movement tests that form part of the examination, including:

1. The movement of the pain-sensitive structures in the vertebral canal and intervertebral foramen and neural linked movements.
2. Physiological spinal movements.
3. The tension in soft tissue and the quality of movement of the intervertebral joint by palpation assessing the accessory movements.
4. The passive range of physiological movement of single intervertebral joints.

**Table 6.9**  Assessment of arm and leg muscles with isometric tests

| Muscle | Nerve root and reflexes | Method |
|---|---|---|
| Flexion of head on upper neck, rectus capitis anterior | C1 | The patient attempts to flex his head on his upper neck against the resistance applied by the physiotherapist's hand under the chin and on the forehead. |
| Extension of head on upper neck, rectus capitis posterior major and minor with obliquus capitis superior | C2 | While the patient attempts to extend his head on his neck the physiotherapist resists the movement by holding the occiput in one hand and the chin in the other. |
| Lateral flexion, scalene muscles | C3 | The patient attempts to flex his head and neck laterally while the physiotherapist resists the movement by placing one hand on the shoulder and the other on the same side of the patient's head and face. |
| Hitching scapula, trapezius and levator scapula | C4 | The physiotherapist applies resistance over the acromioclavicular joint area while the patient endeavours to elevate his shoulder girdle. |
| | | SUPINE |
| Abduction of arm, deltoid | C5 Biceps jerk | The patient holds his arm abducted 45° from his side and the physiotherapist applies resistance to the lateral aspect of the arm just above the elbow. |
| Elbow flexion, biceps | C6 Biceps and brachioradialis jerks | The patient holds his supinated forearm flexed at the elbow to 90°. Resistance is applied against the anterior surface of the forearm just above the wrist. |
| Elbow extension, triceps | C7 Triceps jerk | The patient holds his elbow flexed to 90° and resistance is applied against the dorsum of the forearm just above the wrist. |
| Extension of thumb, extensor pollicis longus | C8 | The patient flexes his elbow to 90° and supinates his forearm to mid-position and holds his extended thumb away from the palm pointing towards his face. Resistance is directed against the thumbnail towards the little finger. |
| Interphalangeal flexion, flexor digitorum profundus | C8 | The patient flexes his elbow to 90° and supinates his forearm to mid-position. The physiotherapist stabilizes his forearm and curls his fingers into his palm so that the patient in clenching his fist squeezes the physiotherapist's fingers. She tests the power of his long finger flexors by resisting terminal interphalangeal flexion. |
| Intrinsic action of the fingers | T1 | The patient flexes his elbow to 90°, extends his wrist, extends his fingers at the interphalangeal joints and flexes them at the metacarpophalangeal joints. The physiotherapist attempts to separate his fingers while the patient squeezes his extended fingers together. He then separates his fingers and she attempts to squeeze them together. |
| | Motor supply in the leg is tested standing, supine and prone lying | |
| | | STANDING |
| Plantar flexion, gastrocnemius | S1 | The patient stands on one leg rising on to his toes and lowering while the physiotherapist holds his hands to maintain balance. |

(*continued*)

**Table 6.9** (*contd*)

| Muscle | Nerve root and reflexes | Method |
|---|---|---|
| | | SUPINE |
| Hip flexion, iliopsoas | L2 | The patient holds his flexed hip and knee at 90° while resistance is applied just above the knee. |
| Knee extension, quadriceps | L3 Knee jerk | The physiotherapist threads one arm under the patient's lower thigh to place her hand on the opposite thigh. While the patient holds his leg just short of the fully extended position, resistance is applied against the front of the leg just above the ankle. |
| Dorsiflexion with inversion, tibialis anterior | L4 Knee jerk | The patient holds his foot in dorsiflexion and inversion while the physiotherapist applies resistance against the dorsomedial surface of the proximal end of the first metatarsal. |
| Big toe extension, extensor hallucis longus | L5 | The patient holds his foot and toes dorsiflexed while resistance is placed against the nail of the big toe. |
| Toe extension, extensor digitorum longus | L5 (and S1) | The patient holds his foot and toes dorsiflexed whilst resistance is applied against the dorsal surface of all toes. |
| Eversion, peroneus longus and brevis | S1 Ankle jerk | The patient is asked to keep his heels together and hold the soles of his feet twisted away from each other. The physiotherapist applies resistance against the lateral borders of the feet, pushing them towards each other. |
| Toe flexion | S2 | The patient flexes his toes over the pads of the physiotherapist's fingers. She resists his action of flexing his toes maximally. |
| | | PRONE |
| Knee flexion, hamstrings | L5 and S1 | The patient holds his knee flexed to 90° while the physiotherapist applies resistance behind the patient's heel. |
| Hip extension, gluteus maximus | L4 and L5 (S1 and S2) | The patient holds his hip extended with the knee bent while the physiotherapist applies a downward resistance just above the knee with one hand and palpates the gluteal mass medially with the other hand to assess firmness. |

OTHER NEUROLOGICAL TESTS
(as applicable)
1. Babinski;  2. Clonus

## Movement of pain-sensitive structures in the vertebral canal and intervertebral foramen, and neural linked movements

To be able to flex the spine fully and touch the toes requires free movement of the spinal cord, lumbosacral nerve roots and their investments. If forward flexion is restricted, it may be that the intervertebral joints are stiff or it may be that there is loss of movement of the structures in the canal or foramen. The tests that can be applied to move the structures in the vertebral canal without also moving the intervertebral joints are few in number.

Straight leg raising tests the free movement of the low lumbar and sacral nerve roots and their sleeves within the vertebral canal and intervertebral foramen. Although straight leg raising restricted to 40° can be

**Table 6.10**  Nerve-root origin for motor supply (M) and related peripheral nerve supply (P)

| Movements | Muscles | | Cervical | | | | | | | | | T |
|---|---|---|---|---|---|---|---|---|---|---|---|---|
| | | | 1 | 2 | 3 | 4 | 5 | 6 | 7 | 8 | 1 |
| Respiratory | Diaphragm | | | | P | M | P | | | | |
| Neck | Short flexors | | M | P | P | | | | | | |
| Flexion | Long flexors | | P | P | P | P | P | P | P | P | |
| | Sterno-mastoid | | P | M | M | P | | | | | |
| | Short extensors | | M | | | | | | | | |
| Extension | Long extensors | | | | P | P | P | P | P | P | P |
| | Trapezius  upper | | | P | M | M | | | | | |
| | middle | | | P | M | M | | | | | |
| | lower | | | P | M | M | | | | | |
| Scapula | | | | | | | | | | | |
| | Levator + rhomboids | | | | P | M | M | | | | |
| | Serratus anterior | | | | | | M | M | P | | |
| Gelno-humeral | | | | | | | | | | | |
| Ext. rot. | Infraspinatus | | | | | P | M | P | | | |
| Abduction | Supraspinatus | | | | | P | M | P | | | |
| | Deltoid  Post. | | | | | | M | P | | | |
| | Deltoid  Mid. | C | | | | | M | P | | | |
| | Deltoid  Ant. | | | | | | M | P | | | |
| Flexion | Coraco-brachialis | MC | | | | | | P | M | | |
| | Pec. Major Clav. | | | | | | P | P | P | P | P |
| | Stern. | | | | | | P | P | P | P | P |
| Internal rotation. | Subscapularis | | | | | | P | M | | | |
| adduction and | Teres major | | | | | | P | M | P | | |
| extension | Latissimus dorsi | | | | | | P | P | P | | |
| Elbow | | | | | | | | | | | |
| Extension | Triceps | R | | | | | | P | M | P | |
| Flexion | Brachialis | MC + R | | | | | P | M | | | |
| | Brachioradialis | R | | | | | P | M | | | |
| Supination | Biceps | MC | | | | | P | M | | | |
| | Supinator | R | | | | | P | M | P | | |
| Pronation | Pronator teres | M | | | | | | M | P | | |
| | Pronator quadratus | M | | | | | | | P | M | P |
| Wrist | | | | | | | | | | | |
| Extension | Extensors carpi rad. | R | | | | | | M | P | | |
| | Ext. carpi ulnaris | R | | | | | | M | M/P | P | |
| Flexion | Flexor carpi radialis | M | | | | | | | M | P | |
| | Flex. carpi ulnaris | U | | | | | | | M | P | |
| | Palmaris longus | M | | | | | | | M | P | P |
| Fingers | | | | | | | | | | | |
| Extension | Extensor digitorum | R | | | | | | | M | P | |
| | Flexor superficialis | M | | | | | | | P | M | P |
| | Flex. profundus    Lat. | M | | | | | | | | M | P |
| Flexion | Flex. profundus    Med. | U | | | | | | | | M | P |
| | Lumbricals 1, 2 | M | | | | | | | P | M | P |
| | Lumbricals 3, 4 | U | | | | | | | | M | P |
| | Opponens + Flex. V | U | | | | | | | | M | M |
| Abduction | Abductor dig. min. | U | | | | | | | | M | M |
| | Dorsal interossei | U | | | | | | | | M | M |
| Adduction | Palmar interossei | U | | | | | | | | M | M |

(continued)

**Table 6.10**  (*contd*)

| Movements | Muscles | | 1 | 2 | 3 | 4 | 5 | 6 | 7 | 8 | T 1 |
|---|---|---|---|---|---|---|---|---|---|---|---|
| **Thumb** | | | | | | | | | | | |
| Extension | Extensor pollicis L. | R | | | | | | | M | P | |
| | Extensor pollicis B. | R | | | | | | | M | P | |
| | Abductor pollicis L. | R | | | | | | | M | P | |
| Abduction | Abductor pollicis B. | M | | | | | | | | M | M |
| | Opponens pollicis | M | | | | | | | P | M | M |
| Flexion | Flexor pollicis L. | M | | | | | | | | M | M |
| | Flexor pollicis B. | M + U | | | | | | | | M | M |
| Adduction | Adductor pollicis | U | | | | | | | | M | M |

| Movements | Muscles | T 1–6 | T 7–12 | L 1 | L 2 | L 3 | L 4 | L 5 | S 1 | S 2 | S 3 |
|---|---|---|---|---|---|---|---|---|---|---|---|
| **Respiratory** | Diaphragm C 3, 4, 5 | P | P | | | | | | | | |
| | Intercostals | P | P | | | | | | | | |
| **Trunk** | | | | | | | | | | | |
| Extension | Sacrospinalis Thoracic | P | P | | | | | | | | |
| |     Lumbar | | | P | P | P | P | P | P | P | P |
| Side flexion | Quadratus lumborum | | P | P | P | P | P | | | | |
| Rotation | External oblique | P | P | | | | | | | | |
| | Internal oblique | P | P | | | | | | | | |
| Flexion | Rectus abdominus | P | P | | | | | | | | |
| | Transversus abdominus | P | P | | | | | | | | |
| **Hip** | | | | | | | | | | | |
| Adduction | Adductors | O | | | P | M | M/P | | | | |
| | Iliopsoas | | | P | M | P | | | | | |
| Flexion | Sartorius | F | | | M | P | | | | | |
| Abduction | Tensor fasciae latae | SG | | | | | P | M | P | | |
| and Inst. Rot. | Gluteus med. and min. | SG | | | | | P | M | P | | |
| Ext. Rot. | External rotators | O | | | | | P | M | P | | |
| Extension | Gluteus maximus | IG | | | | | | P | M | P | |
| **Knee** | | | | | | | | | | | |
| | Semimembranosus | S | | | | | P | P | M | P | |
| Flexion | Semitendinosus | S | | | | | P | P | M | P | |
| | Biceps | S | | | | | | P | M | P | |
| Extension | Quadriceps | F | | | P | M | M/P | | | | |
| | Vastus medialis | F | | | P | M | M/P | | | | |
| **Foot** | | | | | | | | | | | |
| | Extensor dig. longus | DP | | | | | P | M | P | | |
| Dorsiflexion | Extensor dig. brevis | DP | | | | | | M | P | | |
| Toes and | Extensor hal. longus | DP | | | | | | M | P | | |
| ankle | Extensor hal. brevis | DP | | | | | | M | P | | |
| Inversion | Tibialis anterior | DP | | | | | M | P | | | |
| | Tibialis posterior | T | | | | | P | P | | | |
| Plantar flexion | Gastrocnemius | T | | | | | | M | P | | |
| | Soleus | T | | | | | | M | P | | |
| Eversion | Peronei longus & brevis | SP | | | | | | M | M/P | P | |
| | Peroneus tertius | DP | | | | | | M | P | | |

(*continued*)

Table 6.10    (contd)

| Movements | Muscles | T | T | Lumbar | | | | | Sacral | | |
|---|---|---|---|---|---|---|---|---|---|---|---|
| | | 1–6 | 7–12 | 1 | 2 | 3 | 4 | 5 | 1 | 2 | 3 |
| Toe flexion | Flexor dig. longus | T | | | | | | | P | M | P |
| | Flexor hal. longus | T | | | | | | | P | M | P |
| | Lumbricals | | | | | | | | | P | M |
| Abduction | Medial plantars | | | | | | | | | P | M |
| and adduction | Lateral plantars | | | | | | | | | P | M |

C = Circumflex nerve; DP = Deep peroneal nerve; F = Femoral nerve; IG = Inferior gluteal nerve; M = Median nerve; MC = Musculocutaneous nerve; O = Obturator nerve; R = Radial nerve; S = Sciatic nerve; SG = Superior gluteal nerve; SP = Superficial peroneal nerve; T = Tibial nerve; Th = Thoracic; U = Ulnar nerve.

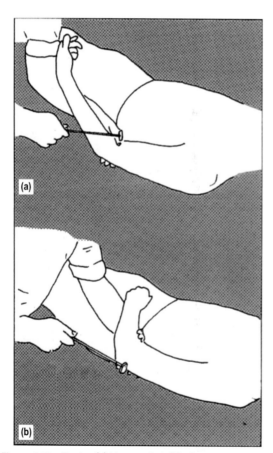

(a)

(b)

Figure 6.21    Testing (a) biceps reflex; (b) triceps reflex

indicative of nerve-root restriction from herniated disc material (Charnley, 1951), pain at full range can indicate some interference with the painless movement of the structures in the canal or foramen. Gross limitation

of passive knee flexion while the patient lies prone can similarly be a sign of restriction of movement of one of the nerve roots of the lumbar plexus, while any reproduction of pain with an almost full range of movement may indicate mild interference and should be noted. For the cervical and upper thoracic canals, if flexion of the head and neck provokes pain in the erect sitting position, adding pelvic flexion and lumbar slumping will move the canal structures caudally without altering the cervical and upper thoracic intervertebral relationships.

Care is required when testing straight leg raising, because minimal restriction may be missed if the test is not done correctly or if it is not repeated two or three times in quick succession while watching carefully for any abnormality of pelvic movement or difference in tension when compared with movement of the other leg. When raising the leg, the knee must not be allowed to bend and the pelvis must not be allowed to rise from the examination couch or hitch towards the shoulder on the side being tested. The leg being tested should be held in a slight degree of hip adduction, keeping the medial malleolus slightly lateral to the median sagittal plane, while lateral rotation at the hip must be prevented. It is possible to increase the tension on the lower lumbar and sacral nerve roots, their rootlets (Macnab, unpublished observations) and their sleeves when testing straight leg raising by passively dorsiflexing the patient's foot while holding his leg at the limit of straight leg raising. The tension may be further increased by fully flexing his head and neck while in the straight leg raising and ankle dorsiflexion position.

Another aspect relevant to the straight leg raising test is that, as there is an increase in intradiscal pressure when the patient sits or stands compared with when lying (Nachemson and Morris, 1964), this may effect a discrepancy in the degree of limitation of straight leg raising performed in the standing and lying positions. Testing in both positions can therefore be of value.

Movement of the dural investments of the spinal cord can also be effected in the supine patient by passively flexing his head and neck. As an example, a patient may have gluteal pain for which examination findings do not clearly identify the lumbar spine or the hip as being the cause. If passive flexion of the head and neck while the patient lies supine reproduces the gluteal pain, and particularly if the range of movement is limited by the pain, restriction of movement of pain-sensitive structures in the vertebral canal is identified as the cause of the pain. This test is used for the thoracic and lumbar spines. Maximum tension can be exerted on the canal structures if the patient sits slumped with his chin on his chest.

To test the movements of the cervical or thoracic nerve roots or their sleeves by applying tension is not so clear cut. However, in the cervical spine, information of a similar nature may be gleaned when the patient is afforded relief of symptoms by placing his hand on his head (thus relieving tension on the fifth cervical nerve root), or supporting his elbow in his other hand in a sling-like fashion (to relieve tension on the seventh cervical nerve root). Conversely, tension can sometimes be increased by protracting the shoulder and stretching the arm across in front of the body.

The work by Breig (1978) presents considerable scope for thought regarding positions and movements of structures in the vertebral canal, and this is discussed in Chapter 10. In the preface to the fifth edition of this book, reference was made to the work being carried out by Elvey, related to movement of nerves in the cervical area, and this too is discussed in Chapter 10.

There is a further test for movement in the cephalad/caudad direction within the vertebral canal and the intervertebral foramen, and this tests movements within the full length of the spine. The test is called the 'slump test'.

## Slump test

The test is called the slump test for two reasons. The first is that when the patient is sitting and the examiner wants him to adopt the position described below (point 2), most patients respond accurately and quickly to the instruction to slump. The second reason is that the action of adopting the test position parallels a test used by architects and engineers for assessing

the consistency of wet concrete and also called the slump test.

With the patient sitting on the examination couch, the therapist proceeds as follows:

1. The patient is asked to sit well back until the posterior knee area is wedged against the edge of the examination couch so that uniformity of the test position is maintained. In this erect sitting position, he is asked to report any pain or discomfort (*Figure 6.22*).

2. He is then asked to let his back slump through its full range of thoracic and lumbar flexion, while at the same time preventing his head and neck from flexing. Once he is in this position, gentle over-pressure is applied to the shoulder area so as to stretch the thoracic and lumbar spines into full flexion. The direction of pressure is a straight line from T1 to the ischial tuberosities, as though increasing the convexity of a bow by shortening its string (*Figure 6.23*). Any hip extension that might take place, as would be the case if the convexity increased markedly, must be prevented by bringing the patient's shoulders

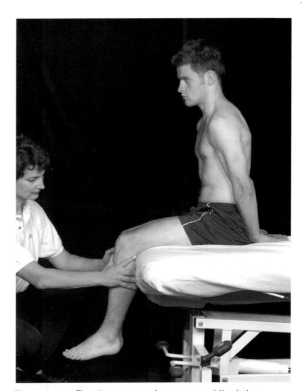

**Figure 6.22** The slump test: pain response while sitting well back

closer to his knees. Any pain response in this position is noted (*Figure 6.24*).

3.  Having established a 90° hip flexion angle he is asked to flex his head and neck fully, approximating his chin to his sternum. Sufficient over-pressure is applied to the neck flexion position to ensure that the whole spine from head to ischial tuberosities is on equal stretch. The range with pain response is recorded (*Figure 6.25*). Next, the over-pressure maintaining the head and neck flexion is maintained by the physiotherapist's chin (*Figure 6.26*) and then her left hand is free to palpate his spine (*Figure 6.27*).

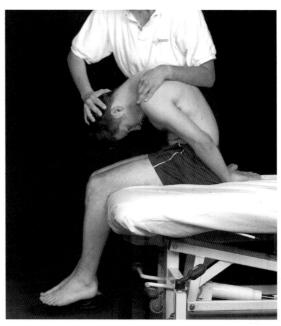

**Figure 6.25**    Fully flexed spine, from head to sacrum

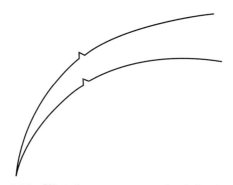

**Figure 6.23**    Effect of over-pressure on spine during slump test

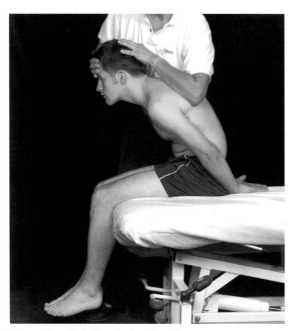

**Figure 6.24**    Fully flexed spine, from T1 to sacrum

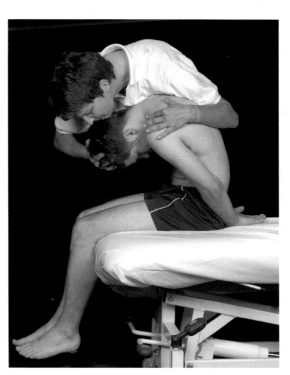

**Figure 6.26**    Maintenance of over-pressure with physiotherapist's chin

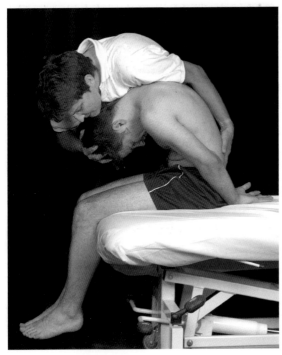

**Figure 6.27**    Palpation of spine while maintaining over-pressure at the cervical spine.

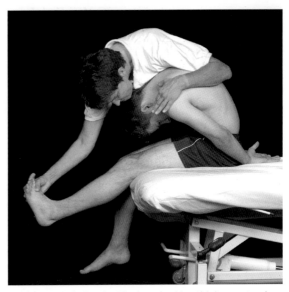

**Figure 6.29**    Active dorsiflexion of ankle, with knee extension and spine over-pressure

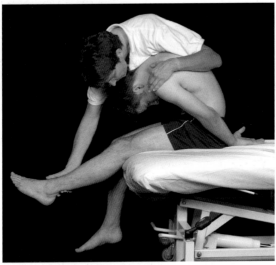

**Figure 6.28**    Knee extension with entire spine under over-pressure during slump test

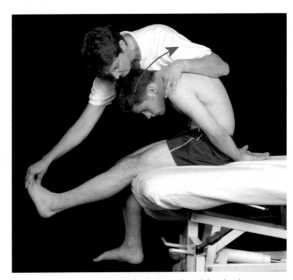

**Figure 6.30**    Raising of neck to neutral position in slump test

5.  The next step is to add active dorsiflexion of the ankle to the knee extension and note the pain response (*Figure 6.29*).

6.  While the neck flexion to knee extension position is maintained, and being sure that the symptoms are stable and consistent, the physiotherapist retains the same over-pressure to thoracic and lumbar flexion while at the same time releasing some of the neck flexion, allowing the patient's head to be raised to the neutral position (*Figure 6.30*) or extended (*Figure 6.31*). He is asked to state clearly

4.  With the whole spine maintained in flexion with over-pressure, he is asked to extend his left knee as far as possible, and while he is holding it in this position the range and pain response is noted (*Figure 6.28*).

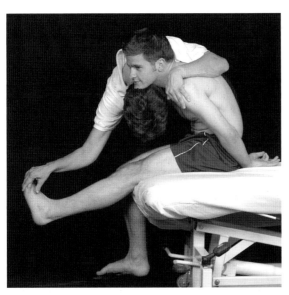

**Figure 6.31**    Head and neck extended in slump test

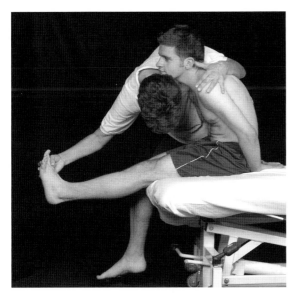

**Figure 6.32**    Assessment of further knee extension and ankle dorsiflexion with head and neck extended

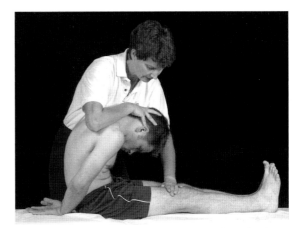

**Figure 6.33**    The slump test in the long-sitting position

what happens to the symptoms. In the fully slumped position he may not have a full range of knee extension. If he is unable to extend his knee fully he is then asked, when neck flexion has been released, if he can extend his knee further. In this new position the range is noted and any pain response recorded (*Figure 6.32*).

This test is effective for all levels of the spine, and should form part of the examination for cervical disorders just as much as for lumbar disorders. When firmer over-pressure is required for the assessment, the procedure can be carried out in the long-sitting position – that is, with the patient sitting on the couch with his legs stretched straight in front of him (*Figure 6.33*).

In making a judgement as to the findings of the test, *the pain responses, particularly in relation to releasing the neck flexion component, are the most important*. A pain-free lack of 30° of knee extension can be normal, as can pain felt centrally at the T9, T10 level (Maitland, 1980b).

An immediate relief of the symptoms on releasing neck flexion indicates involvement of the canal's pain-sensitive structures and, although there may be some restriction of knee extension due to hamstring tightness, this range would be unaffected by releasing the neck flexion. Having extended the cervical spine, which slackens the canal structures, the patient may then be able to gain further extension of the knees. Again, this clarifies the extent to which hamstring tightness is restricting knee extension. There may be some hamstring restriction as well as a canal component to a patient's symptoms. With a patient who is generally very mobile, it is necessary to reach full flexion by getting his head down between his knees. If he is very stiff, this will not be possible and one can expect the canal structures also to be tight. This is seen in people who can, on flexion in standing, hardly reach their knees (they may even comment that at junior school they had difficulty touching their toes), and this stiffness will remain regardless of their exercising. If the source of this restriction is neural, cervical flexion and extension will change the symptomatic response, while in the flexed position. Although some people cannot fully straighten their knees in the slumped position, it does not mean that the range is abnormal; it may be normal *for them*. It is the pain response and the change in knee extension with the release of neck flexion that is important.

**Variations of slump positions** When the slump test is negative although the information gained during the subjective examination indicates involvement of the canal structures, then the test can be taken one stage further by substituting cervical extension for the cervical flexion that may reproduce the symptoms. Only rarely has this been found to be neurally positive, but it can be a useful finding, and used as an asterisk, when the usual test is negative.

The pain-sensitive structures in the vertebral canal have a supporting role with spinal movements of lateral flexion and rotation. This therefore demands, where there are either unilateral symptoms or bilateral (or central) symptoms with physiological or accessory provocative joint signs, that the slump test should be performed incorporating lateral flexion, rotation or the two combined (*Figure 6.34*) (Maitland, 1984).

> Depending on the patient's symptoms and signs, sometimes side flexion or rotation, or a combination of the two movements, should be incorporated into the slump test

There are two options. Begin either by starting the test with lateral flexion (or rotation) and note the pain response; then add the stages of the slump test as already described. The second option is to start in the slump position and then add the lateral flexion (*Figure 6.34*) or rotation.

When the added rotation or lateral flexion provokes the symptoms, neck flexion should be released to assess the symptomatic behaviour. This is the most incriminating aspect of the test. If, however, releasing the neck flexion effects no change, the slump position can be maintained while the lateral flexion (or rotation) is minimally released and any alteration in pain response is noted. If the pain is diminished by releasing lateral flexion (or rotation), the test is not necessarily positive; the diminished pain response may be due to releasing one component of the combined spinal joint position. Therefore, in this new minimally reduced lateral flexion (or rotation) position, changes of the slump knee extension and neck flexion release need to be reassessed. If they result in reducing the provocation still further, it would seem that the canal structures are implicated. This action is essential for differentiating between joint and canal structures.

**Cervical slump** Another slump test, which is primarily used for cervical or upper thoracic disorders, is the cervical slump test, which is performed with the patient in the erect sitting position. He is first asked to flex his head and neck to the point where the cervical symptoms first begin (or first begin to increase). With the head/neck held in this position, he is asked to flex his lumbar spine by pelvic flexion. (It is often necessary for him to be taught how to perform the pelvic movement separately.) The earlier in the lumbar flexion range that the cervical symptoms increase, the more positive is the finding that the canal structures are involved in his disorder; also, the less easily the disorder will respond to conservative non-invasive management.

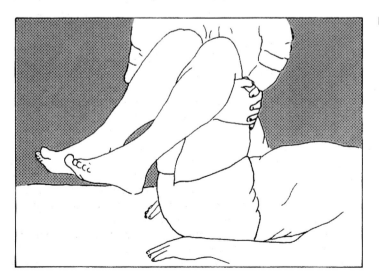

Figure 6.34 Passive lumbar lateral flexion

The cervical slump test is primarily used for cervical or upper thoracic disorders

The slump test is rarely chosen as an initial treatment technique. It can frequently and safely be assumed that there is likely to be irritation of the canal structures due to abnormal movement. This is certainly so in the low lumbar spine. Treatment of the joint and reassessment of the slump findings will indicate if slump treatment techniques are necessary. If, on reassessment, the joint movements improve but the slump findings do not, then the slump may be the element that provokes the symptoms. It is possible to predict how someone will recover from soreness provoked by stretching painful soft tissue structures, but the canal structures do not recover at the same rate; they are much slower. Therefore, when the slump test is used as a technique, care must be taken on the first day and assessment over 24 hours is then necessary to determine whether the strength of the technique needs to be changed. If it is performed vigorously, an interval of 2–3 days should be left between treatments for soreness to settle so as to make accurate reassessment possible to determine how much has been gained.

The slump test is rarely chosen as an initial treatment technique. Treatment of the joint signs and reassessment of the slump findings will indicate if slump treatment becomes necessary

There are situations, however, when neck flexion in the slumped position (without knee extension) causes severe sharp pain in the back. Neck flexion in slump may then be chosen as the first treatment movement.

**Neural linked movements**   Breig (1978), during 1960, was probably the first to make the important impact needed in the area of adverse mechanical tension in the central nervous system. This work has been taken up by Elvey since 1978, and extended by Butler (1991) for the manipulative physiotherapists.

Breig has clearly shown the need to compare the range and pain responses of cervical movements performed in sitting, left side lying, right side lying, and prone lying. These comparisons should be investigated when the patient's symptoms and history indicate the possibility of a neural component.

Butler has gone further, explaining test movements to include the peripheral nervous system (entrapment neuropathy and other affected abnormalities of peripheral neural movement). He makes the essential point of specific examination techniques and treatment methods for every clinician who practises as a manipulative therapist.

For the upper limb, the 'thoracic outlet' test remains a primary procedure. It includes arm traction (shoulder girdle depression), which provokes the arm symptoms (Phillips and Grieve, 1986). Added to this, Butler (1991) describes three other basic tests, the first making use of cervical lateral flexion (contralateral and ipsilateral) with the limb stabilized to compare the symptomatic changes. This is also Elvey's basic test. The second basic test utilizes shoulder depression and either a median nerve bias (Figure 8,5F, as shown in Butler's book) or a radial nerve bias (Figure 8,6D). The third has, as its final stretch position, shoulder depression plus abduction and lateral rotation, with elbow flexion and wrist and fingers in extension, so that the patient's hand reaches the side of his face. The head and neck can be placed in contralateral flexion at the beginning of the procedure or as the final movement (Figure 8,10,G, as shown in Butler's book).

For the lower limb there is straight leg raising (*see Figure 12.63*) with the foot in different positions, such as dorsiflexion, plus inversion and eversion (similarly with plantar flexion) and also with hip adduction. The second basic position is in prone lying, where the knee is flexed and, if necessary, adding hip extension.

## Passive physiological intervertebral movements (PPIVMS)

It is necessary to describe briefly the less specific passive movement tests for sections of the spine, even though they are relatively obvious.

The physiological movements of flexion, extension, lateral flexion and rotation in sitting and standing can be repeated passively in the nonweightbearing position. This very general test of movement is only required when it is necessary to determine whether load through the joint makes any difference to the pain felt on movement.

The physiological movements of the spine are tested passively in the lying position. The techniques, except for lumbar lateral flexion and lumbar rotation, are obvious and do not require description. Lateral flexion in the lumbar spine, however, is performed by the physiotherapist supporting the patient's flexed knees and hips at a right angle and pivoting his feet away from her. When hip rotation reaches the limit of the range, the pelvis tilts laterally and lateral flexion then takes place in the lumbar spine. Lateral flexion in the opposite direction is tested by pivoting the patient's feet in the opposite direction (*Figure 6.34*). Rotation is produced by flexing one of the patient's hips and knees to a right angle, and carrying the knee across the patient to rotate his pelvis and lumbar spine with his leg.

## Intervertebral tests by palpation

In relation to examining the normality or otherwise of intervertebral movements, the most important techniques are those that follow. A patient's physiological movements may appear normal, yet the palpation tests for intervertebral movement will reveal joint signs in appropriate positions. If a patient has nerve root pain, and when this pain is felt only in the distal extent of the dermatome, then the patient's symptoms can frequently be reproduced by the specific physiological movements described on page 133. These tests are the sustained positional tests and the quadrant tests, and the test movements reproduce the symptoms by altering the relationships of pain-sensitive structures in the intervertebral canal. Under these circumstances, passive tests of movement of the intervertebral segments can be negative. In contrast to this, if the patient has symptoms arising from the intervertebral joint, in the absence of any abnormality of movement of the pain-sensitive structures in the vertebral canal, then the tests by palpation will always be positive. They may be difficult to ascertain, but if the directions of movement are tested properly as described in the following section, positive signs of pain, restriction or muscle spasm will be found in one or more directions of the palpation movement. It is also necessary to point out that testing physiological movements either actively or passively does not involve the accessory movements of the intervertebral joints, whereas the palpation movement tests can be directly related to the accessory movements.

> The palpation movement tests can be directly related to the accessory movements

Some readers may question the accuracy of the palpation in determining the intervertebral joint responsible for a patient's syndrome. Jull *et al.* (1984), in the report of a research project, said:

> *The conclusion that can be drawn from this study at this point, is that manual diagnosis, by a trained manipulative therapist, can consistently and accurately determine the offending level in cases of spinal pain mediated by medial branches of the dorsal rami. In this respect manual diagnosis is as accurate as radiologically controlled diagnostic blocks.*

## General palpation routine

> The general palpation routine should consist of:
>
> - Positioning joints in their mid-position for range and comfort
> - Assessing for changes in temperature or evidence of sweating
> - Assessing for soft tissue changes, superficial to deep, general to localized
> - Assessing for bony anomalies, e.g. spinous process position and relative depth
> - Checking for movement anomalies (PAIVMS) – general comparisons of mobility, and early, mid, late range
> - Assessing the pain response to soft tissue palpation and PAIVMS
> - Completing movement diagrams

A palpation examination is performed in the following sequence. First, the patient must be so positioned that there is no lateral flexion or rotation, and so that the spine lies in its natural mid-flexion/extension position (i.e. lying prone or supine for the cervical spine). To make the palpation examination as objective as possible, the examiner should make it clear to the patient that she does not wish it to be a painful procedure. However, the patient should understand that he should not comment (verbally or non-verbally) on when the examination is, or is not, causing discomfort or pain, until later in the procedure – when the examiner has determined which are the normal and abnormal findings in the relevant areas, he will be asked to compare the symptomatic with the asymptomatic sites.

Over recent years there has been considerable discussion and investigation into the validity of palpation examination reliability. More recently, Jull *et al.* (1993) have summarized the work that has been done relating hypomobility and pain response to the source of a patient's symptoms. There is no doubt, in the author's mind, that the manipulative physiotherapist can assess abnormalities of supportive tissues, the shapes and positions of bony prominences and of intersegmental movement. However, it is also necessary to be able to relate these abnormalities to the patient's symptoms and the disorder.

To gain the patient's confidence, the therapist should use the hands and fingers in a general manner over the relevant part of the back as a soothing, circular-type massage during which a general impression can be gained as to the state of the superficial soft tissues. This need not take longer than a few seconds, and is invaluable in gaining the confidence of the apprehensive patient or the patient with extreme tenderness.

The palpation examination of the spine includes the following tests:

1. Skin sweating and temperature.
2. Soft tissue changes.
3. Position of vertebrae.
4. Movement of vertebrae.

When the spine is being examined, the patient lies prone and the skin is checked for sweating and temperature. Palpation for muscle spasm and general tissue tension then follows. Finally, before testing intervertebral movement, the positions of the vertebrae should be assessed in relation to adjacent vertebrae. Not too much importance should be placed on abnormalities found in this latter assessment, as they are only relevant if they can be verified by radiography. As there are some differences in procedure for testing different levels of the spine, each will be described separately in the chapters for each section of the spine. Description of the tests of movement then follow.

Palpating the soft tissue associated with the abnormal intervertebral segment reveals information that cannot be gained in any other way. Even when all other physical tests are negative, palpation is positive. Grieve (1989) comments strongly on this issue. The texture of the tissues differentiates between old tissue changes and new tissue.

## Palpation examination

### Skin sweating and temperature

Any excessive sweating relevant to the level of the spine under examination is found by wiping the hand just once over a wide area, with the main attention being at the paravertebral area. Relevant findings should be noted and assessed at following treatment sessions for changes to the findings. Excessive sweating is not a common finding, but when it is noted it adds to the other examination findings in identifying the level of the spine involved in the disorder.

Examination for temperature changes (mainly increased temperature) is far more important than sweating, and has implications that cannot be ignored. We are taught that inflammation is indicated by 'red, hot, swelling', but redness and swelling are not common with spinal disorders. Warmth or heat, on the other hand, is quite common, and it immediately makes the examiner think of an inflammatory component. However, the warmth, when it is found, does not indicate whether it is a mechanical response or a response to an active disease process. These two differences can only be determined by other general health indicators, or by the responses to the first two mobilization

treatments. The mechanical warmth will disappear or be markedly diminished by the beginning of the second treatment session; it may even disappear by the end of the first treatment session. The response to an active medical condition will not change favourably over two treatments, and such a response could well mean that the disorder is not in the province of the physiotherapist.

> Warmth created by a local mechanical disorder will disappear after two sessions of mobilization. Heat from an active inflammatory disorder will not change significantly over the two mobilization sessions

The best method of examining for warmth is not the same as is usually taught; that is, using the back of the hand is not the best way to feel many of the temperature changes. It is better to place the full breadth of the palm over an appropriate area and keep it in that position for a few seconds to gauge the temperature. The palm is then placed and retained on various sites above and below the symptomatic area and moved from right to left. This procedure is repeated over these sites, comparing the different temperatures until a decision is made.

It is difficult to describe the differences in the kinds of heat/warmth that can be felt. However, experience teaches that the relevant variety is one that is felt to come from deeper within, rather than being just on the surface. From the 'within' situation, it seems to build up and work its way towards the surface, and the palm can feel this difference.

> The warmth/heat most relevant to the manipulative physiotherapist is felt to come from within, working its way to the surface

The flat palm method can then be modified by using mainly the hypothenar eminence to determine the superior and inferior margins of the area of warmth. The area can be further defined if the warmth is felt to be localized to the vertebral column. The method then is to use the pad of the thumb placed transversely over the lamina on one side of the vertebra (mainly in the interlaminar area), with the tip of the thumb reaching the inter-spinous space. The same process of retaining the position until the temperature is gauged is used. The positions are then changed so that the levels above and below as well as the left and right of the column can be compared (Lando, 1994).

### Soft tissue changes

These changes are to be found in the ligamentous, capsular, muscular and connective tissues as thickening or muscle spasm. Palpation of them can reveal tenderness.

Palpation continues by using the full length of the pads of the middle and ring fingers of each hand in the interlaminar-trough area (from the lateral surface of the spinous process to the lateral margin of the articular pillar from C1–C7). The technique involves moving both hands in rhythm with each other, moving the skin up and down with the pads of the fingers as far as the skin allows, while gently sinking into the muscle bellies and other soft tissue. The purpose is to feel for areas of thickness, swelling and tightness in the soft tissue, and also for any abnormalities of the general bony contour. Having performed two or three up and down movements in the area, the fingers should be made to slide caudad 20–30 mm and the process repeated. This is then continued, moving down over the related area. A particular level may be returned to if an abnormality is felt there.

Once the general and more gross impression has been gained through the full pads of the fingers or thumbs, the procedure should be repeated but this time using the tip of the pad of only one digit of each hand and emphasizing the examination to the areas where discrepancies from the normal have been found.

A reasonably accurate determination of the *site* and *type* of tissue abnormality should be made so that a more detailed determination can be made later.

The most common findings at this stage of the examination are:

1. General tightness of muscle tissue along almost the full length of the spine.
2. Local areas of thickening immediately adjacent to one or more spinous processes.
3. Local areas of thickening in the mid-laminar-trough area.
4. Soft thickening over the posterior articular pillar at one or more intervertebral levels.
5. Hard bony thickening and prominence over the zygapophyseal joints.
6. Tightness of the ligaments or localized thickening of a section.

> The older the soft-tissue changes, the tougher they are; the more recent they are the softer they are

The abnormalities of 'feel' in ligamentous, capsular and connective tissues are that the older they are the tougher they feel; and the more recent they are, the softer they feel. For example, palpating old capsular

thickening around the apophyseal joint will be like pressing against leather; there are even variations in the hardness of the leathery feel. Thickening from more recent stresses will be softer or spongier, and this may overlie an older leathery feeling. Thickening within the muscular tissue is usually more diffuse, and rarely feels like hard leather. Nevertheless, when thickening is present it has a stringy feel if it is 'old', and a smoother feel if it is 'new'.

It is necessary to explain to the patient that he should only comment on tenderness if he feels that palpation is excessive, or that to continue palpation will lead to increased symptoms the following day. Explain that when the examination is finished he will be asked for his comments as to what he feels with pressure being applied to the anomalies that the examination has elicited. *It is essential for the therapist to realize that just because an area is thickened or stiff, it does not have to be either painful or the source of a patient's symptoms.* It can, however, be the reason for an adjacent segment to be overworked and thus become painful. By referring to *Table 6.3* (planning the physical examination), it can be seen that the 'thickening/stiffness' becomes the Part two rather than being the *source* of the symptoms (Part one of the planning sheet). The stiffness then fits in as part of the treatment in that it requires the segment to be made more mobile so as to lessen the work required of the adjacent segment. In other words, it is treated as the *cause* of the source rather than the source itself. The discussion raises another issue; the patient has sought treatment for the symptoms, and is probably unaware of the reasons(s) behind them. If the patient has had recurring episodes of the same symptoms, the cause of the source can be explained to him, and the requirements of appropriate treatment (that is, to clear the assumed cause as well as treating the source) will be understood by him.

> A thickened or stiff area does not need to be painful or the source of a patient's symptoms

### The ideal, average and abnormal spine

The ideal spine consists of intervertebral joints that are normal in every respect. The average spine consists of one or more segments that are imperfect but have no symptoms of major consequence. The abnormal spine is both disadvantaged and symptomatic enough for the person to seek treatment.

1. *The ideal spine.* The ideal spine consists of a series of intervertebral motor segments (i.e. interbody and zygapophyseal joints with all of their supporting

ligamentous and motor structures) that are normal in every respect; that is, none is disadvantaged in any way by injury, wear and tear, structural anomaly or disease. Each motor segment is perfect.

2. *The average spine*. The average spine is *not* ideal, and does not consist of a series of ideal motor segments. One or more of them are abnormal in some way, even if they are not causing any symptoms of major consequence. The joint or joints may be imperfect because of:
   a) Congenital or acquired structural anomalies
   b) Degenerative changes
   c) Disease processes or changes resulting from trauma.

   Although the average spine is defined as having no symptoms of major consequence, this needs qualification. Some people have no symptoms whatsoever, while others have minor symptoms of a kind that they accept as normal (Maitland, 1982b). The three kinds of imperfection in the average spine are explained as follows:
   • There are people whose spine is disadvantaged by a congenital or acquired structural anomaly. Examples are a cervical bifid spinous process lacking one of its processes, thoracic or lumbar spinous process inclining towards the left or the right (*Figure 6.35*) or a congenital fusion between the second and third cervical vertebrae, which is not uncommon. Such anomalies are of themselves painless, but they do indicate either asymmetry or that more stress is placed on adjacent intervertebral segments.
   • Despite the presence of intervertebral degenerative changes due to wear and tear, old trauma or old disease processes which are not totally inactive, some people do not have any symptoms whatsoever. Within this group some spines, when palpated or stretched, are painless and some have a minor degree of pain or discomfort. Also within this same group of patients with degenerative intervertebral joints there are people who do have a degree of symptoms that are classed by them as being normal. When their spines are palpated or stretched, they always have a degree of pain (as compared with the previous group, which are either painless or complain only of discomfort). Of these subdivisions, group (1) (i.e. the ones with congenital or acquired structural anomalies) is quite different in kind from group (2) (those with anomalies associated with degenerative disease or traumatic changes), and should be regarded to be so. These patients are only 'disadvantaged' because in all other regards the individual segments fit the ideal group.

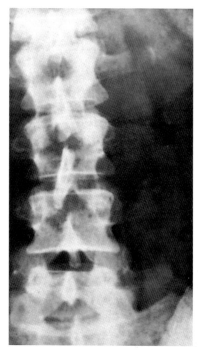

**Figure 6.35** Spine disadvantage by deviant lumbar spinous process (Reproduced from (1982) *The Australian Journal of Physiotherapy*, **28**, with kind permission of authors and publishers.)

   • The third group includes people whose spines show evidence of joint changes due to disease process or trauma and who do have symptoms, for which they may or may not have had adequate treatment, yet who accept these symptoms as being normal for them, despite the fact that the symptoms interfere with their normal life. On examination their joint movements are painful when stretched, and palpation findings are obvious.

3. *The abnormal spine*. The abnormal spine is defined as being a symptomatic spine for which the person seeks treatment. On examination, significant comparable signs will be evident on palpation at the appropriate intervertebral levels. The title 'abnormal' is used to signify an abnormal degree of symptoms rather than abnormal joints – which, as has been stated, may be totally painless.

This labelling into groups highlights important clinical connections between symptoms and examination findings, which can be assessed by the palpation examination. The value of having the different groupings enables therapists to recognize the differences between palpation findings that relate to a patient's symptoms, and those that are not necessarily related. Such differences can then also be related to treatment expectations. For example, it is possible to recognize, through the interpretations of the palpation findings, that the realistic goal of treatment may be a minimally symptomatic 'average' state or a pain-free 'average' state rather than an 'ideal' state.

Unfortunately, very few people over the age of 40 years have a total complement of 'ideal' intervertebral joints. Most people, for one reason or another, fit into one of the 'average' groups. If a group of 40-year-old people who had no pain or discomfort and considered their necks to be normal were examined by palpation, abnormalities would be found in nearly all.

The question is, when such a person has a spontaneous onset of vertebral pain and seeks treatment for it, how does the examiner differentiate between the findings that relate to the present problem and the findings that would have been present before the spontaneous onset of the neck pain? A similar difficulty arises when attempting to determine the degree of disability that can be attributed to a recent injury and the degree that is attributable to pre-existing yet painless 'average' joint findings.

*New or old tissue changes*. If an intervertebral joint suddenly becomes painful for no obvious discernible reason, it is still most likely that tissue changes have occurred. If these recent tissue changes have occurred in an 'ideal' joint, the only findings that will be detected by palpation examination will be of the 'new' or 'recent' kinds – as with, for example, a sprained ankle.

If these recent tissue changes have occurred in an asymptomatic 'average' cervical joint, then on examination by palpation there will be new tissue changes superimposed on the older 'average' tissue changes.

Success in differentiating between the new and old changes makes the prognosis, related to both the success of present treatment and the likelihood of future recurrences, easier to assess. This is an examination skill that can be taught.

If these recent tissue changes have occurred in a symptomatic 'average' segment, there will be 'recent' tissue changes superimposed on the changes that were already painful when stretched or palpated. Because the patient had symptoms before the exacerbation, the palpable tissue changes will not be as 'old' as those in the pain-free 'average' group. Differentiation between the 'new' and 'old' changes under these circumstances is much more difficult.

The ability to differentiate between these tissue changes is difficult to teach to inexperienced practitioners, but a method of thinking and assessing can be taught, which will provide a basis for developing the necessary skill.

## Bony anomalies – position of vertebrae

Bony points and interspinous spaces are palpated next. The tip of the thumb of each hand is used to palpate the bony outline of the spinous processes first.

There are two important planes in which to assess the position of the spinous processes; the first is that they should lie centrally in the sagittal plane, and the second is that they should lie roughly along an arc of a single sagittal circle. That is, the spinous processes should change evenly along the normal lordotic or kyphotic curve. However, normal variations with regard to depth or prominence should be allowed for when interpreting the positions in this plane.

With regard to bony anomalies, the features that can be determined by palpation include abnormal deviation of a spinous process from the central line without or with vertebral rotation; absence of one process of the bifid spinous process; abnormal position of one cervical vertebra relative to its neighbour; and osteoarthritic osteophyte formation of the margins of the apophyseal joints.

The abnormalities of deviation of spinous process and positions of vertebrae can be confirmed by X-rays. If a positional finding is longstanding, the shape of the associated vertebrae will have changed from their symmetrical appearance to accommodate the changed positions. The articular pillar abnormalities that indicate osteoarthritic (-otic) findings are readily determined by palpation, and can also be confirmed by X-rays. If the changes are 'old' and totally inactive, the bony margins of the exostoses will be hard and clean without any sign of soft or leathery covering.

Common findings are discussed in the relevant chapters.

## Movement abnormalities

Movement is assessed by using pressure through the tips of the thumbs against the spinous processes first. Two or three oscillatory postero-anterior movements are performed at each level in turn, moving fairly quickly up and down the spine, until a general impression of comparative movement (both quality and range) is determined.

The movements created by pressure on the spinous processes can be assessed even more finely by varying the direction of the pressures, inclining them left, right, cephalad and caudad. Combinations of these inclinations can also be used. Not only should the direction of the pressure be varied, but the precise point of contact on the spinous process should also be varied. This will produce a change in the movement occurring at the intervertebral segment.

The same procedure is carried out over the articular pillar at each level, comparing both the relative movement of adjacent levels, and the movement found at one intervertebral level on the left with the movement at the same level on the right.

Similar variations of direction and contact are applied to the articular pillar as described above for the spinous processes. However, one of the most useful test movements in the spine is achieved when thumb pressure is applied in a combined postero-anterior and medial direction. This direction of movement produces a maximum sliding of the apophyseal joint immediately under the thumbs. If this direction of movement is performed throughout its total range from maximum foraminal opening to maximum foraminal closing, a very valuable assessment of flexibility and quality of movement at the apophyseal joint is readily obtained. Also, by varying the hand and finger positions these postero-anterior pressures can be performed in such a way as to produce a rotary movement or a lateral flexion movement.

> Movement abnormalities of the intervertebral motion segments include hyper- or hypomobility, through range or end of range resistance, stiffness and spasm. Such abnormal physical findings can be depicted on a movement diagram

Movement abnormalities consist of the following: hyper- or hypomobility; abnormal quality of movement through range; stiffness and spasm. Such abnormalities can all be determined by the palpation being applied in a manner that produces intervertebral movement. Abnormalities of movement should be qualified in terms not only of the available range of movement, but also by any change in the normal free-running movement through the range up to the end of the available range. This may be disturbed by such factors as arthritic change, stiffness in supportive capsular and ligamentous structures, or by protective muscle spasm.

In making determinations, it is important to point out that a hypomobile joint or a hyper-mobile joint is not necessarily a painful joint. Nevertheless, the quality of movement and range of movement must be appreciated before attempting to relate the abnormalities found to the possible cause of the patient's symptoms.

An 'old' hypomobility has a hard end-feel at the limit of the range, with movement before the limit of the range being a smooth friction-free movement. A 'new' hypomobility, on the other hand, has stiffness occurring earlier in the range, building up in strength

of resistance until the end of range is reached; that is, there is 'resistance through range'. When crepitus is present during movement, it will be painless if it is unassociated with presenting symptoms and painful if it is associated.

In 'ideal' joints, when the synovial joint surfaces are strongly compressed and moved, the movement will be painless (Maitland, 1980a). There are circumstances when pain is experienced during a large amplitude of the range, and it is sometimes possible to heighten this pain by holding the joint surfaces firmly compressed while moving the joint through the same amplitude of the range.

Having made the determinations regarding tissue thickenings, bony prominences, quality of movement and ranges of movement, it becomes necessary to relate the pain responses to these determinations. Not only is it necessary to know which movements either provoke the pain for which treatment is sought or produce local pain only, but it is also necessary to determine whether the sensations are felt to be superficial or deep. It may be necessary to apply firm pressure to obtain an accurate determination.

A stiff joint does not necessarily cause pain; it may well, however, be responsible for an associated joint becoming painful. The same applies to thickened tissues.

> The pain response felt by the patient during palpation of tissue and movement is most important

The pain response felt by the patient during the palpation examination of tissues and movement is most important. The pain or discomfort may be felt either through range or at the end of range; it may be felt deeply or it may reproduce a patient's referred symptoms.

Superficial and deep local pain can occur in both 'new' and 'old' situations. Severe pain felt by the patient when only moderate pressure is applied to a soft tissue, or is applied to produce movement, is always 'new'. When a patient has referred pain that can be reproduced by palpation examination, the indication is that it is associated with a 'new' disorder.

### Movement of vertebrae

Testing movement by palpation involves techniques that are used for treatment as well as examination. The test seeks information not only of range, but also of the 'end-feel' of the range, the behaviour of the pain throughout the range and the quality of any resistance or muscle spasm that may be present. Such information is determined both for the physiological movements and for the accessory movements of gapping, rocking and shearing or gliding. Detailed description of the techniques is given in the chapters on the different sections of the spine.

The passive intervertebral movements are produced by pressure against palpable parts of the vertebra, and these pressures should be applied at the right speed to appreciate the movement of the vertebra in relation to adjacent vertebra. If the pressure is applied as a single slow pressure, the vertebral movement will not be appreciated at all; if it is applied too quickly, it can be interpreted only as shaking. However, if the pressure is applied then relaxed and reapplied, and this is repeated two or three times a second, the amount of movement that can take place will be readily appreciated. It is also important that the test should consist of no more than two or three oscillations before moving quickly on to the next vertebra. If too many oscillations are employed on a vertebra before changing to the next one, comparisons of range are less accurate.

When examining movement, the first pressures should be applied extremely gently. When a section of the spine is being moved in this way, no more than two or three gentle pressures are applied to each vertebra in turn. If there is no pain response to the gentle movements, the amplitude and depth of the movement is increased, again with only two or three pressures applied to each vertebra. The testing should be repeated more deeply until pain or abnormality is detected or until the movement achieved indicates that the joint has a painless range in this direction. If pain is produced during movement, or if physical resistance or protective muscle contraction is encountered during the movement, their extent should be assessed. Occasionally a full assessment may not be possible until the second examination, because pain with movement may not be evident until the joint has reacted to the first examination (D plus 1).

> Sometimes a full assessment may only be possible at the second examination, when the structures have reacted to the first examination. This is called the 'D plus 1' assessment

The costovertebral joints are tested in the same manner as described for the intervertebral joints, except that the pressure is directed through the angle of each rib in turn.

The four primary directions in which the pressures are applied to the vertebrae are:

1. Postero-anteriorly on the spinous process (*Figure 6.36a*).

2. Postero-anteriorly on the articular pillar (*Figure 6.36b*).
3. Transversely on the lateral surface of the spinous process (*Figure 6.36c*).
4. Anteroposteriorly on the bony area of the articular pillar.

The test can then be further defined to determine the joint disturbance in greater detail by varying the direction of the above four movements (as follows), and by varying the point of contact with the vertebra.

1. *Varying the inclination postero-anteriorly on the spinous process.* The direction of these movements can be varied between an inclination towards the patient's head (*Figure 6.37a*) and an inclination towards his feet (*Figure 6.37b*).

2. *Varying the inclination postero-anteriorly over the articular pillar or transverse process.* This test can be varied in two ways. First it can be inclined towards the patient's head or towards his feet, as stated above. The second variation is to incline the postero-anterior pressure laterally, away from the spinous process (*Figure 6.38a*) or medially towards the spinous process (*Figure 6.38b*).

3. *Transverse movement against the spinous process.* This can be varied by inclining the direction of the movement towards the patient's feet, towards his head or, even more importantly, through an arc which ends as a postero-anterior movement against the lamina or articular pillar of the same side of the vertebra (*Figure 6.39*).

*Figures 6.40–6.42* show the direction of the movement applied to the processes illustrated in *Figures 6.37–6.39*.

When testing movements by palpation techniques, the vertebra should be thought of as being a sphere that can be moved in any direction (*Figure 6.43*).

Similarly, when moving one vertebra by, say, a transversely directed movement against its spinous process (*Figure 6.44*), the moving effect it has on other sections of the vertebra should be visualized (*Figure 6.45*).

Having visualized the directions of movements of the vertebra being moved, it is easier to visualize what happens to the vertebra above and the vertebra below (*Figure 6.46*).

As well as varying the angles of pressure applied to the vertebrae, the point of contact at the intervertebral joint should also be varied. For example, if the C2/3 joint is being examined by postero-anterior unilateral vertebral pressure on the left, the point of contact should be varied by pressure on C2, then on C3 and lastly on the C2/3 joint line. These tests, carried out effectively, will reveal not only the particular intervertebral

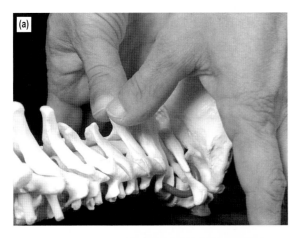

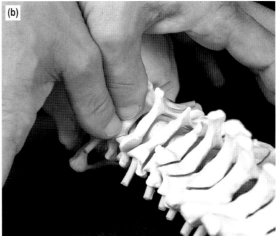

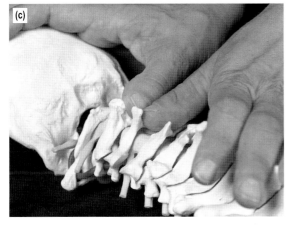

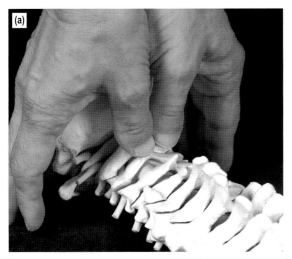

**Figure 6.36**    (*a*) Postero-anterior pressure on the spinous process.
(*b*) Postero-anterior pressure on the articular pillar.
(*c*) Transverse pressure on the lateral surface of the spinous process

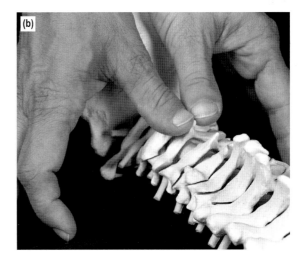

**Figure 6.37**    Postero-anterior pressure on the spinous process. (*a*) Inclined towards the patient's head. (*b*) Inclined towards the patient's feet

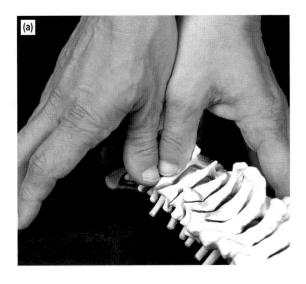

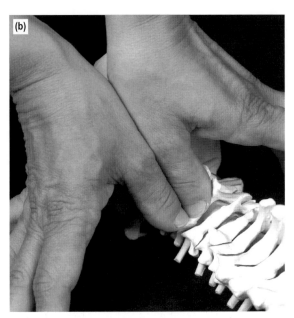

**Figure 6.38**  Postero-anterior pressure on the articular pillar. (*a*) Inclined laterally away from the spinous process. (*b*) Inclined medially towards the spinous process

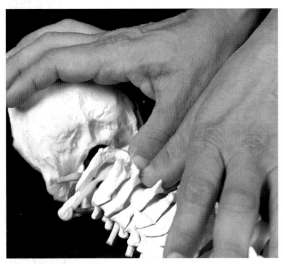

**Figure 6.39**  Transverse pressure against the spinous process inclined postero-anteriorly

joint at fault and the movements of the joint that are affected, but also the manner in which each movement is affected.

*Responses to the movements.* There are three variables to be considered when determining the manner in which joint movement is affected: pain, muscle spasm and physical resistance. It is important to realize that each of these factors, when present, may follow one of many different patterns. Pain, for example, may be present only when joint movement is stretched to the limit of the range; or the opposite may be the case, the joint being too painful even when it is at rest. It may vary in other ways too; if pain starts early in a range of movement, it does not always worsen in the same pattern when the joint is moved further. For example, the pain felt during movement may be quite moderate until approaching the limit of the range, when it suddenly increases to become severe. On the other hand, the pain may increase in intensity considerably in the first part of the movement, and then maintain a steady degree of pain until the limit of the range is reached (*see* Appendix 1). Different patterns of behaviour of pain require different treatment techniques.

Physical resistance of the type offered by contracted fibrous tissue can also vary considerably in its presentation. Movement before the limit of the range may be perfectly free, with resistance being felt at the limit of the range. The amplitude and strength of this slight resistance also vary widely (*see* Appendix 1). These variations also influence the type of treatment technique used.

Muscle spasm is the third variable in normal joint movement. The range of movement may be limited by very strong muscle spasm, or the spasm may be of a type that is evident only if a joint movement is performed in a particular way. For example, if the joint is moved slowly and carefully, no muscle spasm is felt, but if the movement is quick and jerky, spasm protects the joint from movement that would be painful. Movements used in treatments, therefore, must be modified to suit

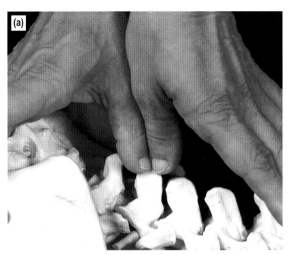
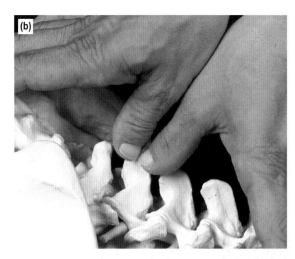

Figure 6.40    Postero-anterior central pressure inclined caudad and cephalad

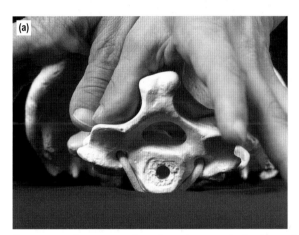
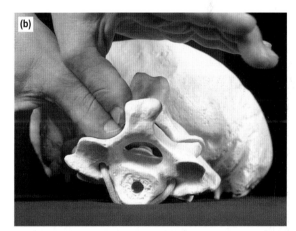

Figure 6.41    Postero-anterior unilateral pressure inclined laterally and medially

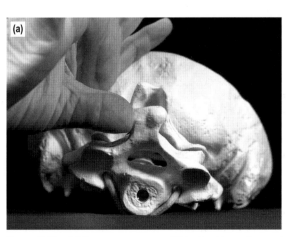
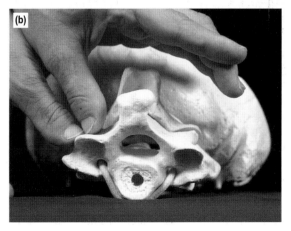

Figure 6.42    (a) Transverse pressure. (b) Inclined to postero anterior

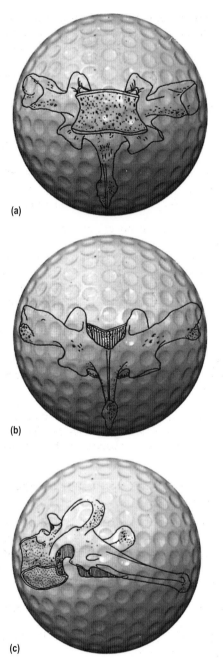

**(a)**

**(b)**

**(c)**

**Figure 6.43** Three views of a vertebrae in a golf ball to assist visual realization of its spherical dimension. (*a*) Anterior view. (*b*) Posterior view. (*c*) An angled view

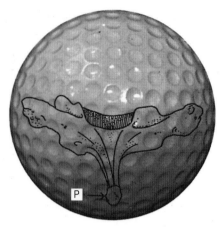

**Figure 6.44** Transverse pressure (P) on the spinous process

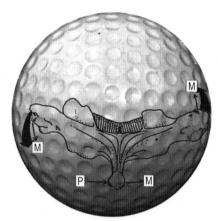

**Figure 6.45** Direction of movement (M) of the sections of the vertebra affected by transverse pressure (P)

the particular combination of behaviour of the pain, resistance and spasm (*see* Appendix 1).

When any of the passive movements are found to be painful, the physiotherapist should endeavour to assess at what stage in the range the movement becomes painful. She should then determine how the intensity or area of pain varies if the movement is carried further into the range. If pain is not too great and the movement can be carried further, an assessment of the possible range should be made. When physical resistance prevents a full range being achieved, the type of resistance (that is, whether it is a protective muscle spasm or just tightness of inert structures) should be noted.

These tests will provide information about joint disorders that is more valuable than that determined by testing in any other way. Details regarding learning to feel these factors found on joint movement, and a method of recording them diagrammatically for purposes of communication and teaching, are explained at length in Appendices 1 and 2. It is sufficient to say that an extremely valuable and detailed assessment of intervertebral joint movement can be made by this examination.

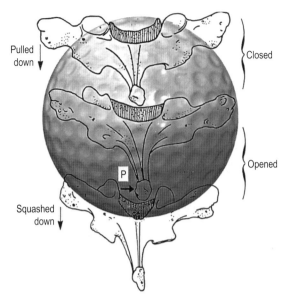

**Figure 6.46** Movement of one spinous process affects adjacent vertebrae. P = transverse pressure

When testing these movements it is necessary, when an abnormality is found, to make three comparisons:

1. With movements to the joints above and below the one being tested.
2. With movement of the joint on the opposite side.
3. With what would be considered to be normal for that joint.

As tests vary for different levels of the spine, each level will be described separately in the relevant chapter. However, relevant information in general terms is as follows.

Many of the procedures that constitute intervertebral joint movement tests have been outlined in the relevant chapters. Other tests (passive physiological intervertebral movement) assess only range. No one aspect of examination technique can be considered in isolation. In fact, it is the combined findings with different tests that give the final information about movement. However, the preceding tests by palpation techniques are the most important, as they reveal the range, pain, resistance and muscle spasm for each intervertebral joint tested. They also test accessory movements as well as the physiological movements. These tests can also be used as very effective treatment techniques.

> To understand and treat joint disorders, it is important to recognize the different relationships between the behaviour of pain, resistance and muscle spasm within a range of movement. They can best be appreciated by depicting them in a movement diagram

To understand and treat joint disorders, it is important to be able to recognize the different relationships between the behaviours of pain, resistance and muscle spasm within a range of movement. They can be best appreciated by depicting them in movement diagrams. An interesting parallel can be drawn from C. P. Snow's (1965) comment on geography and economics:

> *Geography would be incomprehensible without maps. They've reduced a tremendous muddle of facts into something you can read at a glance. Now I suspect economics is fundamentally no more difficult than geography except that it's about things in motion. If only somebody would invent a dynamic map.*

If the words 'passive movement' are substituted in the quotation for the word 'economics', the movement diagram could well be the 'dynamic map'. Appendix 1 describes the theoretical background of the movement diagram, and then explains the details of how a movement diagram can be compiled for any test movement, whether it be cervical extension, postero-anterior pressure on the spinous process of C4, or combined movements.

Regarding these appendices, it is essential to appreciate that the movement diagram is intended to serve only two purposes. These are:

1. To enable the novice to analyse what her hands are feeling when moving a joint passively
2. For use as a means of communication and teaching.

### Passive physiological movements of single intervertebral joints

Description of the specialized test is different for each individual spinal joint. There are two important occasions when examination requires an assessment of flexion, extension, lateral flexion and rotation as they exist at a single intervertebral joint:

1. When the preceding examination has shown that the faulty joint is stiff but not painful.
2. When a joint has suddenly become fixed in an abnormal position.

The information found on examination is also used in assessing improvement in the range of movement that may result from treatment. To estimate the range, the examiner moves the intervertebral joint through a full range of movement between palpable parts of the two adjacent vertebrae. This movement is compared with the following:

1. Movement found at the joint above and below.
2. Movement found on the opposite side.

3. Movement that can be expected to be normal for that particular joint in that particular patient, considering his age, build, disorders, etc.

Description of the method for testing each spinal joint from the occiput to the sacrum is given in the chapters for each section of the vertebral column. These movements are tested:

- Through the range available
- By stronger pressure at the end of the range, to discern the fullest range possible and to determine the 'end-of-range feel'. The oscillatory test movement is performed somewhat more slowly than the oscillatory mobilization treatment technique.

## DIFFERENTIATION TESTS

Differentiation tests help to sort out the source of the patient's symptoms. Tests may help to determine:

- Whether the symptoms arise from the spine or a peripheral joint
- Which spinal level is the source of the symptoms
- Whether symptoms arise from the neural structures or intervertebral structures
- Whether symptoms arise from the spinal joints or pain-sensitive structures of the vertebral canal or intervertebral foramen.

Differentiation tests are special tests used during physical examination to sort out the source of a patient's symptoms under certain difficult circumstances. There are four reasons for performing differentiation tests for vertebral problems:

1. It may be necessary to determine whether a pain disorder is arising from the spine or from a peripheral joint.

2. It may be necessary to determine, when pressure on T7 reproduces a patient's symptoms, whether the symptoms are arising from the joint between T7/8 or T6/7, especially when the same pressure on T6 and T8 is painless.

3. When it is necessary to separate the symptoms arising from the neural elements from those arising from the musculoskeletal structures. They frequently occur together, whereupon skilled examination is required to determine whether the neural component is intrinsic and primary, or whether it is secondary to other extrinsic elements provoking an irritative effect on the neural elements.

4. It may be necessary to determine whether a pain is arising from the spinal joints or the pain-sensitive structures in the vertebral canal or intervertebral foramen.

### Differentiating pain from the spine and from the peripheral joints

A patient may have gluteal symptoms, and routine examination may not clearly reveal whether they are caused by a hip disorder or by a spinal disorder. However, in some circumstances tests may be performed which clearly differentiate between them. These circumstances are that either (i) the patient may be able to demonstrate a movement, or that (ii) the examiner may find a movement that incorporates concurrent movement of the spine and the hip and reproduces the symptoms. A differentiation test can be used under such circumstances, and it can have four parts – that is, four different but related tests. Each test can be performed in isolation, and the finding of any one can be confirmed by each of the three remaining tests.

### Example

*Part 1.* Examination shows that, when the patient stands and twists his trunk fully to the right, this position reproduces his right buttock pain (*Figure 6.47a*). This is the kind of circumstance referred to above that can be used to differentiate between the hip and the spine as the source of the pain.

1. The patient is asked to lift his leg off the floor and to keep it raised while still rotated to the right. He then rotates further to the right and over-pressure is added to be sure his pain is still reproduced (*Figure 6.47b*).

2. He then places his hands on the physiotherapist's shoulder for balance, which leaves her hands free. The buttock pain must still be present in this position (*Figure 6.47c*).

3. The physiotherapist then stabilizes the patient's pelvis, retaining the reproduced right buttock pain (*Figure 6.47d*). The patient is then asked to:

   *Rotate his lumbar spine to the left, that is, derotate the lumbar spine (Figure 6.47e). State whether his right buttock pain remains unchanged (which will be the case if the pain is caused by a hip disorder) or decreased (which will be the case if the pain is caused by a spinal disorder).*

*Part 2.* From the stage 3 position given above, the physiotherapist stabilizes the patient's pelvis to prevent it rotating, and asks him to twist his trunk still further to the right (*Figure 6.47f*).

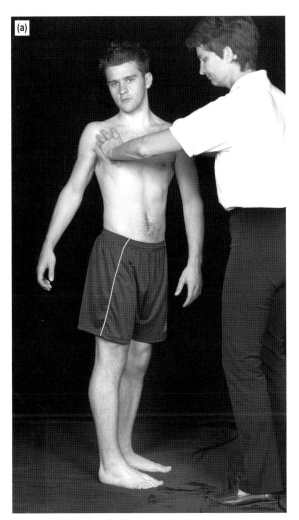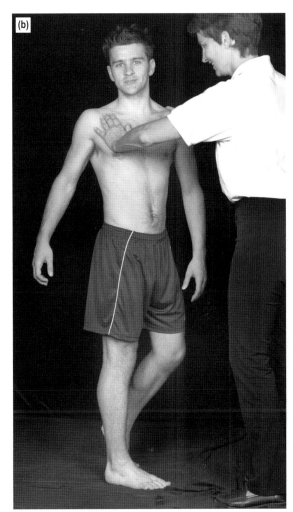

**Figure 6.47**    Differentiation test, spinal and peripheral joint pain, part 1. (*a*) Rotation to the right. (*b*) Patient balancing on right leg and over-pressure added

If the buttock pain is caused by a hip disorder, the pain does not change. If the buttock pain is caused by a spinal disorder, the pain will increase.

*Part 3.* With the patient standing on his right leg, his hands on the therapist's shoulders, and with her hands over the iliac crests laterally, he is asked to twist his pelvis to the right (on his right leg) without any spinal rotation. If the pain arises from the lumbar spine the test movement will be painless, but if it arises from the hip, the movement will reproduce the pain.

*Part 4.* With the patient standing balanced on his right leg and his pelvis held motionless, he is asked to twist his body to the right. If the pain is caused by a spinal disorder the right buttock pain will be reproduced, but if it is a hip disorder the test movement will be painless.

## Differentiating symptoms arising from intervertebral levels

The second differentiation is used when, for example, transverse pressure directed towards the right on the left side of the spinous process of T7 reproduces left-sided symptoms although the same movement applied to T6 and T8 is painless. The question then arises, does the fault lie at T7/8 or T7/6? The steps taken to differentiate are as follows, and to simplify the discussion it is assumed that the left-sided symptoms arise from T7/6:

1. The therapist applies the transverse pressure to T7 with her left thumb until the left-sided symptoms are reproduced. The vertebra is then held in a constant position in relation to T6 (*Figure 6.48a*).

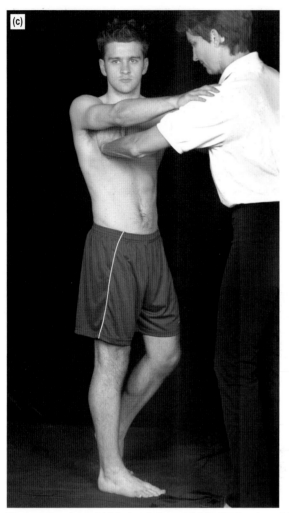

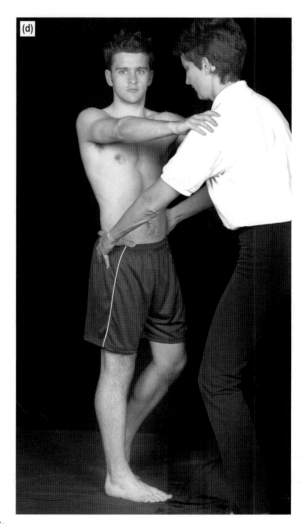

**Figure 6.47** (contd) (c) Patient balanced. (d) Stabilizing the pelvis

2. With her right thumb, the manipulative physiotherapist carefully applies transverse pressure to the right on the spinous process of T8. Because the symptoms are T7/6 in origin, there will be no change in the pain response because the position of T7/6 has not changed (Figure 6.48b).

3. She then changes the direction of her transverse pressure on T8 from left to right to right to left. Again there will be no change in the pain response, because the position of T7/6 has not changed (Figure 6.48c).

4. She now changes her hand position so that her right thumb pushes transversely on T7, directed towards the patient's right, until the symptoms are again reproduced (Figure 6.48d).

5. With T7 held stationary in relation to T8, she now gently applies transverse pressure towards the

right on T6 with her left thumb. Even gentle pressure will result in a lessening of the reproduced left-sided symptoms because the pressure between T6 and T7 has been released (Figure 6.48e).

6. If the transverse pressure against T6 is reversed, the pain will be increased (Figure 6.48f).

## Differentiating symptoms from a joint and from the neural structures

A patient may have right buttock pain which is provoked by full-range forward flexion from the standing position; overpressure is applied (Figure 6.49a). The pain may be caused by movement of the lumbar spine or by movement of the pain-sensitive structures in the vertebral canal or intervertebral foramen.

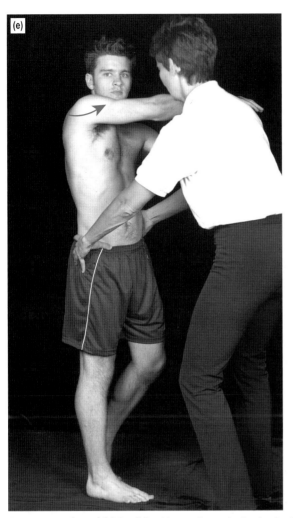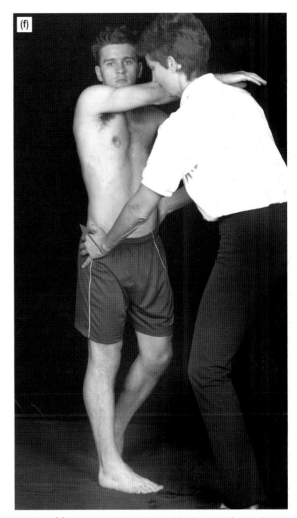

**Figure 6.47** (contd) (e) Retaining hip rotation and releasing lumbar rotation. (f) Part 2: retaining released lumbar rotation and increasing hip rotation

One differentiating test is to ask him, while in the fully flexed position (*Figure 6.49a*), to flex his chin to his chest and assess the change in symptoms. If there is no change in the symptoms, over-pressure should be applied to the neck flexion and the symptoms reassessed (*Figure 6.49b*). If the buttock pain is increased by the neck flexion, the disorder must have some degree of canal/foramina component; if symptoms do not change, the disorder would seem to be free of any canal/foramina component. One point to remember, however, is that in this position his foot is not dorsiflexed.

The 'slump tests' can also be used to differentiate between a joint component and a neural component.

## Differentiating symptoms from both neural and musculoskeletal sources

One of the most difficult kinds of differentiation occurs when neural tests are positive as well as joint tests.

One of the most difficult kinds of differentiation, which is relatively new and very much harder than the previous differentiations, is trying to differentiate a person's problem *when neural tests are positive as well as joint tests*. It is very often only on reassessment of treatment results that differentiation of the contributing structures can take place. The treatment of Mrs C. serves as an example.

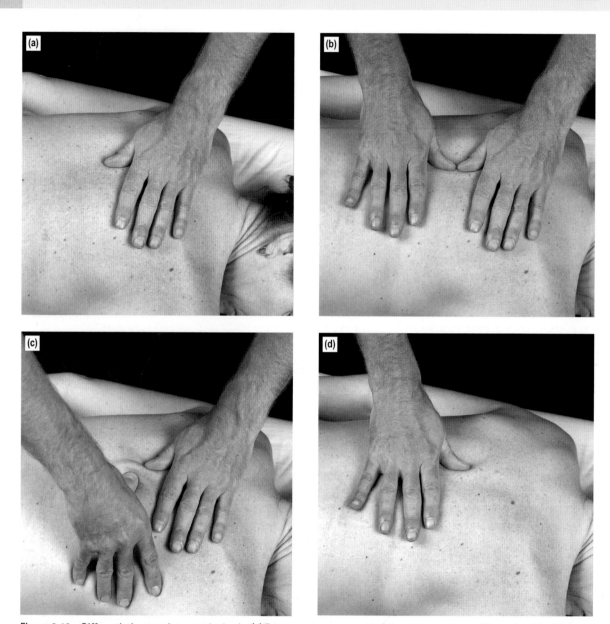

**Figure 6.48** Differentiation test, intervertebral pain. (*a*) Transverse pressure pushing the spinous process of T7 to the right. While maintaining the T7–T6 relationship: (*b*) gently add transverse pressure to the right against the spinous process of T8; (*c*) add transverse pressure to the left against the spinous process of T8. (*d*) Transverse pressure pushing the spinous process of T7 to the right. While maintaining the T7–T8 relationship, gently add transverse pressure

### Example

Mrs C. has pain in her neck and pain in both scapula areas with the right side being worse than the left; pain can spread into both arms but tends to be more in the left than in the right.

On examination of Mrs C.'s cervical spine, cervical flexion was restricted by about 15 per cent and gave pain in the T1–T3 area centrally. The pain was not increased by adding slump to the thoracic and lumbar spine, by adding knee extension (single legs or both together), nor did it provoke any other symptoms. Her range of rotation to the left was 30 per cent less than what would be her full (over-pressure) range, and it very easily produced her left-sided neck pain spreading down and laterally in the left supraspinous fossa area but not reaching the shoulder nor provoking any

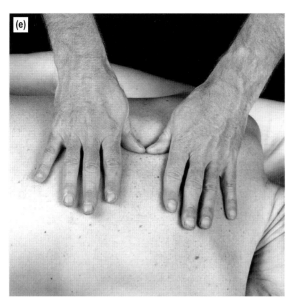 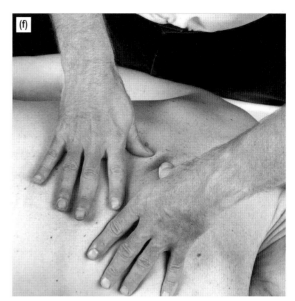

**Figure 6.48**    (*contd*) (*e*) to the right against the spinous process of T6; (*f*) to the left against the spinous process of T6

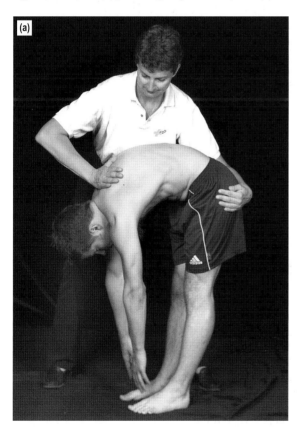 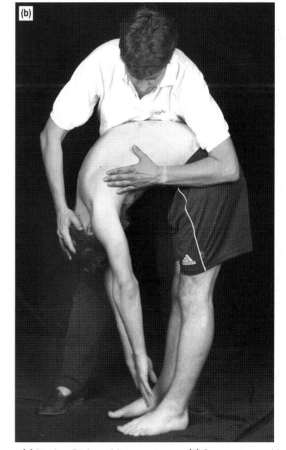

**Figure 6.49**    Differentiation test, vertebral-canal and joint symptoms. (*a*) Lumbar flexion with over-pressure. (*b*) Over-pressure added to neck flexion

arm symptoms. Rotation to the right lacked only 20 per cent of her range of movement, but it provoked left-sided neck and upper scapular symptoms. If this movement was carried further she then had a reproduction of her right scapular pain, which spread from the base of her neck down to approximately T4/5. Her range of extension lacked 35 per cent of normal range, and it provoked left-sided scapular pain and central upper thoracic pain. When testing the upper limb neural movements with both arms, the left arm was distinctly positive in that it lacked elbow extension range, and there was tingling throughout her hand and anterior elbow but no cervical symptoms. Adding SLR to this provoked neck, scapular and arm pain as well as pain in the fingers on the left side.

Palpation examination revealed a prominent thoracic spinous process of T3 (which is common), and the spinous process of T4 was set more deeply. Palpation caused local pain at both levels, but at T3 it was a sharper, more surface pain, and at T4 it was a deep central pain.

Twelve months prior to her having treatment, her symptoms were present on waking (rather than wakening her), with pain in the whole of the cervical area, and she had no ability to turn her head to either side without causing pain. She had had a motor vehicle accident in 1986 when she, as the passenger, was in a car that was hit from in front and she hit her head on the windscreen. She had suffered symptoms of variable intensity but right-sided only, and she had not responded to any of the treatments the doctors and physiotherapists had administered. Over the 3 weeks prior to seeking manipulative physiotherapy treatment, the symptoms had been gradually increasing; they were now in the right side of the arm as far as the elbow. The only guiding indication for her problem being neural rather than joint was the fact that arm symptoms were very vague in their distribution, and there were no nerve-root irritation signs on examination. However, Mrs C. also had the cervical signs and symptoms of a joint component, so it was the aim of the initial treatments to be oriented towards the cervical sign, and assessment was repeatedly performed for both the cervical indicators and the neural indicators. The initial treatment was oriented towards the cervical spine and the T3/4 area (treatment was the palpatory direct type of technique, which produced a very quick response to all cervical movement but did not produce any change in the neural movement asterisked signs). Having proved this, the treatment was then switched to treating the neural movement restrictions and their pain responses. The technique chosen was the first of the three standard tests (Butler, 1991), and although these showed changes in the neural signs by about 20–30 per cent, there were no changes to the cervical signs. However, when neural signs have been present for a long time they tend to be more difficult to treat. The techniques were changed around in various ways, but without any favourable effect – Mrs C. would lose the gain in the neural signs on examination within 24 hours. This pattern did not alter.

The next step was to position the patient supine with her head laterally flexed to the right and her right arm held in the positive number 1 classical position. She was then treated by double leg straight leg raising, gradually pushing the range of the straight leg raising until it reached the maximum extent of pain to which I was prepared to carry it. As this was unsuccessful in inducing improvement in either neural or joint signs, the technique was changed to having her lying supine but with both legs propped up into straight leg raising positions and then using the cervical lateral flexion technique to reproduce her arm symptoms. This was also unsuccessful, so I then changed the treatment so that she was in the same position but the elbow flexion–extension technique was used. This was also disappointingly unsuccessful. On the same day, with her lying normally supine, with one medium-sized pillow, the technique of unilateral pressures on the left-hand side of her neck and into her scapula and elbow areas provoked deep, local pain when pressure was on the articular pillar of C5–C7. She was able to guide me as to the angle for applying the pressure, and the main point was C6/7. While performing the technique Mrs C. spontaneously commented that she felt this was the right thing to do because while she was lying there (with her left arm in the number 1 position) it was markedly improving.

On reassessment, there was improvement symptomatically and her cervical movements improved, although not to the ideal end-result. However, the neural tests also improved. The technique was performed twice, and she gained improvement on both occasions.

Over several treatment sessions Mrs C. made good progress with current mobilizing techniques, and she was totally free of thoracic pain. From 5 pm onwards in the evening she would develop symptoms in the region of the first rib on both sides, with the right being greater than the left; sometimes she would have symptoms generally in the whole of the upper limb on the same side as the first rib symptoms, but never on both sides together. She also commented that it was difficult to turn her head to the right on these occasions.

My intention on that particular treatment day was to differentiate between the sources of symptoms – that is, how much was neural, how much was low cervical and how much was upper thoracic. On physical examination, using the upper limb neural test, there was restriction of elbow extension causing symptoms in the elbow and spreading down the forearm and into the fingers.

On placing Mrs C.'s head in a position of either lateral flexion and rotation to the right or a combination of lateral flexion and rotation to the right, and then adding the neural test, the symptoms in the arm would increase dramatically and her range of elbow extension would be limited by another 10 per cent. Lower cervical extension was limited and caused pain in the area of both supraspinous fossae. Forward flexion was not restricted, but she felt the symptoms medially in the region of the first rib on both sides, which spread up both sides of the cervical area to the occiput. The symptoms were equal on left and right. Her range of rotation to the left was 65 per cent, causing symptoms in the left supraspinous fossa and the left side of her neck, whereas rotation to the right was 75 per cent, and it also caused pain in the same left-sided area although it was less severe than when the rotation was to the left. She had a full range of cervical lateral flexion to each side, each causing a pulling pain in the supraspinous fossa area on the opposite side. Using combined movements, with lateral flexion to the right being the 'primary' movement and adding rotation to the right, these movements provoked equal supraspinous fossa symptoms. At no stage during this examination was there any reproduction of pain in her right thoracic area spreading from approximately T2 down to T4/5 slightly to the right of the midline, which had been one of her primary symptoms in the earlier treatments and could be reproduced quite readily with cervical movements.

The treatment technique at this stage was performing the left upper limb neural test movement with Mrs C.'s head in the normal straight position and laterally flexed to the right, in all three positions, using the elbow extension upper limb neural movement as the treatment technique. The effect was producing no improvement in the neural test movement, but it did produce some improvement in the cervical rotation and movement. However, flexion again began to provoke some symptoms in the right thoracic area between T1 and T3. This gave me an indication of the effect of using the upper limb neural movement. I then changed to producing a PA movement on the right-hand side against the first rib. In this position, I was sometimes able to provoke symptoms in her forearm extending from the elbow to the fingers of her left arm. On reassessment, the cervical movements had improved considerably but the upper limb neural movement was unchanged. This told me that the first rib area played a part in the cervical component that had no effect in the upper limb neural component.

I then lay Mrs C. prone with her head fully laterally flexed to the right and her left arm in the upper limb neural position, which was the same as the testing position. In that position I performed unilateral PAs on the first rib and transverse process of C7, directing the movement in a PA direction plus a caudad inclination. This produced only local pain and no thoracic or arm pain. Following this, all areas had improved subjectively and the physical range of movement in both cervical and thoracic and neural tests was improved. I then repeated the technique but in a much fuller lateral flexion to the right for her head, which I held in this position with my knee. The technique produced local symptoms that spread throughout her left arm, particularly at the elbow and fingers. On releasing the PA part of the technique, the symptoms provoked by the technique were as just described on the first rib area. The technique resulted in an improvement of all components; the thoracic symptoms on cervical flexion had gone completely, her low extension was full range and asymptomatic, and her left arm neural test was almost asymptomatic as well as having a full range. She commented, 'My whole arm feels so much lighter'.

The fact that the last technique produced symptoms in the supraspinous fossa and throughout the arm to the fingers indicated that the upper limb neural test findings were definitely positive, with the source or point of restriction of movement being that the left neck angle. The result of the differentiating routine of sorting out the problem indicated that the arm symptoms were secondary, not primary, and that the cervical findings were positive. Also, positioning her in the lateral flexion position and using the palpatory technique indicated that this was the main source of the right thoracic pain; the pain in the left and right supraspinous fossae and the left arm in particular all had their origin at C7 on the left and the adjacent first rib at the costotransverse junction.

This was the best treatment response we had had throughout her treatment, and it only remains to be seen how much of the improvement she retains.

## Radiographs

From the physiotherapist's point of view, an examination cannot be considered complete unless certain facts have been clarified. For example, if radiographs have been taken the physiotherapist should endeavour to see them so as to be more aware of the state of the spine being treated. It is important to be familiar with the radiological appearance of the normal spine – for example the contour and position of vertebrae, and the size and appearance of disc spaces and intervertebral foramina. This knowledge helps the correlation of congenital and developmental abnormalities with physical findings. The physiotherapist should find out if the patient has had an extended course of steroid therapy, and should know the extent of any osteoporotic changes caused by such treatment. Although it is the province of the medical practitioner to exclude from manipulative treatment patients with signs of cord or cauda equina compression, it is our responsibility to be aware of these dangers.

## OVERVIEW

### PHYSICAL EXAMINATION (P/E) – VERTEBRAL/GENERAL FORMAT

*Observation*
+correct/overcorrect deformities and effects

*Present pain*

*Functional demonstration/tests*
+differentiation

*Brief appraisal*

*Active movements (standing/sitting)*
(Other joints; quick tests)
Active movement: move to pain or to limit, e.g. F, E, LF (L) (R), ROT (L) (R) + over-pressure if necessary
When applicable ('if necessary' tests), e.g.: combining more movements; quadrants; compression/distraction; vertebral artery; differentiation; slump; at speed, sustained, repeated, etc.

*Supine, Side lying, Prone*
e.g.: neurological examination; NF, ULNT, LLNT; passive peripheral joint tests/other joints; isometric tests; palpation examination (temperature, sweating., soft tissues, position of vertebrae, PAIVMS); PPIVMS

*Check case notes for relevant tests*

*Asterisk as you go*

*Instructions to patient*

# Chapter 7

# Principles of techniques

There are two ways of manipulating the conscious patient. The first, better thought of as mobilization, is the gentler coaxing of a movement by passive rhythmical oscillations performed at the beginning, within or at the limit of the range; the second is the forcing of a movement near the limit of the range by a sudden thrust. The difference between these two techniques may seem negligible when comparing a strongly applied mobilization with a gentle manipulative thrust, but there is an important difference: the patient can always resist the mobilization if it should become too painful, whereas the suddenness of the forceful manipulation prevents any control by the patient.

There are two forms of manipulation:

1. Passive rhythmical oscillations in different positions of a range of movement
2. Manipulative thrusts near the limit of a range of movement

In this book, strong emphasis has been placed on the relatively greater importance of examination and assessment skills when compared with the techniques of treatment. Nevertheless, there are times when a technique fails to help a patient, not because it was the wrong choice of technique, but because the technique was not executed skillfully.

The techniques described in this book are intended to be a basis from which innumerable variations can be derived. **There is no limit to the number of different techniques that can be used in treatment, and the techniques described should be seen as a basis only and recognized as forming only the tip of the iceberg.**

It is important that techniques of mobilization should be mastered before manipulation is attempted.

The techniques presented have been kept to a basic minimum, but it should be *very clearly understood* that there are no SET techniques to cover all needs, and that the way the methods are described is not meant to be seen as the way they MUST be performed. They can be adapted from this basis to suit the needs of the manipulative physiotherapist, as well as those of the patient. One of the most important features of the concept that this book attempts to establish is that techniques are not used in any set, rigid pattern, but should be varied, modified, reversed or new ones invented until they achieve the intention of their selection.

## A TECHNIQUE IS THE BRAINCHILD OF INGENUITY

As skill develops with practice and experience, the physiotherapist sometimes finds that starting positions other than those described are easier, and she may make changes to suit her own needs.

The most important factor in achieving effective mobilization is learning to sense or 'feel' movement. It can be likened to the way in which one feels for the meshing of cogs in the gearbox of a car when manually changing gears (*Figure 7.1*); the movements taking place inside the gearbox cannot be seen, but they can be sensed. The vertebral column is similar. Until this 'feel' is learned by repeated practice, treatment by mobilization will not be fully effective.

With every technique, it is the physiotherapist's body that must produce the movement. The physiotherapist's hands, thumbs or fingers should never, under any circumstances, be the prime movers; their muscles must work eccentrically, not concentrically. Whatever the part of the arms or body that is *transmitting* the movement to the intervertebral joints, it should not be the thumb muscle *producing* the movement. This principle is the one main element that will make learning 'feel' possible. In fact, with every

technique performed, the further away from the contact point that the movement can be produced, the finer will be the 'feel'. It should also be said that the further away from the contact point that the movement is produced, the more comfortable it will feel to the patient. In, for example, cervical lateral flexion, the manipulative physiotherapist's upper trunk, arms and hands transmit the lateral flexion to the patient's head and neck, all being figuratively cemented together, while the lateral flexion movement is produced by her lower trunk and legs. Similarly, when using thumbs to perform central PAs (mobilizations in a postero-anterior direction) on say C4, the flexors of the thumbs work only eccentrically in transmitting the pressure that produces the PA movement of C4, the pressure itself coming from the manipulative physiotherapist's body.

When using techniques such as cervical lateral flexion, the manipulative physiotherapist must hug the patient's head between her two hands, her arm alongside his head and her trunk against his head. Her other arm should hug firmly against her trunk, so that the patient's head and her upper body and arms can be 'cemented' together and will at all times move as a unit during the technique. This hugging principle applies equally to using central PA pressures in the cervical spine, but obviously the mode is different. Performing techniques by 'remote control', so to speak (i.e. the physiotherapist is at a distance from the patient), produces poor techniques and poor feel.

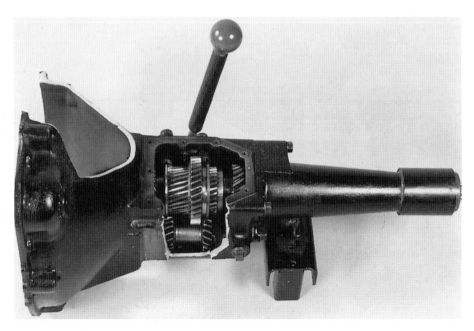

**Figure 7.1**   Cut-away view of a manual gearbox

Many people seem to believe that treatment by passive movement necessarily involves stretching, but this is not always so. However, treatment is always involved with movement, whether it is stretching or not; hence the importance of feeling movement. Almost all of the techniques involve oscillatory movements, but if the rate of oscillation is too quick or too slow it will be impossible to gain any feel of movement at the joint. Instead, the movement will feel like shaking or stretching respectively. Although it would be wrong to try to establish any set rate, some guiding figures seem reasonable and therefore a rate of two or three oscillations per second is offered as a guide. Variations from this rhythm are discussed later (*see* p. 176). The importance of learning to feel movement cannot be emphasized too much, for without this 'feel' examination will be less informative and treatment less effective.

> Gaining 'feel' of the movement is essential in order to perform a technique adequately

When practising techniques on one another, physiotherapists should pay attention to details of positioning and rhythm. Once learned, these skills have to be modified when applied to patients – no two patients have the same build, nor do they have the same joint abnormalities.

> When practising techniques, attention should be paid to many details – positioning, rhythm of the movement, speed, grading of movements, contact of the hands, modification to the patient's structures, etc.

To produce maximum movement of a normal joint in any one direction when practising, it is easier to gain the fullest range, with least effort for the physiotherapist and without strain to the model, if this joint is positioned as near as is available to the mid-position of all its other ranges. A clear example of this is seen in the normal metacarpophalangeal joint of the index finger. If the maximum distraction movement with least effort is desired, the starting position should be midway between the normal limits of flexion, extension, abduction, adduction and rotation. To put the joint at the limit of any one of these ranges will severely limit the range of distraction movement. When applying this principle to the cervical spine, it is clear that if the head and neck are kept in normal alignment the lowest cervical intervertebral joints will be much nearer their extended than their flexed position. Therefore, when using the techniques of longitudinal movement,

rotation, lateral flexion or traction (and in a smaller measure this applies to the techniques involving pressures to the vertebrae), it is necessary to position the neck in some degree of flexion in order to gain the mid-position between the limits of flexion and extension for the lowest cervical intervertebral joints. Exactly the same principle applies to the techniques of traction, longitudinal movement and rotation in the lumbar spine. When movement is desired in the lower joints the lumbar spine should be positioned towards flexion, and when the upper lumbar joints are being mobilized the position of the lumbar spine as a whole is towards extension.

> Clinical tip: To produce maximum movement of a normal joint in any one direction when practising, it is easier to gain the fullest range, with least effort for the physiotherapist and without strain to the model, if this joint is positioned as near as is available to the mid-position of all its other ranges

In Chapter 9, watching for disturbances in the normal rhythm of movement is emphasized. This is equally important when performing cervical and lumbar rotation techniques. During treatment, mobilization is directed to the faulty joint even though the adjacent joints are also rotated. Therefore, during the rotary mobilization, distortion of the movement should be watched for, and if the faulty joint is the cause of such distortion, the movement should be performed only up to this point and not carried beyond it.

Techniques that involve pressure against some part of the vertebra require special care. The thumbs, fingers or the hand, working eccentrically, are the only medium through which the concentric movement of the physiotherapist's body is transmitted to the vertebrae to produce movement. If the intrinsic muscles of the hands are used to produce the pressure, the technique will immediately become uncomfortable both to patient and to physiotherapist; the hands will become tense and all possibility of 'feeling' the movement will be lost. A study of the diagrams will show how the shoulders are positioned above or behind the hands, and how the joints from the shoulders downwards act as a series of springs. Every effort should be made at the beginning to observe these points.

When performing techniques that involve direct pressure on palpable parts of an individual vertebra, two basic sets of circumstances can exist:

1.  The technique may be used in the treatment of a stiff joint with the intention of increasing its range. Movement is produced by thumb pressures against

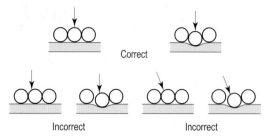

Figure 7.2    Direction of pressure on spinous processes

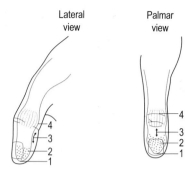

Figure 7.3    Right thumb; four contact points

the vertebrae (*see* pp. 155–156), and the direction chosen should be in the direction that is stiff.

2.  These same techniques can be used in the treatment of pain rather than stiffness. Under these circumstances, the method is to produce as large an amplitude of movement as is possible with the gentlest of pressure and without feeling any degree of stiffness. If postero-anterior pressures are used on the spinous process, care must be exercised to find the right position for the supporting fingers as well as the right direction for the arms and thumbs to be on top of the movement. This can be likened to applying pressure on top of one of a series of balls set in rubber (*Figure 7.2*). If the direction of the pressure or the point of contact of the pressure is off-centre, the movement produced will not be a pure postero-anterior movement. During performance of the technique this will be felt as uneven pressure under the thumbs or sliding on the spinous process.

> Treatment techniques can be used in two basic sets of circumstances: the treatment of stiffness, or of pain rather than stiffness. The method of the technique will differ depending on its objective

The starting positions are also important, since they must allow the patient to relax completely and the physiotherapist to work effectively with the minimum of effort. Relaxation of the physiotherapist's hands is essential, for it is impossible to feel through hands that are tense.

When using techniques involving direct pressures on the parts of the vertebrae, it is essential that they are not performed painfully. There is a difference between the technique being painful and the technique reproducing the local pain. If the patient feels soreness or superficial pain with the technique, then it is necessary for the contact point of the thumb to be modified. *Figure 7.3* shows four sections of the thumb that can

be used to transmit the pressure to the vertebra. They are:

1.  The tip of the thumb. This produces the small contact area needed to define clearly the angle and the contact point of the technique that relates findings to the disorder.

2.  The palmar joint of the tip of the thumb. If the technique provokes local pain when used with contact point number 1, contact point 2 makes more use of the soft palmar joint of the tip of the thumb. This lessens the soreness produced by the thumb.

3.  The palmar surface of the central area of the distal phalanx. The technique used can be made more comfortable still by using this area. Obviously it is not as informative as the others, but it is (or can be) the best and most comfortable way of transmitting the palpatory technique to the vertebra.

4.  The anterior surface of the base of the thumb. The use of this contact point lessens the contact area of the technique in 1 above, but is less informative.

I should acknowledge the idea given to me by Miss Jeanne-Marie Ganne in 1965 when I was preparing a lecture for the Chartered Society of Physiotherapy's 1966 Congress (Maitland, 1966, 1970b). One of the goals for the paper was to describe the different amplitudes of passive movement treatment that could be used. It was Miss Ganne who gave me the idea of depicting the original diagram for the different grades of movement. Many novel innovations have been made since then (*see* Grieve, 1981), but the credit for the basis of the movement grades must be Miss Ganne's.

When using the cervical techniques of lateral flexion and rotation, relaxation and finer control will be obtained if the physiotherapist cradles the patient's head between her arm and chest so that she hugs it.

Each of these techniques, when practised on the normal spine or when used in treatment, can be performed in different positions in the range as well as using

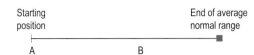

Figure 7.4    Depicting a range of movement

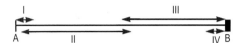

Figure 7.5    Grades in a normal range having a hard end-feel

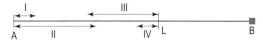

Figure 7.6    Grades in a hypomobile joint. L = Pathological limit of range (hard end-feel)

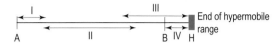

Figure 7.7    Grades in relation to a hypermobile asymptomatic range. B = Range of movement beyond normal average range. N = Normal hypermobile range

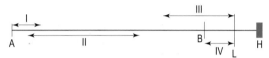

Figure 7.8    Grades in a hypermobile range with slight limitation and hard end-feel

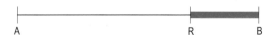

Figure 7.9    Depicting a soft end-feel. R = Beginning of resistance

movements of small or large amplitude. Application of technique in treatment will be discussed in Chapter 9, but for the sake of learning the techniques on the normal spine, the types of movement are divided into four grades.

*Grade I*    A small-amplitude movement near the starting position of the range
*Grade II*    A large-amplitude movement that carries well into the range. It can occupy any part of the range that is free of any stiffness or muscle spasm
*Grade III*    Also a large-amplitude movement, but one that does move into stiffness or muscle spasm
*Grade IV*    A small-amplitude movement stretching into stiffness or muscle spasm.

These grades can be depicted diagrammatically against a line representing a range of movement from a starting or resting position to the end of an average normal end of range (*Figure 7.4*). This line can be represented by any chosen movement, and although the end of the range is always the same, the starting position can be any position of choice. The reason for the thickened point B is explained on page 453. For example, cervical rotation of the supine patient is most easily considered as starting from the position where the nose faces forwards at right angles to the trunk. Obviously, the end-position will be full rotation with the nose facing approximately over the shoulder.

Different joint movements have a different feel at the end of range. For example, elbow extension has a hard end-feel and elbow flexion has a softer, springy end-feel. In the representations for the different grades, a hard end-feel has been assumed. The arrows, marked for each of the four grades, depict the amplitude of each of the movements and the positions they occupy in the range (*Figure 7.5*).

---

Different movement directions have a different end-feel, to which the grades of movement will be adapted

---

When pathology or a physical disorder limits the range of movement and the end-feel is hard, the grades are also reduced in range (*Figure 7.6*).

A hypermobile movement, which has a hard end-feel and which is asymptomatic and normal for that person, would have grades of movement such as those in *Figure 7.7*.

When a hypermobile range is affected by some disorder that causes a slight limitation yet still has a hard end-feel, the grades of movement would be represented as in *Figure 7.8*. It is important to realize that this stiffness still permits a range of movement that is beyond the average normal range, yet in relation to its normal hypermobile range it is still hypomobile.

As was pointed out earlier, the end-feel may be softer and extend over a part of the range of movement. Taking knee flexion as an example, the resistance to flexion may commence at R even though the end of the average normal range is still at B (*Figure 7.9*).

Grades III+ and IV+ under the circumstances of soft end-feel may be depicted as in *Figure 7.10*.

This allows the stronger or gentler techniques that are taken into resistance to be depicted (*Figure 7.11*).

The soft end-feel also provides the opportunity to show that grade II movements never reach into resistance; they are always resistance-free movements (*Figure 7.12*).

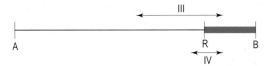

**Figure 7.10**   Grades III and IV under a soft end-feel

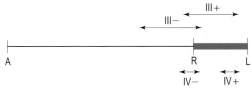

**Figure 7.11**   Depicting techniques taken into resistance in grades III and IV under a soft end-feel

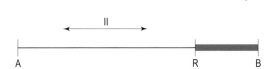

**Figure 7.12**   Grade II movements are always resistance-free movements

Learning to control the gentleness of grade I movements is as important as learning to control the smoothness of rhythm with grades II and III; and all of these need far more emphasis than grade IV. A fitting description for grade I postero-anterior pressure on a spinous process is to say that if a fly were between the therapist's thumbs and the spinous process, it would not be squashed by the technique. That such gentleness can be effective in treatment is hard for some people to believe. Nevertheless, when pain severely limits movement, a technique as gentle as this grade I example can be effective.

In fact, many people (including manipulators) do not appreciate or believe that it is possible to determine such a fine degree of movement or resistance. Those who wish to be convinced would do well to read Evans' research findings (Evans, 1982). He states:

*The accuracy of palpation, and the delicacy with which passive mobilization techniques can be performed by skilled therapists, has long been acknowledged.*

In a recent study to investigate the accuracy of palpation findings (Evans, 1994), an instrument was made to simulate the movement the therapist might expect to find when using her thumbs on a spinous process and examining movement in the postero-anterior direction. The instrument had a plunger which moved

4.0 mm vertically, and was able to measure movement throughout that range more accurately than could be determined by a dial gauge resolving to 0.01 mm. The plunger was controlled electromagnetically, so that mechanical cues from strings, weights or friction were avoided. Resistance to the plunger movement could be introduced at any point by the electromagnetic control system (*Figure 7.13*).

Using a task where the therapist was required to detect the onset of a subtle resistance ($R_1$) at some point within the range of movement of the plunger, the standard deviation for $R_1$ estimation by experienced manipulative therapists was 0.16 mm. Untrained subjects had a standard deviation of 0.79 mm. When asked to perform the smallest grade I oscillatory movement on the plunger, the mean amplitude of oscillation was 0.02 mm for the experienced manipulative therapists, and 0.10 mm for untrained subjects.

Although these are results from a preliminary investigation, and a great deal more research needs to be done, it is obvious that the accuracy that may be obtained by palpation and passive movement techniques is remarkably fine.

## RHYTHM

The rhythm of mobilization can be varied in many ways, ranging from a slow gentle movement to a sharp staccato movement or a sustained position without any oscillation at all.

Staccato techniques are used to make a stiff joint move to the limit of its maximum range before its neighbouring joints have time to start moving. It is obvious that to use such a rhythm the joint disorder must be chronic and not markedly painful. If the symptoms from the joint are minimal, the speed of the staccato technique can be likened to the staccato notes produced on the violin by plucking; if the symptoms are moderate, the staccato technique can be likened to the staccato notes produced with the bow on the violin.

When a joint disorder is quite painful, the oscillatory movement should be performed smoothly and evenly so that the moment when the oscillation changes from 'pressure-on' to 'pressure-off' cannot be determined.

> Rhythm of movement varies from smooth gentle techniques to sharp staccato movement or to a sustained position without any oscillation at all. The rhythm is selected depending on the objective of the technique

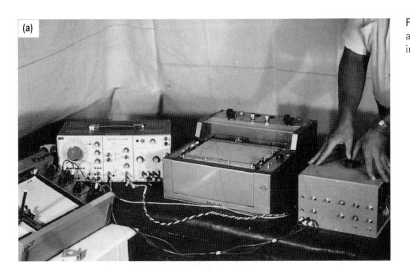

(a)

Figure 7.13 Palpation skills. (*a*) Plunger and recording equipment. (*b*) Measuring instruments

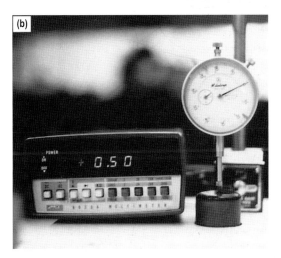

(b)

Using the simile of the violin again, the violinist can play a prolonged note in such a manner that if the listener closes her eyes, she is unable to tell when the bow changes from the up-stroke to the down-stroke. Also, the speed of the forward direction is the same as the speed of the backward direction. Under nearly all other circumstances, the comparative speed in each direction is different. The forward direction (pressure-on) is always faster, even if only fractionally so, than the backward direction (pressure-off). It is a valuable experience for every practising manipulative physiotherapist to have performed an oscillatory cervical rotation of 30° amplitude performed on her, first applied with the rotation movement faster than the de-rotation, and then with the de-rotation faster than the rotation. In this way she can feel the difference between them.

There are three exceptions to this general rule of pressure-on being faster than pressure-off:

1. When pain is experienced as a consequence of movement in a releasing direction.

2. When the spinous process is abnormally deep set and painful when postero-anterior pressure is applied. Under both of these circumstances the 'pressure-off' part of the oscillation should be distinctly faster than the 'pressure-on'.

3. The third exception is when a technique is used as a slowly increasing sustained pressure into either muscle spasm or strong resistance, when the pain provoked by the pressure is quite intense. While the technique is performed at the moment when the pain is about to increase suddenly and sharply,

the pressure should be instantly released, even if only by a millimetre, so as to avoid the sharp increase. This new position is then held for as long as feels reasonable for the intensity to have subsided. The manipulative physiotherapist determines this by closely communicating with the patient. Whereupon the movement is then slowly taken further into the range until the next small 'backing off' is required.

Another facet is that it is possible, by altering the rhythm, to treat with anteroposterior movements by applying postero-anterior pressures. This is achieved by putting the emphasis of the oscillatory movement on the release of the pressure-off rather than on the postero-anterior direction itself. In other words, the speed of the release of the pressure-on (i.e. pressure-off) is faster than the slow, deliberate *application* of the postero-anterior pressure (i.e. pressure-on). This particular rhythm is also used when a patient's pain response is felt on the release component of postero-anterior pressure movements. In other words, the speed of the release of the pressure-on (i.e. pressure-off) is faster than the slow, deliberate application of the postero-anterior pressure (i.e. pressure-on). This particular rhythm is also used when using pressure movements.

## RELEASE PAIN

Pain experienced as a result of this pressure-off situation can be referred to as release pain. This can be experienced actively, as when an arthritic joint is moved to its limit and then released from the limit.

There are three aspects to this, and the first involves time. The amount of time that the limit of the movement is sustained will influence the intensity of the release pain. Secondly, the range of movement in the releasing direction can alter the pain response. For example, if the neck is turned to the left and the releasing movement involves de-rotation to neutral but without stopping the movement is continued to involve some rotation, the right pain may be experienced after the neutral position has been passed. Thirdly, the speed of the releasing movement can influence the pain experience. The more quickly the movement is done, the more pain can be felt. The relative speeds of the 'pressure-on', 'pressure-off' are dictated by the pain response intended. Usually, the further the 'pressure-on' is taken into the range, and also the faster the 'pressure-off' is performed, the greater is the pain so provoked.

Release pain can similarly be experienced as a result of passive movement.

As a treatment technique, a postero-anterior pressure may cause pain and by sustaining that pressure

(using the time aspect already mentioned) the release pain can be useful as an assessment guide or asterisk indicating improvement or worsening.

If the release pain intensity is lessening even though the PA pressure is being sustained for the same length of time, the patient's asterisk movement will show improvement.

## TREATING PAIN-THROUGH-RANGE

When treating pain (that is, treating a pain-through-range situation with grade II movements), the amplitude of the movement must be as large as the symptom response will allow; the greater the pain, the slower and smoother should be the rhythm. The changes that can be made to advance this technique (without altering the patient's position) are to:

1. Make the amplitude larger.
2. Take the movement into a degree of discomfort.
3. Increase the speed of the oscillation while still retaining its smoothness.
4. Make the oscillation slightly staccato.

## TREATING END-OF-RANGE PAIN

When treating pain that is present only at the end of range, or when treating stiffness, the technique should be a small-amplitude staccato movement at the limit of the range. The treatment movement stretches the joint structures to the limit of their range, and is held there firmly by the manipulative physiotherapist for as long as 5 minutes. The staccato small-amplitude overpressures are applied for a time and at a strength dictated by how chronic the disorder is and the degree of discomfort intended to be produced by the stretch.

The pressures referred to above are not performed on only the one vertebra, even if it is only movement of that single vertebra that reproduces the patient's symptoms. If T8 is the vertebra at fault and postero-anterior pressure is the oscillatory treatment technique, the treatment movements would, at least, be applied to T7 and T9 as well. This is only a general rule, and is open to wide variations. However, when the pressures are used to treat a somewhat stiff T8, the rhythm of the technique would be similar to the following: four oscillations on T8, four on T7, then four on T8, then four on T9, T8, T7, and so on.

## TREATING MUSCLE SPASM

When using a technique that is a painful movement protected by muscle spasm, the rhythm is mainly a sustained position rather than an oscillation. The technique is slowly taken in to the point where pain is felt and muscle spasm resists further movement. This technique position is then held still, waiting for the level of pain to lessen to allow the spasm to decrease. The waiting time can be as long as 1 minute, but is usually in the order of 10–20 seconds. The technique is then nudged a fraction further and held at that position to wait again for pain and spasm to allow further movement. During this slow process, some tiny slow oscillatory movement is interspersed: no more than three or four oscillations at a time, and without much of an increase in pain.

When spasm limits the available range of movement, the rhythm of the technique used is a very slowly applied pressure and there is no oscillation other than a tiny release component when the spasm minutely but sharply increases. This pressure is sustained with such precise control that the patient has confidence in the manipulative physiotherapist's skill in predicting the moment to release the pressure and in knowing how slowly to increase the 'pressure-on'. It also enables the patient to gather strength for the next sustained pressure.

## LATENT PAIN RESPONSE

When a patient, during the physical examination, is found to have a latent pain response (*see* p. 63), the duration of sustaining a technique is frequently directly proportional to the timing of that latent pain response. The longer it takes to provoke symptoms on sustaining a test movement with firm over-pressure at the limit of the range, the longer the treatment technique should be sustained. *This is an important principle.*

## CHANGING DEPTHS OF RHYTHM

### SMOOTH RHYTHMS

Once a rhythm has been chosen, it can be performed at different depths in a range. The depth of a smooth, even rhythm used to treat pain is changed in response to pain felt during the technique; that is, the technique is moved back in the range to avoid pain. Similarly, if it is intended that the technique should be performed as close as possible to the point in the range when pain begins, it is necessary occasionally to carry the rhythm a fraction further into the range to see that the position of the oscillation is correct. If the technique is successfully changing the symptoms and signs, the pain may recede, allowing the rhythm to be taken deeper into the range by increasing the range of movement.

## STACCATO RHYTHMS

Staccato techniques can be used as a broken rhythm; that is, a sequence of four staccato movements can be followed, after a small rest, by two movements, then five, then one, then three and so on. This provides the manipulative physiotherapist with a good 'feel' of the movement, and avoids any anticipation by the patient as to when the movement is going to be applied – thus avoiding any 'muscle holding'.

For example, if the treatment technique of choice is lumbar rotation done in side lying, the technique may be done as a IV to treat end-of-range softness, and this may cause some pain. By interrupting the rhythm with a III of large amplitude, he cannot predict the change in rhythm and amplitude of movement, and this interrupts his attempts to 'help'.

## MANIPULATIONS

Rhythm is also important in relation to manipulative techniques. Obviously manipulative techniques are performed with speed, but even though the end-position of the manipulative movement is constant for a particular set of conditions, the starting position may vary. Once the position to perform the manipulation has been adopted, and it is determined that the desired symptom response is felt when the stretch position of the technique is tested, the stretched position can be eased. The decision is then made as to whether the manipulation is performed from the stretch position or from a position where the stretch has been slightly but significantly released. Whichever is chosen, the manipulation is taken to the same end-position. From the stretch position the amplitude is tiny; from the released or eased position the amplitude is larger, but only because it is starting from a position further back in the range, not because it is going further into the range.

## RHYTHM/SYMPTOM RESPONSE

Following examination and assessment, a particular technique may be chosen with the deliberate intention that it should reproduce a calculated degree of local discomfort. This may be the choice for two reasons:

1. It is anticipated that the symptoms will decrease as the technique is continued, and that they may completely disappear. If this does occur during the performance of the technique, the patient's movements and symptoms should show improvement when reassessed.

2. It provides further valuable objective examination information to know the effect of repeated movement in a particular direction that is painful. For example, if a particular movement is performed with a constant rhythm and the movement is painless at first but an ache develops and worsens over a period of say 20 seconds, it is obvious that the state of that joint disorder is worse than if the movement had caused discomfort at the beginning but had become painless within 20 seconds.

> It is important that, with every technique, the manipulative physiotherapist must be fully aware at all times of the effect the technique is having on the patient's symptoms *while the technique is being performed*

Regarding using postero-anterior movements on a spinous process (say L4) that is prominent and painful, the rhythm of the technique should be adjusted to reduce the pain. This may be achieved in a variety of ways:

1. The rhythm may be tiny in amplitude so that the movement through range, being smaller, will not provoke as much 'through-range pain'. The 'through-range pain' will be far less, though *movement* of the joint, which is an essential part of the treatment, will still be taking place.

2. The speed of the oscillation should be reduced to a speed of approximately one oscillation per 2 seconds. This will also lessen the amount of pain with the treatment technique because it is reducing the amount of movement of the joint of a unit period of time.

3. Because the amplitude is tiny and the speed of oscillation is slow, the pain will be less and the patient will be able to relax more readily and therefore the technique will be able to be taken deeper into the range.

4. By being able to go deeper into the range, the technique will be more effective in producing improvement, and in fact it will be noticed during the application of the technique that the physiotherapist will be able, quite quickly, to go more deeply into the range without provoking any increase in pain.

The reverse would happen if a larger amplitude were used and the rate of oscillation were two or three oscillations per second. If the amplitude is too big and the speed too great, then the joint will become more sore with the treatment, thus aggravating the patient's symptoms and indicating to the physiotherapist, incorrectly, that postero-anterior movement is not the right technique to use.

From all that has been said so far, it should be clear that performing a technique well is more than just carrying out a manoeuvre with mechanical excellence. Like the soloist playing her part in, say, a violin concerto, the manipulator needs to be deeply, totally and emotionally involved in the technique she is performing. When she mobilizes a joint by a particular manoeuvre, she needs to block out from her mind all other distracting influences – she needs to try to put herself inside the joint structures she is moving and feel a part of them.

## MANIPULATION

The point has already been made that a mobilization, even though it may be done firmly, does not consist of a sudden movement. A sudden movement or thrust constitutes a manipulation. There are two types of manipulative techniques: those that are the same as the mobilizations already described but performed much more rapidly; and those that localize the manipulation as much as is possible to one intervertebral joint to free its range of movement. Whatever type is used, it is always a quick movement of very small amplitude. Strong traction is unnecessary and, in some instances, is a distinct disadvantage. If it is applied strongly, it lessens the range available for the manipulation. *Some manipulators believe it provides a safety factor. This is false: safety is provided by gradual progression of the strength of the technique coupled with continual assessment.*

### TYPE 1

During treatment by mobilization, the improvement rate may slow down even though the early mobilizations were methodically increased in depth and produced adequate progress. Under these circumstances it may be necessary to alter the technique to include a sudden movement near the limit of the range. Such an over-pressure is usually only necessary in the mobilizing techniques of postero-anterior unilateral vertebral pressure in the thoracic region; postero-anterior central vertebral pressure in the thoracic and lumbar regions; and rotation in the cervical and lumbar regions.

### TYPE 2

Where an almost painless limitation of movement, which is presumed to be the cause of a patient's symptoms, cannot be sufficiently improved by mobilization or the manipulative techniques described above, the manipulation must be localized to the one joint. This manipulation aims at directly restoring movement to the faulty inter-vertebral segment.

## MANIPULATION UNDER ANAESTHESIA (MUA)

Following the issue of the third edition of *Vertebral Manipulation*, a very constructive review was published which emphasized the importance of MUA. In that review, and in subsequent correspondence with the author, the reviewer advocated acknowledgement in the text of the existence of 'manipulation under anaesthesia' (MUA) as it is used widely by doctors and by some physiotherapists, and with this view the author heartily concurs.

Bremner (1958) provides evidence of the effectiveness of MUA in the treatment of lumbosacral strain. Probably the same applies to any local pain and stiffness of spinal origin; it certainly does in the cervical spine. Cyriax (1980) sets out clearly the indications and contraindications for MUA and the same for manipulation (Cyriax and Cyriax, 1993).

A patient's condition may be improved initially by mobilization and manipulation, but a stage may be reached where the rate of progress stops. MUA may then be indicated. The build of the patient, or a degree of voluntary muscle contraction that prevents manipulation while a patient is conscious, may well make MUA the treatment of choice. The reviewer rightly asserts that in 'determining management of difficult and unresponsive cases it proves very profitable for the doctor and physiotherapist to confer'.

If a patient can relax completely, the end-feel of the range of movement being manipulated is the same whether he is manipulated consciously or under anaesthesia.

Care must be taken not to manipulate under anaesthesia too vigorously. Rather than trying to achieve a full range of movement in one manipulation, it is often better to manipulate more gently on two or more occasions. In a second article (Bremner and Simpson, 1959), Bremner advocates 'follow-up' physiotherapy after an MUA has been carried out.

The degree of success of an MUA will be known within 2 or 3 days. If the patient gains complete relief from his symptoms, follow-up treatment is unnecessary. However, if the symptoms do not improve sufficiently, passive mobilization will be required. When radiological evidence of joint changes (which account for some of the stiffness) is present, the patient should be taught to perform daily mobilizing exercises. When there is instability, stabilizing exercises should be performed daily.

It is important to bear in mind that follow-up treatment should only be given selectively and not routinely for all patients.

Where manipulation of the conscious patient has failed, MUA may be successful. The converse is also true. Sometimes, as evidenced by the reviewer, patients may require a balance of both.

## SUMMARY

To summarize the need for manipulations as means of quick thrust techniques or manipulations under anaesthesia in clinical situations, my clinical experience has taught me that whereas a decade or so ago I considered that of the patients who did respond to passive movement treatment 85 per cent only required mobilization and 15 per cent required manipulation, now these percentages have changed to 98–99 per cent and 1–2 per cent respectively.

# Chapter **8**

# Selection of techniques

Patients referred for or seeking manipulative physiotherapy are considered in two distinct groups. First, there are those who have suffered an injury of some kind, whether due to a fall, direct blow or the post-surgical situation. The second group includes patients whose symptoms have appeared spontaneously or following a trivial incident such as lifting a suitcase out of a car or turning sharply. Patients in the second group have symptoms, signs and histories that are readily recognizable. Patients of the first group have had injury to normal tissues and can present with any configuration of symptoms and signs; however, some of their symptoms and signs may fit parts of the patterns of the second group. It is to this second group – where

**Table 8.1**  Sequence of selection of techniques

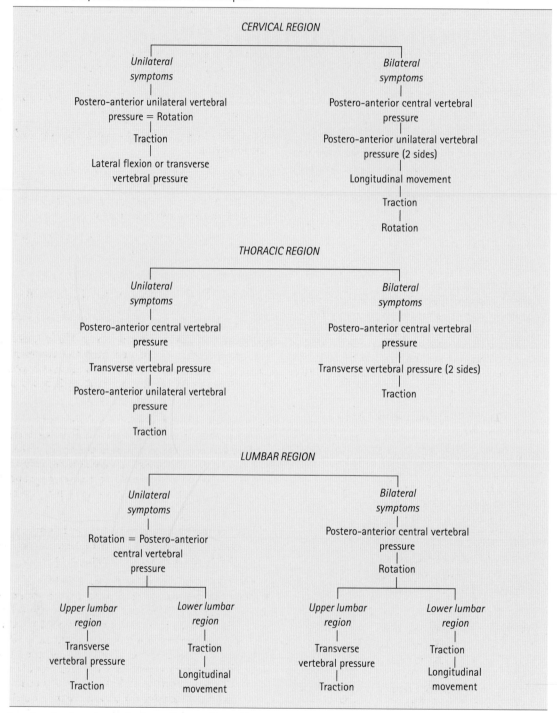

In each region the order may be changed by removing traction from its designated position and placing it anywhere in sequence. The remaining techniques are then used in the same order as shown in this table.

'selection' and 'prediction' are clearest – that the whole of this chapter is applied.

> Manipulative physiotherapy is not only a matter of learning and applying techniques. It is a matter of knowing *when* and *how* to use *which* technique, how to *adapt* the technique to the particular situation of the patient

In earlier editions of this book two tables were provided as guidelines for the selection of treatment techniques. One table listed a sequence of selection based on when the patient's symptoms were distributed unilaterally or bilaterally (*Table 8.1*), and the second table related specific techniques to their primary uses in each section of the spine (*Table 8.2*). These tables are useful as an oversimplified basis for selection of techniques. To set down, in written form, guidelines for the selection of techniques is difficult. The subject is not merely a matter of deciding when to select a particular mobilization or manipulation, or even when to change from one technique to another; it also includes decisions regarding the rhythm, amplitude and strength of the technique and the position in range in which the technique should be performed. Finally, there is of course the duration of application of the technique(s) (summarized in *Table 8.3*).

Item D in *Table 8.3* – the manner and duration of the technique – refers to:

1. The position in the available range of movements in which the technique should be performed.
2. The firmness or gentleness of the movement.
3. The amplitude of the movement.
4. The speed of the movement.
5. The rhythm of the movement, ranging from 'gentle' to 'staccato'.
6. The desired pain response, or absence of pain, during the performing of the technique.
7. The length of time the movement should be continued.

Over the last 10 or more years, the skills associated with the selection and progression of techniques have grown concurrently with the growth of knowledge in anatomy, neurophysiology, biomechanics, pathology and diagnosis, together with refined examination and assessment skills. Probably the greatest growth has occurred in the following four areas:

1. The clearer recognition and interpretation of different patterns of patients' symptoms, signs and histories.

2. The recognition of the different types of pain, and different patterns of behaviour of that pain (Butler, 1999).
3. Predictable responses.
4. Refinement of assessment skills. The analytical assessment of the site, quality and behaviour of the patient's pain plus the concurrent recognition of the neuro-musculoskeletal structures involved are areas of important growth.

'Selection', as discussed in this chapter, is divided into the following:

1. General aspects for selection technique.
2. Aspects of the technique itself.
3. The relation of selection to the diagnosis and presenting symptoms and signs.

A useful additional reference to selection of techniques appears in Magarey (1986).

## SELECTION – GENERAL ASPECTS FOR SELECTING TECHNIQUES

Presuming one knows all the kinds of techniques that are available for use in treatment (*see* comment on page 5, and the test related to techniques in Chapter 7), the selection of a particular technique is based upon the following three integrated parts:

1. *Current knowledge of pathological disorders and injury of the vertebral column*. This knowledge includes known and proven facts, realizing that there is much still unknown. Of greatest importance is knowing the structures that can cause pain and the different patterns of pain response that can occur during test movements.

2. *Diagnosis*. The diagnostic title is important, but needs to be closely related to the history when considering the selection of techniques (p. 196).

3. *History, symptoms and signs* (pp. 199–200).
   a) With regard to the history, and knowing the diagnosis of the patient's disorder, the aspects directly associated with the selection of the treatment technique are: the onset and progress of the disorder; the stage of the disorder when the patient seeks treatment; the degree of stability of the disorder at the time he seeks treatment; and the irritability or severity of the disorder.
   b) The symptoms include the areas and types of pain of which the patient complains, the circumstances under which he feels them and the way it may limit him to pursue activities of his life.

**Table 8.2** Mobilizing techniques and their uses

| Technique | Primary uses |
|---|---|
| | *CERVICAL REGION* |
| Longitudinal movement | Frequently of value in presence of a spasm deformity |
| Postero-anterior central vertebral pressure | Bilaterally distributed symptoms. Bony changes from all causes; muscle spasm. Not for severe symptoms |
| Postero-anterior unilateral vertebral pressure | Unilaterally distributed symptoms particularly if middle or upper cervical in origin. (Direct the push downwards on the side of pain) |
| Transverse vertebral pressure | Unilaterally distributed symptoms. Bony changes from all causes. (Direct the push towards the side of pain) |
| Anteroposterior unilateral vertebral pressure | Unilaterally distributed symptoms. (Direct the push on the side of pain) |
| Rotation | Most valuable – usually the first technique used. Unilaterally distributed symptoms. (Rotate the head away from the side of pain) |
| Lateral flexion | Unilaterally distributed symptoms. Often used to restore rotation. (Flex away from the side of pain) |
| Flexion | Minor symptoms in the presence of intervertebral flexion restriction |
| Traction | Any cervical condition – severe arm pain with markedly limited neck movements |
|     Traction in neutral | Upper cervical conditions |
|     Traction in flexion | Lower cervical conditions |
|     Intermittent variable traction | Gross radiological degenerative changes |
| | *THORACIC REGION* |
| Posterior-anterior central vertebral pressure | Usually the first technique used. Bilaterally distributed symptoms; unilaterally distributed symptoms if poorly defined or widespread |
| Transverse vertebral pressure | Unilaterally distributed symptoms. (Direct the push towards the side of pain and mobilize adjacent rib) |
| Posterior-anterior unilateral vertebral pressure | Unilaterally distributed symptoms. (Direct the push downwards on the side of pain and mobilize adjacent rib) |
| Traction | Widely distributed symptoms especially if radiological degenerative changes are present; when pain is not aggravated by active movements |
| | *LUMBAR REGION* |
| Postero-anterior central vertebral pressure | Bilaterally distributed symptoms. (Equal in usefulness with rotation.) Bony changes from all causes |
| Postero-anterior unilateral vertebral pressure | Unilaterally distributed symptoms particularly if middle or upper lumbar in pressure origin. (Direct the push downwards on the side of pain) |
| Transverse vertebral pressure | Unilaterally distributed symptoms. More useful for upper lumbar spine than lower. (Direct the push towards the side of pain) |
| Rotation | Often the first technique used. Unilaterally distributed symptoms. (Rotate the pelvis forwards on the side of pain) |
| Longitudinal movement | Two legs Bilaterally distributed symptoms of lower lumbar origin |
| | One leg Unilaterally distributed symptoms of lower lumbar origin |
| Flexion | Bilaterally distributed symptoms of a chronic nature in the presence of flexion restriction |
| Traction | Gradual onset of symptoms. When pain is not aggravated by active movements |
| Intermittent variable traction | Gross radiological degenerative changes |
| Straight-leg raising | Unilateral limitation of straight-leg raising without extreme pain |
| | For symptoms of a chronic or stable nature arising from the nerve root. (The technique is not used as a first technique) |

Table 8.3    Guidelines for the selection of technique

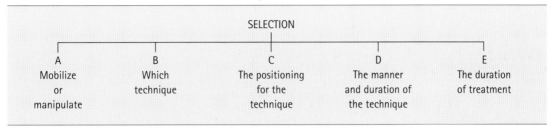

| | | SELECTION | | |
|---|---|---|---|---|
| A | B | C | D | E |
| Mobilize or manipulate | Which technique | The positioning for the technique | The manner and duration of the technique | The duration of treatment |

c) The signs refer to the complete physical examination findings, but the aspect most important to the selection of techniques is the manner in which the patient's symptoms can be reproduced and varied by the examination test movements of the structure(s) causing the patient's symptoms.

Before relating the selection of particular techniques to these three integral parts, it is necessary to discuss each of them in depth. To some readers this may seem tedious and to others unnecessary, but as the authors believe that the whole process of treatment is based on 'cause and effect', the importance and influences of the integral parts must be thoroughly understood. A discussion of selecting techniques will follow.

## CURRENT KNOWLEDGE OF PATHOLOGICAL DISORDERS

There are three aspects to consider:

1. Movements and the related range/pain response.
2. Pain-sensitive structures and their patterns of pain.
3. The pathological disorders and injury.

## MOVEMENTS

### Physiological movement considerations

The movements referred to include movements of the vertebrae and their functional structures, movements of the structures in the vertebral canal and intervertebral foramina, and movements of all the neural components. Movements of the vertebrae include movements of the intervertebral disc, the neurocentral joints of Luschka and the zygapophyseal joints, while movements of the foraminal and canal structures include movements of the spinal cord, the dura, the vessels, the nerve roots and their dural investments (Breig, 1978).

The least complicated *gross* movements are flexion, extension and longitudinal movement cephalad and caudad (that is, long-axis extension or axial extension),

and straight leg raising. Each of the joint movements can be performed while the joint is positioned in various degrees of lateral flexion and rotation. Additionally, longitudinal movement can also be performed with the joint positioned in various degrees of flexion and extension (plus degrees of lateral flexion and rotation). Similarly, the movements of flexion and extension can be performed in various positions of longitudinal movement either cephalad or caudad.

In most levels of the spine the gross movement of lateral flexion includes a component of rotation, and similarly the movement of rotation includes a component of lateral flexion (White and Panjabi, 1978). For example, it is believed that if the normal lumbar spine is positioned in flexion and is then laterally flexed to the left, the lateral flexion will include a degree of rotation to the left. Similarly, if the normal lumbar spine is positioned in extension, the movement of lateral flexion to the left is combined with rotation to the right. If these two statements are correct, then there must, of necessity, be a position between lumbar flexion and extension when lateral flexion to the left will not include any rotation. However, in this flexion/extension position, the available range of lateral flexion will be more limited than if the position of flexion/extension were altered so as to allow rotation to take place. In the cervical spine (C2–C7), lateral flexion and rotation occur to the same side regardless of the amount of flexion and extension.

The transverse axis around which flexion and extension take place, like the sagittal axis for lateral flexion and the longitudinal axis for rotation, is not in a single fixed position; there is an 'instantaneous' axis of rotation for each phase of a movement. These varying axes are discussed in depth by White and Panjabi (1978).

There must also be a difference as to what takes place in the intervertebral joint when lateral flexion (say of the lumbar spine) is performed from above downwards (that is, asking the patient to bend his trunk to the right), compared with being performed from below upwards (asking the patient to hitch his right hip upwards towards his right shoulder; *see* p. 349 and *Figure 12.6*). There must be a difference, because patients frequently have different pain responses depending on whether the movement is carried out from the top downwards or the bottom upwards.

The pain-sensitive structures in the vertebral canal and intervertebral foramina can be moved in either a cephalad or caudad direction. Also, the canal structures can be moved or approximated towards any desired surface of the canal, either by standing or lying the patient in different positions (for example, lying him on his left or right side, prone or supine); or by positioning the intervertebral joints in flexion, extension, lateral flexion or rotation while producing the cephalad or caudad movement of the canal structures. This subject is dealt with fully by Breig (1978).

Tests for the pain-sensitive neural elements from the CNS (central nervous system) to the periphery rely on movement tests/range/pain-response manoeuvres, as do 'joints', but the skills are different. The two main physiotherapists to explore this continuing subject, R. Elvey (Perth, Western Australia) and D. Butler (Adelaide, South Australia), have evolved procedures in the field of recognition and treatment by passive movement. To understand and learn from their contribution it is necessary to understand Elvey's articles and Butler's book (Butler, 1991).

There are tests designated for different peripheral nerves (Butler, 1991). These give the examiner the means of differentiating between a radicular spinal referred pain and the pain from a peripheral neural pain (intraneural, perineural, extraneural).

## Range/pain response to movement

This is determined by the many test movements of the JOINTS and the CANAL/FORAMINA and neural structures. There are three considerations:

1. Stretching or compressing pain.
2. The pain may present as a pain-through-range situation, and end-of-range situation or a combination of both.
3. When a patient has spinal pain and referred pain, movements may provoke the local pain, the referred pain, or both.

### Stretching or compressing pain

> With active testing there are three passive end-of-range pain responses: a compression feeling, a stretch feeling or a feeling of pain

When pain of intervertebral joint origin is felt locally yet unilaterally, examination movements may reproduce this pain by either stretching or compressing the faulty structure. For example, if the patient has pain on the right side of the T10–T12 area, this pain may be provoked by lateral flexion to the right, which would be a compressive type of pain response, or it may be provoked by lateral flexion to the left, which would be a stretch response. However, under the latter circumstance the patient may feel that the response is just a stretching feeling, or he may feel it as a pain. We therefore have three end-of-range pain responses.

### End-of-range or through-range pain

These descriptive titles are self-explanatory. A patient will feel pain only when he moves the part at fault to the end of its range of movement. The pain may occur only in one direction of movement, in many different directions, or only in one direction that is a combined movement – such as combined extension plus lateral flexion to the right and rotation to the left (as at the end of the swing for a right-handed golfer).

A through-range pain is commonly associated with symptoms that are felt constantly by the patient. On examination of the movements, pain is felt well before the end of the range of the test movement and the pain tends to increase in intensity as the movement is carried further into range. An area or arc of pain or an ache can also be considered to be through-range in nature.

### Local and referred pain

When a patient has referred pain, the pain response to test movements of the intervertebral joint, the canal/foramina or neural structures is extremely important. The pain responses that are of greatest significance in the selection of techniques are as follows:

1. Test movements, even if restricted, may provoke only local spinal pain without making any difference to the referred pain either at the time of the test movements or as a latent pain response. This movement response can be handled firmly with safety.

2. Test movements may provoke an ache, a lancinating pain, or tingling in the referred area. Such a response demands respect, and provoking the responses should be avoided during early treatment and daily activities.

3. Test movements may provoke distally referred symptoms as an immediate response to the movement without provoking any spinal pain. Though it may be necessary to provoke the pain slightly with a treatment, it should be done only if the pain reverts to its prior level on releasing the technique.

4. When referred pain is provoked by a test movement, the pain may start distally and spread proximally,

or *vice versa*. Neither is a favourable response to movement, and should be avoided.

5. A test movement may need to be sustained before the referred pain is provoked. If the latent period is long and the symptoms chronic, the treatment technique should be sustained. If the symptoms are acute, provoking should be avoided.

6. The referred pain provoked by a test movement may linger even after the test has been completed, or it may disappear immediately on completion of the test movement. Lingering referred pain requires considerable respect, whereas immediate loss of pain on releasing the technique permits firmer techniques.

7. A test movement may be painless, yet once it is completed the patient may experience the referred pain as an after-effect from the tests movement. Such a response demands gentleness of technique, short treatment sessions followed by a rest period and very careful assessment over each 24-hour-period following treatment if worsening of the disorder is to be avoided.

> With referred pain, special attention needs to be given to the pain responses during test movements before the application of treatment techniques

## PAIN-SENSITIVE STRUCTURES AND THEIR PAIN PATTERNS

The following is an endeavour to relate the pain that a patient may experience to the pain-sensitive structures of the intervertebral segment. The lists that follow must NOT be seen as being infallible, complete or exact. There is still much that is unknown about pain, and many existing theories in the experiments directed towards relating areas of referred pain to pain-sensitive spinal structures are still contested.

In the intervertebral segment, the common structures that cause symptoms can be divided into two main groups. First, there are the joints and their supportive structures; and secondly there are the pain-sensitive structures in the vertebral canal and intervertebral foramina and the neural disorders.

The intervertebral JOINT structures are:

1. The intervertebral disc (Bogduk *et al.*, 1982).
2. The ligamentous structures between adjacent vertebrae and the capsule of the zygapophyseal joint, and the intrinsic muscle attachments.
3. The zygapophyseal joint.
4. The bones.

5. The periosteum, fascia, tendons and aponeuroses.
6. The arteries and arterioles.
7. The epidural and paravertebral veins (points 2–7: Wyke, 1976).

The particular pain-sensitive structures in the vertebral CANAL and intervertebral FORAMINA referred to in this text are:

- The dura.
- The nerve root sleeve.
- The nerve roots and their rootlets (Macnab, 1989; personal communication).

When any of the above structures (excluding the nerve root or its sleeve) cause pain, that pain may be felt locally but may also be felt in a referred area. However, the referred pain has different characteristics for some of the different structures. The local and referred pain from the joint and canal structures are as follows.

### The intervertebral joint structures

#### The intervertebral disc

(*See*: Kellgren, 1939; Inman and Saunders, 1944; Sinclair *et al.*, 1948; Hirsch *et al.*, 1963; Mooney and Robertson, 1976; Glover, 1977; Bogduk, 1980a, 1980b; Grieve, 1988; Groen *et al.*, 1990; Bogduk and Twomey, 1991; Kakamura *et al.*, 1996.)

Pain from disorders of the intervertebral disc is commonly distributed in broad areas with ill-defined margins (Hirsch *et al.*, 1963). In the lumbar spine it may be a broad band across the back, or it may have an ill-defined gluteal distribution to which the patient is only able to point by using his whole hand over the buttock. If questioned, he is unable to palpate a particular spot to demonstrate the distribution. This pain may also spread into the upper posterior or posterolateral thigh and lower abdomen. In the cervical spine the pain area is also broad and vague, either across the suprascapular areas or over an ill-defined area of one scapula (Cloward, 1959). Such pain may also spread vaguely into the upper arm. The distribution of discogenic pain may be central, unilateral, bilateral symmetrically or bilateral asymmetrically.

Pain or aching arising from a discogenic disorder within an intact outer annulus fibrosus (with the exception of symptoms that have been mild over a long continuous period without change) has a quality about it that makes it more difficult to bear than pain or aching arising from ligamentous disorders. This discogenic pain is commonly more distressing, wearing, sickening and depressing.

The intervertebral disc does not usually refer symptoms into the distal part of a limb unless other pain-sensitive structures are also involved in causing the pain.

Discogenic pain of recent origin or recent exacerbation has two features. The first is that the symptoms are felt to be deep and poorly localized and often cause a sickening or nauseous response. The patient can increase, decrease or eliminate the symptoms by adopting certain postures. When a patient adopts a position that puts the intervertebral joint towards the limit of one range of movement and sustains this position for some time, he will find that to reverse it will be difficult and require time (a few seconds); he will not be able to change position sharply (e.g. standing erect after a prolonged interval of slumped sitting).

The second feature is that, even when movements are restricted by discogenic pain, the point in the range at which this pain is felt will vary depending upon the speed of the movement. Linked with this feature are the facts that there will be a pain-through-range component to the symptoms and there may be a summation of pain, a relief of pain, or latent pain that follows a sustained position. Although these features may occur with other structures than the disc, the qualities of the discogenic features are characteristically more unpleasant, slower to occur and more lingering.

Discogenic pain may be provoked either by stretching movements or by compressing movements (see p. 188).

### The ligamentous and outer capsular structures

Pain is almost always felt locally at the site of the faulty structure, and can usually be specifically pointed to by the patient. Areas of referred pain from these structures are poorly defined. Although the referred pain can spread into the distal area of a limb, this distal referral is ALWAYS of less intensity than the more proximally referred area of pain. It is uncommon to be able to provoke the referred pain during a consultation by any particular position or movement.

Local symptoms arising from these structures can always be provoked by movement in one of the following three ways:

1. A movement that stretches the structure may provoke a sharp pain.
2. A movement that stretches the structure may cause a pulling stretching feeling at the site of the symptoms.
3. Stretching movements may be painless, but a movement that compresses the structure may reproduce the local symptoms (see p. 188).

### The zygapophyseal joint

The zygapophyseal joint should be thought of in two categories, intra-articular and periarticular. The joint is subject to the same changes as any synovial joint. There are, for example, the osteoarthritic type disorders (Harris and Macnab, 1954; Figure 8.1) – degenerative, post-traumatic, non-infective disorders – and mechanical disorders from intrusion of structures into the joint such as exist with a loose body, a meniscus entrapment and synovial membrane entrapment (Figure 8.1).

Though there may be radiological evidence of osteoarthritic joint changes, the joint can be quite pain free or it may be extremely painful. The extent of radiological change is no indication of the amount of pain. The arthritic hip can cause referred pain in the knee without there being any pain in the area of the hip or thigh. The zygapophyseal joints have these same three similar properties.

Pain from the zygapophyseal joint can therefore present: (1) in an acute phase when the pain, which is always felt locally and may spread, is quite severe; (2) in a pain-free phase; or (3) in a chronic phase where there may be no local pain, yet referred pain may be felt in a distant localized area (Dwyer et al., 1990). An example of this is a patch of abdominal pain, which may arise from the appropriate thoracic zygapophyseal joint (Lewitt et al., 1951; Bogduk, 1978).

### Referred pain

Pain from ligamentous and capsular structures as well as from the zygapophyseal joints can be referred into areas distant from their source.

Structures that are well distant from the nerve root can cause this somatic referred pain when injected with an irritant (Kellgren, 1939; Inman and Saunders, 1944; Sinclair et al., 1948; Feinstein et al., 1954; Hockaday and Whitty, 1967; Mooney and Robertson, 1976; McCall et al., 1979).

When the space in the vertebral canal and intervertebral foramina is severely narrowed, the pain-sensitive structures are far more easily compromised and they then cause referred radicular pain, with or without neurological signs or changes.

The disc itself can cause referred pain, an example being the referred pain felt by patients during discography. This can occur even when the discogram does not indicate any fissure extending into the outer layers of the annulus fibrosus. Any damaged disc can impinge against the posterior longitudinal ligament or the dura and thereby cause referred pain. Also the disc, as it is herniating or when it herniates, can impinge upon the nerve-root sleeve, the nerve root or the rootlets, and cause referred pain. The characteristics of the referred pain from these different sources have been stated above.

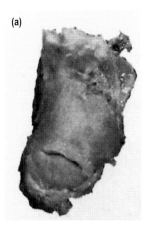

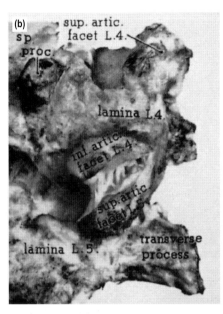

**Figure 8.1** (*a*) An inferior articular facet from a third lumbar vertebra showing a fissure fracture running across the inferior pole of the facet. (*b*) Dense adhesions in a posterior joint. The specimen was photographed from behind and the lips of the posterior have been opened as far as possible, showing a dense mass of adhesions passing from one articular surface to the other. (*c*) Degenerative changes in the posterior joints. (*d*) A posterior joint showing a loose body connected to the synovial membrane. The inferior articular facet of the vertebra above is shown below the loose body lying between the articular surfaces (Reproduced from Harris, R.I. and Macnab, I. (1954) *Journal of Bone and Joint Surgery*, **36B**, 304–322, with kind permission of authors and publishers.)

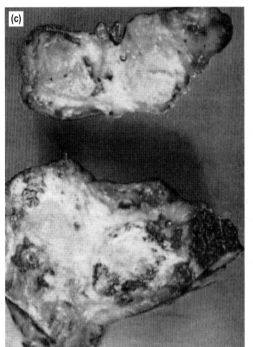

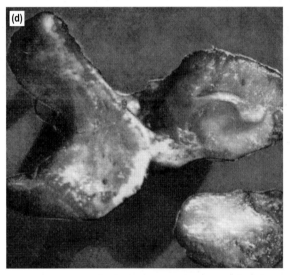

Discogenic/nerve-root referred pain has three clinical features:

1. It can be a lancinating pain felt throughout the full length of the referred distribution and lasting only a fraction of a second.
2. If a particular weight-bearing position of the spine is adopted and sustained, pain may first appear locally, followed a few seconds later by a spread of the pain into the nearby area of referral and, if sustained longer, spread throughout the full area of the referral. This order may be in the reverse sequence.
3. Following movements of the vertebral column in one or more directions, a surge of pain is felt by the patient to build up in the referred area of pain distribution.

*Surge of pain* – Little or no pain may be felt during examination of test movements, but within 4–5 seconds after completing the movements, the patient experiences an intense surge of pain which may last as long as 10 seconds before showing signs of subsiding, and taking another 4 seconds to return to normal.

## PAIN-SENSITIVE STRUCTURES IN THE VERTEBRAL CANAL AND FORAMINA

The structures referred to in this text are the dura, the nerve-root sleeve, the nerve root and its associated nerves.

### The dura and nerve–root sleeve

The site of pain from these structures depends upon which section is at fault. If the mid-line part of the dura anteriorly is affected, the pain will probably be felt centrally. If the lateral extent of the nerve-root sleeve causes pain, there may also be vague referral of symptoms to an area similar to the one to which the nerve root, which it embraces, would refer (Edgar and Park, 1974). However, the distal pain is never greater than the proximal pain. Pain arising from the nerve-root sleeve is not referred into the foot. Paraesthesia is never present.

### The nerve root and associated nerves

The symptoms are often felt only in the distal part of the dermatome. Allowing for pre- and post-fixed plexuses and for neural anomalies (Angoli, 1976; *Figure 8.2*), each nerve has specific areas of symptoms (*see* pp. 108–109; Ethelberg and Rüshede, 1952; Keon-Cohen, 1968; Nathan and Feuerstein, 1970; Bernini *et al.*, 1980).

The manner in which the pain disturbs or disrupts the patient's rest and activities and the manner in which the pain is changed by the physical examination test movements also add to the information required to make a diagnosis. For example, a man may have pain in his lower back radiating into his right buttock, thigh, calf and foot in a distribution that suggests that the nerve root and its sleeve investment are the origin of his pain. On examination of this patient's movements, lumbar extension initially causes back and buttock pain; however, if the position is sustained for 15 seconds the pain gradually spreads down his leg and into his foot. Such a behaviour of pain can be interpreted diagnostically as incriminating the intervertebral disc, as the disc is probably the only structure that can move in such a way as to produce this kind of latent pain response.

## PATHOLOGICAL DISORDERS AND INJURY

The total text relating to the selection of techniques is divided into two parts. The first, which appears in this chapter, is related to patients having the pathological disorders and injuries that are common and are seen frequently. The remaining parts appear in the chapters dedicated to each individual section of the spine.

In this chapter, the disorders (both pathological and injury) are related to:

1. The commonly seen disc disorders, both when the disc causes symptoms and when it causes symptoms in conjunction with the pain-sensitive structure in the vertebral canal and intervertebral foramina.
2. The commonly seen ligamentous and capsular presentations resulting from sprain and strain.
3. The zygapophyseal joints with their presentations of 'arthritic/arthrosic' and capsular disorders.

### The herniating or herniated disc

#### The disc

The intervertebral disc continually undergoes change throughout life as a normal process. It changes from a strong, mobile, resilient structure in early life to a far less mobile structure, which has little or no recuperative powers when damaged (De Palma and Rothman, 1970).

The normal age changes can be distorted by such influences as sustained end-of-range positions both at work and at home, excessive, heavy or jarring demands on the disc, and unguarded movements.

The common sitting position of sustained lumbar flexion is one such bad influence; but when the added insult of the joggling or vertical vibration that occurs in a car, bus or tractor is superimposed, the influence is even greater. These are influences that plague all modern societies (Kelsey and Hardy, 1975; Troup, 1978; Frymoyer *et al.*, 1980; Twomey and Taylor, 1994).

There are two further influences that modify the otherwise normal disc changes. The first of these is the damage that accompanies the knocks, bumps, falls and injuries that take place in our youth, but which are soon forgotten because any damage that does occur repairs very quickly. The damage, however, leaves its scars and weaknesses and predisposes to more rapid disc degeneration or intradiscal fissuring. Structural anomalies (e.g. spondylolysis) or asymmetries (e.g. alternating tropisms) can compound the above effects.

The intervertebral disc changes that take place as described above can occur asymptomatically. They may, however, result in a 'weak link', which can give way when placed under load or stress.

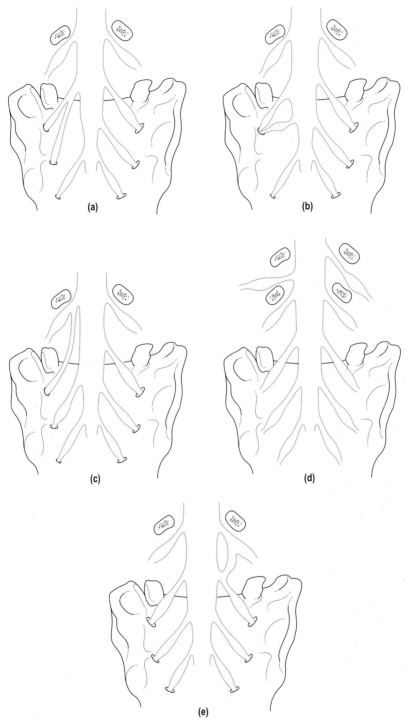

**Figure 8.2**    Anomalies of the pattern of lumbosacral nerve roots. (*a*) Common origin S1–S2; (*b*) common exit S1–S2; (*c*) Y-shaped division L5–S1; (*d*) transverse course L4; (*e*) interradicular corrections (Reproduced from Agnoli, A.L. (1976) *Journal of Neurology*, **211**, 217–28, with kind permission of author and publishers.)

By following the patterns of symptoms that occur from time to time, some assessment of what is happening in the intervertebral disc can be made. It is possible to determine whether the intervertebral disc is progressively degenerating without any likelihood of ever compromising the vertebral canal or intervertebral foramen, or whether it is progressing towards an eventual interference with the canal or foraminal structures. With the former, each episode is accompanied by pain in roughly the same area each time, and the pain does not spread further (in the case of the lumbar and cervical spine) than the buttock or scapula. With the latter, however, progressive episodes cause pain that spreads further and further into the limb. This may occur over two or three episodes, over several episodes, or during a single episode.

With the progressive changes taking place in the intervertebral disc there are accompanying changes in the zygapophyseal joints and the supporting ligamentous structures, all of which can cause pain and can, in part, be responsible for recurrent episodes of pain.

It is these two kinds of disc disorders that are so common in our modern societies, and it is in their conservative management that the manipulative physiotherapist has so much to offer. The discussion on selection of techniques will be directed at these two disorders only, but it is necessary to mention other discogenic situations that are not uncommon.

A disc can rupture for no obvious reason, causing sudden severe pain. The disc can also be infected, calcified, or present with a vacuum phenomenon. Among other intervertebral disc disorders are the juvenile disc, the herniation of disc material into the body of the vertebra and the primary posterolateral protrusion.

There has been a vast increase in the understanding of disc pathology and research over recent years. Keeping up with this growth requires keeping up with current literature.

## The herniating and herniated disc

Once the annulus fibrosus is weakened or contains deep fissures, the outer wall of the annulus can bulge and interfere with the structures in the vertebral canal and intervertebral foramen. A bulging disc will probably not interfere with the nerve root unless canal stenosis exists at that level. This bulging or herniating disc will cause symptoms that are ill defined, yet vaguely match parts of all of a dermatome. How far the pain is referred into the limb depends upon the degree of irritation provoked in the structures in the canal and foramen. It is important to recall that the pain experienced in this distal segment of the dermatome will not be greater than that experienced more proximally unless the nerve root is directly involved (*see* pp. 189–190).

**Table 8.4**

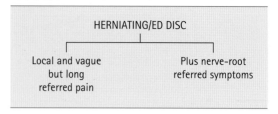

If the herniating progresses to a herniation – that is, the disc material extrudes (and may even become sequestrated) into the canal or foramen – both canal and foramen can become more seriously involved. When prolapsed material begins to compress a nerve root, examining straight leg raising will show limitation of range, and distal dermatomal paraesthesia may be present. This statement should not be interpreted to mean that limited straight leg raising only implicates the nerve root; Mooney and Robertson (1975) have clearly shown the effect the test has on the zygapophyseal joint. Neurological changes include loss of sensation, muscle weakness and reflex changes. A herniated disc involving the nerve root will, if it also involves other pain-sensitive structures, cause pain throughout the limb and may include neurological signs or changes. The distally referred pain is often of greater intensity than the proximal pain (*Table 8.4*).

## Rate of progression

> A rapid, relatively easily progressing disorder requires care in assessment and treatment

It is important to be able to recognize the intervertebral disc disorder that is likely to progress towards herniation with a possible final involvement of the adjacent neural elements. When this condition is recognized by the history of the patient's complaint, it is then vital to be able to assess the rate and ease with which this progression is taking place. Obviously, the more rapidly and the more easily it is progressing, the more care is required in treatment and of assessment (*see* history, pp. 118–121).

## Stability of the disorder

> The stability of the disorder has an influence on the intensity of assessment and treatment

It is important to know how stable the disorder of the disc is when the patient attends for treatment.

**Table 8.5** Symptoms and signs in herniating or herniated disc, and with intact outer annulus fibrosus

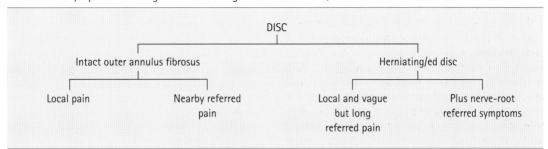

For example, the rate of progression of the disc disorder over the past 4 years may be rapid, yet at the present time the symptoms (and therefore the disorder) may be quite stable, its stability being indicated by the fact that the patient is, for example, able to continue with manual work without worsening the disorder. Under these circumstances the presenting situation is a stable one and, although the usual care is taken, firm techniques will therefore probably be needed to alter the situation and encourage recovery.

### Relationships

Once a disc has herniated and irritates or compresses the nerve root and the other pain-sensitive canal structures, the symptoms and signs can present in many different combinations (*Table 8.5*).

There can be pain in various areas, pain of varying intensities in the various areas, paraesthesia, neurological signs and neurological changes. There is no one single pattern of pain and neurological signs for a herniated disc/nerve-root situation. Most patients suffering nerve-root pain also suffer pain concurrently from other intervertebral structures.

Examining the movements of such patients can be very informative and important. For example, a patient with pain in his buttock, posterior thigh and calf, and with tingling along the lateral border of his foot and the lateral two toes, must have involvement of the first sacral nerve root. His history may clearly indicate disc herniation. His movements may nevertheless be limited by pain, but this pain may be only buttock pain and no test movements will reproduce the rest of the pain or paraesthesia. The techniques of treatment and prognosis would be different (this is discussed later) if his movements were limited by calf pain and increased tingling in the foot, especially if these symptoms had a component of latency or summation (Weber, 1994).

### Ligaments and capsules

This aspect of intervertebral joint disorders also applies as much to the disc as it does to the zygapophyseal joint

and the supportive intervertebral ligaments. However, for the purpose of this text, sprain and strain are considered in relation to the ligamentous-type structures because, from the point of view of selection of techniques, almost the same guidelines apply whichever structure is sprained or strained.

*Sprain* – This occurs following an incident that injures by sudden movement. In the text of this section, the only kind of incident that injures as a sprain is the trivial incident, such as tucking the sheets under a mattress while making a bed, turning suddenly to see what caused a sudden noise, or an unguarded type of movement such as the jarring that occurs when walking and not seeing a small downwards step in the path. More major incidents and traumas are not considered here.

*Strain* – This occurs when a faculty or part of the body is overtaxed. It may be due to bad postural positions at work or at rest as well as to overuse and abuse in sport or work.

The sprains referred to are not caused by more major trauma. The effects of sprains and strains on periarticular and ligamentous structures present in one of two ways, and on examination will exhibit the following:

1. Stretch response:
   a) Producing local stretch pulling
   b) Producing pain.
2. Compress response – pain is provoked during test movements performed in compressing directions.

Both of the above tend to be symptomatic at or near the end of a range of movement if chronic. The 'stretch' pain and the 'compress' response may, if of recent onset, exhibit a pain-through-range phenomenon.

### Local pain, presentations of ligaments, capsular and chronic discogenic disorders

In the early stages of overuse types of strain, the patient may feel symptoms only intermittently. Under these circumstances, although the stretch or compress phenomena will still be evident on examination, the test movements that will qualify the phenomena will need to be combined movements, and they will often be associated with the functional overused movement that the patient can demonstrate as being the painful activity.

The symptoms resulting from sprain and strain on the intra-articular structures (i.e. of the zygapophyseal joint) are quite different from the above. The symptoms will include aching and, on examining movements, pain will begin comparatively early in the range and will continue, frequently increasing, until the limit of the range is reached. This is the definition of the phase 'through-range component' as used in this text. Other aspects of the zygapophyseal joints were discussed earlier (*see* p. 190).

The periarticular disorders usually present with an 'end-of-range' pain, whereas the intra-articular disorders, excluding the intrusive disorders mentioned, present with a 'through-range' pain.

## DIAGNOSIS

In the preceding section it has been indicated how the area and behaviour of a patient's pain can assist in formulating a diagnosis in terms of the structures that may be involved. When patients develop symptoms either spontaneously or following a trivial incident (that is, no direct trauma has been involved), the history of the progression of the disorder over the years also assists in formulating a diagnosis; there is a characteristic history for a postural ligamentous pain, as there is also for a degenerating, a herniating or a herniated intervertebral disc.

This progressive history over the years also provides information that determines the stage that the patient's disorder has reached in relation to the worst possible stage of progression of that disorder. This is discussed in Chapter 6 (*see* pp. 121–122).

The subjective and physical examination of the patient carried out at the time of seeking treatment must also aim at determining the stability of the disorder at that particular time. The degree of stability of the disorder has a very decided influence on the selection of techniques, and therefore will be discussed later in this chapter.

The selection of technique is guided by the diagnosis, with particular reference to:

1.  The pathological and mechanical changes involved.
2.  The manner in which the diagnosis manifests itself in terms of the patient's symptoms and abnormalities of movement.

This relationship – that is, the diagnosis/symptomatic presentation – is the primary, all-pervading and never-ceasing guide to the selection and modification of techniques throughout treatment. True though this statement is, the term 'diagnosis' needs to be qualified.

Patients having a diagnosis of 'disc herniation with nerve-root irritation' may have different patterns of symptoms and signs. Six examples of different patients may help to make this point clear, as it is very important when relating the selection of treatment techniques to the diagnosis:

- The first patient may have pain radiating from his lower back to his posterior thigh, while another may have pain radiating down the full length of his leg from his lower back to his big toe.
- The second patient may have neurological changes, while another with similar symptoms may not.
- The third patient may have marked limitation of straight leg raising and forward flexion with a full pain-free range of extension, while another may have a full range of both forward flexion and straight leg raising yet have his range of extension grossly limited by calf pain.
- The fourth patient may have an ipsilateral list, as compared with another who has a contralateral list.
- The fifth patient may have symptoms that are chronic, while another's may be more recent and more severe.
- The sixth patient may have pain that is more severe proximally, while another has the severe pain distally.

YET ALL HAVE THE SAME DIAGNOSIS.

Besides having differing clinical presentations when it arises from 'disc herniation', 'nerve-root irritation' may arise from other sources. Macnab (1971) reported having made a diagnosis of disc herniation with nerve-root irritation demanding surgical intervention in 842 patients. Of these, 68 had negative disc findings at surgery; the nerve-root irritation arose from one of five other sources. Although a clinical diagnosis of disc herniation was proven to be wrong in 8 per cent of cases, this is a very small percentage; however, the fact is significant. The point being made here about diagnosis and its relation to selection of manipulative techniques is that, even when a diagnosis of 'disc herniation with nerve-root irritation' is made, it is the presenting symptoms and signs, linked with the progressive history of the disorder, that guide the selection of manipulative techniques – not the bald title of the diagnosis.

It is the presenting symptoms and signs linked with the progressive history of the disorder that guides the selection of manipulative techniques rather than the bald title of the diagnosis

It is important to recall that referred pain can arise from other structures than the nerve root (*see* pp. 190–192).

Diagnosis is defined in Butterworth's *Medical Dictionary* as follows:

*The art of applying scientific methods to the elucidation of the problems presented by a sick patient. This implies the collection and critical evaluation of all the evidence obtainable from every possible source and by the use of any method necessary. From the facts so obtained, combined with a knowledge of basic principles, a concept is formed of the aetiology, pathological lesions and disordered functions which constitute the patient's disease. This may enable the disease to be placed in a certain recognized category but, of far greater importance, it also provides a sure basis for the treatment and prognosis of the individual patient.*

This definition, which refers only to pathology, should be expanded to include similar wording to cover the purely mechanical joint disorders that occur. These patients are not sick, as defined in *The Concise Oxford Dictionary*, but they are in pain and may be disabled. To cover the mechanical disorders, the definition should be expanded to read:

*It also implies the art of applying scientific methods to the elucidation of the problems presented by a patient suffering pain from a mechanical disorder. This implies the collection and critical evaluation of all the evidence obtainable from every possible source and by the use of any methods necessary. From the facts so obtained, combined with a knowledge of basic principles, a concept is formed of the aetiology and disordered functions that constitute the patient's disorder. This may enable the disorder to be placed in a certain recognized category but, of far greater importance, it also provides a sure basis for the treatment and prognosis of the individual patient.*

There is another feature of diagnosis which is important and is covered in the definition of aetiology:

*Aetiology – the science of the investigation of the cause, origin and development of vital phenomena.*

The importance of the aetiology component of diagnosis is critical in the selection of manipulative techniques when treating patients in group (1), the disc/nerve root group (*see* pp. 205–206). The following example will help to clarify the importance.

The original cause of a patient's pain arising from a lumbar intervertebral disc may have been a very trivial incident when he was in his late teens. The pain spontaneously disappeared, but he noticed that over the ensuing 10 years he had episodes that occurred more easily and seemingly, at times, without any incident. Gradually his pain spread from being in his back only at first, to being referred into the buttocks and posterior thigh in later episodes. For no explainable reason he was then free of pain for 5 years. After a period of unusual and heavy work, he developed pain that spread to his calf. Palliative treatment and discontinuing his heavy work effected complete relief of pain. Two years later (his present episode) he wakened one morning with a dull pain in his calf and tingling along the lateral border of his foot to the two lateral toes. Even on persistent questioning, he could not think of any reason for the onset. When he sought treatment he had had the symptoms for 3 weeks. Following 3 weeks of palliative treatment and anti-inflammatory medication, his symptoms were unchanged. He was referred to an orthopaedic specialist, who recommended manipulative physiotherapy. On questioning and examination it was found that the symptoms were stable and not influenced by activities, even playing sport (non-competitive tennis).

The 'cause' and 'origin' part of the aetiology of the disorder are reasonably recognizable. The 'development' part of the aetiology is also fairly clearly assessable. But there is a third related component which should perhaps be included in the definition of 'aetiology', which is, perhaps, even more important, and that is the degree of stability of the disorder at the time of commencing treatment.

This episode began in an unreasonable manner, indicating that care during treatment will be essential if the disc's integrity is to be maintained. The repeated episodes indicated a progressive deterioration of the disc towards an eventual herniation. The current presentation indicates that the disc is herniating (if not already partially herniated).

However, as previous episodes have become symptom free, it can reasonably be hoped that, with proper manipulative physiotherapy treatment, the same endresult may be achieved. Special care with treatment and with assessment is required because of the progressiveness of the disorder.

## PRESENT STABILITY COMPONENT

The present stage of the disorder indicates a stable situation because the patient is able to play tennis without worsening his symptoms and, despite the tennis, his present symptoms have remained unchanged for 3 weeks. Therefore, techniques may require firmness for them to be successful. (Further deterioration may be lessened by proper treatment and instruction in 'back care'.)

Aetiology is also important to the diagnosis of other disorders, but there the emphasis lies more in the progressiveness of the disorder and its origin rather than in its present stability – the exception being, of course, the stage of any inflammatory destruction.

These expanded definitions meet the requirements of the manipulative physiotherapist.

The concept enunciated in *Vertebral Manipulation* from the first edition has hinged upon the continual assessment of the patient's symptoms and signs from the beginning of treatment to the end. This concept has been further emphasized in succeeding editions. By basing treatment on symptoms and signs, useful treatment may be effected while the medical profession and its scientists continue to work towards understanding more in regard to diagnostic titles. The concept has proved to be acceptable, and has even provided manipulative physiotherapists with a basis from which to contribute towards understanding more about diagnosis. It is pleasing therefore to see the following definition in Butterworth's *Medical Dictionary*. The bracket is the author's insert to include mechanical disorders as explained above.

*Diagnose – To recognize the presence of a disease [or mechanical disorder] by examination and assessment of the symptoms and signs.*

Although the diagnosis as defined and its symptomatic presentation are the primary, all-pervading and never-ceasing guide to the selection and modification of techniques throughout treatment, the making of an informative diagnosis is not always possible. Two different situations commonly exist. With the first, although a doctor referring patients to a manipulative physiotherapist may not be able to give an informative diagnosis, he may be able to say, 'this patient's problem is musculoskeletal'. Such a diagnosis can be adequate. With the second situation, although the disorder is thought to be mechanical, there may also exist the possibility that

metastases or an inflammatory process may be involved. The problem of incomplete diagnosis can be overcome by treating the patient with judicious manipulative physiotherapy on the basis that the disorder has, at least, a mechanical component. The analytical assessment will determine the diagnosis in retrospect.

What information does the manipulative physiotherapist ideally want from the doctor's diagnosis? First, she wants to know what the doctor thinks is the cause of the patient's disorder and what led him to that decision. It is often this latter part, the doctor's reasoning that leads him to the diagnosis, that is the most valuable for the manipulative physiotherapist. Secondly, she wants to know what the doctor considers is the present stage and likely prognosis of the disorder. The doctor's answers to these two questions will provide all the important information that is needed, even if an informative diagnostic title cannot be given.

> The most useful information the physician can give is:
> - The cause of the patient's disorder and the reasoning leading to the diagnosis
> - The present stage and likely prognosis of the disorder

The information and knowledge that lead the doctor to being able to make the diagnosis include 'knowns', 'thought to be knowns', 'unknowns' and 'speculations' (*see* pp. 6–7).

Although the specialist manipulative physiotherapist is highly skilled in neuromusculoskeletal examination, it is not in the patient's best interest for her to take responsibility for areas of diagnosis and medical examination that are beyond her scope of practice. This is of particular importance when manipulation is the treatment and the diagnosis is in doubt.

## Selection – diagnosis

To discuss the selection of techniques in relation to diagnosis it is necessary to separate patients' disorders into four groups (*Table 8.6*). Each of the four groups applies to all sections of the spine, but some disorders are more common in particular sections.

The discussion regarding selection of techniques in this chapter relates to general principles. Aspects of

**Table 8.6**   Aspects of pain that influence selection of a technique

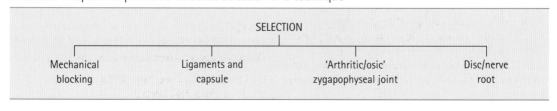

| | | SELECTION | | |
| --- | --- | --- | --- |
| Mechanical blocking | Ligaments and capsule | 'Arthritic/osic' zygapophyseal joint | Disc/nerve root |

selection of techniques that are relevant to particular sections of the spine are discussed in their chapters. The same applies to discussion concerning the management (as compared with the techniques that might be selected) of instability and hypermobility disorders, juvenile disc prolapses, primary postero-lateral protrusion and spondylolisthesis. The four groups are as follows.

### Blocking of joint movements

*The first group* is affected by the mechanical blocking of intervertebral joint movement. Examples of such mechanical blocking of movement in peripheral joints are a torn and displaced medial meniscus in the knee, or a loose body in the knee. Mechanical blocking is not uncommon in the cervical and lumbar spines. This group, involving mechanical blocking, has been given many diagnostic titles, many of which are unacceptable. Whatever the cause of the blocking or locking may be, the history, symptoms and signs are readily recognizable and specific techniques are selected to restore movement. Movement of the intervertebral joint is blocked; canal movements are not usually affected.

### Ligamentous and capsular strain or sprain

*The second group* includes patients whose symptoms arise from the ligamentous-type structures that support the intervertebral segment, including the capsule of the zygapophyseal joint. They present in many different forms, but there is always a compatible relationship between the patient's symptoms and either intervertebral joint movement and its pain response, or movement of pain-sensitive structures in the vertebral canal and intervertebral foramen and its pain response. The pain responses with movement may be felt only at the end of a range of movement, or they may be felt through the range of movement up to the end of the range. As has been mentioned earlier, the pain may be local or referred.

### Zygapophyseal joint arthritis/arthrosis

*The third group* includes patients where symptoms arise from the 'arthritic/arthrosic' zygapophyseal joint in either the chronic or the more painfully acute phase. The symptoms felt by the patient may be local or referred where comparisons were made with the 'arthritic' hip being painless yet causing referred pain in the knee.

### Intervertebral disc/nerve root

*The fourth group* includes those patients whose symptoms arise from an intervertebral disc that is progressively deteriorating. The diagnosis is a confident prediction that the intervertebral disc is both faulty and progressively worsening, with the possibility of eventual nerve-root involvement. The disc may only disturb movement of the intervertebral joint, but at a later stage of the disorder, movements of the canal structures may also be affected. When they are affected, the conduction of the nerve root may also become affected. However, it must be realized that a patient may develop severe radicular pain without any alteration to the conduction of the nerve. For the purposes of this chapter, this group relates to the patient whose pain is severe and in whom it is known that the intervertebral disc is in danger of affecting the integrity of the nerve root.

### Selection – pain

There are many aspects related to pain that influence the selection of a technique and the manner in which the technique is performed (*Table 8.6*). In the text so far, the kinds of referred pain have been stated, as has been the difference between end-of-range pain and through-range pain. However, pain may also be latent and it may have the capacity to summate or linger. The disorder causing the pain may or may not be extremely irritable (*see* p. 117). All such aspects of pain must have a meaning, and they certainly have an effect on the manner in which the selected technique is performed (*see* C and D, *Table 8.3*). These aspects are discussed on pages 201–203.

## HISTORY, SYMPTOMS AND SIGNS

The third integrant part (*see* Chapter 6) consists of:

1. The history.
2. The symptoms – that is, the circumstances under which the patient feels the particular areas and types of symptoms.
3. The signs – that is, the manner in which the patient's symptoms can be reproduced and varied by physical examination.

## HISTORY

The three main features of history are:

1. The onset and progress of the disorder throughout its history.

2. The stage of the disorder at the time when the patient seeks treatment.

3. The degree of stability of the disorder at the time when he seeks treatment.

They apply equally to the mechanically blocked movement and the sprain/strain disorders of the intervertebral joint, as they do to the commonly seen and more serious problems of the intervertebral disc and nerve root.

## SYMPTOMS

The areas and types of a patient's symptoms and the circumstances under which he feels them can in an important way influence the selection of a treatment technique. For example, the patient may have pain in his lower back, right buttock and right posterior thigh, extending to his knee. He comments that the position that provides him with greatest ease is to lie on his left side with hips and knees flexed and his right knee resting on the bed. To lie on his right side increases his buttock and leg pain. This may indicate that he should be positioned lying on his left side and that the pelvis might be rotated towards the left as the technique.

Any comments the patient makes about his symptoms can only be used in the selecting of treatment techniques when the physical examination findings match the manner in which the patient is affected by his disorder.

## SIGNS

The signs refer to the physical examination findings. They indicate whether canal movements are involved, whether nerve conduction is impaired and whether the symptoms have a stretch or compress component, and they help to confirm the degree of irritability of the disorder.

While diagnosis is all-important, the manner in which the patient's symptoms can be increased or decreased is equally significant. With regard to selection of technique, the following example should explain the importance of examination findings as compared with the importance of the diagnosis.

Two patients diagnosed as having 'disc herniation with nerve-root irritation' may have left scapular and arm pain. However, one has cervical movements that are markedly restricted by severe increasing scapular and arm pain. The other has full movements, but it is found that, if his head and neck are sustained in a stretched position of combined rotation to the left plus lateral flexion of his head to the left, only faint scapular

pain can be produced without there being any changes in the arm pain. The technique chosen for treatment of the first patient would have to be a position and a movement that relieved the symptoms so as not to damage the structures causing his pain; whereas the second patient may require a firm sustained technique that provokes a calculated degree of the scapular symptoms to improve the disorder and the pain it causes.

Examination of movements consists of three distinct parts:

1. Examination of movements of vertebral canal and intervertebral foramina structures.

2. Examination of physiological movements of the intervertebral segments, which infers:
   a) Routine anatomical movements (flexion, extension, lateral flexion and rotation, also as part of a functionally demonstrated movement).
   b) Expanded physiological movements into combinations of movements grouped together in varied sequences.
   c) Sustained positions, distraction and compression.

3. Examination by palpation techniques, which infers:
   a) Assessment for temperature changes and sweating of the skin surface.
   b) Soft-tissue assessment for muscles.
   c) Soft-tissue assessment of the interspinous, laminar trough and zygapophyseal joint areas.
   d) Accessory movements in standard directions.
   e) Accessory movements in varied inclinations.
   f) Accessory movements in varied inclinations in different physiological positions.

Selection of techniques related to these components is considered largely from the point of view of which finding best fits the patient's disorder. In other words, if a 'combined' physiological test movement completely reproduces a patient's local symptoms while palpation and canal findings are vague, the combined physiological movement would be chosen as the treatment technique. It should be pointed out, however, that canal movements, even when found to be directly related to the patient's disorder, should not be used as a first choice but should be used after physiological and accessory movements have served their usefulness.

### Components of recognizable regular patterns

At the beginning of this section on selection of techniques, the statement was made that the greatest advance made in manipulative physiotherapy in recent years is in the clearer recognition of patterns of pain, patterns of movement, and histories. These are detailed on pages 133–136 and 185–196.

There are certain history–symptom–sign presentations that are readily recognizable, and their response to particular treatment techniques is predictable.

The history of the degenerating disc is readily recognizable, particularly if the patient has had several episodes. The progression of a disc disorder to producing nerve-root irritation or compression is equally recognizable.

When a patient presents with a recognizable regular pattern of episodes, and the pattern of symptomatic response to examination movements is also of a matching regular pattern, the two together strengthen and confirm the pattern.

When the movement patterns are regular, the selection of techniques is clearer and the response to treatment is more predictable (*see* pp. 133–136, by Brian Edwards).

There will obviously be many times when a patient's history or movement signs only partly fit a regular pattern, there being other components of the disorder that present with irregular patterns. Under these circumstances, though the selection of technique may be directed towards the regular recognizable pattern, the response to treatment will obviously be less predictable.

The history of the locked intervertebral joint is another example of a recognizable history, and on examination it is found that the movement signs also fit a regular pattern. Under these circumstances again, the treatment response from a particular technique is predictable.

There are many times when a patient's history is not clear, and under these circumstances there is no regular pattern. However, on examination the movements may fit a regular pattern. For example, cervical lateral flexion to the left and rotation to the left may both reproduce the patient's left-neck pain. Both of these movements produce a closing down of the left side of the intervertebral joint. Cervical extension also closes down the left side of the joint posteriorly. Therefore, if the disorder lies in the left-sided structures posterior to the transverse axis of extension and extension also reproduces the pain, the pattern of movement will be a regular recognizable pattern. When such a patient is treated with the selection of techniques based on the recognizable pattern of movement findings, the treatment response should be predictable. If the treatment expectation is not achieved, the reason for the irregular response may lie in the history of the patient's disorder implicating other structures.

Among the mechanical disorders there are many recognizable patterns of examination findings. In the degenerative zygapophyseal joint disorders and the discogenic disorders it is the history that gives the main information with regard to the regular pattern. When trauma is involved in the onset of the patient's problem, he may present with an historical progression of his symptoms which *partly* resembles one or more aspects of a recognizable pattern; the movement signs found on examination may also fit parts of one or more regular patterns, besides having some movements which do not fit any pattern.

Brian Edwards (pp. 133–136 and 221–222) deals in depth with aspects of these mechanical regular patterns.

## SELECTION – ASPECTS OF THE TECHNIQUE ITSELF

We now need to consider what 'selection' aspects regarding the *technique itself* require decision (*Table 8.3*). The aspects are:

1. Mobilize or manipulate.
2. Direction of movement.
3. Position in which the directed movement would be performed.
4. The manner of the technique.
5. The duration of the treatment.

## MOBILIZE OR MANIPULATE

Except in the case of the mechanical blocking or locking of intervertebral joint movements, to mobilize is a better and wiser selection than to begin treatment by manipulating. The exceptions to this statement would be rare. However, it is usually necessary to manipulate when the intervertebral joint movement is locked.

> In most clinical cases it is wise to begin treatment with mobilizing techniques rather than manipulation. On rare occasions of, for example, locked joint movements, the physiotherapist may progress to a manipulation if mobilization does not work in the first treatment session

With disorders other than locked movement it may become obvious, after at least the first treatment, that a manipulation in the direction of the limitation may be required.

An irritable joint disorder may sometimes be better treated by a single, gentle manipulative thrust, because repetitive mobilization may only serve to irritate the disorder further.

When a selected large-amplitude movement is not being as effective as expected, it may be more effective if preceded by a manipulation. Similarly, when either sustained or intermittent traction is being used, it may be more effective if preceded by a manipulation.

## THE DIRECTION OF MOVEMENT OF THE TECHNIQUE

The direction of movement, particularly of a mobilizing technique, is guided by the purpose of the technique. The following list indicates the factors that may influence the selection.

1. *Should the aim be to open one side of the intervertebral space?* To do this implies widening the intervertebral disc space between adjacent vertebrae on the opened side, and also widening the intervertebral foramen on that side. Times when this might be a choice are when the patient has nerve-root pain and marked canal/foramen signs on examination.

2. *Should the aim be to stretch contracted structures that have become painful?* When ligamentous-type structures are strained and cause local pain (or even referred pain of the type described on p. 190) they often need to be stretched, in a controlled manner, to become full range and pain free. Whether this is so can be determined only by performing the stretching technique gently and at a constant rhythm during the performing of the technique. If discomfort lessens during the technique, it is the correct selection. A worsening pain response extending progressively over a period of 20 seconds of the gentle stretching technique says 'stop'. However, the full answer as to whether the contracted structures should be stretched or not can only be made by assessment of changes that take place as a result of the treatment over a 24-hour interval.

3. *Should the aim be to avoid provoking any referred pain, or is it better to provoke the very smallest amount?* When considering this approach, provoking referred pain is acceptable when the referred pain is chronic, when it is unlikely to be nerve root in origin, when distally referred pain is not provoked on examination, and when there are no signs of neurological deficit.

4. *Should the aim be to move in a direction that moves the canal/foramen structures rather than the joint structures?* At the time of the initial examination of a patient, spinal movements may provoke relevant referred pain, and movements of the canal structures may also provoke the same relevant pain. The direction of movement chosen initially should be one that moves the joint and leaves the canal structures relatively undisturbed. Only when these

have failed should canal movement techniques be used. There are exceptions to this rule, as with all rules. One exception is when the patient's symptoms are localized to the spine or nearby, rather than being referred into the limb. This is especially so if the symptoms are chronic and are more difficult to reproduce by spinal movements than by canal movements.

5. *Should a physiological movement or an accessory movement using direct contact with the vertebra be selected?* The choice depends upon which of the two produced the most significant findings. That physiological movement techniques can make marked changes to the palpation findings and that accessory movement techniques can clear physiological movement restrictions must always be kept in mind when making these decisions.

6. *Should an effort be made to determine whether a particular painful movement of the structure which is at fault needs to be hurt in order to make it recover its pain-free range?* Sometimes a patient becomes symptom free with treatment, yet there may be one remaining examination test movement that is painful. It may be important to free this movement of its pain in the interests of prophylaxis. On the other hand, the history of the patient's disorder may indicate that it is highly unlikely that it could be made pain free.

## POSITION OF THE INTERVERTEBRAL JOINT IN WHICH MOVEMENT WILL BE PERFORMED

The answers to this aspect of selection are clearly linked with points 1–5 in the above section. The following descriptions are related to that section by using the same reference numbers.

1. *To open one side of the intervertebral segment*, the choice of position is determined by two factors. The first is related to known biomechanics and the second is the pain response felt by the patient once he is placed in the determined position. For example, to open the right side of the C6/7 space the patient's 'neckon-trunk' position would be a combined position of flexion, lateral flexion left and rotation left. However, the amount of the flexion, lateral flexion and rotation, or the emphasis on one of the three directions, depends on the pain response desired. If the aim is to avoid pain, then the amount of flexion, lateral flexion left and rotation left is modified until the pain-free position is found. To take this discussion further, once in this position, the direction of movement selected

(see above section) would be to mobilize into further flexion or rotation left or lateral flexion left, whichever produced the desired response.

2. *The same comments apply to the 'positioning' as have been listed for 'direction' in the above section.*

The technique direction and the positioning of the joint are two separate components, yet are selected on virtually identical criteria. If, for example, the aim of the technique is to avoid any provoking of discomfort or pain, then the 'position' must be a pain-free position and the technique movement must be pain free. If the aim is to reproduce the symptoms, then the 'position' chosen must either provoke some degree of the symptoms or put the joint or canal structures in a position where the technique direction does reproduce the symptoms.

An unusual example of 'positioning' and 'movement direction' will help clarify their interrelationship. A patient had right scapular pain, which could be reproduced on examination by the slump test (*see* pp. 144–149) as well as by joint movements. Joint movement techniques initially produced improvement in both the patient's symptoms and joint signs, but without any improvement in the slump test signs. At this stage, 'joint techniques' failed to gain any further changes. It was then decided to:

1. Use canal (neurodynamic) techniques based on the examination findings.
2. Use the 'positioning' and 'direction' to reproduce the symptoms.

So the slump test 'position' was adopted, and the component of the slump test that most provoked the scapular symptoms was the 'direction' chosen.

The favourable effect of the technique was dramatic and lasting. The *position* for the technique was sitting with legs stretched out in front with knees extended. The cervical, thoracic and lumbar spines were held fully flexed, and the trunk was flexed forward at the hips until a strong stretch was felt by the patient in the hamstring area. His right leg was raised and held supported in this position, and knee flexion prevented.

The *direction* for the technique used was maximum ankle dorsiflexion. This movement reproduced his scapular pain severely with each stretch.

## THE MANNER OF THE TECHNIQUE

Two features play an important part in this context. They are:

1. Whether the problem is a pain limiting movement near the beginning of range or

pain-through-range problem and exacerbation is to be avoided at all costs, or

2. Whether pain is not a major concern and is an end-of-range problem with faulty structures which can be handled firmly without exacerbation.

*When pain is to be respected and the problem is one that limits movement early in range or is a pain-through-range one:*

1. The position, in the available range, in which the technique should be performed should be free of discomfort.
2. The technique should be very comfortable and comforting.
3. The amplitude should be as large as can be performed provided it is free of any discomfort whatsoever.
4. The speed should be slow.
5. The rhythm should be smooth.
6.* The duration of the technique must be short, initially until the 48-hour response is assessed.

It is in this area that grade I and II movements are so valuable. As pain decreases, grade III movements may be used. Point (5) refers to the rhythm of the technique; 'rhythms' are discussed in detail on page 176.

*When stiffness is dominant, and the faulty structures are not weakened by trauma or disease:*

1. The end-of-range position should be chosen.
2. The technique should be firm.
3. The amplitude should be mainly small, but should be interspersed with some larger amplitude movements.
4. The speed can be quicker.
5. The rhythm needs to be somewhat staccato.
6. Discomfort should be respected, especially if there is any indication of summation of symptoms during the performing of the technique.
7.* The duration can be longer, though active movements should interspersed between the passive mobilization.

It is sometimes difficult to decide just how firmly the grade IV movement should be performed. The decision is based on the relationship between the following:

- The newness or oldness of soft-tissue changes (the older they are, the firmer the pressure).
- The relationship between pain on movement and the resistance felt on movement (the closer the relationship in terms of strength and position in range, the firmer the pressure).
- The 'irritability' response from the previous treatment (the less 'irritable' the response, the firmer the pressure).

## DURATION OF TREATMENT

Although related to the selection of techniques in that the amount of changing from one technique to another is governed by the amount of treatment that can be administered at one session, the duration of treatment is discussed more fully under 'application of techniques' (*see* p. 219). There is an optimum amount that can be achieved at one treatment session, and the number of times a technique can be repeated at one session may be limited by the same factors asterisked in 6* and 7* above.

## SELECTION – RELATED TO DIAGNOSIS AND PRESENTING SYMPTOMS

Before treatment is undertaken, the manipulative physiotherapist must first know the diagnosis of the patient's disorder, both from her own knowledge and from knowing the referring doctor's processes of reaching the diagnosis. The second essential is for the manipulative physiotherapist to determine exactly all of the details that form the examination of the history, the symptoms and the circumstances under which the patient feels them, and the signs (that is, the test movement findings relating pain response to range of movement) (*Table 8.7*). Obviously, all other aspects of examination to cover contraindications to treatment must also be responsibly examined, both subjectively and physically.

In the preceding text it has been emphasized that accurate informative diagnosis is often extremely difficult or even impossible to achieve. Reference has been made, too, to the fact that often the diagnosis can be made only in retrospect, once the effect of particular treatment procedures is known; hence the great importance of analytical assessment. Nevertheless,

**Table 8.7**   Relationships governing selection of technique

| First compartment 'Theoretical and speculative' | Second compartment 'Clinical presentation' |
|---|---|
| Diagnostic title | History, symptoms, signs |

very specific decisions relating to selection of technique can be based on diagnoses subdivided into the four groups suggested on pages 198–199 and summarized in *Table 8.8* below.

## MECHANICAL BLOCKING

Mechanical blocking occurs most commonly in the cervical spine, somewhat less commonly in the low lumbar spine, and is uncommon in the thoracic spine.

In summary, if the mechanical blocking occurred very easily (and has done so in the past and been followed by spontaneous unlocking), mobilizing techniques that open the intervertebral space on the blocked side should be used first. If these fail, a manipulation to open the blocked side will be used.

## LIGAMENTS AND CAPSULE, AND 'ARTHRITIC/ARTHROSIC' ZYGAPOPHYSEAL JOINT

The common presentation of disturbances fitting the above headings are often impossible to tell apart at a once-only examination. The ligamentous and capsular group, made symptomatic by minor sprain, or strain from new-use, misuse, overuse, abuse or posture (as distinct from traumatic causes), can be 'end-of-range' problems or 'pain-through-range' problems. The 'pain-through-range' ligamentous group usually causes pain localized to the vicinity of the structure causing the pain. The progressive 'arthritis' disorder is also usually a 'pain-through-range' problem, with the main pain being felt locally.

The ligamentous 'end-of-range-pain' group may cause referred pain, but it will be of the vague kind, decreasing in intensity the further it refers (*see* p. 190). The chronic 'arthritis' zygapophyseal joint disorder can also present as an 'end-of-range' problem and cause referred pain. (*see* p. 190).

There is one other presentation; the patient experiences his pain intermittently as a sharp pain associated with movement. The pain is always a localized pain

**Table 8.8**   Selection of technique based on subdivisions of diagnosis

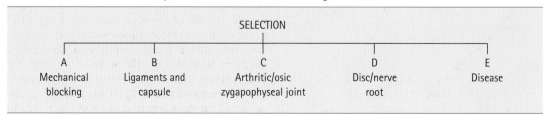

| | | SELECTION | | |
|---|---|---|---|---|
| A | B | C | D | E |
| Mechanical blocking | Ligaments and capsule | Arthritic/osic zygapophyseal joint | Disc/nerve root | Disease |

and never a referred pain. The patient may not be able to reproduce the pain consistently with a particular movement.

For the initial selection of techniques, specific differentiation as to the source of the symptoms is not an issue; however, when improvement stops or is too slow, differentiation is necessary. The text that follows applies to pain and stiffness arising from ligaments and capsules. Additional comments, which apply to the more chronic 'arthritic/arthrosic' (that is intra-articular) zygapophyseal joint problems, follow.

## SELECTION

The passive movement techniques from which a selection can be made in the treatment of intervertebral joint disorders are as follows:

1. The physiological movements of:
   a) Flexion and extension.
   b) Lateral flexion.
   c) Rotation.
2. The group accessory movements of:
   a) Distraction.
   b) Compression.
3. The localized accessory movements, which can be produced by direct pressure being applied to palpable parts of a vertebra or two adjacent vertebrae.

The directions of the pressures that produce these accessory movements are:

- Postero-anterior central or unilateral vertebral pressures.
- Anteroposterior central or unilateral vertebral pressures.
- Transverse vertebral pressures.

The directions of the above pressures can be varied by inclining the directions of the pressures medially, laterally, cephalad and caudad, and also by varying the points of contact minimally.

All of the above movements can be used in different grades and rhythms, and they can be combined in many varied sequences, often related to the patient's functional demonstration or injuring movement. The movements can be used to treat five groups of presentation as follows:

1. Pain.
2. Stiffness.
3. Pain associated with stiffness.
4. Momentary jabs of pain.
5. Disorders directly related to a specific diagnosis.

These groupings parallel those in the companion book *Peripheral Manipulation* (Maitland, 1990).

Because the severity of local and nearby referred symptoms can vary so widely, it is more helpful when dealing with the subject of selection of techniques if the selection is first related to the two extremes of severity. The first extreme to be described will be the pain-limiting movement at the beginning of range of the pain-through-range situation (group 1), where pain is severe and inhibits the patient's movements – there is no stiffness or muscle spasm limiting movement. The other extreme is where the patient complains of stiffness, not pain, although pain is provoked when the stiff movements are stretched (group 3). This is the end-of-range situation, where pain is minimal.

## GROUP 1 – PAIN

These patients have severe pain-limiting movement, rather than it being limited by any other factors. The techniques that can be used are as follows.

### Accessory movements in a part of the range that is totally free of any pain or discomfort

The joint to be treated must be positioned in a totally symptom-free position (*see* examples below). The amplitude of the movement should be the largest possible amplitude that can be achieved painlessly. To make the amplitude large, it may be necessary to start from a point well back in the range. The rhythm of the movement must be smooth and slow.

The following example may serve to make these points clear. If a patient has severe mid-cervical pain and the chosen treatment movement is postero-anterior central vertebral pressure, the patient's head and neck should be in a pain-free position. This can be achieved with the patient prone or supine.

To achieve a large amplitude for the postero-anterior movement, particularly if the patient is lying prone, it may be necessary to lift the patient's mid-cervical area posteriorly with the fingers (*Figure 10.61*) so that the postero-anterior movement has its starting point further back in the range.

If the patient has severe left neck pain that is easily reproduced by extension, rotation left and lateral flexion left, then the symptom-free position will be a combination of flexion (midway between erect and full flexion), lateral flexion right (midway between erect and full lateral flexion right) and rotation right (midway between straight and full rotation right). Under these circumstances the first choice may be to use postero-anterior unilateral pressure on the left, but the unilateral pressure may need to be inclined laterally to avoid provoking discomfort. If this technique cannot be performed painlessly, transverse vertebral pressure from the right side is used.

As the patient's symptoms improve, so the treatment movement can be moved further into the range and the position of the patient's head may be carefully changed towards the painful restriction. The technique may also be advanced to a stage where the large-amplitude movement is taken into a degree of discomfort.

## Physiological movements

When physiological movements are used to treat pain, they too must be performed without provoking pain or discomfort. As with the accessory movements, the intervertebral level being treated must be positioned painlessly in a mid-position for all other directions of movement. That is, if lateral flexion left is to be used to treat right-sided pain arising from the C5/6 level, then the C5/6 joint should be supported in a painless position midway between the limits of its flexion/extension ranges, its rotation ranges midway between being compressed and distracted. The lateral flexion treatment movement should be in the painless direction, and the large, slow, smooth amplitude must end before the onset of any discomfort. As the patient's symptoms and movements improve, the technique may be taken into a known and controlled degree of discomfort. Further progression is achieved by changing the position of the head and neck in which the physiological movement is performed until full range is possible in all positions.

When the patient's movements are markedly restricted by bilateral or central pain, the amplitude of the treatment movement may have to be extremely small to avoid discomfort. Relating this to using lateral flexion or rotation, the movement would be a very slow, smooth, gentle, oscillatory movement from approximately 5° lateral flexion left to 5° lateral flexion right, or 5° rotation left to 5° rotation right. Longitudinal movement, although not truly a 'physiological movement' as defined in this text, would also be a useful technique under these circumstances. It would be equally smooth, slow, small and gentle.

As the patient's symptoms and movement signs improve, so the treatment movement can be taken further into the range and the amplitude of the movement thereby increased. A later progression, as mentioned above, is that the movement can be taken into a controlled degree of discomfort.

## Progression

The initial choice between selection of one of the accessory movements and one of the physiological movements is decided by which of the two can be performed with the largest amplitude most comfortably for the patient.

The first progression is being able to move the same technique at the same speed, but now into a controlled degree of discomfort. If it is the right stage of treatment to be doing this, the discomfort will lessen while the technique is being performed. The amplitude of the technique may then be increased until large-amplitude movements are possible.

The next progression is to change the position of the joint by moving it towards the painful direction, but not so far that the position is painful or a large amplitude of treatment movement is not possible.

There is one other method of treating pain, which is described later. It is quite different in concept to the foregoing; for this reason it is kept separate.

## GROUP 2 – STIFFNESS

This category relates to patients who seek treatment because stiffness limits normal function, or because a stiff joint is slightly painful when stretched strongly. They are not seeking treatment because of severe pain, but because they have difficulty in reversing the car or are losing their full golf swing. There are many other similar circumstances. When one is examining their movements, all movements are restricted. When their movements are stretched, they are either pain-free or minimally painful.

The selection of techniques for such problems is to use two kinds of stretching movements, alternating from one to the other. After selection of the primary movement needing to be stretched (e.g. cervical rotation right because the patient has difficulty seeing where he is going when reversing the car), the first kind of movement is the physiological movement of cervical rotation right as an oscillatory stretching movement at the limit of the range. This should be performed for approximately a minute or so, varying between strong and gentler strengths. The second kind of movement involves accessory movements (again stretching and oscillatory movements of varying strengths) while the cervical spine is positioned at the limit of the range of rotation right. All directions of accessory movement should be utilized. Following the accessory movements, the rotation right technique is repeated. And so the routine continues, alternating accessory movements at the limit of the physiological range with the primary physiological movement. The same principles can be used in conjunction with any primary physiological movement.

Sometimes a patient may have a restricted range of movement, where the restriction is caused by one particular accessory movement rather than the physiological movement itself. This is determined during the examination, when the ranges of accessory movements are assessed at the limit of the stiff movement. On such examination, the particular accessory movement will be found to be stiffer than the remainder, and if all are stretched equally strongly the primary accessory movement will not only be less 'giving' but will also cause greater discomfort.

The following points should be taken into consideration when performing the techniques:

1. The biomechanics of the intervertebral joints are such that lateral flexion and rotation can occur together. Therefore in that part of the spine between C2 and C7, when one is performing rotation right, it may be necessary also to stretch the head and neck in the direction of the coronal plane – that is, stretch the patient's chin towards his right shoulder at the same time.

2. Whereas the accessory movement of postero-anterior unilateral vertebral pressure may need to be inclined laterally when treating pain; when treating stiffness it will need to be directed medially.

3. In treating pain, the techniques are performed gently, slowly and smoothly. In treating stiffness, the accessory movements should, for part of the total treatment time, be performed in a staccato manner so as to emphasize the impetus of the movement to the one intervertebral level.

4. The stretching technique can be expected to cause soreness, but this soreness is easily resolved by performing the same movement(s) as large-amplitude movements in the same directions as those used during treatment but this time performed just nudging at, or just short of, the limit of the range, until the soreness goes.

With this group of patients, the manipulative physiotherapist often fails because she is not prepared to be firm enough with her mobilization techniques.

## GROUP 3 – PAIN WITH STIFFNESS

Having discussed the two extremes of presentation – all pain and no stiffness, and all stiffness and no pain – we now come to the third group of patients, where pain and stiffness occur together. This is the largest group and the most challenging to treat. These patients will have pain, either as a constant symptom or as a pain on movement. In both examples the movements will have an element of stiffness. On examining the movements, there will be a relationship between the point of onset of the pain in the range and the limit of the available range. There should be a 'matching' comparison between the symptoms of which the patient complains and the findings on examining his spinal movements. Patients having constant symptoms will have pain commencing early in a range of movement, and the pain will continue and increase until the limit of the range is reached (i.e. a pain-through-range situation). With the majority of disorders that cause a patient to have pain only on movement, he will have this pain provoked at the end of the available range of an appropriate movement (i.e. an end-of-range-pain situation).

In addition to the patient having through-range pain or end-of-range pain, there is another feature to be clarified. With the patient who worsens with pain at the end of range, it is necessary to determine whether the restriction of the movement is the dominant factor or whether pain is more dominant.

The use of the movement diagram (*see* Appendix 1) explains this clearly.

When pain is the dominant factor, $P_1$ will start before $R_1$ and even if it is $R_2$ that limits movement, $P'$ ('P prime', prime being an engineering and mathematical term) will be very high on the $R_2L$ vertical line above L.

When stiffness is the dominant element, $P_1$ may start before $R_1$, after $R_1$, or at the same point in the range as $R_1$, but $R_2$ will be the factor that limits the available range, while $P'$ will be at any level on the $R_2L$ vertical line above L, well below $R_2$. However, the more dominant the stiffness factor, the lower $P'$ will be on the $R_2L$ vertical line.

When pain is by far the more dominant element, the choice of techniques will be identical with that already described above for 'pain'.

Within this 'pain with stiffness' grouping there is another method of treating pain, which was referred to on page 206–207 but not described there because of its different concept. It is only applicable when a patient's pain is directly related to the stiffness, and it involves pushing into the resistance until the desired degree of pain is provoked. In the description of the method there will be some readers, including experienced practitioners, who will say, 'But that is treating stiffness, not pain'. This is incorrect, because the intention is to provoke a calculated symptomatic response and the movement is taken into the resistance until this response is achieved. The treatment movement is not limited or controlled by the resistance; it is controlled by the pain response. The following is an example of *treating pain* by pushing the selected technique firmly into the stiffness.

A man had left suboccipital pain, which could develop into left-sided headaches. On examination he was found to have marked limitation of atlanto-axial rotation to the left, and movement in this direction reproduced the left suboccipital pain. The initial treatment sessions used techniques described above under the heading of treating 'pain', but they did not alter the patient's symptoms or movement signs. The decision was then made to 'treat pain by moving into stiffness'. The particular variety of technique does not matter at this stage, except to say that it was a small-amplitude, slow, oscillatory stretch, localized to atlanto-axial rotation to the left. The point of importance is that, although a degree of stretch was applied, the strength of the technique was *governed by* the intended severity, quality and site of pain being produced. It was not ruled by the strength of the resistance in any way at all.

The goal of the treatment technique is to eliminate that severity, quality and site of pain so that *it* cannot be reproduced irrespective of what happens to the resistance.

When stiffness and pain are equally dominant, it is important for the less experienced practitioners always to limit the initial techniques to those already described for treating 'pain'. It is only when these fail to improve the patient's symptoms or his test movements that using techniques for treating stiffness should be considered. When stiffness is by far the more dominant element, the technique will be the same as has been described above for 'stiffness'. The only differences will be the following:

1. Initially *only* the accessory or physiological movements will be used, not both, either because the amount of treatment should be limited at the beginning, or so as to make assessment of the value of the relative techniques more effective.

2. It is necessary to decide whether the most painful and restricted (i.e. primary) accessory movement near (not at) the limit of the primary physiological range should be selected, or whether the most painful and restricted (i.e. primary) physiological movement should be selected.

3. The firmness and rhythm of the techniques may need to be modified in response to respecting the discomfort felt during the technique. The discomfort felt during the performing of the technique at a constant rhythm and position in the range should lessen, or at least remain unchanged; it must not be allowed to continue worsening.

4. Initially, a stretching technique should not reproduce a patient's referred pain.

Clinical experience shows that some structures that have been sprained or strained need, at some stage, to be hurt in a controlled manner to set the healing processes in motion. Perhaps this fact bears some relationship to the mechanical measures resorted to in order to stimulate union in un-uniting fractures. When such a technique is being performed, the patient will often spontaneously say, 'It's hurting but it's a nice hurt'. Such a comment nearly always means that the right choice of technique has been made, but proof lies in the assessment. Other painful disorders decidedly object to being hurt. If the first steps in selection are to choose techniques for treating 'pain' described earlier, and to progress to treating pain only by using a technique that provokes pain as described above, no wrong steps will be taken. There is no method of determining whether the patient's disorder requires to be hurt to make it heal, other than to use the technique provoking minimal discomfort for a very brief time and then to assess its effect over 24 hours. Therefore, this means that when first using a technique that provokes local pain:

1. The discomfort must be kept at a minimum.

2. The technique must be performed slowly and smoothly with the patient totally relaxed.

3. During the first few oscillations of the technique, performed at a constant rhythm and position in the range, the manipulative physiotherapist must know:
   a) If the hurt is only slight and in rhythm with the technique, in which case the technique is continued for another 10 seconds; if the hurt in rhythm is increasing, STOP.
   b) If the technique is causing an ache, irrespective of whether it is also causing a hurt in rhythm, STOP.
   c) That the technique is continued only if the hurt decreases or remains unchanged.

4. The technique is performed only for a maximum of half a minute before reassessing the patient's symptoms and signs.

5. It is important to remember that it is better to do only a little treatment and make use of the 24-hour assessment and find that nothing has been gained, than it is to do a little too much and find later the patient was much worse half an hour after treatment.

It is the 24-hour period that is the most informative and useful of the types of assessment.

## GROUP 4 – MOMENTARY PAIN

This patient experiences his pain as a sudden momentary jab, which occurs unexpectedly. It is always associated with movement, although the movement may be so minimal that the patient is not aware that there has been a movement.

The selection of technique under these circumstances is entirely dependent upon the examination defining the movement(s) that provoke this pain. The movement is usually a combined movement and position, which includes an accessory movement involving direct contact with a palpable part of the vertebra. The treatment technique selected is the accessory movement in the combined position that reproduces the 'momentary pain'. The technique is nearly always a strong grade IV movement followed by gentle grade III movements to relieve any treatment soreness.

## GROUP 5 – ARTHRITIC/ARTHROSIC ZYGAPOPHYSEAL JOINT

The definitions of arthritis, arthrosis, spondylitis and spondylosis appear to vary. Synovitis or any intra-articular mechanical inflammatory process will present as a pain-through-range situation, and if it is to be treated by passive movement techniques rather than other methods of orthopaedic medicine, the *initial* selection of techniques and progression of treatment are identical with those already described in detail under the heading of treating 'pain' (p. 205).

The zygapophyseal joint can be responsible for patches of referred pain without there being any pain in the vicinity of the zygapophyseal joint. In the examination of an arthritic hip that is causing referred knee pain, it will be painful locally if stressed, and frequently will reproduce the knee pain. Similarly, if the arthritic zygapophyseal joint that is responsible for a patch of referred pain is stressed, it will be painful locally and sometimes reproduces the referred pain. Selection and progression of techniques are identical with those described for treating the pain-with-stiffness group. However, within this category of disorder, there are two further ways in which techniques may be advanced.

### First way of progressing

When mobilization has reached the limit of its effectiveness, manipulation of the kind that is localized or emphasized at the one faulty intervertebral level should be selected. It must stretch the zygapophyseal joint, and should be followed by a repeat of the end-of-range mobilization, using both small- and large-amplitude movements.

### Second way of progressing

When the symptoms are believed to be arising from an intra-articular disorder yet there is no synovitis, the initial progression of techniques is the same as referred to above. However, when such mobilization has

ceased to produce an acceptable rate of progress, the technique selected must move the zygapophyseal joint through a large amplitude while its opposing surfaces are compressed together. During the performance of the technique, if the right selection has been made, the patient will be aware of local discomfort. A validating examination procedure is that, if the movement is continued but the compression is gradually reduced until minimal distraction is applied, the local discomfort goes (Maitland, 1980).

A simple example which explains the features described is that of the elderly patient with left-sided occipital headaches in conjunction with marked 'arthritic/arthrosic' changes of the left atlanto-axial joint. The physiotherapist, standing behind the seated patient, cups her clasped hands over the patient's head and supports his back with her thorax. She is then in a position to rotate his head to left and right (through an arc of 25° to each side) and at the same time *gradually* increase the pressure on the crown of his head.

This pressure should be gradually increased, until the patient is aware of left-sided suboccipital discomfort and perhaps even a reproduction of the occipital pain. If the 50° rotation is continued and the compression through the crown of the head gradually released, the patient's left suboccipital discomfort and the occipital pain will decrease and disappear.

One may liken the zygapophyseal joint to the osteoarthritic hip in that it can present as a very painful disorder, having both local and referred pain, or it can present as a stiff joint which, if subjected to a sustained and progressing stretch, will demonstrate the rough bone-on-bone 'chinking' noise so typical of the chronic osteoarthritic hip.

In the latter group, improvement in functional range can often be achieved if the technique is directed at stretching the direction of movement causing the functional loss.

In the former group, where the pain is the problem, selection follows the same pattern as that described for treating pain (p. 205).

## DISC/NERVE ROOT

When the intervertebral disc is responsible for repeated episodes of symptoms, the state of the disc can progressively worsen in one of two basic patterns (*see* p. 194). The first is that it progressively degenerates and causes symptoms from its own structure, and because of stresses it places on other structures associated with the mechanics of the intervertebral joint. The second is that it progresses and herniates into the vertebral canal or foramen and irritates or compresses the neural structures, causing referred pain into the limb, usually accompanied by neurological signs and changes.

There are three presentations:

1. Severe and disabling symptoms sufficient to indicate that surgery is contemplated.
2. Less severe symptoms which, though severe, do not prevent continuing light work.
3. Chronic remnants of nerve-root symptoms.

## SEVERE AND DISABLING SYMPTOMS SUFFICIENT TO INDICATE THAT SURGERY IS CONTEMPLATED

Such a situation can be expected to exhibit the following features:

1. The patient's pain will be worse with continued weight bearing.
2. There may be an accompanying deformity or list.
3. Movements will provoke limb pain and paraesthesia, and these may summate or surge.
4. The patient may have pain even when lying, but he can probably adopt some positions that are less painful than others, even if this relief lasts only a short time.
5. There will probably be associated neurological signs and neurological changes.

In relation to the selection of techniques, the technique obviously must not irritate the existing symptoms. This means that a position has to be selected that relieves the symptoms, and the movement chosen must further relieve the symptoms.

The 'position' may be one the patient can adopt himself, or it may be a position that he cannot adopt himself. An example of each will serve to explain what is meant.

The example of the first position is a patient with a left S1 nerve-root pain. He may be able to relieve his calf pain and lateral foot tingling by lying on his right side with both hips and knees flexed, but with his left knee resting on the bed. Once he is in this position, the selection of the treatment technique will be found by the manipulative physiotherapist performing slow, small-amplitude movements in, say, a rotary direction, endeavouring to increase the movements without provoking any discomfort in the leg. To achieve this, small adjustments may need to be made to the angle of the rotation, incorporating lateral flexion or flexion/extension. It may be found that rotation cannot be performed painlessly, and under these circumstances a lateral flexion, flexion or extension movement may be the pain-free movement that can be gradually increased.

And so the treatment techniques are modified and advanced. Such patients would also be asked to adopt the position many times during the day, and even asked to attempt some movement similar to the mobilizing technique, with the instruction that it should be stopped when and if pain is provoked.

An example of the second position is as follows. A similar patient may not be able to find a sufficiently successful position for pain relief, and the selection of technique under these circumstances may well be to choose very gentle traction. He may be reasonably comfortable lying supine on the treatment couch with his hips and knees supported in flexion; then, by adding the gentlest of longitudinal traction, his symptoms may be further relieved (this response may be an indication for his treatment being constant hospitalized traction; *see* p. 388). The traction, distraction, longitudinal movement (or whatever word is used to describe it) is an accessory movement position, and cannot always be adequately performed by the patient himself.

The description of treatment by traction is described in the relevant chapters concerning the sections of the spine.

Positioning and traction as discussed here are currently going through a phase of being referred to as 'three-dimensional traction'.

## LESS SEVERE SYMPTOMS WHICH, THOUGH SEVERE, DO NOT PREVENT THE CONTINUING OF LIGHT WORK

The essential features are as follows:

1. The patient is able to be ambulant for all or most of the day.
2. There will be certain movements or positions that positively increase his referred symptoms, and others that lessen them.
3. There may be no accompanying deformity on standing or trunk movements.
4. Though movements may provoke referred symptoms, they will not have a latent quality, or, if present, will be of short duration and not severe.
5. There may be associated neurological signs without neurological changes.

Selection of techniques, as directed by this kind of presentation, must all be associated (at least initially) with positions, directions of movement and quality of movement that avoid pain. They should produce an improvement in the patient's symptoms and restricted movements of both canal and intervertebral joint structures. Examination of spinal movements, making particular use of combining movements in various ways, forms a vital part in selecting the technique that should be used. For example, if a patient in this category has a right discogenic C7 nerve-root disorder, it may be found that while he is lying supine, if his head and neck are flexed 60°, laterally flexed to the left 30° and rotated to the left 40°, his right forearm symptoms decrease. However, if the position is maintained, the symptoms do not further decrease. While maintaining this combined position, the manipulative physiotherapist should gently increase each direction of the combined position, and find the one she should use as the mobilization technique.

Mobilizing into the pain-free directions *must* be the first choice. However, there are times when this approach does not produce the desired progress. Under these circumstances, the technique should be changed to one that can be controlled to provoke an assessable minimal degree of discomfort. When such an approach is selected, little should be performed at the first session because it is the 24-hour response that provides the information upon which adjustments to the technique so selected should be made.

When these approaches fail, the next choice should include moving the canal structures. This may be achieved in conjunction with moving the intervertebral joint, or may be performed with the joint stabilized in a pain-free position. The first application of the technique should provoke only the most minimal of referred symptoms for a very limited time, and an assessment after 24 hours then provides the essential information to guide progression of the technique. If the disorder has worsened in any way, the technique must be discontinued.

## CHRONIC REMNANTS OF NERVE-ROOT SYMPTOMS

This state is not dissimilar (in terms of treatment selection) to referred pains of other origins in the spine, but with one essential proviso. The chronic disc/nerve-root situation does have a damaged intervertebral disc as its source, and has nerve-root involvement even in the absence of severe nerve-root pain, neurological signs or neurological changes. It is therefore necessary to know that:

1. The history is in a stable and safe phase.
2. The current behaviour of symptoms shows that the present stage is totally stable.
3. If there are any neurological signs or changes, that they are old, stable and certainly totally unlikely to deteriorate.

The other essential features are that:

4. The referred pain, even with the distal dermatome, is minor, does not restrict activities, and basically is of 'nuisance value' only.
5. Examination movements will provoke any of the referred symptoms only if the test movements are performed with firm overpressure and sustained.
6. If canal movements are restricted, they are restricted by stiffness rather than by pain.
7. Any protective-type deformities, which may be seen on standing or during movement, exhibit stiffness when corrected and do not cause any referred pain.

Under these circumstances, the skilled manipulative physiotherapist selects techniques that reproduce the patient's symptoms. Initially, these will be *joint* movements, as distinct from *canal* movements, and will be determined by examination movements that incorporate various combinations of the physiological and accessory movements.

If such techniques are performed and progressed to being firm in the position that most produces the symptoms, and yet ceases to improve or is still too slow, the techniques should be changed to those that move the canal structures (as distinct from the joint) and reproduce the patient's symptoms.

Neurological changes are not, of themselves, as some would have us believe, a contraindication to treatment by manipulation. Nevertheless, they should provide diagnostic information, which then governs the selection of all the details concerning the technique chosen to treat them.

## SUMMARY OF SELECTION

There are three associated requirements for selecting techniques in treatment. The first is as follows.

A decision regarding selecting the initial technique cannot be made until the following information has been determined from the examination of the patient:

1. The diagnosis.
2. The prognosis.
3. The present degree of stability of the disorder.
4. The manner in which the disorder affects the patient and his daily activities.
5. The site of the symptoms and the symptomatic responses associated with ranges of movement:
   a) 'End-of-range' or 'through-range' pain.
   b) Severe or 'nuisance-value' symptoms.
   c) Recent or chronic.
   d) Movements produce only local pain even in the presence of referred symptoms.

**Table 8.9**    Principles of treatment associated with different diagnosis

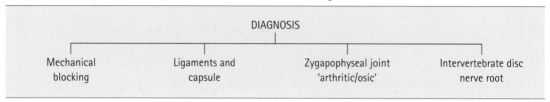

| | | DIAGNOSIS | | |
|---|---|---|---|---|
| Mechanical blocking | Ligaments and capsule | Zygapophyseal joint 'arthritic/osic' | Intervertebrate disc nerve root | |

e) Movements produce referred symptoms indicating the structure at fault and its degree of damage.

6. All other important examination findings associated with contraindications, cautions and nerve conduction – taken as read.

The second requirement is to know that the *main* BASIC joint techniques are rotation, lateral flexion, palpation techniques and longitudinal movement (which includes traction), and the *main* BASIC canal techniques are straight leg raising and 'slump' techniques, and ULNTs (*see* pp. 144 and 249).

The third requirement is a clear understanding of the principles of treatment associated with the different diagnoses (*Table 8.9*), which are described on pages 192–197.

From a framework based upon the above three areas of knowledge, the following list of thoughts is considered so as to arrive at the selection of the techniques:

1. How much gentleness (i.e. related to the symptoms, the diagnosis and the examination findings) must be exercised?
2. Is mobilizing to be the first choice, or should the joint be manipulated as in mechanical blocking?
3. Is the joint to be treated first, or the vertebral canal/intervertebral foramina structures?
4. Is the problem a pain-limiting movement early in range 'through-range pain', an 'end-of-range-pain' problem or momentary pain?
5. Should 'opening' the intervertebral joint be a first consideration?
6. Should the initial techniques be directed towards treating 'pain' or treating 'stiffness'? (the elements described under 'the manner of the technique' on p. 203).
7. Should the positioning and technique be in a 'symptom relieving' direction?
8. Should the technique provoke local symptoms or referred symptoms?
9. Should the technique be devised around the position in which the patient can relieve his symptoms, or should it be devised around the end-of-range or momentary pain position and movement that provokes his pain?

10. Should the technique be a palpatory accessory movement? Should it be performed in conjunction with a physiological movement or position?
11. Should the technique be primarily a physiological movement, either in solo or conjunction with other physiological movements and positions?
12. Should the pain-sensitive structures in the vertebral canal and intervertebral foramen be moved instead of the intervertebral joint, or in conjunction with an intervertebral joint technique? What should the pain response be during the technique?

After the initial technique has been selected, the possible effect it should have on the patient's symptoms and signs, both during and after the technique, must be calculated. If the response is not as expected, the technique should be repeated and, if the anticipated response is still not achieved, then an assessment needs to be made as to why it failed. What was the particular aspect of the patient's symptoms and signs that failed to improve? Perhaps the technique should be repeated but the position changed. Perhaps the same questions listed above should be reexamined, and the next technique decided upon for selected reasons.

Every technique used must be selected for a particular reason, and the selected technique must be expected to produce certain changes. If the expectations are not achieved, the reason could be that:

1. The technique was ineffectively performed.
2. The reason behind the selection was wrong.
3. The communication channels are not open – this could be the reason why the technique was ineffectively performed or the reasoning was wrong (refer to Chapter 3).
4. The disorder is too stable to be affected by the particular technique selected, and another should be chosen.

When progress in the patient's symptoms and in his movement signs ceases, a reappraisal of the whole problem should be made and the reasoning behind a new selection of technique reconsidered – and so the process continues until a final conclusion regarding the value of the treatment is reached.

# Chapter 9

# Application of techniques

(with a contribution by **B. C. Edwards,** OAM, BSc(Anat), BAppSci(Physio), Grad Dip Manip Th, MMPAA FACP Hon DSc (Curtin) (Specialist Manipulative Physiotherapist))

Manipulative physiotherapy techniques are only valuable as a form of treatment if accompanied by accurate repeated assessment. In this way the correct choice of technique direction, grade, speed, rhythm and duration will be made. Furthermore, experience in predicting the possible outcome of treatment will be gained. The assessment should take place before, during and after each technique is performed

Many people believe that to use manipulation as a form of treatment requires only the learning of techniques. *This is a dangerous mistake, and could not be further from the truth.* This same thought is also, unfortunately, carried into some of the courses on manipulation – this is deplorable. Obviously it is important that the techniques must administer movement properly, but even a technique performed well may do harm or fail completely if the wrong movement is selected or if it is done at the wrong depth or rhythm. The choice of a technique and the changing from one technique to another is determined by repeated accurate assessment of the patient's symptoms and signs before, during and after each application of a technique, and from treatment to treatment. This routine must be rigidly adhered to if the treatment is to be objective and safe at all times. However, safety and guidance for changing from one technique to another are not the only reasons for continually assessing symptoms and signs; it is by this means that the manipulator gains experience in predicting the possible outcome of treatment.

When a particular technique does not produce any change it should be repeated perhaps more firmly, and if it still fails to produce any change then the technique should be discarded. When a patient says his symptoms have improved as a result of the treatment, or if any of the signs show improvement, the same technique should be repeated. Repetition would be indicated if only one of the signs had shown improvement, provided of course that none of the remainder had been made worse. When the symptoms or signs are made worse by a technique, it should not be repeated. However, it may be attempted again at a later stage of treatment (more gently perhaps) when, provided there has been an alteration in joint signs, it may be useful. Care needs to be taken in assessing symptoms, because a patient may say that his symptoms are worse when in fact the pain may be of a different nature, being a response to stretching rather than a worsening of the existing symptoms. Further questioning about the onset of the worsening symptoms and the area and behaviour of these symptoms is important (*see* Chapter 6, pp. 108, 120). In such cases it is unlikely that the symptoms have been made worse if there is no associated deterioration in the signs. It can be that there was no change in symptoms following the previous treatment for 2 days, and on the third day the intensity increased. It must be clarified as to whether the intensity has worsened or the area of symptoms has spread peripherally. In the case of nerve-root (or radicular) symptoms, the patient may perceive a worsening because the intensity has increased although the peripheral symptoms have in fact disappeared. So we know that these are signs of resolution. On the other hand, if on the third day the intensity increased, further questioning of 'why do you think it got worse?' or 'what happened around that time for it to get worse?' may reveal that the patient performed an unusual task/activity prior to the worsening of their symptoms.

The physiotherapist must develop the ability to assess and weigh up the evidence accurately.

## TREATMENT ASSESSMENT

> If rapid improvement is expected during the initial examination and treatment, the change from one technique to another can be made more quickly. If slow improvement is expected, it would be wrong to change from one technique to another until it is clear the technique is not being effective

Although it has been suggested that two applications of a mobilizing technique are sufficient to show the value of a technique, this is not always so. The whole point of assessing between techniques is to have a means whereby their effect can be measured. During the initial examination of a patient, the physiotherapist should assess whether it will be possible to bring about quick improvement in the patient's condition or whether the progress is likely to be slow. If quick progress is possible, changes from one technique to another can be made more rapidly. For example, when a technique is producing improvement, if it is thought that the rate of improvement is slower than might be possible, a change or addition of technique may increase the rate of progress. When it is known that improvement will be slow, it may be wrong to change from a technique until it has been used for two or more treatment sessions. *Each technique must be used until proven to be ineffective at changing the patient's signs and symptoms favourably.*

The question is, how much improvement in a patient's signs is enough to justify continuing to use a particular mobilization technique? This is difficult to learn except through practical experience based on continual assessment of changes produced by the technique under various conditions. Subtle clues from the patient can be useful here too: 'I don't think that manipulation you did last time has helped my pain', or 'I don't feel any better but I think you've hit the spot, and if you push a bit harder I think that's what it needs'.

The therapist can also explore the body's capacity to inform by asking the patient directly whether he thinks a particular technique is making him better. For example, he may say: 'I think the first thing you did to me will get me better quicker than the second technique'. Obviously some patients will show a greater rate of change than others. It has been found (Maitland, 1957) that as pain is referred increasingly further from the source, treatment takes longer and is less likely to be successful (*Table 9.1*). As the survey summarized in this table consisted of 220 patients preselected by medical practitioners it cannot be expected to be precise, and it is not the author's wish that it should be accepted as anything more than an approximate guide. Because the results from treatment of cervical syndromes follow a somewhat similar pattern, the survey can help the student to know how much treatment a particular patient may need.

The routine of treatment is as follows:

1. The patient is first assessed for his response to the previous treatment session. The questioning is not as easy to carry out effectively as some may think. Great care must be taken to avoid misinterpreting the patient's words and it is essential to be critical of one's interpretations. C/O (complains of) asterisks should be used as continual evaluation of the patient's symptoms and his perceived disability.

2. The second assessment consists of comparing the important movement signs with those that were evident before. These findings are recorded as set out in *Table 9.2* (P/E asterisks).

Table 9.1    Results of treatment

| Symptoms | Patients relieved (percentage) | Average length of successful treatments (days) |
|---|---|---|
| Back pain: | | |
| Without protective scoliosis | 96 | 4.5 |
| With protective scoliosis | 91 | 6 |
| Back to buttock pain: | | |
| Without protective scoliosis | 95 | 4 |
| With protective scoliosis | 95 | 4 |
| Back to knee pain: | | |
| Without protective scoliosis | 96 | 5.7 |
| With protective acoliosis | 60 | 11 |
| Back to foot pain: | | |
| Without protective scoliosis | 91 | 7 |
| With protective scoliosis | 50 | 9 |
| Pain with neurological changes* | 54 | 9 |

*Pains with neurological changes referable to the third lumbar nerve root were more difficult to relieve than those from the sacral nerve roots and both of these were more difficult to relieve than were all others of lumbar origin.

Table 9.2    Symbols

| | |
|---|---|
| | Central postero-anterior pressure (PAs)  ✗  with a Ⓛ inclination |
| | Central anteroposterior pressures (APs) |
| | Unilateral PAs on Ⓛ  ◀  with a medial inclination |
| | Unilateral APs on the Ⓛ |
| | Transverse pressure towards Ⓛ |
| | Rotation of head, thorax or pelvis towards Ⓛ |
| | Lateral flexion towards Ⓛ |
| | Longitudinal movement (state cephalad or caudad) |
| | Unilateral PAs at angle of Ⓡ 2nd rib |
| | Further laterally on Ⓡ 2nd rib |
| | Unilateral APs on Ⓡ |
| CT ↗ | Cervical traction in flexion |
| CT ↑ | Cervical traction in neutral (sitting) |
| IVCT ↑ | Sitting |
| IVCT ↗ | Lying |
| IVCT ↗ 10 3/0 15 | Intermittent variable cervical traction in some degree of neck flexion, the strength of pull being 10 kg with a 3-second hold period, no rest period, for a treatment time lasting 15 minutes |
| LT | Lumbar traction |
| LT 30/15 | Lumbar traction, the strength of pull being 30 kg for a treatment time of 15 minutes |
| LT crk 15/5 | Lumbar traction with hips and knees flexed; 15 kg for 5 minutes |
| IVLT 50 0/0 10 | Intermittent variable lumbar traction, the strength of pull being 50 kg, with no hold period and no rest period, for a treatment time lasting 10 minutes |

3. Following the assessment, a technique is chosen for reasons that should be stated and recorded.

4. The technique is then performed, and any favourable or unfavourable symptomatic response during its performance should be noted. If necessary, the technique will be adapted to the response of the patient.

5. Following the treatment technique, the patient's symptoms and signs must be reassessed in a way that will endeavour to prove the value of the technique that has just been used. If the improvement is adequate the technique is repeated, but if there is not adequate improvement then a change in technique is made. The new technique is applied for the required time and another assessment made. Unless the patient's symptoms are minimal the number of mobilizations between assessments is limited to approximately four per session, each lasting anything from 8 seconds to 2+ minutes.

> If the amount of improvement from a particular session is exceedingly favourable (75 per cent or better), there is only one inherent danger; the thought process tends to tempt the therapist into doing the same technique somewhat more strongly or for a longer time. However, when pain is the patient's main complaint, such changes should NOT be made. It is far better to do nothing for 48 hours to see if the improvement is retained (or if even more improvement occurs, in which case defer the treatment until it reaches a plateau). The other alternative is to repeat the treatment without any change to strength or duration of technique, or repeat the technique but for less time and with less strength

It is important to remember that there is an optimum amount of improvement that can be achieved in any one day. It is therefore necessary to realize that the amount of treatment that can be given at any one session is limited, and the treatment must therefore be balanced if the optimum advantage is to be gained from changes in technique. This clinical knowledge can only be learned by practice under supervision.

Although it is possible to have some idea of whether a quick or slow progress with treatment might be achieved, it is necessary to give some examples of what can constitute adequate improvement of signs with the successful application of a technique. The following figures are not intended to be taken too literally, and are offered only as a guide. With a patient who can be helped quickly these changes should be expected after each technique, but with slower examples the same changes should not be expected in less than two or three sessions. The minimum improvements that justify repeating a technique are increases of 2.5 cm (1 inch) of forward flexion in the standing position, 5° of straight leg raising or 5–10° of trunk or cervical rotation.

There are many pointers that may be found on examination to indicate that a slow rate of progress can be anticipated, and these may appear singly or in combination. The pointers can be considered under the headings deformity, movements, and pathology.

## DEFORMITY

> There are certain protective deformities, patterns of movement restriction and recognizable pathologies which, in general, respond more slowly to treatment

The four points given here relate mainly to low lumbar discogenic disorders, but can be thought of at other levels of discogenic problems.

1. A patient whose pain radiates to one leg and who also has a protective list displacing his shoulders towards the side of pain (ipsilateral list) is certain to be much slower in his response to conservative treatment than if he had a contralateral list.

2. A patient who has a protective-type list that alternates from side to side is always difficult to help. The more easily the scoliosis can be changed, the harder it is to help him.

3. When a patient with low back pain exhibits marked spasm of the extensor muscles to limit the movement of forward flexion, his condition can be expected to be difficult to help. This lordotic type of muscle spasm can be bilateral or unilateral. Occasionally a patient is seen who has an ipsilateral list combined with a unilateral lordotic type of muscle spasm. When these two factors are combined, the response to treatment is likely to be even more difficult.

4. A patient who has a lumbar kyphosis is usually fairly easy to help with mobilization unless the degree of kyphosis is in excess of 30°. Under these circumstances it is almost impossible to help him conservatively unless rest is part of the treatment.

## MOVEMENTS

1. When a patient with pain in his back and leg has a marked restriction of forward flexion and straight

leg raising on the painful side, he is likely to be difficult to help (Charnley, 1951).

2. A patient may have limb pain, and extension of his neck or back may reproduce some of this limb pain. However, if the range of extension is markedly limited and this movement reproduces the distal area of the pain, then the patient's disorder is likely to be very difficult to help.

3. When a patient's movements in all directions are very limited and these movements produce sharp pain, then the degree of severity and restriction indicates the slowness with which the patient can be expected to respond to treatment.

4. A patient with thoracic or lumbar pain may have the sign where passive neck flexion is very limited while reproducing the thoracic or lumbar symptoms. The more the movement is restricted by pain, the more difficult it is to relieve his symptoms.

5. It is common for patients with gross arthritic or spondylitic changes to have localized aching. Their movements, although generally stiff, are not painfully restricted by this aching. These patients are reasonably easy to help. However, if the patient with these radiological changes has a localized joint lesion of comparatively recent origin, then he is certain to be slow in his response to treatment.

6. A patient having bilaterally distributed pain from his lower back into both legs of symmetrical distribution and equal severity provoked by minimal extension is certain to be difficult to help.

## PATHOLOGY

> Clinical tip: During treatment, severe nerve-root pain may remain the same for several days before the patient notices any reduction in his symptoms

1. Severe nerve-root pain is always a concern in its response to treatment. Initially it may be 7–10 days before the patient is aware of any lessening of the pain. The total treatment time is longer than that for referred pain from other sources. There are three nerve roots that seem to respond less readily to conservative measures than others: L3, which is harder to help than S2; and in the cervical area, C8.

2. A primary posterolateral protrusion is always slower in its results, although it can usually be helped (Cyriax, 1982).

3. Patients whose symptoms arise from an unstable spondylolysis or spondylolisthesis are always difficult to help with mobilization. Also, their response to treatment is not as complete as that of patients with similar symptoms from other sources. Functional postural modes must be taught, and exercises are essential.

4. Patients whose symptoms arise directly from trauma are always more difficult to help because the extent of damage is greater. A particular form of trauma that should also be included in this category is the post-surgical patient who has not responded as well to surgery as was expected.

5. One particular group of patients is always difficult to help due to the type or extent of pathology involved. Any young patient, adolescent or juvenile, who has not recovered from his symptoms without requiring treatment, will always be difficult to help. Young people have extremely good powers of recovery, and therefore almost without exception any junior who has pain that lasts long enough for him to have been through medical channels to the manipulative physiotherapist is likely to be far slower in his response to treatment than his adult contemporary with similar signs. If young patients have any neurological changes, the therapist should monitor these over a long period.

## DEPTH OF MOBILIZATIONS

> The depth of the mobilization technique will be determined by pain, muscle spasm and resistance, and their relationship to one another

At first it is difficult to know how firmly mobilizations should be done. Any technique used for the first time should be performed gently, so that the movement produced at the intervertebral joint seems too small to cause any change in the patient's symptoms or signs. Gentle technique is particularly important in the presence of severe pain, neurological changes or muscle spasm. The factors that guide the depth at which a technique is performed are the irritability of the disorder, the increase in pain with test movement, muscle spasm, and pathological contraindications. The severity and relative position of these factors in the range of movement are the important guides.

## PAIN

Pain on movement is perhaps the most important guide to how deeply a technique should be performed, and pain that is localized to the vicinity of the joint must be considered separately from referred pain. When the pain is localized to the joint, the mobilization should be done in the range that is pain free but the movement should be carried up to the point where pain begins. Where pain is felt at the beginning of the range, the mobilization must be performed with very small rhythmical movements (grade I, see pp. 174–175). As this technique increases the range of pain-free movement, the mobilization can be performed further into the range (grade II). A stage may be reached when it is necessary to carry the movement into the pain to reach the resistance. This is necessary when progress with this technique has slowed down and changes of technique have not effected progress.

> Care must be given when a mobilization technique produces a pain that is referring into a distant segment, and assessment must be scrupulously repeated

Greater care is necessary when a mobilizing technique produces pain that is referred into a distal segment. To begin with the movement must be performed in the painless part of the range, and a very careful assessment should be made of its effect immediately following the technique and 24 hours later. Provided the symptoms or signs have not been made worse, the technique can be repeated. It may even be necessary to increase the movement minimally to the point where discomfort in the referred area can be felt. Assessment must be scrupulously repeated. While performing a mobilization that does cause distal discomfort, the physiotherapist must continue the technique at a fixed amplitude and position in the range whilst assessing any change in discomfort. If referred symptoms increase without any increase in technique, the amplitude and position in the range of the mobilization must be reduced. Assessment over 24 hours, or on the day following a further gentle mobilization in the same range, will clearly show whether the technique should be continued. Frequently it is necessary to provoke discomfort very gently to produce an improvement in movements and subsequent lessening of symptoms.

When pain is found to be in the last quarter of the range of the mobilization it is likely that the technique can be taken through pain, whether it is a local pain or a referred pain, up to the limit of the range or up to any physical resistance that may be restricting movement.

## RESISTANCE

When a resistance can be felt the choice will be between a large- or a small-amplitude movement (grade III and IV, see p. 175). The small-amplitude stronger movements are used in the treatment of end-of-range pain. They tend to produce local soreness, but though this grade of movement may be necessary, larger amplitude movements will lessen the soreness. Large-amplitude movements are used when pain is felt through a large part of the available range and if pain is felt through range while the end of range may accept some over-pressure without discomfort.

> Small-amplitude movements will be used in the treatment of end-of-range pain. Sometimes treatment soreness can be lessened by large amplitude movements

When a patient has pain in an arc of movement, or if it is a catching pain, the mobilization chosen should be performed in a large amplitude (grade II or III).

To summarize, severe pain must be handled gently and movements must be small, without provoking extra discomfort – usually grade I. When there is very little pain but there is restriction of movement, grade IV movements can be used and in fact are frequently the only movements that will help. Gentler grade III movements will relieve any local soreness produced by the grade IV movements.

## SPASM

There are many varieties of muscle spasm, but the one referred to here comes into effect in response to pain. When a mobilization produces a quick muscle contraction, the technique must be performed more slowly and at a depth that avoids the spasm. If pain is used as the guide to the depth for performing the technique, spasm will be avoided because pain starts earlier in the range than the spasm. As the signs improve, the depth at which the mobilization is performed may need to be increased to a point in the range that fails to provoke spasm. Because mobilization can effect prompt improvement, an occasional oscillation should be taken further into range to elicit spasm to ensure that the technique is being performed deeply enough. Careful technique in this way can be expected to produce quite rapid increases in the range of spasm-free movement. The presence of such spasm in a patient is not a contraindication to mobilization, and in fact the opposite is true; the technique to choose is the one that would cause the protective spasm if done too strongly.

Muscle spasm that limits a range of movement and is always present at that point in the range, no matter how gently or slowly the technique is performed, is spasm of another kind from that described above. Techniques in treatment can be done as described above, up to the point where spasm begins. Naturally all spasm must be respected, but this variety, which is so strong that further movement is prevented, must never be forced. The spasm described in the foregoing paragraph, however, can be avoided if the technique is done more slowly or gently. No attempt should ever be made with any technique to force a way through spasm. This can be confused with the patient's active 'holding' or resisting a movement because of pain. In this situation, keep the mobilizing short of pain and occasionally increase the depth of the technique to test where pain begins.

> All spasm registered during a movement must be respected, handled gently and never be forced

## DURATION AND FREQUENCY OF TREATMENT

The amount of treatment that can be given on the first day should be considered separately from that of subsequent treatment sessions. On the first day, a full examination of the patient and any treatment given adds to the load being exerted upon what is presumably a faulty structure. Also, the first stretching of a joint appears to cause more reaction than subsequent stretches.

> The duration of the first treatment session should be less than subsequent treatments, as the first stretching of a joint appears to cause more reaction than subsequent stretches. With this in mind, adequate warning of a temporary increase in symptoms should be given to the patient after the first treatment session. The duration of treatment at subsequent sessions depends on the response to the previous treatment

The first day's treatment therefore should be less in regard to the number of mobilizations given. At the end of this first treatment the patient should be given adequate warning of the temporary increase of symptoms that may follow, to allay fears that can arise from an unexpected increase in pain. The number of mobilizations that can be given in subsequent treatments depends on the reaction to the previous sessions. If there is no undue reaction and the patient's symptoms

and signs are not severe, much more can be done than if the reverse is the case. It should be remembered, however, that there is an optimum that can be achieved at any one treatment, and to continue mobilizing a joint beyond a certain length of time will cause increased soreness and regression. Obviously this optimum will vary with different joint conditions, but the amount of treatment is approximately three or four mobilizations of a joint lasting approximately 30 seconds each. With extremely painful joint conditions this should be halved, and when symptoms and signs are minimal it can be increased.

Treatment must be sufficiently frequent to be able to assess changes resulting from the treatment so as to avoid the complications created by the patient's intervening activities. For this reason, if the patient asks 'Should I continue taking my tablets?' or 'Should I cut down on my activities?', the physiotherapist should say, 'In the initial stages of treatment I want to assess, as exactly as I can, the effect of my treatment. With this thought in mind, continue doing whatever you have been doing so that I will have a better chance of telling that whatever changes take place are due to what I am doing and not to what you have changed doing or not doing, as the case may be'.

> If treatment is perpetuating joint soreness or if there is no improvement over a number of treatment sessions, then treatment might be discontinued temporarily in order to decide whether treatment is having any long-term effects or not

Frequently a stage may be reached in treatment when it is difficult to tell whether it should be continued or stopped. The difficulty of assessment may be because treatment is perpetuating joint soreness, or it may be because a stage has been reached when assessment from treatment session to treatment session does not clarify the effectiveness of the treatment techniques. Under either of these circumstances, treatment might well be discontinued temporarily and a reassessment made in 7–14 days. Depending on whether the signs have shown further improvement, treatment may or may not need to be re-instituted.

There is one final point that occurs quite commonly and should not be forgotten. A patient may be treated over 10–14 days without producing any noticeable change in symptoms or signs. A 2-week break from treatment is then advisable, because there are times when the improvement is evident in the third week. This happens sufficiently often that its possibility should not be forgotten. The patient should therefore be asked to telephone and report any change so that assessment and advice can be formulated. With this thought in mind, it is a good policy for referring doctors to review patients 2 weeks after treatment ends. Such timing gives a more accurate assessment of the effect of the treatment.

## MOBILIZATION V. MANIPULATION

> Manipulation is rarely chosen at the beginning of treatment, and certainly 'never' in presence of a very painful joint or muscle spasm.
> It is a cardinal rule **never** to thrust forcibly through protective spasm

The question now arises as to when mobilization is used and when manipulation is used. Manipulation is rarely chosen at the beginning of treatment, and certainly never in the presence of a very painful joint or a joint whose movement is protected by muscle spasm. One of the cardinal rules of treatment of passive movement is that a movement must never be forcibly thrust through protective spasm. Manipulations are usually progressions from mobilizations that have increased in strength and shown clearly that further increase is necessary. Grades of mobilizations have been discussed (*see* p. 175), and a manipulation is similar to a grade IV mobilization in amplitude and position in the range; it differs only in speed. A grade IV mobilization is an oscillatory movement that the patient can prevent if he chooses to do so, whereas the movement of the manipulation is so quick it cannot be prevented by the patient. Because there is this link between the two procedures, it is perhaps an advantage to consider manipulation as a grade V movement.

> A manipulation is similar to a grade IV mobilization in amplitude and position in range. The difference lies in the speed

One of the occasions when manipulation might be used early in treatment is when a stiff and almost painless joint is responsible for minor symptoms. However, whether manipulation is used or not will depend partly on whether it is believed that an attempt must be made to increase forcibly the range of movement of the joint. In most circumstances, the symptoms can be relieved by mobilization without having to resort to manipulation.

> In most clinical circumstances, symptoms can be relieved by mobilization without having to resort to manipulation

It is not always possible, nor is it necessarily advisable, to aim for restoration of a full range of movement. For example, in the presence of degenerative or arthritic changes or when adaptive shortening has taken place in response to postural deformities, it will be impossible to regain the full range of movement that would exist in an unaffected spine. Also, a limitation of movement may be present to protect an otherwise unstable intervertebral joint. It is not always in the best interests of the patient to continue manipulative treatment/ mobilization or manipulation techniques in an effort to produce a full range of movement beyond the stage where symptoms have been relieved. In practice, approximately 85 per cent of patients successfully treated will respond to mobilization, leaving 15 per cent requiring the stronger manipulative techniques.

If mobilization is being used successfully in treatment, the patient should show marked improvement within 4–5 days. However, if there has been progress but it has not been as great as expected, then manipulation should probably form part of the treatment. Under these circumstances the treatment would commence with mobilization, which would be followed by manipulation and then completed by more mobilization. Similarly, manipulation might be used as a forerunner prior to the administration of traction. Under these circumstances it is intended that the increased movement obtained by the manipulation would assist the effectiveness of the traction. So it can be seen that manipulation may be used separately or in conjunction with mobilization.

Manipulation differs from mobilization in its effect on an intervertebral joint. If it is done vigorously, it must have some traumatic effect. The tissue reaction from the trauma influences the treatment plan, which normally aims at producing the quickest result possible with the minimum discomfort to the patient. As a joint should not be manipulated until all soreness from previous manipulations has gone, it may not be possible to manipulate until 2–3 days after the first manipulation. This soreness tends to increase, and it can result in a break of 4–5 days before the third manipulation and another 5–7 days before the fourth manipulation can be given. However, it should not take more than four or five manipulations to gain the maximum possible improvement in the range of movement of a joint. By allowing the soreness to subside, progress may be more accurately assessed. Although symptoms should be the ultimate guide to treatment, intervertebral movement should be checked each time for improvement.

Crack-like sounds coming from joints of the spine may be heard during manipulation, but they are only of significance in treatment when the joint is being manipulated to restore its movement. When there is almost no movement in an intervertebral joint, early attempts to manipulate it will possibly produce little more than a forcible stretch on the joint. However, when the movement has improved a little, the manipulation is more likely to produce a 'crack', which indicates an increased range of movement. This crack is different from the tearing sound associated with rupturing adhesions.

## MOVEMENT PATTERNS

by B. C. Edwards, OAM, BSc (Anat), BAppSci (Physio), Grad Dip Manip Th, MMPAA, FACP, Hon DSc (Curtin) (Specialist Manipulative Physiotherapist)

Within the patterns of movements described above, parts of patterns can be present. For example, irregular patterns of movement, which may be the result of trauma, may have regular patterns or even parts of regular patterns of movement present. This means that even when irregular patterns of movement are found during examination of a patient's movements, thought must be given to deciding whether they have any regular pattern components that may be forming part of the irregular pattern and thereby indicating a recognizable regular component to part of the patient's disorder.

The recognizing of different patterns of movement can assist in predicting:

- The result of treatment.
- The manner in which the symptoms and movement signs may improve.

Regular patterns of movement tend to respond to treatment in such a way that the least painful movement will improve before the most painful. For example, if right lateral flexion of the cervical spine in neutral produces the patient's right suprascapular fossa pain and this pain is made worse when the movement is done in extension, then right lateral flexion in neutral will improve before right lateral flexion in extension.

One can also expect that the treatment technique of right lateral flexion done in flexion (found on examination to be the painless position) is unlikely to make the symptoms worse.

The response in the case of irregular patterns of movement is not as predictable, and the improvement

in the symptoms may appear in an apparently random fashion.

When choosing the technique, care must be taken that the correct grade of movement is chosen in relation to the reproduction of pain, spasm or restriction of movement (*see* Chapter 8).

Most examinations of the cervical, thoracic and lumbar spinal joints are carried out in the upright position. However, most treatment techniques are done with the patient prone, supine or in side lying. Because of the altered weight distribution and position of canal structures when adopting the positions of supine, prone or side lying, there may be some alteration in the pain response when the same movements are compared with those in the upright position. It is important, therefore, that if the technique is to be chosen that produces particular symptoms in the upright position, the treatment position adopted must be adjusted to produce the same signs and symptoms.

There are two alternatives:

1. Examine for patterns of movement in the position in which the treatment is to be carried out.
2. Perform the treatment in the upright position.

## SELECTION OF TECHNIQUE

There are basically two types of passive movement techniques; physiological and accessory. Not only may the physiological movements be combined, but also the accessory movements may be done in a combined physiological position. It is usual to find with regular patterns that the accessory procedures of, say, postero-anterior unilateral vertebral pressure will be found to produce most symptoms when performed in the combined position that produces the increased symptoms than when done in the neutral position. However, with irregular patterns this may not be the case.

The recognition of regular (or irregular) patterns of movement can help in the selection of technique. The aspect of technique in which combinations of movement assist are:

1. The sequence of obtaining the direction.
2. The direction.

## SEQUENCE OF OBTAINING THE DIRECTION

It is important to assess accurately which movement of the examining movements is the significant movement either in reducing or in increasing the symptoms. This can be considered the primary movement of the examination. For example, if the patient complains of left leg pain extending down to the calf, the calf pain is increased when the patient extends the lumbar spine, and other movements of the lumbar spine do not alter the calf symptoms, then extension may be considered to be the primary movement of the examination. When using combined movements, one examines the effect of lateral flexion to the right and left performed in extension. If, for example, left lateral flexion done in extension increases the left calf pain, it is necessary to assess the effect of doing left lateral flexion first and then performing extension, and compare this with doing extension and adding in left lateral flexion. The difference in the sequence of the movements may be important in terms of the reproduction of the patient's symptoms. The technique of extension may be performed in left lateral flexion, or the technique of left lateral flexion may be performed in extension.

Similarly, in the cervical spine if flexion is the primary movement producing, say, right suprascapular pain and this same pain is increased when left rotation is added, it is necessary to assess the effect of performing flexion first and then adding rotation, and compare this with the effect of performing left rotation first and then adding in flexion.

## The direction

The direction of movement refers to the direction in which the oscillatory procedure of mobilizing or the thrust of manipulating is performed, and it is the last movement of the combination.

## FOR REGULAR PATTERNS

When a patient presents with regular patterns of movement, the technique chosen is usually the one that is found on examination to be the most painful direction of movement, but it is performed in the least painful way. For example, a patient has right suprascapular pain and on examination right lateral flexion of the cervical spine reproduces the right suprascapular fossa pain; this pain is made worse when the movement of right lateral flexion is done in extension and eased when it is done in flexion. Similarly, if right lateral flexion is sustained while producing the right suprascapular pain, then the pain eases when flexion is added and increases when extension is added. When each of these movements is done in extension the pain is worse but it is eased when flexion or right rotation is performed in flexion, and is progressed to performing the movement in extension.

Similar principles can apply when using accessory movements. Considering the same examples as above, it will be found that unilateral postero-anterior pressure on the right side of, say, the C4/5 interlaminar joint will produce maximum symptoms when the cervical spine is put in the position of right lateral flexion and right rotation. If the unilateral postero-anterior movement on the right is the primary finding it would be used as the treatment technique, starting by performing the technique in neutral and progressing to the most painful combined position.

## FOR IRREGULAR PATTERNS

The direction of movement chosen for irregular patterns of movement would similarly be the most painful direction of movement done in the least painful way, or, if the disorder is one of extreme pain or high irritability, the least painful direction of movement would be used as the technique in the least painful combined position. However, if combining of movements is not part of any obvious pattern, the chosen direction for the treatment technique would be in the least painful direction. For example, on examination right lateral flexion produces right suprascapular pain and this pain is eased when done in flexion. The chosen direction is right lateral flexion done in extension. However, the response to treatment will not be as predictable.

Performing the technique in the least painful position may improve the most painful examination movement – right lateral flexion done in flexion. On the other hand, the movement of right lateral flexion done in extension may deteriorate. In other words there may be a random response to the technique.

## CONTRAINDICATIONS

It is a cardinal rule that movements must never be forcibly thrust through protective spasm

The possibility of serious damage resulting from manipulation, particularly cervical manipulation, is often emphasized when this form of treatment is discussed. Although deaths have occurred (Smith and Estridge, 1962), it must be realized that if the number of manipulations carried out daily by lay manipulators is compared with the mortality rate, the danger is extremely small (Brewerton, 1964). Coupled with this is the fact (Liss, 1965) that similar damage resulting in death can occur with daily activities. With care of application and the continual assessment of the patient's symptoms and signs advocated in this book serious damage is almost impossible, especially if it is realized that patients with serious pathological conditions are excluded from manipulative treatments by the medical practitioner.

> The manipulative physiotherapist should always ask the question, 'Can I do harm?' throughout the examination and treatment process

There are many considerations influencing contraindications to manipulations. For example, some medical conditions may be considered contraindications because manipulation is potentially harmful, while other conditions may be considered contraindications in the sense that the conditions are unsuited to or unlikely to be affected by the treatment. On these grounds, the doctor will exclude such conditions as Paget's disease, rheumatoid arthritis, osteomyelitis, ankylosing spondylitis, malignancy, cord and cauda equina syndromes, and vertebral artery involvement.

> Some conditions may be contraindications to manipulation, but not necessarily to mobilizations

Another consideration is that some conditions may be contraindications to the more forceful manipulations, yet they may not be contraindications to the mobilizations described in this book. In fact, one of the important facets of mobilization is that, by its gentleness and with careful assessment, most of the possible dangers are eliminated and the treatment can be applied more widely. Neurological and radiological changes cover two groups of conditions that may be contraindications to any but the gentle techniques.

## NEUROLOGICAL CHANGES

Pain associated with disturbances of reflex activity, muscle power or sensation due to nerve-root compression are frequently cited as contraindications to manipulation. Patients having these signs certainly should not be manipulated vigorously at the commencement of treatment. However, provided the proper care is taken and the nature of the complaint is appreciated, the gentler mobilizing techniques can be used from the beginning. It may even prove necessary, as treatment progresses, to strengthen and/or sustain the techniques, and eventually but rarely manipulation may be indicated.

Herniated disc material at one intervertebral level in the lumbar spine can cause compressive signs in two nerve roots, but in the cervical spine only one nerve root can be involved. Therefore, a patient with arm pain and neurological signs attributed to two nerve roots has a pathology that is a contraindication to manipulation. Disturbances of bladder or bowel function or perineal anaesthesia are similarly contraindications.

Cord signs are also a contraindication to any form of forceful manipulation. Very gentle mobilizing may be quite safe, but it is unlikely to be of any value. Cervical traction is quite safe also, and although it is occasionally prescribed it is difficult to see how it can effect a favourable change in the cord signs. Gentle techniques may be used to treat intervertebral joint pain when this exists with cord signs, but if gentle techniques fail, forceful measures must not be employed.

## RADIOLOGICAL CHANGES

Osteoporosis and rheumatoid arthritis are two conditions that should preclude forceful manipulation, yet both conditions can be present in a patient who has pain that can be relieved by mobilization. Both conditions present situations where the safety measures detailed in this book are not enough to prevent fracture or serious damage if forceful procedures are used. There are no signs to warn the physiotherapist that an osteoporotic bone or diseased ligament is about to give way under the strain; therefore, forcible manipulation must never be used. However, it is wrong to preclude gentle mobilization.

> Two techniques that should be performed with great care are cervical rotation in the presence of marked rheumatoid arthritis changes, and rib pressure in the presence of osteoporosis

Two techniques require particular care. Cervical rotation in the presence of marked rheumatoid arthritic changes can rupture the transverse and alar ligaments, and cause atlanto-axial dislocation. Rib pressures used to manipulate the costovertebral joints may fracture an osteoporotic rib.

Differential diagnosis can be difficult, and in the early stages of a disease a patient may have symptoms and signs that are believed to be skeletal in origin. This patient may be referred for manipulative therapy. However, if the signs do not follow the usual patterns or if the patient does not improve during treatment, he should be referred back to the doctor. Treatment must not be continued for prolonged periods when only minimal improvement is being gained. Occipital headaches and neck stiffness, even a wry neck, can be the first sign of a subarachnoid haemorrhage or a cerebellar tumour. If such a patient is referred for manipulation before a correct diagnosis is possible, the physiotherapist should send the patient back to the doctor as soon as it becomes clear that the pain and signs do not improve with mobilization.

## VERTIGO

Vertigo is another condition that requires close observation when manipulative treatment is requested. Although vertigo can have a cervical origin (Cope and Ryan, 1959) it is usually only when it is secondary to headache that mobilization techniques will help (Ryan and Cope, 1955). Exploratory movements should be made with cervical techniques before they are used and a technique that causes any feelings of giddiness must not be used.

## HYPERMOBILITY

> 'Hypermobility' can be interpreted as a general laxity of ligaments allowing excessive ranges of movement of all or most joints of the body, which are not necessarily painful, OR as one or more intervertebral joints which are excessively mobile in relation to neighbouring joints

Hypermobility and instability are two words that are frequently used loosely, thus causing considerable misunderstanding. When dealing with spinal problems, the term 'hypermobility' can be interpreted in two distinctly different ways.

The first is illustrated by the patient who has general laxity of ligaments, allowing excessive ranges of movement of all or most joints of the body. This hypermobility is easily detected. Although patients may have hypermobile joints, they do not necessarily have pain from them.

The second kind of hypermobility is particularly evident, and of importance, in spinal problems. Under the circumstances being referred to here, the patient is not generally hypermobile as described above but rather has one intervertebral joint (or more) that is excessively mobile in relation to the neighbouring joints. When such a patient presents for treatment of pain arising from this area, the passive intervertebral movement tests described on pages 360–364 are used to assess which joints are stiff and which are hypermobile. When it comes to treating such a patient, it is

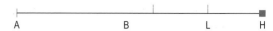

**Figure 9.1** The hypermobile joint movement has become stiff (limited to point L in the range) yet it still appears to be hypermobile because the limited range AL is still greater than the normal average range AB: that is, the range is still hypermobile whilst still being stiff for that joint. A = Beginning of a range of movement. B = End of the normal average range for that movement. H = End of the normal range of the movement when it is hypermobile. L = Limit of range of movement when the hypermobile movement AL is painful or stiff

first necessary to decide whether the pain is coming from the stiff joint or the hypermobile joint. If the stiff joint requires treatment, then reasonable care should be taken to avoid putting excessive strain on the hypermobile joint. However, when the hypermobile joint becomes painful and requires treatment, then the considerations are quite different, as will now be explained.

Hypermobility is generally held to be a contraindication to manipulation. This statement, however, requires clarification. A clinical or radiologically hypermobile joint may become painful in just the same way as a stiff joint or a joint with an average range of movement. There is usually some loss of movement when a hypermobile joint becomes painful. However, its loss of range may be small enough for the joint to still appear hyper-mobile on examination (*Figure 9.1*).

Mobilization is not contraindicated under these circumstances, and in fact it would be the treatment of first choice. Forcible manipulation of a full-range hypermobile joint is another matter. Although there may be occasional circumstances when a further increase of range is advisable, the general rule is that hypermobile joints should not be forcibly manipulated.

> A hypermobile joint is not necessarily unstable. Instability refers to the joint that has laxity of supporting ligaments, permitting the joint to move abnormally in a manner that makes the joint unstable

The above description identifies two kinds of hypermobility. It needs to be pointed out that under neither circumstances is the joint necessarily 'unstable', the movements still being within the patient's muscular control. Instability refers to a joint that has laxity of supportive ligaments, permitting the joint to move abnormally in a manner that makes the joint unstable. The joint does not have to be generally hypermobile for it to be unstable in any one particular direction. Testing of flexion/extension (*see* Chapter 12) indicates how the lumbar spine can be tested in such a manner as to reveal instability in a particular intervertebral joint.

## Instability

Any patient with symptoms arising from either a hypermobile joint or an unstable joint can be treated by mobilizing techniques, and the effect of such treatment assessed as described in Chapter 4. Once the joint has been made symptom free, the patient must be shown exercises to strengthen the muscular support around the hypermobile or unstable joint in an endeavour to add greater support for that joint. If pain is not relieved readily, then stabilizing exercises should be added or substituted early in treatment. If pain is aggravated by mobilizing exercises, they should be discontinued and stabilizing exercises substituted. The addition of supports to make the area more stable should also be considered. It should also be pointed out here that hypermobility does not directly relate to the orthopaedic diagnosis of 'instability'.

Clearly, the dangers of manipulation increase as the strength of the technique increases. Safety measures taken with manipulative treatment must be emphasized if the medical profession is to understand and have confidence in its use. Every effort has been made in this book to emphasize the importance placed on gentleness, with techniques that are only increased in strength as the continual assessment of signs indicates the need for increase. Even then, no attempt is ever made to thrust forcibly through muscle spasm.

*Some people believe that maintaining strong traction while performing cervical and thoracic manipulation is essential for safety, but this can give the physiotherapist a false sense of security. If pain and spasm are ignored because traction is being used, dangers will still exist. Care and assessment, together with knowledge of pathology, provide safety.*

## RECORDING

> Accurate recording is a visualization of the manipulative physiotherapist's logical, methodical evaluation of the cause and effect of all that occurs before, during and after treatment. In this way she can learn the finer points of examination, treatment and assessment

Manipulative techniques and the indications for their use can be taught, but this is not enough. Experience with analytical assessment teaches the finer points of treatment so that the best result is produced in the shortest possible time. The best way to learn from manipulative treatment is to record accurately the cause and effect of all that occurs during and following treatment. This written record should include all of the following elements, in the suggested sequence.

> Writing down the treatment plan facilitates clearer thinking and helps the therapist to learn from the treatment results

1.  It should begin with a summary of the patient's account of changes that have resulted from the previous treatment. Perceptive questioning may be required to obtain the relevant information, and when recording the information it is wise to include a direct quotation from the patient, using his own language and quotation marks. This information must be a *comparison*, not just a statement of facts.

2.  The record should then indicate changes in the important signs from physical examination performed throughout treatment.

3.  Next, today's treatment is planned. The advantage of a written planning stage in relation to the examination of a patient is especially important, and it is even more valuable when recording treatment. Once the changes that have resulted from previous treatment have been assessed, the physiotherapist must choose whether to continue with the same technique, and she must know clearly why she has made such a decision. If she chooses to change to a particular technique, she must know why she has chosen that particular technique. Writing this plan down facilitates clearer thinking and encourages consideration of the next day's treatment.

4.  Treatment is recorded by naming the technique used, stating the grade in which it was used, and *noting any effect it had on the patient's symptoms while it was being carried out.*

5.  Following the record of the technique, and separated from it by a clear and thick vertical line, a record is made both of the assessment of what the patient feels has happened as a result of the last treatment, and also of the physiotherapist's assessment of the changes that have taken place in the patient's joint signs.

6.  When the treatment has been completed, the manipulative physiotherapist will have made many judgements related to what she particularly wants

**Table 9.3**   Record during the treatment

| | | |
|---|---|---|
| C/O | = | Subjective assessment: assessment of what the patient says (use quotations) has happened as a result of the last treatment (comparisons not statements). Check on any asterisked points. With patients whose progress can be expected to be slow, make the comparison over a week rather than over 24 hours. |
| O/E | = | Objective assessment: physiotherapist's assessment of changes in any of the signs resulting from the last treatment. (Asterisked signs.) |
| Plan | = | State which technique is to be used and why. |
| P.P. | = | Present pain. |

R *The treatment*

*Effect after treatment*

(i)  State the technique used.
(ii)  The grade used.
(iii)  The level at which it was done.
(iv)  The number of times it was done.   C/O
(v)  **THE EFFECT IT HAD WHILE BEING**   O/E
**PERFORMED.**

Plan   — State reason for any possible treatment change and note any reminders for next treatment.

**Table 9.4**   Pattern for the mental and physical processes at a treatment session

| | | | |
|---|---|---|---|
| D9 | R × 4: (meaning this is the 4th treatment session of the 9th day from the initial consultation) | | |
| C/O | 'It has improved since I last saw you because I can turn over in bed without pain now' | | |
| Q? | 'No pain with coughing now' | | |
| P/E | ........................ | ........................ | |
| Plan: do xyz because pqr | | | |
| pp (present pain) | ............... | | |
| Rx: | in ........ | C/O | |
| | did ....... | P/E | |
| | (without pain) | | |
| Plan: | Now it is worth assessing to see if, by taking the technique into a small degree of discomfort, the behaviour of pain beyond P has changed | | |
| pp | ...................................... | | |
| Rx: | in ........ | C/O | |
| | did ....... | P/E | |
| | (into sl. discomfort) | | |
| | (in rhythm) | | |
| Plan: | ........................ | | |
| pp | ........................ | | |
| Rx: | ........................ | | |
| | etc. | | |

to assess, and to what she feels she may choose to use in treatment at the next session. These should be recorded. *Table 9.3* summarizes all of the above elements.

In the learning stages, and for clarifying what the mental processes during a treatment session are, the written notes from other than the initial consultation would follow a pattern something like that shown in *Table 9.4*.

**Table 9.5**    Example of writing up a treatment

C/O – 'Moving more freely, but more back pain'
O/E – F same range but less pain and less list
       SLR Ⓛ 40° same 'pressure' in back ↕ L5?ISQ
pp – Slight ache across back
Plan – Repeat last R because improvement is adequate
R – 3 × L/S IV | C/O 'about same'
      No p. | O/E F low 1/3, less list
       | SLR SI imp

     1 × U.S. 1.5 cm² | ISQ
     7 mins. No p. |

Plan – If not further improved do ↕ or LT

> When recording treatment, it is essential to include a statement of how the patient feels *during* the performance of the treatment technique

The 'in' and the 'did' (indid) is Butler's excellent way of teaching the writing up of the treatment technique, but it also needs to include a statement to describe what the patient feels DURING THE TIME THE TECHNIQUE is being performed. The examination findings will reveal positions of comfort or positions that increase the symptoms. The findings will also reveal the movements that provoke the symptoms and the ones that lessen them. The third component is, is it

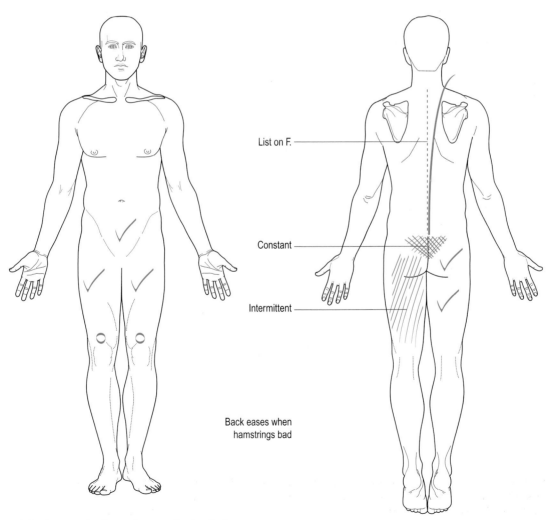

List on F.

Constant

Intermittent

Back eases when
hamstrings bad

**Figure 9.2**    An example of recording examination findings

better to do the movement from the top end or from the bottom up? With this information in mind, all other influencing factors will help in making the decisions concerning:

1. The position in which the patient is placed.
2. The movement technique that will be performed.

Then, it *must* provoke or lessen the symptoms, whichever the clinician decides.

One of the main complaints made about recording treatment in this way is that it is too time consuming; this is quite wrong. Abbreviations will make the task quicker and encourage the omission of unnecessary words. *Table 9.2* offers descriptive symbols that might be used to describe each of the techniques. (Full credit for the origin of these symbols must be given to Miss Margaret Jenkinson, MCSP, of King's College Hospital, London, and agreement on their identification was reached by a group of physiotherapists in England in 1966.) From these basic symbols innumerable variations can be made, but the essence of the symbols should be that they tell, at a glance, what they mean without having to learn them. Grieve (1988, 59) gives many such variations. If the number of times a technique is used is written in numbers and grades are recorded in Roman numerals, the whole procedure can be very quickly recorded once the habit is established.

To enable easy reference to previous treatment and quick retrieval of information, it is suggested that each treatment should be written up as shown in *Table 9.5*. Only by this means can a methodical treatment be given and the steps taken be clearly understood. This will avoid unnecessary waste of treatment time resulting from false impressions.

*Figure 9.2* is an example of the brevity that can be employed to record very detailed information of the examination and treatment of a patient with a lumbar disorder.

# Chapter 10

# Cervical spine

## CHAPTER CONTENTS

## INTRODUCTION

> For examination and treatment purposes, the cervical
> spine can be subdivided into head on neck (upper
> cervical), neck on neck (mid cervical), and neck on
> trunk (lower cervical)

The cervical spine (*Figure 10.1*) is best considered in
three sections: the upper cervical spine (occiput to C3),
which includes the high cervical spine (occiput to C2);
the lower cervical spine (C5–C7); and the area of overlap, the mid-cervical spine (C3–C5).

Disorders of the upper cervical spine frequently
result in headaches. The high cervical spine does not
involve intervertebral discs, whereas the upper cervical
spine also includes the C2–3 intervertebral joint where
there is an intervertebral disc, which needs to be taken
into account. The reason for subdividing the high cervical spine from the upper cervical spine is so that one
particular part of the palpation examination can be
emphasized. The lower cervical spine involves synovial joint structures and the intervertebral disc.

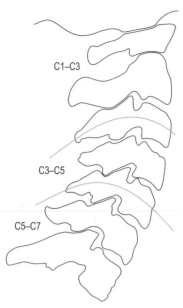

**Figure 10.1** Divisions of the cervical spine

Cervical discogenic disorders (which may also involve nerve roots) occur most frequently in the lower cervical spine. Disorders of the mid-cervical spine are most commonly synovial joint type disorders, and pain from these levels may be referred upwards or downwards.

The canal structures, dural attachments and cervical nerve roots are also potential sources of symptoms and functional restriction in this region.

## SUBJECTIVE EXAMINATION

*Table 10.1* sets out the examination pattern, but certain points require expansion.

> Patients with neuromusculoskeletal disorders of the neck usually complain of pain as well as associated symptoms such as stiffness, headache or dizziness. The site and description of the symptoms often helps to establish the source

### 'KIND' OF DISORDER

The answer to 'Question 1' establishes the 'kind' of disorder the manipulative physiotherapist is dealing with. This forms the basis for the rest of the examination and treatment options.

The 'kind' of disorder in the cervical spine is usually one of pain. This may range from headaches, to

**Table 10.1** Subjective examination

**'Kind' of disorder**
Establish why the patient has been referred for or sought treatment:
1. Pain, stiffness, weakness, instability, etc.
2. Acute onset.
3. Post-surgical, trauma, MUA, support, traction, etc.

**History**
Recent and previous (see 'History' below)
Sequence of questioning about history can be varied.

**Area**
Is the disorder one of pain, stiffness, recurrence, weakness, etc?
Record on the 'body chart':
1. Area and depth of symptoms indicating main areas and stating types of symptoms.
2. Paraesthesia and anaesthesia.
3. Check for symptoms all other associated areas, i.e.:
   (a) other vertebral areas;
   (b) joints above and below the disorder;
   (c) other relevant joints.

**Behaviour of symptoms**
**General**
1. When are they present or when do they fluctuate and why (local and referred).
2. Effect of rest on the local and referred symptoms (associate/dissociate with day's activities; pillow size/content, inflammation).
   Compare symptoms on rising in the morning with end of day.
3. Pain and stiffness on rising; duration of.
4. Effect of activities (beginning of day compared with end of day).

**Particular**
1. What provokes symptoms – what relieves (severity – irritability)?
2. Any sustained positions provoke symptoms?
3. Are quick movements painless?

**Special questions**
1. Does the patient have any associated dizziness (vertebral artery)?
2. Does the patient have bilateral tingling in hands and/or feet, or any gait disturbance (cord signs)?
3. General health and relevant weight loss (medical history).
4. What tablets are being taken for this and other conditions (osteoporosis from extensive steroid therapy)?
5. Have recent radiographs been taken?

**History**
1. Of this attack.
2. Of previous attacks, or of associated symptoms.
3. Are the symptoms worsening or improving?
4. Prior treatment and its effect.
5. Socio-economic history as applicable.
HIGHLIGHT MAIN FINDINGS WITH ASTERISKS
**Planning the objective examination**

local neck pain, and associated scapula, shoulder and arm pain.

A consistent link between the pain and activities involving the neck should be established. For example, the patient may say 'Every time I look over my shoulder I get a sharp pain in my shoulder blade. My arm movements seem fine'.

Occasionally, the patient's main complaint may not be pain. He may have seen the doctor because of dizziness, for example. The manipulative physiotherapist should establish whether there is a relationship between the behaviour or onset of neck symptoms and dizziness.

The manipulative physiotherapist should also be aware that, on occasions, the patient may complain of neck pain in the absence of any comparable signs in the neck. In such cases it is likely that the pain is being referred from elsewhere, such as the shoulder, thoracic spine or viscera.

## AREA OF SYMPTOMS

### Upper cervical spine

When a patient complains of suboccipital pain, the site must be determined with accuracy because it helps determine whether the cause is likely to have arisen from the occipito-atlantal area, the atlanto-axial area, or the area between C2 and C3. The most precise way of determining this site is to:

1. Ask the patient to point to the area of pain with one finger.
2. Replace his finger with yours.
3. Apply pressure and ask, 'Do you mean here?'.
4. If he says 'Yes', the next step should be to vary the angle of the pressure, and also vary the points of contact with the finger until the exact point is decided upon. Tedious as this may sound, it saves considerable time in other aspects of examination; it even directs the path the physical examination may take.

### Lower cervical spine

A second area of pain of cervical origin that is worthy of discussion is pain felt across the suprascapular area. This is a common site of pain, which may arise from the lower cervical spine or the upper thoracic spine. The most helpful information is obtained by determining whether the symptoms:

1. Start in the lower cervical spine and then spread downwards and laterally to the shoulders (*Figure 10.2*).
2. Spread from shoulder to shoulder across (approximately) the T2 level without spreading into the neck at all (*Figure 10.3*).

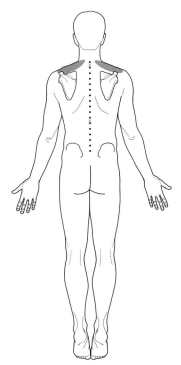

**Figure 10.2**  Distribution of pain of lower cervical origin (C5–7)

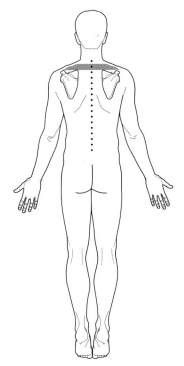

**Figure 10.3**  Distribution of pain of upper thoracic origin (T1–2)

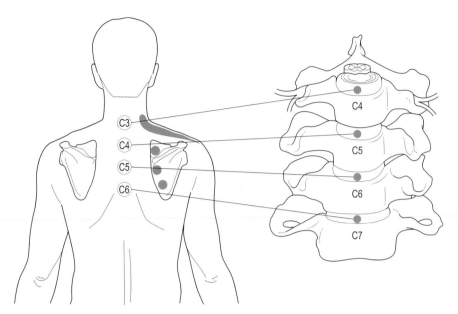

**Figure 10.4** Discogenic pain, referred from anterior surface of lower cervical discs (Reproduced from Cloward, R. B. (1959) *Annals of Surgery*, **150**, 1052–64, with kind permission of author and publishers.)

This gives a guide as to whether the symptoms arise from C5–7 or from T1–2.

It is important to know that both lower scapular area symptoms and vague T3–7 symptoms may arise from the lower cervical spine (*Figures 10.4 and 10.5*). To the clinician at least, these symptoms may relate to those areas of pain discussed by Cloward (1959).

When the patient has stated where his problem lies, the manipulative physiotherapist should question him as to whether he has symptoms in any other areas associated with the cervical spine. If these are checked and found to be asymptomatic, the relevant area on the body chart should be ticked. To do this has two purposes. The first is that it makes the examiner carry out the checking, and the second is that she then has proof that he did not have symptoms in a ticked area when she first asked him.

She must also determine the MAIN area of the symptoms and record them as being 'MAIN' on the body chart.

To add to this, Dwyer *et al.* (1990) and Dreyfuss *et al.* (1994) have carried out valuable research, which has helped the manipulative physiotherapist to identify potential sources of referred pain in the cervical region (*Figure 10.6a* and *10.6b*).

## BEHAVIOUR OF SYMPTOMS

As symptoms are rarely constant and unvarying for 24 hours of the day every day of the week, their behaviour must be established. The common cervical musculoskeletal symptoms, having a spontaneous onset, follow fairly regular patterns and are worsened by activity and by cervical movements. The patients frequently waken with temporary neck stiffness, even though their pain is less. Patients who have been involved in an accident will not have regular patterns of behaviour of the symptoms.

When symptoms are aggravated by movements, the exact movements must be determined. If symptoms are worse on wakening, the height and content of the pillow should be determined (*see* Appendix 4).

## SPECIAL QUESTIONS

Certain questions must be asked to determine whether the spinal cord and vertebrobasilar system are likely to be involved in the disorder. These are listed in *Table 10.1*. However, dizziness requires special consideration, and is discussed on page 242.

## HISTORY

For patients whose present episode began without incident, the development of the symptoms must be determined in detail from the time when they were first felt. It is only by relating this to any past history that the likely effect of treatment can be determined and the future prognosis estimated. On the other hand, when a patient has been involved in trauma the direction and force of that trauma (e.g. the extent and site of the damage to the car is a guide) should be determined

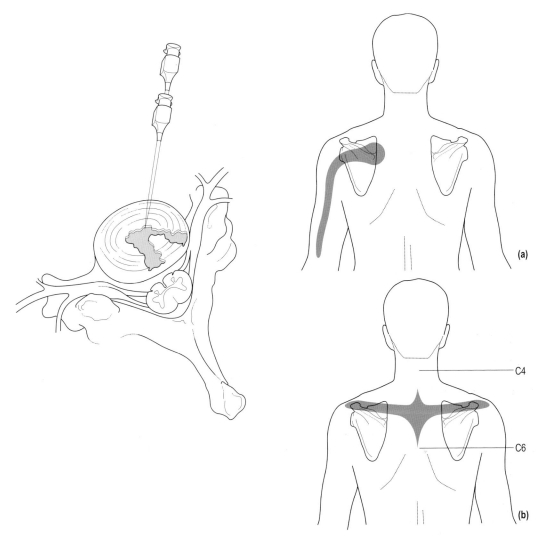

**Figure 10.5**  Discogenic pain. (*a*) Referred from posterolateral surface of cervical discs. (*b*) Referred from central disc ruptures (Reproduced from Cloward, R. B. (1959) *Annals of Surgery*, **150**, 1052–64, with kind permission of author and publishers.)

to enable a mental picture of the forces involved to be formed.

> 'Wry neck' is an asymmetrical neck posture accompanied by pain, and the pain is aggravated by an attempt to correct the protective deformity

The wry neck, as a disorder, is a special entity in the cervical spine, and can have many causes. The first is when a sudden movement has taken place and the patient is unable to return the head to the original forward-facing position. The disorder is commonly referred to as a 'locked joint'. A wry neck can also arise

from a sudden movement that sprains structures in the spine. However, with a sprain the patient can initially return his head to the normal position, even if a wry neck position develops later.

A third variety of wry neck occurs when the patient wakens with his head stuck to one side. The important difference between this disorder and a locked joint is that the patient wakens with it, as compared with a locked joint (Maitland, 1978), which wakens the patient when it occurs.

It is also essential to know the effect of any treatment the patient has had previously, the present degree of stability of the disorder, and whether it is worsening or not.

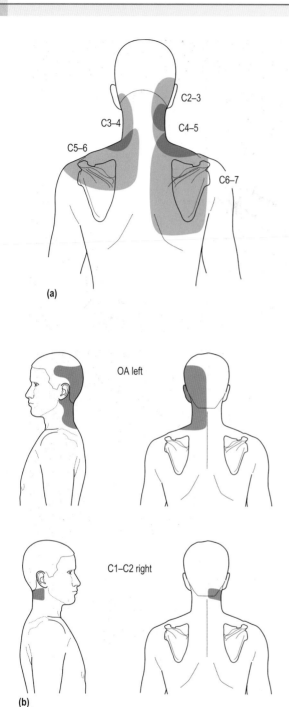

**Figure 10.6** (a–b).
a) Cervical zygapophyseal joint pain patterns (reproduced from Dwyer A., Aprill C., Bagduk N, (1990) cervical zygapophyseal joint pain patterns 1: a study in normal volunteers spine 15(6) 453–457 with kind permission of the author and publisher) and b) Atlanto-occipital and lateral atlanto-axial joint pain patterns (Reproduced from Dreyfuss P. et al (1994). Atlanto-occipital and lateral atlanto-axial joint pain patterns spine 19(10) 1125–1131 with kind permission of the author and publisher.)

## PLANNING THE PHYSICAL EXAMINATION

If a clear subjective picture has been established, the physical examination is much more straightforward. By astute observation, an appraisal can be made of the kind of examination – that is, the vigour of the examination – and the kinds of test movements that will be used.

When the symptoms are severe or the disorder is irritable (*see* p. 117), or if the history indicates a serious disorder (*see* planning sheet, *Table 6.3*), the test movements should be tested up to the point where pain begins. However, when the disorder is chronic and pain is moderate, test movements are taken to the limit of the range. *Table 10.2* is a guide for the physical examination.

## PHYSICAL EXAMINATION

### OBSERVATION

The physical examination should begin with observation. The patient's PRESENT PAIN should also be determined. Subtle clues such as postural alignment faults, protective deformities (and the effects of correcting and overcorrecting them) and longstanding muscle wasting will help to determine the source, contributing factors and stage of the patient's disorder.

### FUNCTIONAL DEMONSTRATION

Analysis of the demonstration by the patient of his functional limitation will establish the degree to which the cervical spine is involved. Wherever possible, differentiation of the functional demonstration will help to confirm the source of the patient's symptoms.

For example, a patient demonstrates that reaching high above his head with his right arm reproduces the pain in the back of his shoulder. Whilst this position is maintained by the manipulative physiotherapist, the patient is asked to take his neck into more extension, right side flexion and right rotation (lower cervical quadrant). If the pain in his shoulder increases the cervical spine is the likely source, especially if further elevation of his arm does not change his pain.

### BRIEF APPRAISAL

Brief appraisal of neck movements and palpation of the cervical spine for tenderness may be of value at this stage to confirm the need for further examination of the cervical spine. Quick active tests of the thoracic spine, shoulder, elbow and wrist and hand would also establish the degree to which these areas are involved.

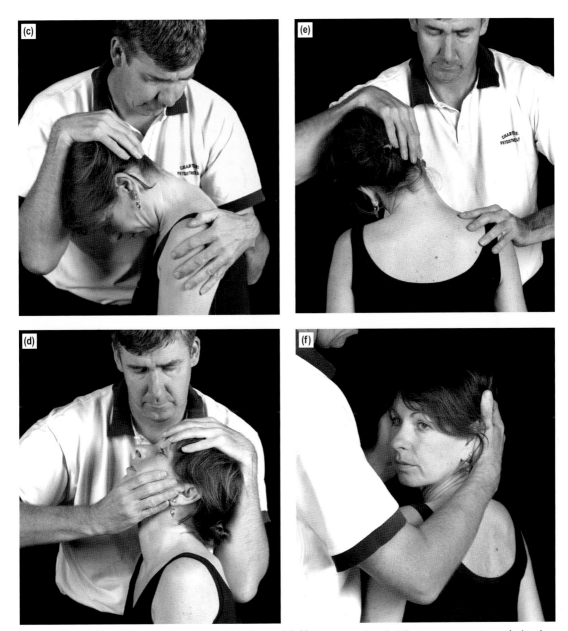

**Figure 10.6** *(contd)* (c) Adding over-pressure to cervical flexion. (d)–(f) show examples of adding over-pressure to cervical active movements. (d) Adding over-pressure to cervical extension (take care!). (e) Adding over-pressure to cervical lateral flexion left (stretch open the joints and structures on the right). (f) Adding over-pressure to cervical rotation

## Active movements

Clinical tip: For consistency in reassessment, it is important to reassess the active movements of the cervical spine (range, symptom response and quality of movement) in the same order each time

The physiological movements are usually tested first. All cervical movements should be watched carefully from the front, as each can reveal useful information (*Figure 10.6 C–F*); the contour of the neck when fully flexed is best seen from behind or above. Care is required when applying over-pressure to certain movements. With cervical **extension**, whether the pressure is applied by lifting under the chin or pressing against the forehead,

**Table 10.2** Cervical spine. Physical examination

**Observation**
Posture, willingness to move head and neck tenderness, swelling

**Brief appraisal**

**Movement sitting**
Other joints (quick tests)
    Move to pain or move to limit
F (flexion), E (extension), LF Ⓛ and Ⓡ (lateral flexion to left and right) and in F and E $Rot^n$ Ⓛ and Ⓡ (rotation to left and right; and in F and E pain and its behaviour, range, countering protective deformity, localizing, over-pressure, intervertebral movement (repeated movement and increased speed)

**When applicable, sitting**
Differentiating between upper and lower cervical.
Sustained E, LF towards pain, $Rot^n$ towards pain (when necessary to reproduce referred pain)
Q, upper and/or lower, and sustained (if F, E, LF and $Rot^n$ are negative)
Compression in slight LF towards pain and minimal E (when necessary to reproduce referred pain)
Distraction (if F, E, LF and $Rot^n$ and Q are negative)
Combined movement tests
Sustained $Rot^n$ each side and F or Q (vertebral artery)
Other vertebral artery tests
Passive physiological intervertebral movement (PPIVM)
C1/2 $Rot^n$
Active peripheral joint tests

**Supine**
Neurological examination (scalp sensation)
Canal tests as applicable
Static tests for muscle pain
PPIVM – F, E, LF, $Rot^n$
First rib
Passive peripheral joint tests

**Prone**
'Palpation'
Temperature and sweating
Soft-tissue palpation (muscle, articular pillar)
Position of vertebrae
Passive accessory intervertebral movement (PAIVM)

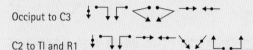

Occiput to C3

C2 to TI and R1

Combined PAIVM with physiological movement positions

**Examination of other relevant factors**

**OTHER TESTS**

Check 'case notes' for reports of relevant tests (X-rays, blood tests)

HIGHLIGHT IMPORTANT FINDINGS WITH ASTERISKS.

**INSTRUCTIONS TO PATIENT**
1. Warning of possible exacerbation
2. Request to report details
3. Instructions in 'back care' if required

---

care should be exercised to prevent it being a movement merely one of traction or compression respectively.

When pain is produced on only one of either **flexion or extension** movements of the neck, it is possible to differentiate between an upper and lower cervical disorder by extending the upper cervical spine while flexing the lower cervical spine. This movement is achieved by asking the patient to poke the chin forward and applying over-pressure (*Figure 10.7*). Similarly, by retracting the head, the upper cervical spine can be flexed while the lower spine is extended. Over-pressure is applied at the end of the range (*Figure 10.8*). Comparison of pain caused by these two movements with that produced by the normal flexion and extension tests can indicate whether it is the upper or lower joints causing pain.

The over-pressure with cervical **lateral flexion** can be performed in two opposite ways. If the pressure is being applied to lateral flexion to the left, it can be used to:

1. Stretch open the joints and structures on the right.
2. Squeeze together the joints and structures on the left.

By varying the place of the ulnar border of the hand, the test can be emphasized at any intervertebral level between the occiput and C7. If the lowest levels are to be tested, the physiotherapist's hand positions are quite different. In lateral flexion to the left she places her right hand against the patient's right parietal area and her left hand over the acromioclavicular area, and then she applies the stretch. The appearance of the head–neck–trunk relationship is quite different too,

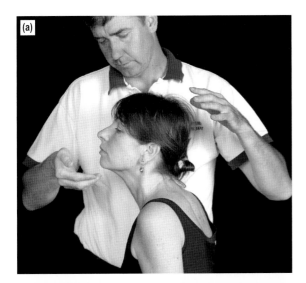

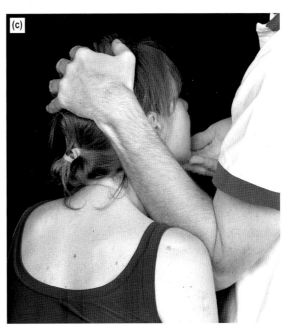

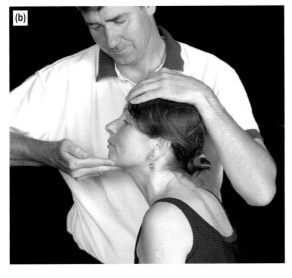

**Figure 10.7**  Upper cervical extension and lower cervical flexion. (*a*) As an active movement. (*b*) Position of hands, and (*c*) position of left forearm for applying over-pressure

with the head-on-neck position being different from the neck-on-trunk position (*Figure 10.9*).

The over-pressure with **cervical rotation** is described in Chapter 11 as part of differentiation of the cervical and thoracic spine in rotation.

## WHEN APPLICABLE TESTS

The cervical 'quadrants' and other combined movements are useful when trying to reproduce minor symptoms originating from the cervical spine, attempting to exclude the cervical spine as a source of symptoms, or as part of establishing a favourable treatment direction

An auxiliary test that may elicit joint signs when active movement tests followed by passive over-pressure are painless is the movement of combined extension lateral flexion and rotation towards the side of pain. The technique for testing the lower cervical spine in this 'quadrant' position varies appreciably from that used for the upper cervical spine.

### Lower cervical quadrant

To test the lower cervical spine for right-sided pain, the neck is tilted back into the right corner until the lower cervical spine is fully extended and laterally flexed to the right (*Figure 10.10*). With extension and left lateral flexion held in this combined position, rotation to the right side is added.

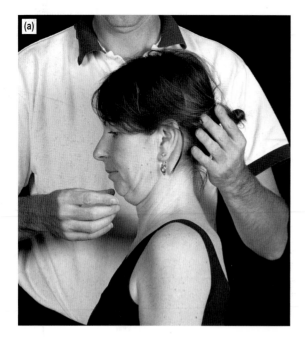

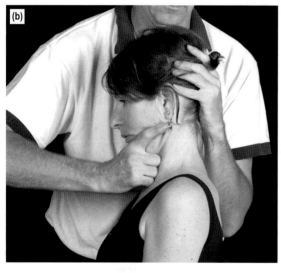

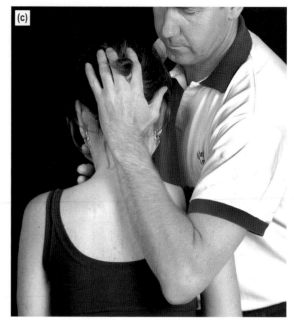

**Figure 10.8** Upper cervical flexion and lower cervical extension. (*a*) As an active movement. (*b*) Position of hands. (*c*) Position of left forearm

## Upper cervical quadrant

To test the left quadrant for the right side of the upper cervical spine, the physiotherapist stands by the right side of the patient and guides his head into extension and applies pressure to localize the movement to the upper cervical joints. This is done by grasping the patient's chin from underneath in the right hand and his forehead in the left. At the same time his trunk should be stabilized by the physiotherapist's arm from behind and her side from in front, while applying pressure through her hands to flex the lower cervical

spine with the head held in extension. While head extension is maintained, rotation to the right is added. The axis of rotation has changed from the vertical when the head is in the upright position to almost horizontal when the head is in full extension. It is the head that is turned, and the technique is to produce oscillatory movements so that the limit of the rotatory range can be felt. When the head is fully turned towards the physiotherapist, she then adds the lateral flexion component. The lateral flexion movement involves tilting the crown of the patient's head towards her and his

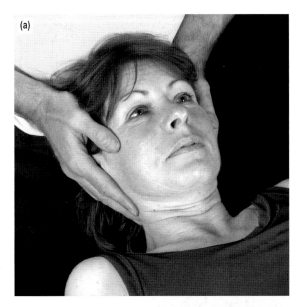

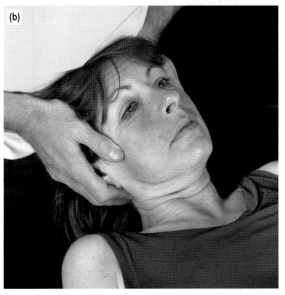

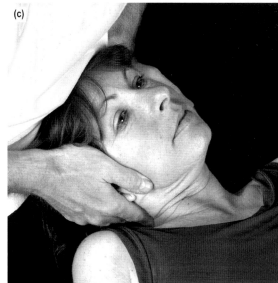

**Figure 10.9**  Cervical lateral flexion. (*a*) Neutral position.
(*b*) Head-on-neck lateral flexion. (*c*) Neck-on-trunk lateral flexion

chin away from her. This movement is also performed in an oscillatory fashion until the limit of the range is reached (*Figure 10.11*). This is a very difficult test movement to carry out accurately, and much practice is necessary to perform it well.

## SEQUENCES OF COMBINING MOVEMENTS

As well as quadrant movements, any other combination of movements can be used in an effort to find test movements comparable with the patient's disorder.

For example, the patient's head can be held in rotation to the left, to which can be added flexion or extension of the head and then lateral flexion of the head to left or right. (It should be pointed out that if, for example, after adopting a position of full rotation to the left, lateral flexion of the head to the left is added, this lateral flexion of the head is not a lateral flexion of each cervical intervertebral segment; for example the C7/T1 joint would be extending rather than laterally flexing.)

There is another very important point that must be remembered during the testing of combined movements

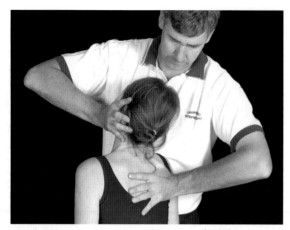

Figure 10.10    Lower cervical quadrant position

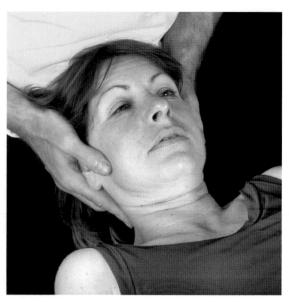

Figure 10.12    Neutral starting position for combining three physiological movements

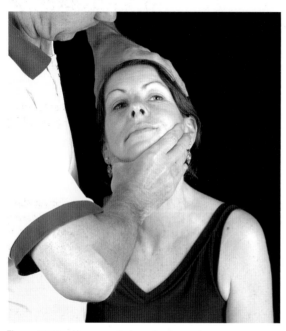

Figure 10.11    Upper cervical quadrant position

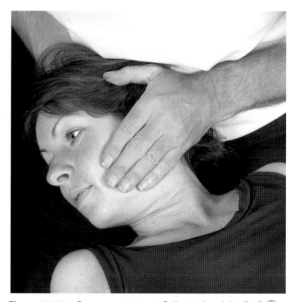

Figure 10.13    Sequence 1, step 1. Full rotation right. Rot$^n$ Ⓡ

starting from a neutral position (*Figure 10.12*). The patient's head is:

1. Fully rotated to the right (*Figure 10.13*) and then, while in that position;
2. His neck is laterally flexed to the right (chin to shoulder), which is a flexion of his head on his neck (*Figure 10.14*) and then;
3. His neck is flexed, which is lateral flexion of his head on his neck, and flexion of his neck on his trunk (*Figure 10.15*).

His head and neck will be in a particular position and have a particular pain response. However, if the sequence of the three movements (the three steps) is changed (to 1, 3, 2; or 2, 3, 1; or 2, 1, 3; or 3, 1, 2; or 3, 2, 1), the end-position and pain response will be different.

Three sequences that differ from the figures of the first sequences described above are 3, 2, 1 (i.e. F + LF Ⓡ + Rot Ⓡ – *Figure 10.16*); 2, 3, 1 (i.e. LF Ⓡ + F + Rot Ⓡ – *Figure 10.17*); and 1, 3, 2 (i.e. Rot Ⓡ 1 F 1

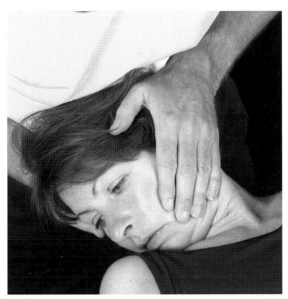

**Figure 10.14**    Sequence 1, step 2. Superimposed lateral flexion of neck to right (that is, chin to right shoulder or flexion of head on neck plus lateral flexion of neck on trunk). Rot$^n$ Ⓡ + LF Ⓡ

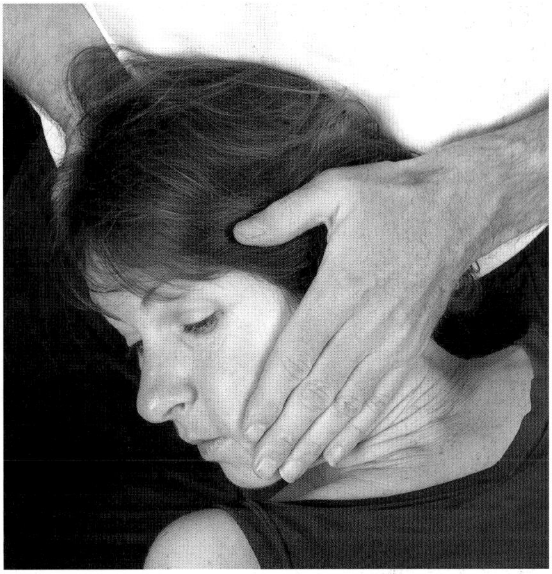

**Figure 10.15**    Sequence 1, step 3, Superimposed flexion of neck (that is, lateral flexion **right** of head on neck plus flexion of neck on trunk). Rot$^n$ Ⓡ + LF Ⓡ + F

LF Ⓡ – *Figure 10.18*). Drawings for the other two possible sequences of the same combinations – LF Ⓡ 1 Rot Ⓡ 1 F (2, 1, 3) and F 1 Rot Ⓡ 1 LF Ⓡ (3, 1, 2) – have not been included. Recognizing that these six sequences all end in the same 'corner position', the innumerable combinations are obviously interminable; after all, compression and distraction movements have not been included, nor have palpation techniques.

The reason for the differences is that as soon as one movement is taken to the end of its range, it immediately limits the available movement in every other direction. The examiner should be prepared to examine any combination of movements, in any sequence, in an effort to find 'comparable joint signs'.

Comparison has been mentioned in relation to narrowing the intervertebral foramina, but compression can also be another of the movements combined with other physiological movements. It is of greatest value in examining the upper cervical spine movements in patients suffering stubborn cervical headaches.

## Movements under compression

### Starting position

The physiotherapist stands behind the seated patient, cups her linked hands over the crown and parietal areas of his skull. His thorax must be stabilized by her abdomen, chest and medial side of her elbows. She

should press her chin against the dorsum of her hands so as to help apply the compressive pressure (*Figure 10.19*).

### Method

While in this position:

1. The therapist applies an axial compression, sustaining it as a grade IV+ 'pressure' for approximately 10 seconds, waiting to ascertain if there is any indication of relevant sensations being provoked. This axial pressure can then be oscillated as a grade IV+ movement, again asking about responses (*Figure 10.19b* and *10.19c*).

2. She then retains the compression and tilts the head on the neck, oscillating it from side to side in the lateral flexion direction through about 15° approximately six times. This movement involves considerable atlanto-axial rotation (*Figure 10.19a* and *b*).

3. She then returns to neutral, retaining the compression, and rotates the patient's head to each side.

4. From approximately 15° of high cervical flexion, a flexion–extension movement (under compression) of 30–40° should be performed. This direction is more difficult to isolate to the high cervical spine than lateral flexion.

5. If the patient's head is placed centrally and under compression, a sharp flick movement in any of the

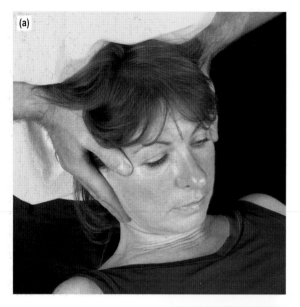

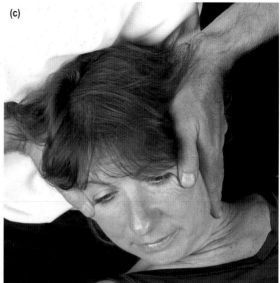

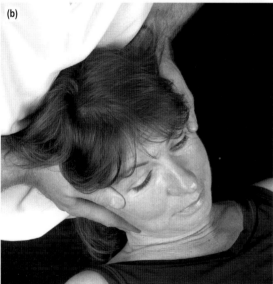

**Figure 10.16** Sequence 2. (*a*) Step 1. Full flexion; F. (*b*) Step 2. Superimposed lateral flexion right; F + LF Ⓡ. (*c*) Step 3. Superimposed rotation right; F + LFR + Rot$^n$ Ⓡ

directions may reveal a pain response even when movements (1)–(3) are symptom free.

## VERTEBROBASILAR ARTERY TESTING

> Vertebrobasilar insufficiency (VBI) is one contraindication to cervical manipulation. Remember that overzealous testing for VBI can also be a cause of vertebral artery compromise. Note that the evidence for and against physical testing for UBI remains conflicting

Reference has already been made to the testing of the vertebrobasilar system (p. 118). Vertebrobasilar insufficiency is one of the contraindications to cervical manipulation, and therefore questions regarding dizziness (especially dizziness associated with either neck movements or neck positions) should be a routine part of the initial investigation. The importance of examining for vertebrobasilar insufficiency cannot be over-emphasized, because it is an unfortunate fact that even when all of the physical tests are negative, during treatment of the cervical spine the system may be sufficiently compromised to cause symptoms.

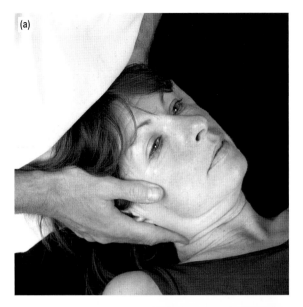

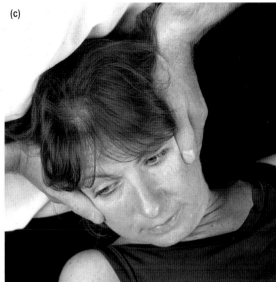

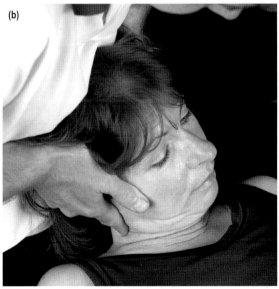

Figure 10.17 Sequence 3. (*a*) Step 1. Lateral flexion right; LF Ⓡ. (*b*) Step 2. Superimposed flexion; LF Ⓡ + F. (*c*) Step 3. Superimposed rotation right; LF Ⓡ + F + Rot$^n$ Ⓡ

There are many instances of complications following cervical manipulation referred to in medical literature (Pratt-Thomas and Berger, 1947; Schwartz and Geiger, 1956; Green and Joynt, 1959; Bladin and Merory, 1975; Krueger and Okazaki, 1980; Shellhas *et al.*, 1980).

De Kleyn and Nieuwenhuyse (1927) were the first to demonstrate that the vertebral artery could be obstructed at the atlas and axis levels by rotation and extension of the head. The vertebral artery enters the cervical spine at the level of C6 and passes through a foramen at each of the transverse processes, where it is closely approximated posterolaterally to the zygapophyseal joints and medially to the neurocentral joints of Luschka. Scheenan *et al.* (1969) demonstrated angiographically that distortion of the vertebral artery was possible by cervical osteophytes, and extension and rotation of the head increased compression of the artery on the side to which the head was rotated. Brain and Wilkinson (1967) showed that rotation of the head may cause compression of the vertebral artery as it passes through the transverse process of the atlas on the side away from which the head is rotated. For this reason, when a patient complains of dizziness, sustained rotation must be assessed to both sides.

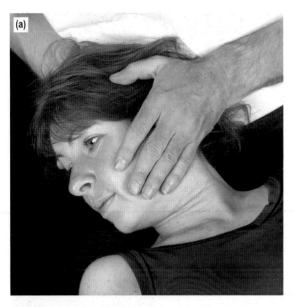

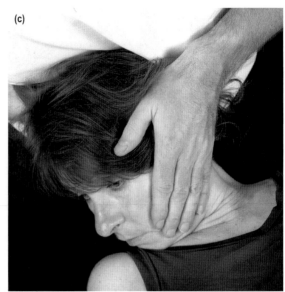

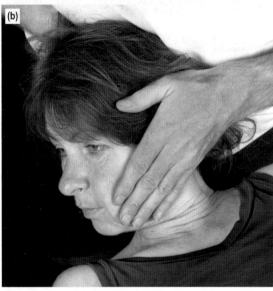

**Figure 10.18** Sequence 4. (*a*) Step 1. Rotation right; Rotn Ⓡ. (*b*) Step 2. Superimposed flexion; Rotⁿ Ⓡ + F. (*c*) Step 3. Superimposed lateral flexion right; Rotⁿ Ⓡ + F + LF Ⓡ

The presence of atheromatous and arteriosclerotic changes complicates the situation, as do marked degenerative changes in the cervical spine. It is important to question thoroughly aspects of the patient's history, which may include onset of dizziness due to changes in position of head, neck or whole body. In particular, middle-aged and elderly patients must be carefully assessed both by the referring physician and by the manipulative physiotherapist for conditions such as hypertension or vascular disease before cervical manipulation is carried out. One should not manipulate the cervical spine unless an X-ray has been taken and viewed critically. Tulsi and Perrett (1975) have shown evidence of erosion and indentation of the pedicle of C4, which they state as being the most common level when compared with other levels between C2 and C6. The phenomenon may be pathological or developmental, and it may be symptomatic or asymptomatic. The manipulative physiotherapist must respect its presence whether it is developmental and asymptomatic or not.

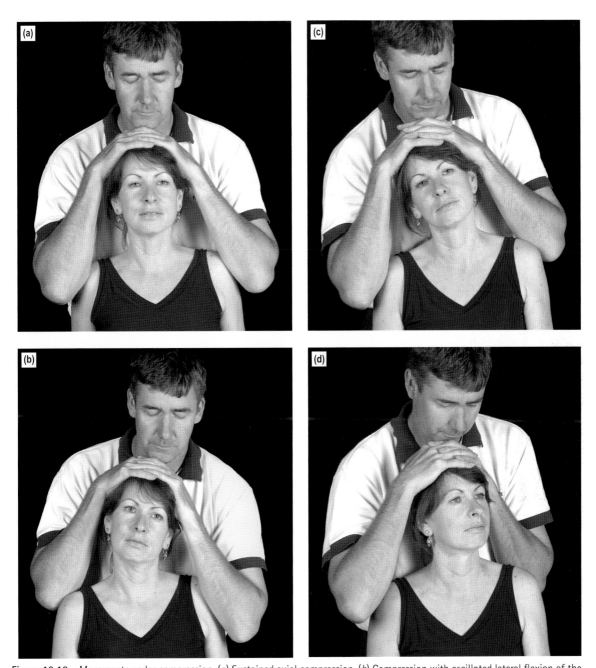

**Figure 10.19**   Movements under compression. (*a*) Sustained axial compression. (*b*) Compression with oscillated lateral flexion of the head on neck to the left. (*c*) Compression with oscillated lateral flexion of the head on neck to the right. (*d*) Compression with rotation to the left

Signs of vertebrobasilar involvement in a patient who has symptoms of dizziness should be assessed in four stages:

1. Initial questioning.
2. Physical tests (*see* p. 247).
3. Symptoms (listed below) provoked during mobilization or manipulation of the cervical spine.
4. Symptoms (listed below) following such procedures.

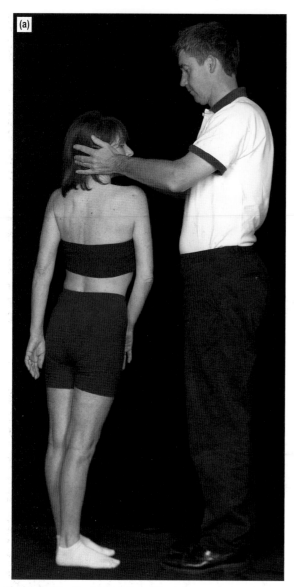
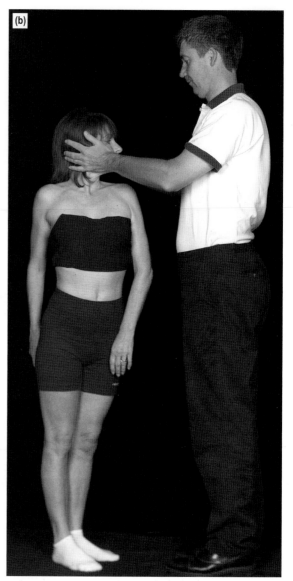

**Figure 10.20**   Cervical rotation without ear movement

The symptoms referred to in (3) and (4) above are:

1. Facial paraesthesia.
2. Diplopia.
3. Blurring of vision.
4. Nausea.
5. Vomiting.
6. Unsteadiness.
7. Nystagmus.

## Initial questioning

The first step is to question the patient effectively regarding any symptoms of dizziness. In order to

understand the kind of symptoms that the patient feels and calls 'dizziness', it is necessary to relate:

1. The history of dizziness to the history of neck symptoms.
2. The presence or aggravation of dizziness by movements of the head and neck.
3. Aggravation of dizziness by sustained positions of the head and neck in relation to the body.

The physical tests and the symptoms (above) both during and after treatment are now described.

## Physical tests

The manipulative physiotherapist may need to expand on the procedures given by Cope and Ryan (1959). When a patient associates dizziness with quick rotary movements of the head and neck, the following examination procedures should be performed.

*Test 1* – With the patient standing, he should be asked to turn his head from side to side several times through the full range while being assessed for dizziness or any of the seven symptoms listed above.

*Test 2* – To differentiate the relationship of the dizziness felt in test 1 to neck movements, rather than to disturbance of the vestibular system, repeated neck rotation should be tested while the head is held motionless, thus eliminating the effect of the middle ear. To achieve this movement the patient stands while the manipulative physiotherapist, standing in front of him, holds his head in her hands. The patient then twists his trunk fully from side to side while his feet and head remain stationary. Thus his trunk rotates under his head without movement of the head (*Figure 10.20*). Dizziness provoked by this test is not caused by vestibular disturbance.

When a patient complains of dizziness with 'positions' of the head rather than 'movement', as well as testing the positions he can quote, the following tests should be performed in the sitting position.

*Test 1* – Rotation to each side. With the patient seated, he is asked to turn his head fully to the left side. The physiotherapist then places her right arm behind the patient's left shoulder so that the right hand is placed over the occiput. The left hand is placed over the right zygomatic arch so that the fingers extend up to the forehead. Pressure is then applied and sustained for at least 10 seconds. The patient is questioned regarding dizziness or associated phenomena both during the technique and again after the position is released, while also watching his eye movements. A period of at least 10 seconds should be given to allow for any latent response from the sustained rotation. The test is then carried out with rotation to the opposite side (*Figure 10.21*).

*Test 2* – Adding extension. The previous position of rotation is adopted, and then the patient's head, relative to his neck, is extended and the position sustained for 10 seconds or more. Again assessment is made of the symptoms both during and after the test movement, allowing time for any latent response. The test is repeated with rotation plus the extension component to the opposite side (*Figure 10.22*).

*Test 3* – Sustained extension. The manipulative physiotherapist stands in front of the patient and asks him to extend his head and neck as far as possible. Gentle over-pressure is applied, and the position is

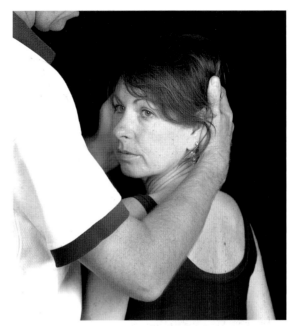

**Figure 10.21**  Sustained rotation test

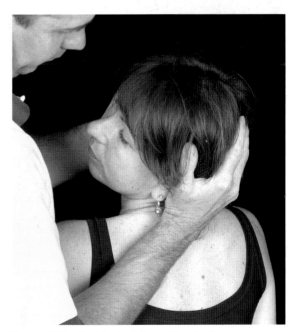

**Figure 10.22**  Sustained rotation, with extension

maintained for 10 seconds. The symptomatic responses are sought as explained above (*Figure 10.23*).

If the tests are positive in the sitting position, there is no need to repeat them in the lying position. However, if this is not the case, then the tests must be performed in the lying position. This is because a

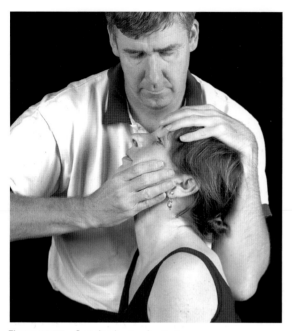

**Figure 10.23** Sustained extension test

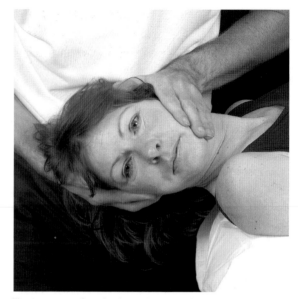

**Figure 10.24** Sustained rotation test, lying position

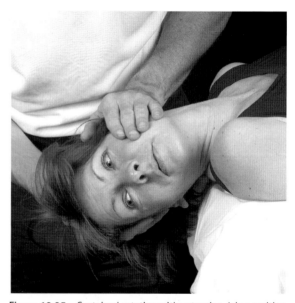

**Figure 10.25** Sustained rotation with extension, lying position

greater range of movement can sometimes be achieved in lying. Tests (4)–(6) are therefore performed with the patient supine.

*Test 4* – Sustained rotation. The patient lies supine with his head and neck beyond the end of the couch. The manipulative physiotherapist holds his head, with her left hand supporting around the head and her right hand around the zygomatic arch. The head is then stretched in rotation to the right, and the position sustained for 10 seconds or more (*Figure 10.24*). The patient is questioned regarding dizziness or any associated phenomena both during the technique and again after the position is relaxed. While in this position of sustained rotation, and also in the next two test positions (5 and 6), nystagmus should be assessed by watching the patient's eye movements as he watches her moving finger.

*Test 5* – Sustained rotation with extension. The above position is adopted, and extension of the head on the neck is added and sustained while assessing symptoms both during and after the procedure (*Figure 10.25*).

*Test 6* – Extension. The patient lies supine with his head and neck extended beyond the end of the couch. The manipulative physiotherapist holds the head in the manner described above, and full extension is performed and assessed (*Figure 10.26*).

## QUALIFIED ASSESSMENT

Careful assessment needs to be carried out when full rotation or extension of the cervical spine is restricted by either pain or stiffness. Under these circumstances, assessment of the vertebrobasilar system CANNOT BE COMPLETE, BECAUSE THE TEST MOVEMENTS CANNOT BE TAKEN FAR ENOUGH TO COMPROMISE THE ARTERY. If there are any positive findings on examination tests, while adopting any treatment technique position, during a treatment technique, or after treatment, manipulative procedures are contraindicated.

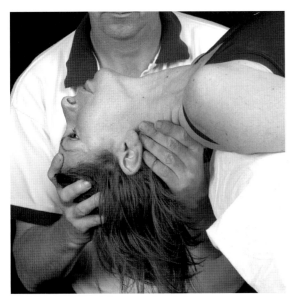

**Figure 10.26**   Extension test, lying position

Whether or not there are any symptoms or signs of vertebrobasilar insufficiency, manipulation, as a sudden movement beyond the patient's control, is contraindicated in every elderly patient who has marked degenerative changes. Techniques must be limited to mobilizations used in continual conjunction with observations and questions related to dizziness.

Grant (1994) has detailed a medico-legal protocol for minimum standards of vertebrobasilar artery testing.

## MOVEMENT IN THE VERTEBRAL CANAL AND INTERVERTEBRAL FORAMINA

### Upper limb neural tests (ULNTs)

Methods for testing for movements of the cervical nerve roots or their sleeves by stretching are not yet clear cut. Nevertheless, helpful information is often gained when a patient spontaneously comments that he achieves relief of his symptoms by placing his hand on his head (assuming the possibility that this position relieves the stretch on the fifth and sixth cervical nerve roots), or by supporting the elbow of his painful arm in his other hand in a sling-like fashion (which perhaps relieves stretch on the seventh cervical nerve root). These positions are spontaneously adopted by patients whose symptoms and neurological changes are in the areas related to the nerve roots stated. Conversely, stretch can sometimes be increased by protracting the shoulder and stretching the arm across in front of the body.

Elvey (1979), at the Western Australian Curtin University of Technology, is continuing the extremely valuable work in the area of defining physical tests whereby certain movements of the arm (neck and leg) cause neural movement in the cervical spine in a similar manner to neural movements such as those achieved by straight leg raising in the lumbar spine. He has shown quite clearly on cadavers at autopsy that, in addition to movement of the shoulder, movement of the elbow when the shoulder is positioned in abduction and external rotation is accompanied by movement of nerve roots in the vertebral canal and intervertebral foramina. He has shown also that movement of the left shoulder and left elbow creates movement of the nerve roots and brachial plexus on the right side of the spine. These tests are so important that all physiotherapists should know and use them, even at undergraduate level. Butler (1991) describes further neurodynamic testing of the upper limbs.

Qualified manipulative physiotherapists know that some patients have shoulder pain that is cervical in origin. When a patient has such shoulder pain, it can frequently be reproduced by the neural tests Elvey and Butler have described. Some of the tests show, by virtue of the behaviour of the pain when cervical movements are coupled with them, that the patient's shoulder pain must be cervical in origin. A number of tests can be carried out. The routine of one of these tests is as follows:

1. a) The patient lies supine with his arm able to be extended freely beyond the edge of the couch. With his arm by his side, his shoulder symptoms are then assessed. The physiotherapist then abducts his arm, without elevation of the shoulder girdle, in a frontal plane posterior to the median frontal plane until the symptoms change (*Figure 10.27*).
   b) She then releases the abduction tension to a position just short of provoking the symptoms. She then externally rotates his arm and supinates his forearm and assesses any change in symptoms (*Figure 10.28*).
   c) She then releases the lateral rotation to a position just short of provoking symptoms, and then she extends his elbow followed by his wrist and fingers to assess whether this reproduces his symptoms (*Figure 10.29*). If the shoulder symptoms are provoked by extension of the hand, the source of the symptoms must be in structures other than the glenohumeral joint.
   d) While maintaining wrist and finger extension, she flexes his elbow and assesses the pain response (*Figure 10.30*).

2. a) If the patient's arm is then put into the position that reproduces the shoulder pain – let us

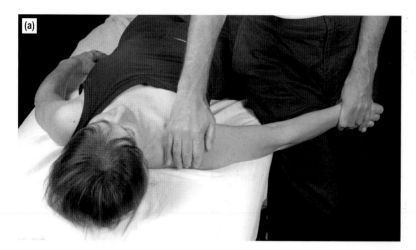

Figure 10.27 (*a*) Abduction arm in test for shoulder pain. (*b*) Abducted

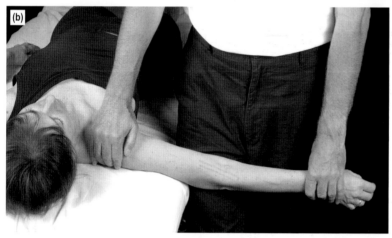

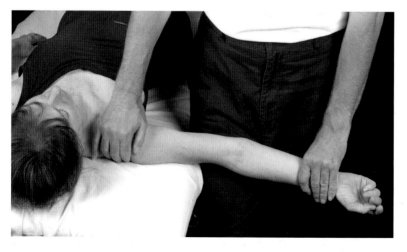

Figure 10.28 Release of abduction tension followed by external rotation

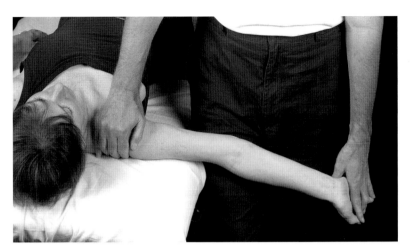

Figure 10.29 Release of lateral rotation followed by extension

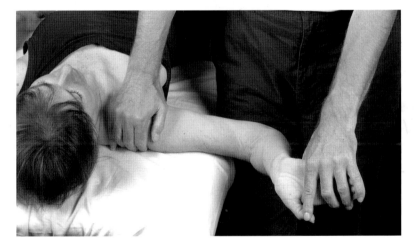

Figure 10.30 Elbow flexion during wrist and finger extension

assume that it is this last step of the test just described above – he is then asked to take his ear towards his painful shoulder and the physiotherapist assesses the changes in his pain response. It is vital that the glenohumeral joint and shoulder girdle be maintained in exactly the same position throughout the test of cervical movements. If this is not done with fine judgement, the test becomes invalid (*Figure 10.31*).

b) The next test is for the patient to take his ear away from his painful shoulder, while again assessing the change in symptom response to the movement (*Figure 10.32*). The other cervical movements can be utilized to determine whether there is a cervical component to the patient's symptoms.

c) The same pain responses are assessed with the cervical movements of flexion (*Figure 10.33*) and rotation towards and away from the side being tested (*Figures 10.34* and *10.35*).

3. To add another component to the tension, double straight leg raising can be included (*Figure 10.36*). Lastly, a further step can be taken by asking the patient to flex his chin on to his chest (*Figure 10.37*).

## SLUMP TEST

The slump test, as described on page 144, should be incorporated into the physical examination when the examination findings of joint movements do not fit the patient's symptoms.

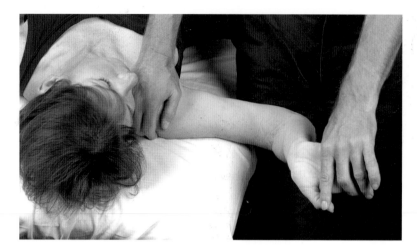

**Figure 10.31**    Assessment of pain response during rotation of the patients head towards shoulder

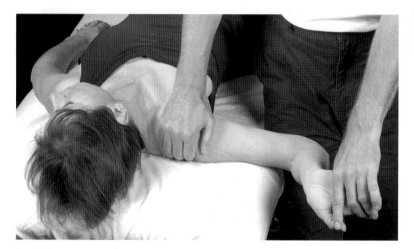

**Figure 10.32**    Assessment of pain response during rotation of patients head away from shoulder

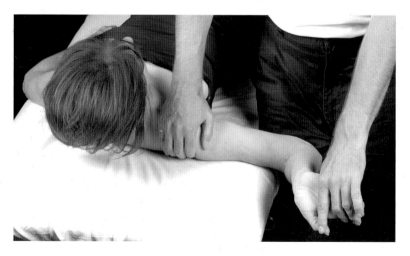

**Figure 10.33**    Assessment of pain response during cervical flexion

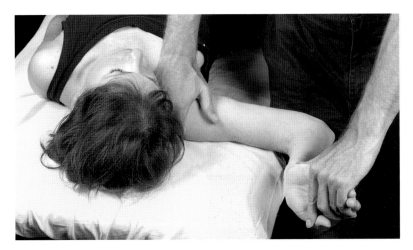

Figure 10.34    Assessment of pain response during lateral flexion towards shoulder

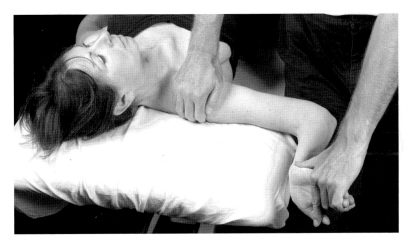

Figure 10.35    Assessment of pain response during lateral flexion away from shoulder

There is another aspect of vertebral canal tests, which is particularly pertinent in the cervical area. Breig (1978) has shown clearly that the pain-sensitive structures in the vertebral canal can lie in different places when the patient is in different positions. For example, during cervical lateral flexion to the left the pain-sensitive structures will be in a different position if the movement is performed with the patient sitting to that when he is lying on his left side, and will be different again if he is lying on his right side. Therefore, if a patient has symptoms and signs that do not fit in with the common musculoskeletal patterns, such tests as described above should be performed. If when doing the lateral flexion to the left a particular site of pain is provoked at 20 per cent of the normal range, yet it is full range and pain free when done in left side lying, and is more severely provoked with minimal lateral flexion to the left while lying on the right side, then there must be some canal structure involvement in the patient's disorder.

## EXCLUDING THE CERVICAL SPINE AS A SOURCE OF SHOULDER SYMPTOMS

To be certain that shoulder symptoms are not cervical in origin, three other tests are mandatory:

1. The first tests the physiological movements of: rotation towards the painful shoulder; extension; and the right low cervical quadrant. These positions should be sustained in an over-pressure position for a short time. If this test reproduces the shoulder pain, then the cervical spine is implicated. If the test produces local cervical pain, the test should be repeated to the other side for comparison, so as to allow a decision to be made on the implication of the cervical spine.

2. The second test is cervical compression with the patient's head in slight extension and lateral flexion towards the side of pain. If it provokes the shoulder pain, the test is positive. If it produces

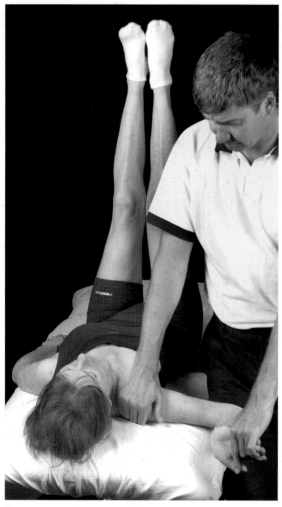

**Figure 10.36**    Assessment of shoulder-pain response during double straight leg raising

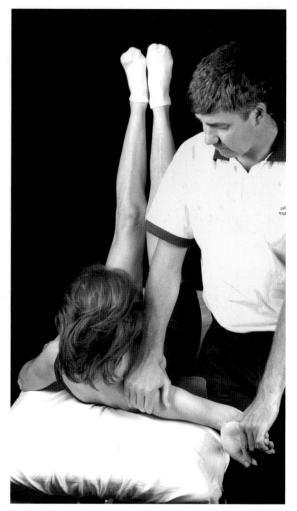

**Figure 10.37**    Assessment of shoulder-pain response during double straight leg raising with neck flexion

pain centrally (at approximately C6) or slightly laterally towards the painful shoulder, comparison should be made by performing the test on the opposite side. If this test also provokes the previous pain, the cervical spine is implicated. However, if the test on this opposite side produces pain on the side of the compression, the decision as to the involvement of the cervical spine rests with the quality of pain on each side. If the pain on the symptomatic side is far greater, deeper, or sharper than on the other side, the involvement of the cervical spine is heightened.

3.  The last and most important test is that the cervical spine from C4–7 should be examined very care-

fully by palpation. If the cervical spine is involved, there will be a marked difference between the painful shoulder side of the cervical spine compared with the opposite side.

## PALPATION

(Adapted from Maitland (1982a), by kind permission of publishers.)

The routine of palpation examination is performed in the following sequence. It is first necessary to have the patient lying prone with his forehead resting in one palm (palms overlapped) and his neck so positioned

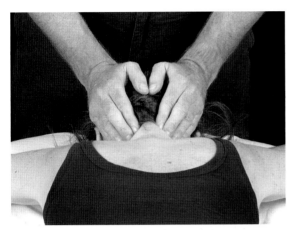

**Figure 10.38**    Soft-tissue palpation with three fingers

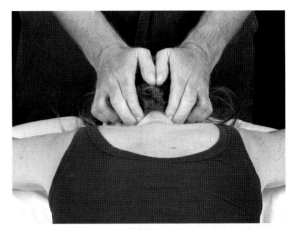

**Figure 10.39**    Soft-tissue palpation with two fingers

that there is no lateral flexion or rotation, and so that the spine lies in its neutral mid-flexion/extension position.

## Areas of sweating and temperature change

The first step should be to palpate the posterior aspect of the neck (especially laterally) to ascertain the presence of any sweating or temperature increase, resulting from an inflammatory disorder or increased sympathetic outflow. A decrease in temperature may also be detectable in cases of 'old', 'cold', chronic arthritic pathology. This is assessed by using the backs of the fingers.

## Soft-tissue changes

To gain the patient's confidence, the second step should be to use the hands and fingers in a general manner over the back of the neck and adjacent supraspinous fossa area in a soothing circular petrissage-type massage, during which a general impression can be gained as to the state of the superficial soft tissues. This need not take longer than a few seconds, and it is invaluable in gaining the confidence of the apprehensive patient or the patient with an extremely tender neck.

To begin the more positive part of the soft-tissue examination, the tips of the middle three fingers (*Figure 10.38*) should palpate the sub-occipital area from the superior nucal line to the atlas. To do this, the pressure of the fingertips should be directed towards the patient's eyes and the tissue palpated by both a medial-lateral movement and a postero-anterior movement. Palpation continues by now using the full length of the pads of the middle and index fingers of each hand in the laminar trough area (that is, from the lateral surface of spinous process to the lateral margin

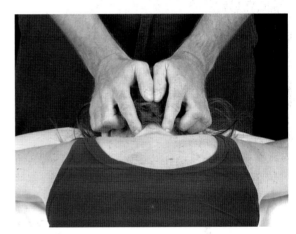

**Figure 10.40**    Soft-tissue palpation with one finger

of the articular pillar), from C1–7 (*Figure 10.39*). The technique involves moving both hands in rhythm with each other, moving the skin up and down with the pads of the fingers as far it allows, while gently sinking into the muscle bellies and other soft tissue. The purpose is to feel for areas of thickness, swelling and tightness in the soft tissue, and also for abnormalities of the general bony contour. Having performed two or three up and down movements in the upper cervical area, the fingers should be made to slide caudad 2–3 cm and the process repeated. This is then continued, moving down the neck in approximately four stages, until the level of C7 is reached. A particular level may be returned to if an abnormality is felt there. Once the general and more gross impression has been gained through the full pads of the fingers, the procedure should be repeated but using the tip of the pad of only one finger of each hand (*Figure 10.40*) and emphasizing the examination to the areas where discrepancies from the normal have been found.

A reasonably accurate determination of the site and type of tissue abnormality should be made so that a more detailed determination can be made later.

The most common findings at this stage of the examination are:

1. General tightness of muscle tissue along almost the full length of one side of the cervical spine.
2. Local areas of thickening immediately adjacent to one or more spinous processes.
3. Local areas of thickening in the largest part of the muscle bulk in the mid-laminar trough area.
4. Soft thickening over the posterior articular pillar at one or more intervertebral levels.
5. Hard bony thickening and prominence over the lateral and posterolateral margins of the articular pillar.
6. Tightness of the ligamentum nuchae, or localized thickening of a section of it.

## Bony changes and position tests

Bony points and interspinous spaces are palpated next. The tip of the thumb of each hand is used to palpate the bony outline of the spinous processes first.

There are two important planes in which to assess the position of the spinous processes: the first is that they should lie centrally in the sagittal plane; and the second is that from C2–6 they should lie roughly along an arc of a single sagittal circle. That is, the spinous processes should change evenly along the normal cervical lordotic curve. However, normal variations with regard to the depth of C3 and the prominence of C6 and C7 should be allowed for when interpreting the positions in this plane.

### C1–2

The patient lies prone and rests his forehead in his palms while the physiotherapist palpates between the spinous process of C2 and the occiput to ascertain whether the posterior tubercle of C1 is palpable. From this point she palpates bilaterally through the relaxed suboccipital muscles, moving laterally until the tip of the transverse process is reached. The relationship that each side of C1 bears to the occiput and to C2 should be assessed. This finding is assisted by also palpating the tip of C1 laterally to assess its relationship to the anterior aspect of the mastoid process.

The spinous process of C2 varies widely in its shape and tubercles. It may have only one lateral tubercle and thus appear to be rotated. If rotation is present, one articular pillar of C2 will be more prominent than the other. X-rays will also show the shape of C2's spinous process.

### C2–7

The spinous processes are unreliable as the sole source of information regarding position of the vertebrae. They frequently lie to one side without there being any rotation of the vertebra, and absence of one or other terminal tubercle of the bifid spinous process is common. However, as they are accessible they are palpated first. If a spinous process is not central, the articular pillar and interlaminar space are then palpated to assess if their position indicates any vertebral rotation or lateral flexion. With practice it is also possible to appreciate a small loss of the normal cervical lordosis, particularly between C2 and C5. Similarly, an abnormal closeness (which is a quite common finding) of the spinous process of C6 to C7 is readily palpable.

The articular pillar is also palpated laterally, and the transverse processes anterolaterally. The age of any soft-tissue thickening found can be assessed by virtue of the hardness or softness of its feel, and zygapophyseal joint exostoses can be clearly felt.

Gauging any anomaly of the position of the vertebra must be done by a correlation of the three findings. The first is the position of the spinous process, the second is the prominence and depression of opposite articular pillars for the same vertebra, and the third is confirmation by X-ray findings. Displacement laterally of a spinous process without any accompanying rotation of the vertebra is common.

The three most common reliable findings are:

1. Prominence of a spinous process associated with limited range of movement and pain.
2. Prominence of a level of the articular pillar.
3. An abnormal closeness of the spinous process of C6–7.

Exostoses associated with the zygapophyseal joints are easy to find. Assessing the relationship of the changes to the patient's disorder depends upon the quality of soft tissue around the joint and also the quality of pain that may be provoked by moving the joint during the palpation examination.

## PASSIVE ACCESSORY INTERVERTEBRAL MOVEMENTS (PAIVMs)

Movement is first assessed by moving quickly up and down the spine, performing two or three oscillations at each level with the tips of the thumbs against the spinous processes and articular pillar. In this way a general impression of comparative mobility can be determined

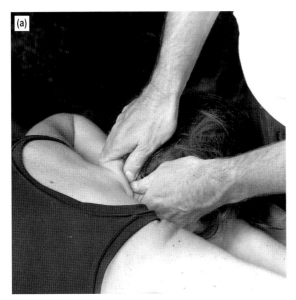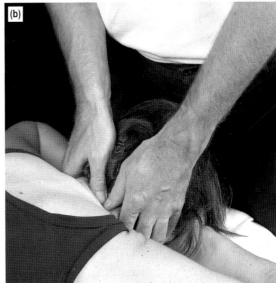

**Figure 10.41**    Unilateral postero-anterior movements. (*a*) Medially ⟋ (*b*) More laterally ⟋

Movement is assessed by using pressure through the tips of the thumbs against the spinous processes first. Two or three oscillatory postero-anterior movements are performed at each level in turn, moving fairly quickly up and down the spine, until a general impression of comparative movement in both quality and range is determined.

The movements created by pressure on the spinous processes can be assessed even more finely by varying the direction of the pressures, inclining them left, right, cephalad and caudad. Combinations of these inclinations can also be used (*see* pp. 157–161). Not only should the direction of the pressure be varied, but also the precise point of contact on the spinous process. This will produce a change in the movement occurring at the intervertebral joint. The same procedure is carried out over the articular pillar at each level, both medially and more laterally (*Figure 10.41*), comparing both the relative movement of adjacent levels, and also that found at one intervertebral level on the left with the movement at the same level on the right.

> Variations in inclination and point of contact will produce a change in the movement occurring at the intervertebral joint or zygapophyseal joint

Similar variations of direction and contact are applied to the articular pillar. However, one of the most useful test movements in the middle and upper cervical spine is achieved when thumb pressure is applied in a combined unilateral postero-anterior and medial direction. This direction of movement produces a maximum sliding of the zygapophyseal joint immediately under the thumbs. If this direction of movement is performed throughout its total range – that is, from maximum foraminal opening (lifting the neck posteriorly and laterally) to maximum foraminal closing – a very valuable assessment of flexibility and quality of movement at the zygapophyseal joint is readily obtained. The technique for the lifting component of this movement is facilitated by hooking the little finger under the patient's chin (*Figure 10.42b*). Also, by varying the hand and finger positions, these unilateral postero-anterior pressures can be performed in such a way as to produce a rotary movement or a lateral flexion movement.

The movement abnormalities that can be found are: limited range or hypomobility; resistance to movement through the range due to crepitus, stiffness or muscle spasm; and different qualities of end-feel.

In making determinations, it is important to point out that a hypomobile joint or a hypermobile joint is not necessarily a painful joint. Nevertheless, the quality of movement and range of movement must be appreciated before attempting to relate the abnormalities found to the possible cause of the patient's symptoms.

### Pain response

The next stage of the examination is the assessment of pain responses. The above stages of examination are

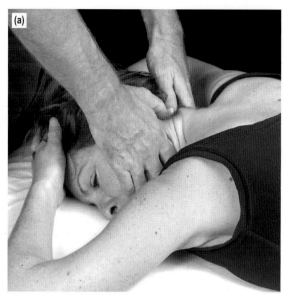 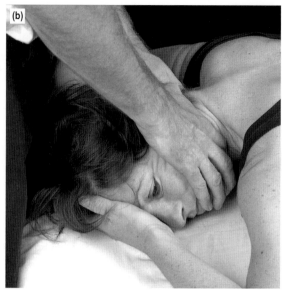

**Figure 10.42** Occipito-atlantal rotation. (*a*) Unilateral postero-anterior movements on the left of C2. (*b*) Hooked fingers increasing O/C2 rotation left

carried out without asking for any comments by the patient, and in fact it is wise to instruct the patient to make no comment about soreness, tenderness or pain until asked for later in the examination.

> In most cases, only after tissue thickening, bony prominences and quality and range of movement have been determined should the patient be asked about any pain response

Having made the determinations regarding tissue thickening, bony prominences, quality of movement and range of movement, it becomes necessary to relate the pain responses to these determinations. Not only is it necessary to know which movements either provoke the pain for which treatment is sought or produce local pain only, but it is also necessary to determine whether the sensations are felt to be superficial or deep. It may be necessary to apply firm pressure to obtain an accurate determination.

A stiff joint does not necessarily cause pain; it may be responsible for an associated joint becoming painful. The same applies to thickened tissues.

Having discussed the general examination procedure and the possible findings, it is now possible to discuss special palpation techniques and the abnormalities that can be found at each of the three sections of the cervical spine, and to indicate what these findings mean to the manipulative physiotherapist.

## UPPER CERVICAL SPINE

For the upper cervical spine, it is important to palpate deeply the soft tissue and the capsular area of each occipito-atlantal joint from posteromedially to laterally. It is possible to discern the degree of such thickening when it is present.

Postero-anterior pressures should be applied along the atlas from the midline to the tip of the transverse process. When the patient's head is fully turned to one side, postero-anterior pressure is applied to the articular process of the axis on the side to which the patient's head is turned. The fingers, hooked under his chin, can pull and apply opposite rotary movement of the occiput and atlas to that produced at C2 by the thumbs (*Figure 10.42*). Assessment of the quality and range of occipito-atlantal atlanto-axial rotation so produced can be assessed in this position and compared with that on the opposite side when the head is turned to the other side. The quality of this atlanto-axial movement throughout its range is fully assessed by positioning the head in different degrees of rotation before applying the thumb pressures (*see* p. 277).

With the patient's head still turned slightly to one side, transverse pressure can be applied to the transverse process of the atlas and a comparison made with the movement available on the opposite side (*see* pp. 283–284, *Figure 10.71*). These pressures can be varied in their directions from posterior through transverse to anterior pressure. While performing these movements, not only is it possible to assess the quality of the movement and its range, but it is also possible to assess the quality of the soft tissue immediately surrounding this area, which is frequently thickened unilaterally.

## Differentiation of symptoms arising from C2–3 or C1–2 apophyseal joints

There is another particularly important test procedure that is used when it is necessary to determine whether a patient's symptoms arise from a disorder of the C2–3 apophyseal joint or the C1–2 apophyseal joint. With the patient prone and the head in the neutral position, postero-anterior pressures are applied, for example, to the left articular pillar of C2 so as to move it in a postero-anterior direction. The quality and range of movement, and the accompanying pain response, are compared with the same features when the postero-anterior pressure is applied with the same strength to C2, but this time with the patient's head rotated approximately 30–40° to the left. If the pain response is greater with the head rotated than it is with the head straight, the disorder is at the C1–2 joint. If the pain response is greater with the head straight, then the disorder is at the C2–3 joint.

The common findings are as follows.

## Suboccipital area

### Soft-tissue changes

Two particularly important findings in the sub-occipital area are generalized thickening and tightening of the suboccipital structures overlying the atlas, and, even more particularly, lying between the atlas and occiput. It is more common for this tightness to lie in the medial two-thirds of the areas, but very occasionally it is felt to be in the lateral half only, and solely on one side.

The second common finding is marked thickening of the capsule and surrounding tissue of one or both atlanto-occipital joints. The thicker and harder the tissues are (as compared with being spongier), the older they are.

The relevance of the findings to the patient's symptoms depends upon two things. The first is the agreement between the chronicity of the history and symptoms of the disorder and the oldness of the tissue changes found on palpation examination. The second is the reproduction of the patient's referred pain or the provocation of a degree of deeply felt local pain compatible with the patient's symptoms when the tissues are palpated firmly.

### Bony anomalies

The common bony abnormalities of the atlas are that it is often felt to be slightly rotated or slightly displaced to one side in relation to the occiput. Before accepting, from the palpation findings, an interpretation of being displaced to one side, the radiological views should be assessed. This is because it is not uncommon for the transverse process of the atlas to be smaller on one side than the other.

To determine whether a positional abnormality is old or new, the X-rays must be viewed to see if bony adaptations to the changed position have taken place. If the positional abnormality is old, the bone will have slightly changed its shape to accommodate to the adopted position.

A palpable rotary anomaly is only of clinical relevance to the presenting symptoms if derotation by palpation provokes deep local pain or reproduces the patient's symptoms. This principle applies to any palpable anomaly. When very strong palpation pressures produce only a small degree of derotation and only local pain, the positional change is probably longstanding.

### Movement abnormalities

The most common movement finding that can be determined by palpation is a difference in the range of movement produced by postero-anterior pressure over the articular pillar at each level. Stiffness at one level should be compared with the other levels and the same level on the opposite side.

Movement abnormalities have more significance than do the more fixed positional changes. The easier it is to push into the stiff range and produce movement, the easier it will be to restore the range. However, it is important that the improvement in range must be accompanied by a concurrent improvement in the pain response during the movement.

## Atlanto-axial C2–3 areas

### Soft-tissue changes

Soft-tissue changes in the C1–2 laminar trough are less common than elsewhere, although it is not uncommon to find thickening of the soft tissue immediately adjacent to one side of the spinous process of the axis. For this finding to be pertinent to a patient's upper cervical symptoms, firm palpation must provoke deep local or referred pain. As mentioned above, the hardness or sponginess of the soft tissues guides the interpretation of the oldness or newness of the changes and their consequent reversibility.

Prominence and thickening around the articular pillar of the C2–3 apophyseal joint is a common finding, particularly in patients suffering from cervical headaches. It is possible to differentiate between 'old' and 'new' in relation to the soft tissue (as explained above), and to relate them to osteoarthritic (-osic) exostoses.

The comparability between the palpation findings and the patient's symptoms is assessed by relating:

1. The pain response while applying pressure.
2. The strength of the pressure required to provoke the pain response.
3. The oldness or newness of the tissue changes.

### Bony anomalies

Osteoarthritic (-osic) exostoses are readily palpable at the C2–3 apophyseal joint. Their relevance to a patient's symptoms is in part indicated by the sharpness of the margins of the exostoses. If they are not sharp or bony, being covered by other soft-tissue thickening, they are more likely to be related to presenting symptoms.

The absence or smallness of one of the processes of the bifid spinous process of the axis is common, as is deviation of the spinous process from the median sagittal plane. The only importance related to such findings when they exist alone is that:

- There must be a reason for the spinous process being shaped thus.
- It indicates the presence of an asymmetrical functional difference, of some kind, at this cervical level.

Such bony abnormalities do not of themselves cause symptoms, but they do indicate that the joint may be disadvantaged if subjected to an asymmetrical unguarded movement.

### Movement abnormalities

With a patient who suffers from cervical headaches, postero-anterior pressure on the spinous process of C2 inclined cephalad is frequently extremely painful locally deeply, and may reproduce the headaches.

It is surprisingly uncommon for the atlanto-axial joint to be limited in range when compared with the frequency of limitation of movement and poor quality of movement at C2–3.

Occurring concurrently with this poor C2–3 movement is the common finding of a prominent spinous process of C3, which is readily palpable.

The common pain response is one of local deep pain felt with movement of the C2–3 joint by pressure directed postero-anteriorly over the C3 spinous process and at the articular pillar.

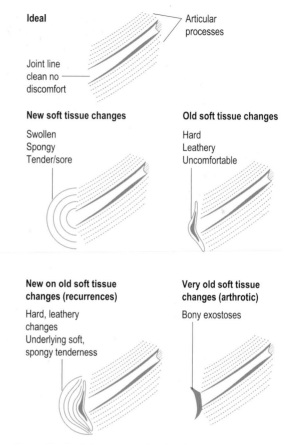

**Figure 10.43** Palpation examination. Soft tissue changes

If the postero-anterior movement applied over the articular pillar is directed medially, the common finding is a noticeable lack of range associated with marked discomfort and poor quality of movement through range (*Figure 10.44*).

Differentiating between pain arising from the C2–3 and the atlanto-axial joints has been described above.

### Indication of findings

It is important to determine, when palpating over the C2–3 apophyseal joint area, the quality of the tissues. Hard bony prominences, indicating osteoarthritic exostoses, are common. When these bony prominences are not covered by soft spongy tissue, the interpretation is that although they indicate osteoarthritic (-osic) changes in the apophyseal joint, the arthritic process is currently inactive and not a source of pain. However, when the tissue overlying the exostoses is thickened, the interpretation is quite different. The thickening varies between two extremes, from being like tough dry leather to being very soft and spongy.

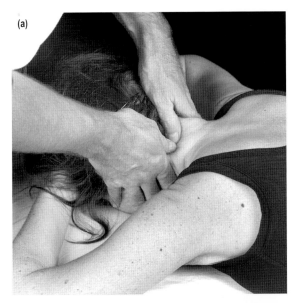

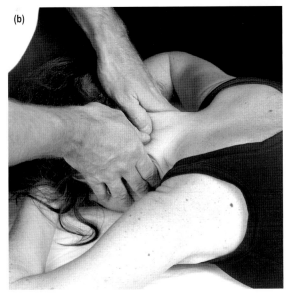

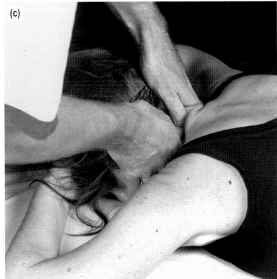

**Figure 10.44**    Unilateral pressure postero-anterior with medial inclination on C2, III. (*a*) Neutral starting position. (*b*) Fully lifted and open position. (*c*) Fully closed postero-anterior movement medially (⤛ C2, III)

The more leathery it is the less likely it is to be causing other than mild local symptoms, whereas the softer it is the more likely it is to be of recent origin and associated with recent symptoms (*Figure 10.43*).

In terms of treatment, the somewhat harder thickening demands firmer treatment. Also, manipulation may need to be introduced more quickly. The goal of treatment is to eliminate totally any soft spongy tissue changes, to lessen the thickness of the harder soft tissue or, under ideal circumstances, to eliminate the thickening, leaving 'clean' bony exostoses which are painless if pushed.

In relation to prominence of the spinous process of C3, the goal is to improve the quality of the movement in its postero-anterior direction, to decrease its prominence, and to eliminate any deep pain response that may accompany the movement.

## MID-CERVICAL SPINE

There are two special aspects of the palpation examination for this section of the spine. First, medially directed unilateral postero-anterior pressure is particularly relevant. The second is that postero-anterior pressures

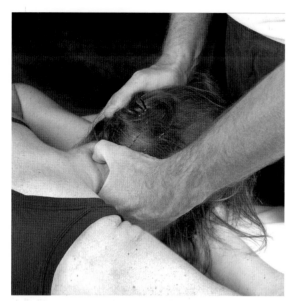

**Figure 10.45**   Palpation between spinous processes and bifid processes

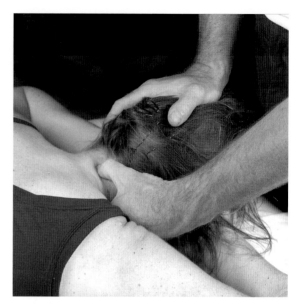

**Figure 10.46**   Medially directed palpation of posterior interspinous space

on the spinous processes need, at times, to be performed through their maximum range. This requires that when performing the postero-anterior movements the fingers should lift the patient's neck so that the movement begins from the maximum antero-posterior position (*Figure 10.44b*).

## Soft-tissue changes

The most common findings in this section of the cervical spine are thickening of soft tissue immediately adjacent to a spinous process or between adjacent spinous processes, and posterolaterally over the articular pillar. The technique for the interspinous palpation is as follows:

1. Palpation using the very tip of one thumb is carried out between adjacent spinous processes, first centrally (with ligamentum nuchae pushed out of the way) then between adjacent bifid processes (*Figure 10.45*).

2. Palpation is carried out between adjacent bifid processes but this time palpating medially against the lateral and posterolateral surfaces (*Figure 10.46*).

3. Following the side of the spinous process the palpation is still directed medially, changing more and more anteriorly until the muscles prevent interspinous contact (*Figure 10.47*).

4. The final step is to direct the palpating pressures medially, but now from beneath (anterior to) the muscle belly, and still into the interspinous area.

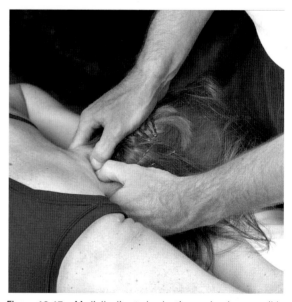

**Figure 10.47**   Medially directed palpation as deeply as possible

This palpation is then continued in the interlaminar trough area, continuing laterally to the articular pillar (*Figure 10.48*).

## Bony anomalies

The common bony anomalies that can be found are of two kinds. The first is a prominence of the spinous process of C3 (associated with headache symptoms), a

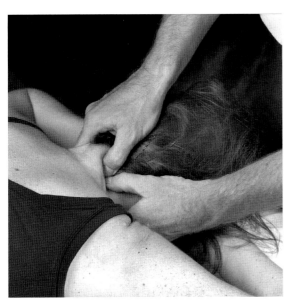

**Figure 10.48** Palpating anterior to the muscle belly for the interspinous and interlaminar space

depression of the spinous process of C3 accompanied by a prominence of the spinous process of C4 (usually related to mid-cervical pain) and, less commonly, a prominence of the spinous process of C5 (usually associated with mid- or lower-cervical symptoms).

The second common finding is the exostoses associated with arthritic change in the zygapophyseal joints. These may be felt over the articular pillar posteriorly or posterolaterally.

### Movement abnormalities

As has been mentioned above, the medially directed unilateral postero-anterior pressures are very valuable. Loss of range of movement and poor quality of zygapophyseal joint movement is readily discernible by this technique.

Large-amplitude postero-anterior pressures on the spinous processes when these are prominent readily shows up their relevance to a patient's symptoms by virtue of the range of movement available and the pain response felt when this movement is pushed to the limit of its range. Pain of two kinds will be provoked. The first and common one is a sharp pain, and the second is a deeply felt sensation.

## LOWER CERVICAL SPINE

There are no special aspects to the palpation examination of this section of the spine. However, the common findings are important.

### Soft-tissue changes

Soft-tissue changes that can be found in the laminar trough and over the articular pillar can readily be determined at the level of C5. If the patient is of a long, slender build, then it is equally easy to feel the changes at the C6 level and sometimes at C7. However, with the majority of people it becomes more difficult to differentiate the findings the further down the spine the palpation is carried. The soft-tissue changes that can be determined are the same as those described above for the middle cervical spine.

Soft-tissue thickening around the 'dowager's hump' is normal, yet it is of importance if the thickening is excessive and is abnormally painful with such techniques as skin rolling or connective tissue massage.

### Bony anomalies

Although the prominence of the spinous process of C5 has been described above, it is extremely difficult at times to determine whether it is the source of scapular or suprascapular symptoms. Most commonly the source is C6, while C7 is more common than is C5. The differentiating factors are first the extent of the bony anomalies, and secondly the pain response to postero-anterior movements. The bony anomaly that occurs most commonly is that the tip of the spinous process of C6 lies very close to that of C7. This leaves a larger gap between the spinous processes of C5 and C6, and gives a feeling of prominence of C5. The pain response is described below.

### Movement abnormalities

Associated with the closeness of the spinous process of C6–7 described above, the movement abnormality is that there is a distinct restriction of movement with postero-anterior pressure applied to the spinous process of C6. The pain response associated with this movement (and the movement may need to be applied quite firmly) is one of deeply felt pain (sometimes described by the patient as a 'nice hurt'). There may also be a spread of pain into the scapular area, or even a bilateral spread. When C7 is the source of the symptoms, the pain response is the same as that described for C6; when C5 is the source of symptoms, pressure on its spinous process, though still provoking a deeply felt pain, less frequently refers pain into the suprascapular area. Transverse pressures against the spinous process of C6 and C7, with varied inclinations, are also of great value in determining which level is the source of symptoms.

Postero-anterior pressures applied unilaterally over the articular pillar will frequently provoke a significant pain response, although relative movements at C6 and C7 are much harder to determine than is the same movement at C5. Nevertheless, they should form part of the examination procedure for symptoms arising from the lower cervical spine, despite the fact that more time is required to discern the findings at this level. It is sometimes necessary to apply these unilateral postero-anterior pressures through the muscle belly, while at other times clearer information is gained if the muscles are pushed out of the way so that the articular pillar, particularly that of C7, can be palpated directly.

## Pain response

Aspects that are of special significance for the lower cervical spine are:

1. The deep local pain referred to above.
2. The common reproduction of referred pain.
3. The clear association of the pain response when pressure is applied to the soft-tissue changes at the spinous processes and articular pillar.

## PASSIVE RANGE OF PHYSIOLOGICAL MOVEMENTS OF SINGLE INTERVERTEBRAL JOINTS (PPIVMs)

The following are the techniques used for assessing the ranges of flexion, extension, lateral flexion and rotation for each level of the cervical spine.

## Occipito–atlantal joint (lateral flexion)

### Starting position

In this examination, the patient lies supine with the crown of his head projecting beyond the end of the couch. Standing at the head of the couch, the physiotherapist cradles the patient's occiput in her left hand and grasps the forehead in her right hand with the fingers pointing towards the right and the thumb towards the left. While the tip of the left thumb is in a position to palpate deeply between the left transverse process of the first cervical vertebra and the adjacent mastoid process, the fingers reach beyond the midline to the right occipital area. Very slight pressure is then applied to the crown of the patient's head by the physiotherapist's abdomen to assist in steadying head movement during examination (*Figure 10.49*).

### Method

Although the patient's head must be laterally flexed to the right, the crown of the head is moved and not the neck. To do this, the physiotherapist's hands combine with a swaying movement of her pelvis to tilt the head. When the upper neck is fully stretched in lateral flexion, the position of the physiotherapist's left thumb, between the transverse process and the mastoid process, must be checked. Care must be taken when producing the lateral flexion movement to ensure that it is a 'head on neck' movement. It is so easy to be misled into performing lower cervical movement without any occipito-atlantal movement.

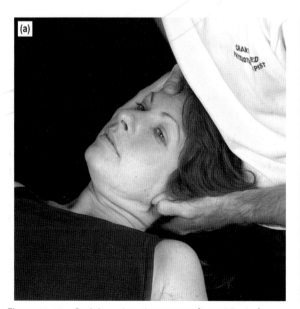
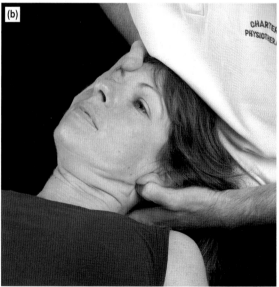

**Figure 10.49** Occipito-atlantal movement (lateral flexion)

As the head and neck are moved back and forth in the inner one-third (approximately 15°) of the lateral flexion range, the thumb can feel the opening and closing of the gap between the two bony points and the resulting changes in tension of the tissues.

## Occipito–atlantal joint (rotation)

The starting position is identical with that described for testing lateral flexion (*Figure 10.50*).

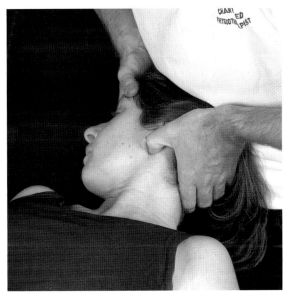

Figure 10.50 Occipito-atlantal movement (rotation)

*Method*

When the patient's head has been turned fully to the right, the position of the tip of the left thumb between the left mastoid process and the left transverse process of C1 must be checked. The patient's head is then rotated back and forth in the inner one-third of the range (approximately 20°) before maximum rotation is approached, when the transverse process is felt to draw nearer to the mastoid process. As the head is brought back towards midline, the transverse process moves away from the mastoid process.

## Occipito–atlantal joint (flexion/extension)

*Starting position*

There is a small amount of movement in the nodding movement of the head. To feel this, the patient lies supine with his head extending beyond the end of the couch. The physiotherapist cradles the patient's head in her lap, holding his occiput in both hands and placing the tips of her thumbs in contact with the tip of each lateral mass of C1 and the antero-inferior border of the mastoid process (*Figure 10.51*).

*Method*

The physiotherapist rocks the base of the patient's skull back and forth through approximately 20°, reproducing the nodding movement. The crown of the head remains comparatively still. With the tips of her

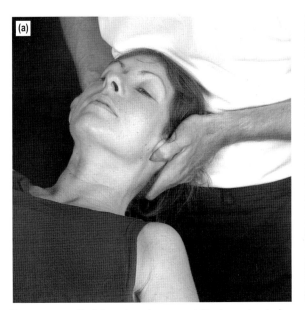

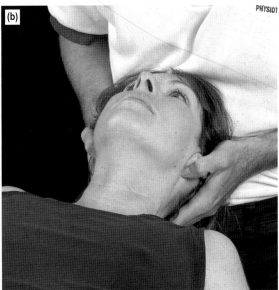

Figure 10.51 Occipito-atlantal movement (flexion-extension)

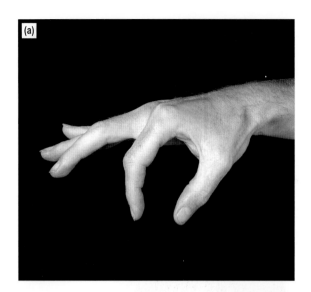

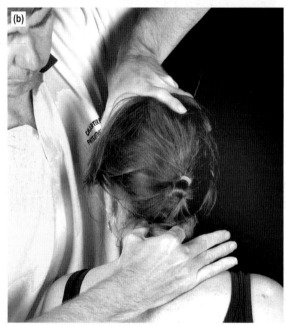

**Figure 10.52** (*a*) Pincer grip. (*b*) Atlanto-axial joint movement (rotation)

chair and the physiotherapist stands slightly behind the left shoulder. She places her left hand over the crown of his head, with the little finger and thumb spreading over the right and left parietal areas respectively and the remaining fingers spreading backwards over the occiput. The hand should be spread to the maximum so that, with her left forearm pointing vertically, the physiotherapist has full control of the patient's head. With her right hand she grasps the spinous process of C2 in a pincer grip (*Figure 10.52a*) between the tip of the index finger and thumb. The paravertebral muscles lie within the circle formed by the finger and thumb (*Figure 10.52b*).

*Method*

Having taken up the position prior to testing the rotary movement between C1 and C2, the physiotherapist should, with her left hand, perform small lateral flexion movements of the head on the neck through approximately 20° (10° to each side). As she tips the patient's head to the left, she should feel the spinous process of C2 move to the right. Similarly, as she laterally flexes his head to the right, she will feel the spinous process of C2 move to the left. By assessing this movement, she should stop at the point where the spinous process of C2 is in the midline. She then rotates the patient's head back and forth from the centre to the left up to the point where the spinous process is felt to move. The lamina of C2 on the left is felt to move backwards against her thumb, and the right lateral surface of this spinous process moves against the pad of her index finger. Once this point has been reached, the patient's head is held still and the range of movement assessed. Although the rotation to the right can be assessed by merely turning the patient's head the other way, it is far more accurate to change sides to repeat the technique to the right.

### C1–2 (rotation) supine

*Starting position*

The patient lies supine with his head extended beyond the end of the couch and cradled in the physiotherapist's right arm (for rotation to the right). With her left hand, she clasps the spinous process of C2 in much the same pincer grip as that in *Figure 10.52a* (*Figure 10.53*).

*Method*

Starting with the patient's head in the straight position, the physiotherapist slowly oscillates his head in rotation

thumbs, she assesses the small movement between the two bony points on each side.

### C1–2 (rotation) in sitting

*Starting position*

To examine the range of rotation to the left between the first and second cervical vertebrae, the patient sits in a

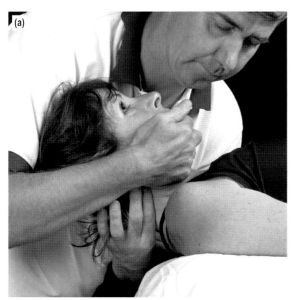 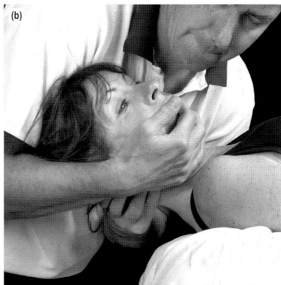

**Figure 10.53**    C1–2 rotation Ⓡ. (*a*) From the straight position. (*b*) Rotated right to where C2 starts to move

to the right while maintaining the grasp of C2's spinous process. By increasing the range of head movement with full range, the point when C2 starts to rotate can be felt through her right thumb and index finger, thereby enabling her to assess the range of C1–2 rotation.

## C2–7 (flexion)

### Starting position

The patient lies supine with his head beyond the end of the couch, while the physiotherapist crouches at the head end of the couch below the level of the patient. She holds the patient's occiput near the heel of her right hand, while the fingers and thumb point forwards over the crown of the head. Her left hand is then placed against the left side of the patient's neck, with the tip of the thumb between the sides of two spinous processes and the tip of the index and middle fingers reaching around the left sternomastoid muscle to the anterior surface of the cervical transverse processes. If movement is to be examined between C3 and C4, the thumb is placed laterally between the tips of the spinous processes of these vertebrae and the index and middle fingers are placed over the anterior surface of the left transverse process of C4 and C5 (*Figure 10.54*). If the ligamentum nuchae proves an obstacle to easy palpation, the tip of the thumb is moved a little away from the centre line to palpate adjacent spinous processes from the side. This palpation can also be

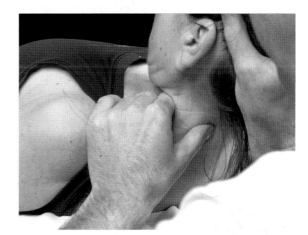

**Figure 10.54**    Intervertebral movement. C2–7 (flexion)

performed at the interlaminar area or at the zygapophyseal joint posteriorly.

### Method

The patient's head is passively flexed by the physiotherapist's right hand with a 'chin into chest' action, while with the tip of her left thumb she feels between the spinous processes for the amount of opening and closing that takes place as the head is moved backwards and forwards through a range of movement of

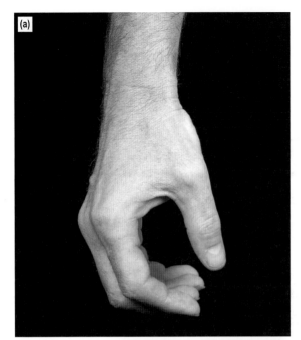

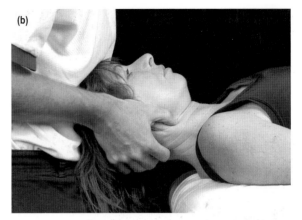

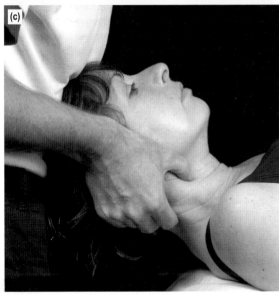

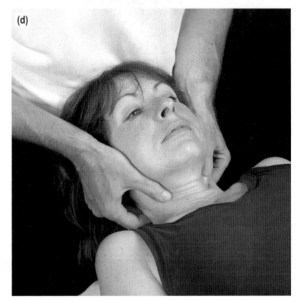

**Figure 10.55** Intervertebral movement. C2–7 (bilateral flexion and extension). (*a*) Pincer grip. (*b*), (*c*) and (*d*) Pincer grip applied at starting position

15–20°. To produce the maximum movement between C3 and C4, the fourth cervical vertebra and those below it are stabilized by pressure against the anterior surface of their left transverse processes. The position of the 20° arc of oscillation within the full range of forward flexion varies with the joint being examined; to examine movement between C6 and C7 the oscillation is performed near the limit of forward flexion range, whereas movement between C2 and C3 must be sought in the first part of the range. Care must be exercised to ensure that

movement is produced at the level being tested, and that the movement is the maximum available.

## C2–7 (bilateral flexion extension)

This is a useful technique because, with the pincer grip on each side of the neck at the one intervertebral level, small variations from the normal range of movement can be finely appreciated.

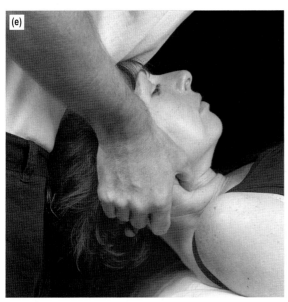

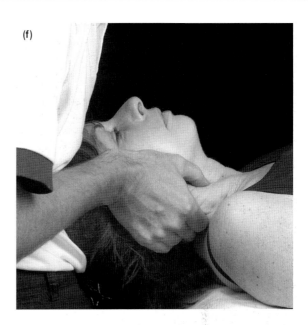

**Figure 10.55** (*contd*) (*e*) Flexion. (*f*) Extension

## Starting position

The patient lies supine with his head extending beyond the end of the couch and supported in the physiotherapist's lap. With the pincer grip (*Figure 10.55a*) she grasps between adjacent transverse processes with her thumb tip medial to the sternomastoid anteriorly, and the tip of her index finger at the same intervertebral level on the articular pillar posteriorly.

## Method

The physiotherapist raises and lowers the height of her lap (by extending and flexing her knees) and thereby flexes and extends the patient's head and thus the neck, producing movement down to (and not beyond) the level of her pincer grip. In this way she can feel the range of movement available.

## C2–7 (lateral flexion, closing)

### Starting position

The patient lies supine with his head resting on the table on a pillow or in the physiotherapist's lap – preferably the latter. The position chosen should facilitate relaxation, and support the head and neck midway between flexion and extension for the joint being examined. In this position, both lateral flexion and rotation are freest.

The physiotherapist places the tip of her index finger into the interlaminar space deeply enough to palpate adjacent laminae. With both hands, particularly the

non-palpating hand, she gives support under his occiput. When the lower cervical movements are tested, this support extends under his neck (*Figure 10.56*).

## Method

Being careful to ensure that intervertebral movement can be felt, and not just the head on the neck, the physiotherapist first laterally flexes the joint fractionally away from her palpating finger then performs the lateral flexion towards her palpating finger and assesses the movement at the interlaminar space. The opposite movement is then performed to assess the closing capacity of the space. By this means the excursion of lateral flexion at that level on that side can clearly be evaluated. The palpating fingertip must remain motionless in the space; thus care must be exercised when that hand is used to produce the lateral flexion of the neck.

## C2–7 (lateral flexion, opening)

### Starting position

This is the same as for the 'closing' test position (*Figure 10.57*).

### Method

With the patient's head cradled in the physiotherapist's lap, she pivots her body (especially her pelvis) on her feet to produce the head and head–neck movement.

Irrespective of the intervertebral level being assessed, the movement starts as a movement of the head, which

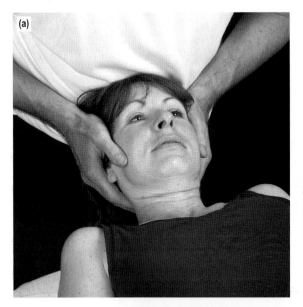

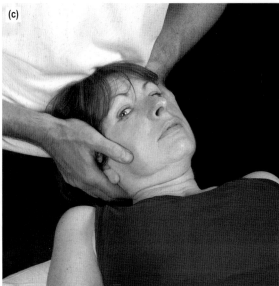

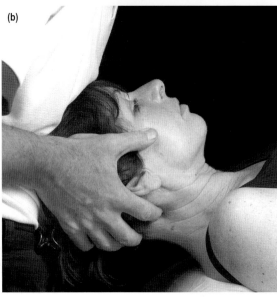

**Figure 10.56** Intervertebral movement. C2–7 (lateral flexion right, closing right side). (*a*) Starting position, slight lateral flexion to left. (*b*) The palpating finger for C2–3 at the starting position. (*c*) oscillating lateral flexion right assessing closing. C2–3 at the closing position

is then continued down to movement of the neck at the level being assessed.

## C2–7 (rotation)

### Starting position

The 'starting position' is identical with that described for lateral flexion, except for the palpating finger. This is carried a fraction laterally, and a slightly broader contact is made. The tip and adjacent lateral margin of

the index finger palpate the margin of the zygapophyseal joint (*Figure 10.58*).

### Method

The head is pivoted, away from the side of palpation, around an imaginary central axis passing through the joint being tested. The physiotherapist's hands produce the movement in a steady oscillatory fashion, giving movement down to the joint but not beyond it.

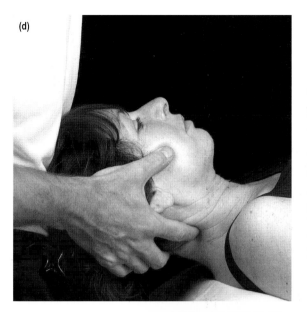

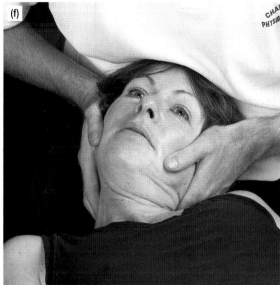

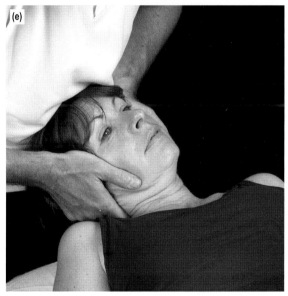

**Figure 10.56** (*contd*) (*d*) C5–6 at the starting position. (*e*) C5–6 at the closing position. (*f*) C5–6 at the opening position

Her palpating finger follows the movement of the joint, assessing the extent of sliding or opening between the two adjacent articular processes. It is not possible to assess the rotation towards the palpating finger, because the muscles obstruct the palpation.

## Occiput–C7 (extension)

### Starting position

The patient lies supine with his head resting on the couch or in the physiotherapist's lap. The physiotherapist stands near his head, supporting under the patient's head and neck down to the level of the joint being tested. She places the tip of both index fingers into the interlaminar space on each side, as described above for lateral flexion (*Figure 10.59*).

### Method

The physiotherapist extends the patient's head and neck down to the level being examined, by lifting under his neck. At the same time, she palpates for closing down of the interlaminar space with her fingertips.

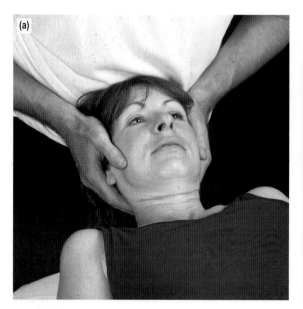

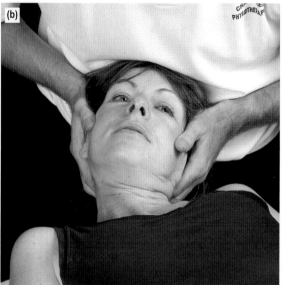

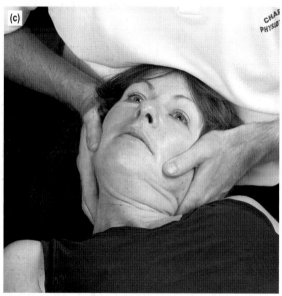

**Figure 10.57** Intervertebral movement C2–7 (lateral flexion, left, opening right side). (*a*) Starting position, head straight and cradled in hands and lap. First movement is small lateral flexion to the right. (*b*) Slow oscillatory lateral flexion to left, palpating movement on right. Appropriate end of range for C2–3 and C3–4. (*c*) Appropriate end of range for C4–5, C5–6 and C6

## EXAMINATION AND TREATMENT TECHNIQUES

Any examination procedure can be used as a treatment technique, and some such techniques have been described on pages 239–271. The techniques that are now described are also used as examination procedures, especially those techniques involving palpation.

## MOBILIZATION

### Longitudinal movement ←•→

*Starting position*

The patient lies supine with his neck level with the end of the couch. His head, supported in the physiotherapist's hands, rests with the joint being treated in a neutral position, approximately midway between full

(d)

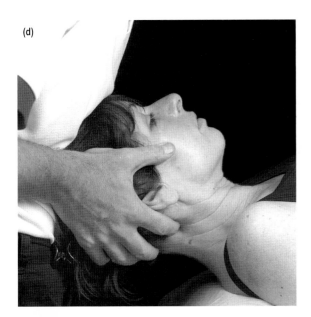

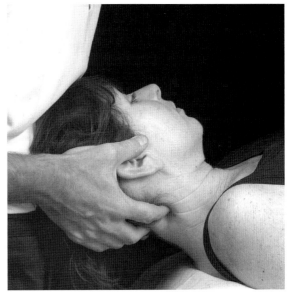

Figure 10.58    Intervertebral movement. C2–7 (rotation)

(e)

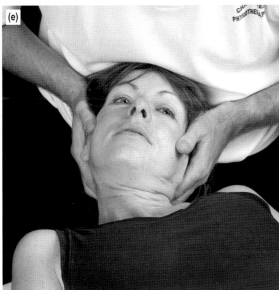

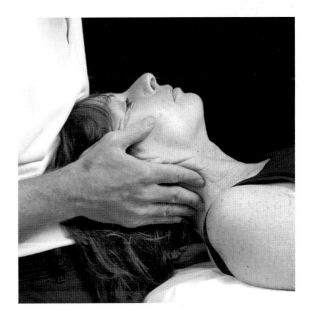

Figure 10.57    (contd) (d) Index fingertip palpating for movement at C2–3; starting position head straight. (e) Index fingertip palpating for movement at C2–3. End of range

Figure 10.59    Intervertebral movement. Occiput–C7 (extension)

flexion and full extension (or as near to it as pain permits).

The physiotherapist stands at the head of the couch with the back of the patient's head cradled in her right hand so that the fingers are spread over the left side of the patient's occiput to behind the left ear, while the thumb is placed behind the right ear. The palm of the right hand is so positioned that the palmar surface of the metacarpophalangeal joint of the index finger lies over the superior nuchal line. This then gives a good grasp of the occipital area of the head. If the lower cervical spine is the only section requiring mobilization, the right hand grasps around the neck immediately above the level being treated. The physiotherapist comfortably grasps the patient's chin with her left hand from the left side, being careful to avoid any

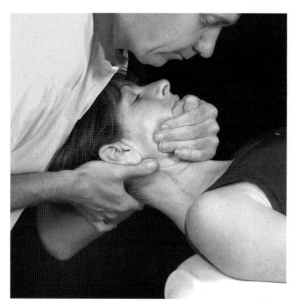

**Figure 10.60**   Longitudinal movement (◄─►)

pressure on the throat. The left forearm lies along the left side of the patient's face.

The physiotherapist, with her feet in a position as if walking and her arms flexed at the elbows, crouches over the patient's head to hold the crown of his head against the front of her left shoulder (*Figure 10.60*).

## Method

The oscillatory movement, elongating the patient's neck, is produced at the intervertebral joints by a gentle longitudinal pulling through the physiotherapist's forearms combined with a slight backward movement of her body, followed by an equally controlled relaxation to the starting position. This is repeated continuously to produce the oscillation.

As the technique is gentle, friction between the patient and couch is sufficient to prevent any sliding of the patient's body.

## Local variations

When this technique is used in treatment of the lowest cervical intervertebral levels, the neck should be positioned in approximately 30° of flexion. Mid-cervical treatment requires a neck position approximately in line with the body. For upper cervical problems, it is the head–neck relationship rather than the angle of the neck that is important. Again, the position must be midway between flexion and extension.

## Precautions

Pain can be produced in the mid-thoracic spine, but this only occurs if the pull is strong or if it is carried out with the spine in too much extension. This over-extended position must be avoided if the patient has an abnormal kyphosis, and consideration must be given to these factors when positioning the patient. A strong pull can irritate an existing thoracic condition, and may in fact cause thoracic pain in a previously pain-free area.

## Uses

This procedure is of particular value in gaining the confidence of the patient. By the assessment of the patient's symptoms and signs afterwards, it can serve as a useful guide as to whether or not it will be easy to relieve the symptoms. Those patients whose symptoms or signs improve markedly with this procedure are likely to respond easily and quickly. It will effect initial improvement in a neck exhibiting a protective deformity such as a wry neck, when the technique should be performed initially in line with the deformity for best effects.

Examples of treatment include pain simulating migraine, page 424; cervical joint locking, page 428; and shooting occipital pain, page 429.

## Postero–anterior central vertebral pressure ↕

### Starting position

The patient lies face downwards. It is usually satisfactory for him to rest his forehead in the palms of his hands, but it may be necessary for the chin to be tucked well in. This is particularly necessary for mobilization of the first and third cervical vertebrae because of their relative inaccessibility. When a patient has a limited range of extension or the movement is painful, an alternative starting position is for him to cradle his forehead in his palms with the arms partially under the chest.

The physiotherapist stands at the head of the patient with her thumbs held in opposition and back to back, with the tips of the thumb pads on the spinous process of the vertebra to be mobilized. The fingers straddle the sides of the patient's neck and head. Balance and steadiness of the physiotherapist's thumbs are gained through the finger position, but it is unnecessary for the fingers to grip firmly.

If too much of the pad is used, the localizing ability will be lost because the spinous processes are so small. However, with strong pressure the bone-to-bone contact may be uncomfortable, and it is then advisable to use more of the pad of the thumb near the tip.

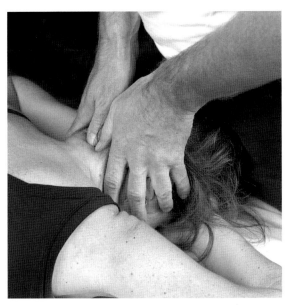

**Figure 10.61**   Posterior–anterior vertebral pressure (↕)

The best position is to have the thumbs in contact with each other on the tip of the same spinous process. A method using one thumb to reinforce the other can be used, but this tends to make a very gentle technique difficult to achieve and certainly detracts from the ability to feel small movements. In the case of the second cervical vertebra, the thumbs can be placed on the upper and lower margins of its spinous process (*Figure 10.61*).

### Method

Extremely gentle pressure will produce a definite feeling of movement, but the tendency always is to use too much pressure.

The alternating pressure should be applied by the arms combined with the trunk. It is impossible to carry out the technique successfully or comfortably by the action of the intrinsic hand muscles. If the patient has considerable pain, thus making this technique difficult to perform, the palmar surfaces of the pads of the fingers can be used to lift the neck into a degree of flexion. This will make the technique possible in a pain-free range.

### Local variations

The degree of pressure required to feel movement in the mid-cervical area is much less than that required at either the second or the seventh cervical vertebra. The first cervical vertebra can rarely be palpated in the midline as a bony surface; however, it is possible to produce movement by pressure through the overlying

muscles and ligaments. The third cervical vertebra is often difficult to palpate owing to the large and sometimes overhanging spinous process of the second cervical vertebra. Palpation of the two vertebrae is enhanced by asking the patient to tuck his head into slightly more flexion.

As was mentioned in Chapter 6 (*see* pp. 157–159), the direction of the central pressure can be angled towards the head or towards the feet. Such changes in direction may be required due to pain or stiffness found with these movements.

The thumbs do not always have to transmit the pressure via their tips, nor do the metacarpophalangeal joints always have to be close to each other. For example, more of the pad of the thumb other than the tip can be the contact point on each of the bifid spinous processes (*Figure 10.62a*). This is achieved by widely separating the metacarpophalangeal joints.

The pressure producing the movement may be delivered through more of the pad of just one thumb while the other thumb stabilizes its position on either the one bifid process, or more broadly across the central line to transmit the pressure through both bifid processes (*Figure 10.62b*).

### Postero-anterior central vertebral pressure as a 'combined' technique

The following description is presented as an example of postero-anterior movement performed with the spinous process mobilized with the joint in a position of combined lateral flexion to the right with extension.

### Starting position

The patient lies prone and the physiotherapist positions his head (and thus the intervertebral level to be mobilized) in the degree of lateral flexion and extension required. She then places the tips of her thumb pads on the spinous process (*Figure 10.63*).

### Method

The oscillatory postero-anterior pressure is applied to the spinous process in the same manner as has been described above.

### Precautions

Mobilizing in the region of the first and second cervical vertebrae, if very excessive both with regard to the length of time and the strength of the pressure, can produce a feeling of nausea. The technique must never be used if it causes giddiness.

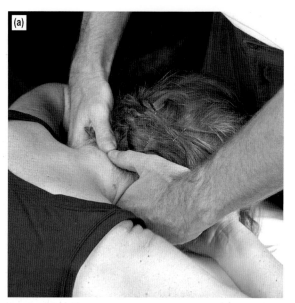
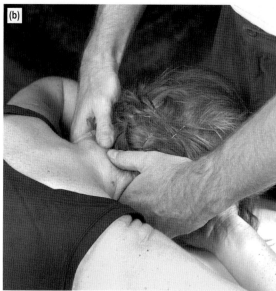

**Figure 10.62** Postero-anterior central vertebral pressure. (*a*) Increased area of thumb contact. (*b*) Using one thumb to transmit the pressure while the other thumb stabilizes its position

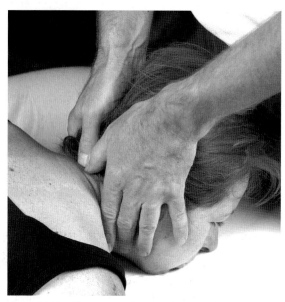

**Figure 10.63** Postero-anterior central vertebral pressure with the patient's head and neck in the combined position of lateral flexion to the right with extension

## Uses

Such a technique would probably be used mainly as a grade IV technique to clear the remaining joint movement signs. However, there is no reason why it cannot be used either as a very gentle grade IV when the movement is painful, or as a grade II when treating pain.

Postero-anterior central vertebral pressure is of most benefit to those patients whose symptoms of cervical origin are situated either in the midline or distributed evenly to each side of the head, neck, arms or upper trunk.

This technique is valuable for patients who have considerable bony degenerative changes in the cervical spine, irrespective of the area to which the pain of cervical origin is referred. While carrying out this procedure on these patients, however, the degree of movement felt is noticeably less than that felt in the normal cervical spine.

The technique is of particular value when pressure over the vertebrae produces even small amounts of muscle spasm. Under these circumstances, the pressure used and the depth of mobilization produced should be just less than that which causes spasm. After using this technique, it will be noticed that a greater depth of pressure can be applied before spasm reappears.

When the C2–3 level is the source of headaches, C3 will be found to be both prominent (that is, easily palpated) and proportionally painful. C4 and C5 are common levels to give rise to midcervical symptoms, and they too are usually prominent and painful at this time.

C6, when it is the source of pain in the upper thoracic or scapular area, is usually found to have its spinous process close to C7, with much thickening filling the interspinous space. Firm mobilization of C6 will cause pain, which is felt to be very deeply situated.

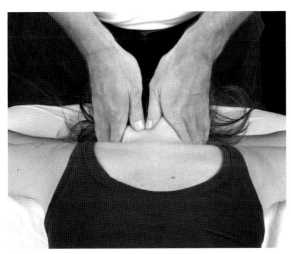

**Figure 10.64**  *Postero-anterior unilateral vertebral pressure*
($\overset{\bullet}{\underset{\downarrow}{\mathsf{\Gamma}}}$ )

Examples of treatment include pain simulating migraine, page 424; and shooting occipital pain, page 429.

## Postero–anterior unilateral vertebral pressure $\overset{\bullet}{\underset{\downarrow}{\mathsf{\Gamma}}}$

### Starting position

The patient lies prone with his forehead resting comfortably on his hands. The physiotherapist stands towards the side of the patient's head. She places the tips of her thumb pads, held back to back and in opposition, on the posterior surface of the articular process to be mobilized. Her arms should be directed 30° medially to prevent the thumbs from slipping off the articular process. The fingers of the uppermost hand rest across the back of the patient's neck and those of the other hand rest around the patient's neck towards his throat. Most of the contact is felt with the underneath thumb (*Figure 10.64*).

### Method

Oscillatory pressure directed postero-anteriorly against an articular process if done very gently will produce a feeling of movement, but to prevent any lateral sliding at the point of contact a gentle constant pressure directed medially must be maintained. If the movement is produced correctly, there will be small nodding movements of the head but no rotary or lateral flexion movement.

As with other techniques involving pressure through the thumbs, this movement must not be produced by intrinsic muscle action.

### Local variations

When mobilizing the first cervical vertebra, the physiotherapist needs to lean over the patient's head so as to direct the line of her thumbs towards the patient's eye. In the lower cervical area, the line is directed more caudally.

The second, third and fourth articular processes are far easier to feel accurately than are the remainder. The first cervical vertebra can be felt laterally, and the lower articular processes can be felt if the thumbs are brought in under the lateral border of the trapezius.

The symbol $\overset{\bullet}{\underset{\downarrow}{\mathsf{\Gamma}}}$ indicates that the unilateral pressure on the vertebra is directly postero-anterior. There are two common variations to this direction that are used in treatment. Under circumstances where pain is quite severe, the direction is angled slightly away from postero-anterior as indicated by the symbol $\overset{\bullet}{\underset{\downarrow}{\mathsf{\Gamma}}}$. The second variation, used when the joint is still and pain is minimal, is to angle the pressure more medially, endeavouring to increase the range. The angle is indicated by the symbol $\leftrightarrow$, and the technique is described on pages 257–258; it is a very important examination procedure, especially for the upper cervical spine.

Also, as was mentioned in Chapter 6, these directions can be varied still further by inclining them cephalad and caudad as indicated by the requirements of pain or stiffness.

### Precautions

The only precaution is to perform the techniques very gently, especially in the upper cervical region. It is seldom realized how effective these techniques can be while still being performed very gently.

### Uses

Application of this technique is the same as for the previous technique, except that it is used for unilateral symptoms on the side of the pain. The medially directed technique is an especially important technique for upper cervical disorders, particularly when aimed at restoring a full range of pain-free movements to prevent or lessen recurrences.

## Postero–anterior unilateral vertebral pressure $\overset{\bullet}{\underset{\downarrow}{\mathsf{\Gamma}}}$ C2, and $\overset{\bullet}{\underset{\downarrow}{\mathsf{\Gamma}}}$ C2 in 30° rotation Ⓛ

When postero-anterior unilateral vertebral pressure is applied to C2 with the patient's head straight, it is the C2–3 joint that is being examined or mobilized when pain is a dominant feature. If, however, the patient's

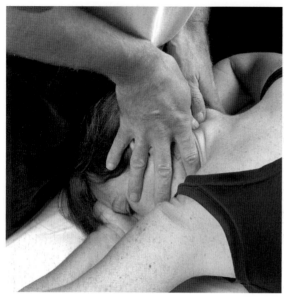

**Figure 10.65** Testing for abnormalities of C1–2 rotation on the left side (↓ ⌐• C2, and ↓ ⌐• C2 in 30° Rotn Ⓛ)

head is turned 30° to the left and the postero-anterior unilateral vertebral pressure is applied to the left side of C2, it is C1–2 rotation that is being examined or mobilized. This is because when the prone patient turns his head to the left C1 is rotated to the left on C2, and postero-anterior pressure on the left articular pillar of C2 further increases this rotation.

When the range of C1–2 is being examined by this procedure, the patient fully rotates his head to the side, thus putting C1–2 on maximum rotary stretch. Further stretch is then added by applying postero-anterior pressure unilaterally on the articular pillar of C2 on the same side as that to which the head is turned (*Figure 10.42*) in cervical palpation examination.

### Starting position

The patient lies prone with his head turned approximately 30° to the left and places his forehead in his palms. The physiotherapist stands at his head and places the tips of both thumb pads, their nails back to back, against the articular pillar of C2 on the left. The articular pillar is found in relation to the spinous process of C2, which will be unchanged from the position it held when the head was straight, and the left lateral mass of C1. Her fingers are spread to each side to stabilize the hands. She holds her thumbs in opposition and directs the long axis of each thumb in a postero-anterior direction and inclined slightly towards the head (*Figure 10.65*).

### Method

The movement is produced by a trunk and arm action transmitted to the thumbs, which act as springs. Although the mobilization is created by a postero-anterior pressure against C2, it is in fact increasing the rotation between C1 and C2.

### Uses

This technique is of value for suboccipital symptoms or headaches arising from the C1–2 joint. It is usually performed on the side of the pain or restriction.

## Bilateral postero–anterior vertebral pressure ↓ ⌐ ↓

### Starting position

The patient lies prone with his forehead in his palms. The physiotherapist wraps her hands, and in particular her thumbs, index fingers and the web between them, comfortably around the patient's neck. The grasp must be comfortable, with the pads of the thumbs reaching the articular pillar and the pads of the fingers reaching as far anteriorly as the transverse processes (*Figure 10.66*).

### Method

The oscillatory movement is produced through the physiotherapist's arms and body, while her hands are kept stable with an evenly distributed pressure around the patient's neck. It is important that the neck and hands move as a single unit.

The technique can be made to be of large amplitude by lifting the patient's neck with the pads of the fingers. It is a particularly comfortable and comforting technique, and is especially useful when more direct contact with the bony parts is very painful, yet movement of large amplitude is desired for the treatment.

## Anteroposterior unilateral vertebral pressure ⌐• ↓

### Starting position

The patient lies supine. A pillow is not used unless the patient has a 'poking-chin' postural abnormality. The physiotherapist stands by his head and makes a broad contact medial to the transverse process of the vertebra to be mobilized with both thumbs. The thumbs should be used with care, as direct bone-to-bone contact can be uncomfortable. She spreads her fingers around the adjacent neck area for stability while positioning her shoulders above the joint being treated (*Figure 10.67a*).

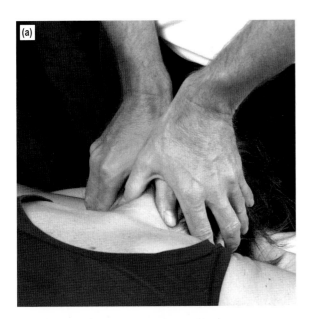

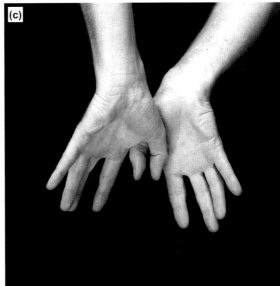

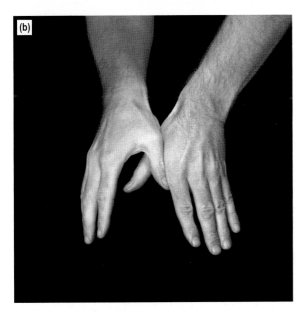

Figure 10.66    (*a*) Bilateral postero-anterior vertebral pressure ( ⌐•⌐ ). (*b*) Hands position. (*c*) Hands position reversed

## Method

The oscillatory anteroposterior pressures are performed very gently, and the movement must be produced by the physiotherapist's arms and trunk. Any effort to produce the movement with intrinsic thenar muscle action will produce discomfort immediately.

This technique is not a comfortable one to use unless great care is taken. Also, the muscles lying over the area make direct contact rather difficult, and care should be taken to see that the thumbs are positioned medial to the transverse process. This means that at some levels the muscle belly needs to be moved to one side.

## Local variations

This technique can be performed either unilaterally or bilaterally, as is shown in the diagrams (*Figure 10.67a* and *10.67b*). The intervertebral level to which one can

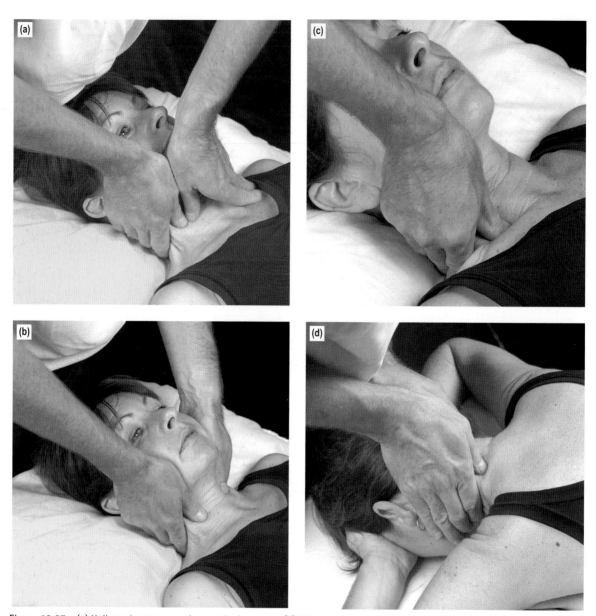

**Figure 10.67** (*a*) Unilateral anteroposterior vertebral pressure. (*b*) Bilateral anteroposterior vertebral pressure. (*c*) Anteroposterior unilateral vertebral pressure in upper thoracic area. (*d*) Anteroposterior unilateral vertebral pressure

reach varies enormously from patient to patient. In the stocky, heavily built patient with a short, thick neck, extending down into the thoracic area is almost impossible. Conversely, in the long-necked, slim person enough space is allowed to reach down to approximately T3 (*Figure 10.67c*). With all patients, the technique can be used as high as C1.

Anteroposterior movement can be produced with the patient lying prone. The patient rests his forehead in his palms, and the physiotherapist grasps around the sides of the neck to hook the palmar surface of the pads of her fingers medial to the transverse process area. It is easy to localize the joint to be mobilized by the accurate placement of the fingers (*Figure 10.67d*).

## Precautions

The only precaution necessary is to avoid discomfort from undue pressure.

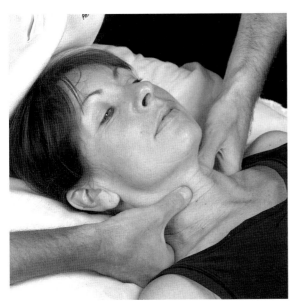

**Figure 10.68** Transverse cricothyroid pressure to the right

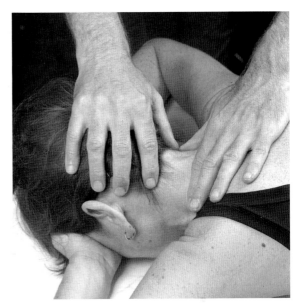

**Figure 10.69** Transverse vertebral pressure (←•—)

## Uses

Application of this technique is reserved for patients whose symptoms, felt anterolaterally, can be reproduced by anteroposterior pressure on the side of the pain. Pain referred to the ear or throat can often be reproduced by this technique. Anterior shoulder pain, scapula pain (Cloward, 1959) and headache associated with irritation of the stellate ganglia of the sympathetic chain may be reproduced by this technique also. Under all these circumstances, the described technique could be the treatment of choice.

## Cricothyroid

Palpation techniques for these non-synovial joints is included here because patients can have throat symptoms that may have a musculoskeletal component either from the vertebral column (particularly C3) or from the cricothyroid articulation.

### Starting position

The patient lies supine with his head resting in the flat position, without a pillow, on the couch. The physiotherapist places her thumb pad at the junction of the cricoid and thyroid cartilages (*Figure 10.68*).

### Method

Movement can be produced in any direction, but in the figure a transverse oscillatory movement towards the right is produced through the pad of the thumb near its tip.

## Transverse vertebral pressure ←•—

### Starting position

The patient lies face downwards with his forehead resting on the backs of his fingers or palms, with a moderate degree of 'chin-in' position to lessen the cervical lordosis slightly.

The physiotherapist stands at the patient's right side with her hands placed over the patient's neck, so that the distal part of the pad of the left thumb is against the right side of the spinous process, with the right thumb giving a reinforcing pressure against the left thumbnail. The fingers of each hand are spread out over the adjacent bony surfaces to provide stability for the thumbs. The part of the thumb in contact with the lateral surface of the spinous process should consist of as much of the pad of the thumb near its tip as it is possible to use; using the hard tip of the thumb causes too much discomfort to the patient and should be avoided. It is essential that the physiotherapist's wrists be in a position to allow for a horizontally directed pressure to be imparted to the spinous process through the thumbs (*Figure 10.69*).

### Method

Only very gentle pressure should be used here, because movement is produced very easily. For the same reason, the amplitude of the oscillations should also be very small. It is necessary, therefore, to judge the direction and pressure finely if a feeling of movement is to be gained.

### Local variations

When applying pressure in this position there is a moderate degree of natural tenderness, which must be considered. This makes it necessary to use as much of the thumb pad as possible to produce the movement without jeopardizing the ability to localize the pressure to the one spinous process.

The second and the seventh cervical vertebrae are the most easily palpated. However, although the lateral surface of the seventh cervical spinous process is superficial, to reach the lateral surface of the second cervical spinous process it is sometimes necessary to get under the paravertebral muscles. The spinous processes of the third to the sixth cervical vertebrae are much smaller, but can be reached by reducing the cervical lordosis with a slightly increased chin-in position of the patient's head. It is sometimes necessary to use each thumb against the same side of adjacent spinous processes to gain sufficient feeling of movement.

### Uses

As with the postero-anterior central vertebral pressure, transverse vertebral pressure is of most value in cases where the cervical spine shows marked degenerative radiological changes. Its greatest application is with unilateral symptoms of cervical origin. This is particularly so if the symptoms do not extend very far from the vertebrae or are ill-defined in their area of distribution when no neurological changes are evident.

When this technique is used for treating pain that is felt unilaterally, it is more likely to produce an improvement if the direction of the pressure is performed from the non-painful side towards the painful side.

### Variations

There are two variations of 'transverse vertebral pressure' that can be used effectively. Both involve pressure at the most lateral aspect of the vertebrae. The first description is for the method applied to the second to the sixth cervical vertebrae, and the second is for the first cervical vertebra.

### Alternative transverse vertebral pressure C2–6 ←•—

### Starting position

With the patient lying prone and his forehead resting on the backs of his fingers or palms, the physiotherapist stands to the patient's right and places the pad of the left thumb against the lateral border of the

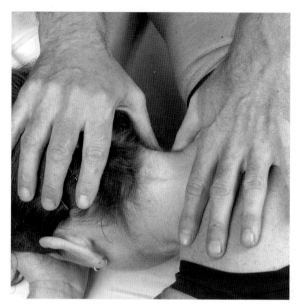

**Figure 10.70**   Alternative transverse vertebral pressure (C2–6 ←•—)

zygapophyseal joint while the pad of the right thumb reinforces the left thumbnail. The fingers of each hand spread out over the left side of the patient's neck on to the head and thorax respectively (*Figure 10.70*).

### Method

With this technique, the supporting fingers are used to apply a lateral flexion movement of the neck around the fulcrum of the thumbs.

The oscillating movement is produced through the thumbs, with the fingers either acting as stabilizers or supplying a counter-pressure by laterally flexing the neck. This counter-pressure is produced by adduction of both glenohumeral joints and ulnar flexion of both wrists. It is poor technique to attempt to produce this counter-pressure by finger flexion. Also, the thumb flexors must not be used as prime movers.

### Local variations

This technique can only be used from the second to the sixth cervical vertebrae, and any sense of movement that can be felt is more general than that felt with the former method.

### Uses

These are the same as for the former method.

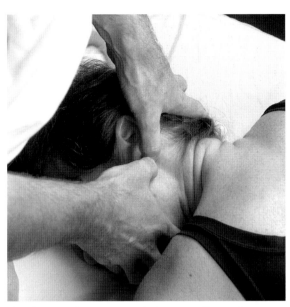

Figure 10.71  Transverse vertebral pressure (C1 →→ )

## Transverse vertebral pressure C1 →→

### Starting position

The patient lies prone with his head turned comfortably to the left. The physiotherapist stands facing the patient's head and places the tip of her left thumb over the tip of the left transverse process of the first cervical vertebra. The tip of the transverse process is found situated deeply between the angle of the mandible and the mastoid process just distal and anterior to the mastoid process. The right thumb points towards the crown of the head, and is placed tip to tip with the left thumb over C1. The fingers of each hand are spread out over the adjacent surface of the crown of the head and back of the neck to stabilize the action of the thumbs (*Figure 10.71*).

### Method

As with the previous mobilizations, the pressure must be transmitted through the body and arms to the thumbs and not by thumb movement only.

The bony prominence is sometimes very difficult to find and it is normally a particularly sensitive area, which sometimes prevents any deep pressure. The sense of movement with mobilization in this area is very small, and frequently it is impossible to feel any movement at all because of stiffness in the joint.

### Uses

It is used for symptoms about the head or upper neck that arise from this level of the cervical spine, whether

they are distributed evenly to both sides or unilaterally. If the symptoms are unilateral, the technique should, as the first choice, be carried out on the non-painful side. This avoids tenderness from the technique, which can confuse the assessment of its effect. If the symptoms are bilateral, the mobilization should be performed on both sides.

## Rotation ↺

### Starting position

The position described is for a 'rotation' to the left. This particular starting position is chosen because it is the most suitable position for learning feel, and because it is the starting position for the manipulative technique described later (*see* pp. 296–297).

The patient lies on his back so that his head and neck extend beyond the end of the couch. The physiotherapist stands at the head of the couch and places her right hand under the patient's head and upper neck, with the fingers spread out over the left side of the occiput and adjacent neck. The thumb extends along the right side of the neck, with the thenar eminence over the right side of the occiput. She grasps the chin with the fingers of her left hand, while the palm of the hand and the forearm lie along the left side of the patient's face and head just anterior to the ear. The patient's head should be held comfortably yet firmly between the left forearm and the heel of the right hand, and also between her left hand and the front of her left shoulder.

When oscillatory movements are being performed near the beginning of the rotation range, the physiotherapist stands head-on to the patient and the occiput is centred in the palm of her right hand. When the movements are performed at the limit of the range, she moves her body to the right until she is facing across the patient, and moves her hand further around the occiput towards the ear. The head should at all times be comfortably supported from underneath. The physiotherapist should crouch over the patient so that she hugs the patient's head. The position of the patient's head and neck may be raised or lowered to position the joint being treated approximately midway between its flexion and extension limits. A position of flexion is shown in the diagrams.

The starting position finally adopted should be the one where the grasp with either arm should be able to perform the movement on its own (*Figures 10.72* and *10.73*).

### Method

The position is taken up by turning the head to the left with a synchronous action of both hands. It is most

(a)
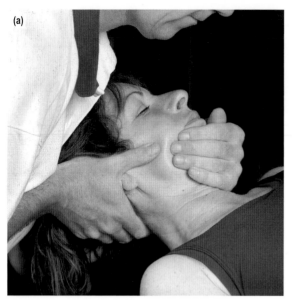

(b)
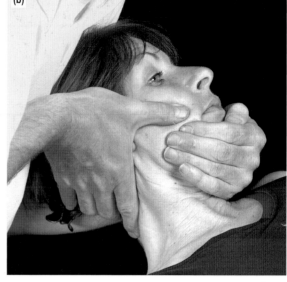

Figure 10.72    (a) and (b) Rotation Grades I and II

important that the fingers of the right hand should produce as much movement of the occiput as the left hand produces with the chin. This turning movement of the patient's head can be likened to the movement of a barbecue chicken as it revolves on a spit. In most other techniques the oscillatory movement is produced by body movement, but with rotation the physiotherapist's trunk remains steady and the rotation is produced purely by the physiotherapist's arm movement. The movement of the left arm is glenohumeral adduction with the elbow passing in front of the trunk.

Particular care needs to be exercised to be sure that a normal rotation is being produced and not a rotation distorted by deformity or muscle spasm. The range at which the oscillation is done should be kept at the limit of the normal movement obtainable.

### Local variations

The upper cervical vertebrae are more readily mobilized with the head and neck in the same plane as the body. To mobilize the lower cervical vertebrae, the neck needs to be held in a degree of neck flexion. The lower the cervical level being mobilized, the greater the angle of neck flexion required for successful movement of that vertebral joint. The level being mobilized can be isolated somewhat by using the index finger of the occipital hand to hold around the vertebra above the joint.

### Precautions

If a patient feels neck discomfort on the side of the neck to which the head is turned during or following this technique, it will readily disappear in a few minutes with active neck movements.

Although it may seem reasonable at times (when the technique is very gentle and symptoms are localized to the neck) to do rotation towards the side of pain, it should rarely be done in this direction as a strong manipulation when pain is referred from the neck.

Rotation should never be used in treatment if it produces any sign of dizziness, and to this end it is wise to do an exploratory rotation before carrying out rotary treatment.

### Uses

Rotation is one of the most valuable mobilizing procedures for the cervical spine. It is frequently the first technique chosen when treating symptoms of cervical origin, and is of greatest value in any unilateral distribution of pain of cervical origin. In such cases, the procedure is carried out with the patient's face being turned away from the painful side.

Examples of treatment include pain simulating cardiac disease, pages 421–422; pain simulating supraspinatus tendonitis, pages 422–423; pain simulating migraine, pages 424; scapula pain, pages 426–427; acute torticollis, page 427; and shooting occipital pain, page 429.

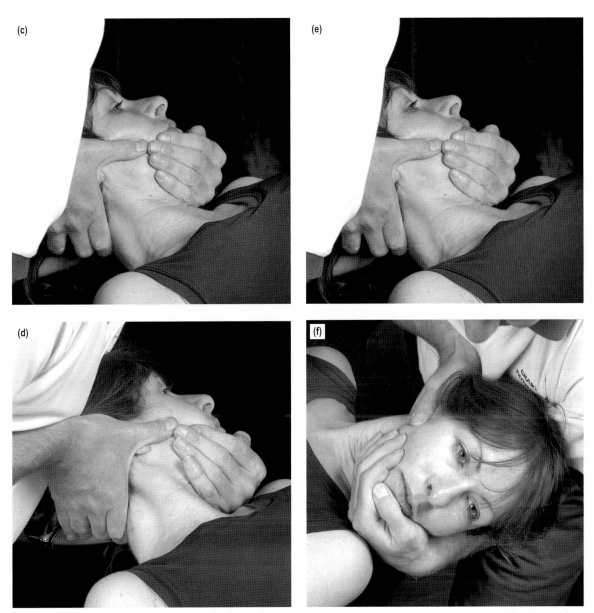

**Figure 10.72**    (*cont'd*)  (c) Rotation Grade III. (*d*), (*e*) and (*f*) Rotation Grade IV

## Lateral flexion

### Starting position

The position described is for a 'lateral flexion' mobilization to the right. This technique is one of the most difficult to do well, and the starting position is best reached in three stages:

1.  The patient lies on his back, with his head and neck beyond the end of the couch.

2.  Initially the physiotherapist should stand at the head end and take up the head and arm position adopted for rotation. This position should then be altered so that her left forearm lies behind the patient's left ear almost under the occiput, and the right hand is brought forwards so that the palm covers the whole of the ear. Slight left rotation of the patient's head will balance it most comfortably until the next stage is adopted. Without permitting any lateral flexion of the patient's head or allowing any movement of the heel of the right hand away from the patient's ear, the physiotherapist moves round alongside the patient's right shoulder to face diagonally across his head. If the right hand is felt in

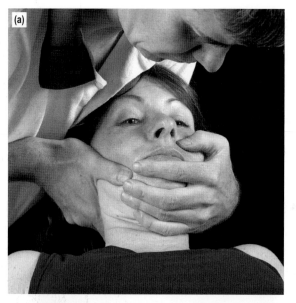

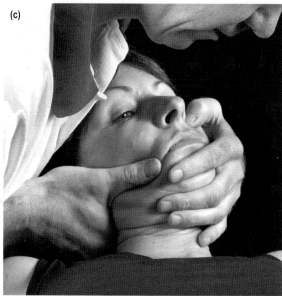

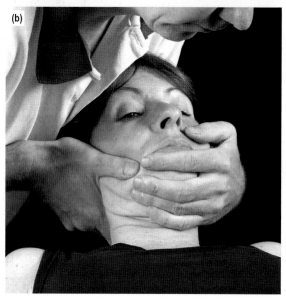

Figure 10.73    Lateral flexion. (*a*) Starting position (b) grade I II (c) grade III IV

position, the physiotherapist's right arm will lie across the front of the patient's right shoulder and her right elbow will be almost in her right iliac fossa.

3.  The final stage involves crouching to hug the patient's head while adopting the required degree of lateral flexion by displacing his neck to the left with the right hand and laterally flexing the head with the left hand and arm. The movement can be localized to a particular intervertebral level by the pressure of the palmar surface of the index finger, just distal to the metacarpophalangeal joint, on the relevant level of the articular pillar. Head rotation is prevented by

the action of the left hand and arm and the right hand. It is imperative that the palmar surface of the right hand remains in contact with the patient if the technique is to be comfortable. If the physiotherapist is properly crouched over the patient, her right forearm will be fixed between her side and the front of the patient's shoulder (*Figure 10.73*).

## Method

The oscillatory movement is produced entirely by body movement, which is a combination of movements in two directions. The physiotherapist rocks her hips gently from side to side to flex his neck laterally, and at the same time employs a forward movement of her right pelvis to displace his neck away from her. These movements are transmitted to the patient's head by a very localized pressure against the articular pillar while his head is firmly hugged.

It is very easy to give an unbalanced pull on the patient's chin, which will result in the patient's face being pulled out of its coronal plane. Care must be taken to control this with the heel of the right hand. If the position of the lateral flexion in the range is correctly maintained, the head will not be any nearer the shoulder at the end of the procedure than it is at the beginning.

### Local variations

Variations in the position of the patient's head in relation to the right shoulder are necessary when localizing the movement at the different vertebral levels. When carrying out lateral flexion at C5 or C6, the neck is taken further into lateral flexion. It may be necessary to depress the patient's shoulder to obtain sufficient space in which to work. When localizing the movement to the first cervical vertebra, the movement becomes a lateral flexion of the head without any marked curving of the neck into lateral flexion.

If lateral flexion is being localized to any of the lower levels, the neck should be flexed, and for the upper cervical levels the neck should be nearer the neutral or straight position.

The feeling of movement is greater in the midcervical spine than it is in either the upper or lower cervical spine, although in all positions the feeling of local movement is possible.

Care must be taken to stabilize the localizing index finger adequately. This is necessary because sliding on the articular pillar causes discomfort. Because of natural tenderness, pressure must be moderate and the palmar surface of the index finger must be used.

### Uses

Lateral flexion is used in patients whose symptoms of cervical origin are unilaterally distributed, either cranially or in the neck, scapula or arm. In such cases, when this mobilization is being used for the first time it is done with the patient's head laterally flexed away from the painful side. It can be used towards the painful side, but this is usually only of value when the associated stiff painful lateral flexion is towards the painful side.

Mobilizing in lateral flexion is often of value in improving a limitation of the patient's active range of rotation.

Examples of treatment include acute torticollis, page 427.

## Cervical flexion (F)

### Starting position

The patient lies supine with his head near the end of the couch. The physiotherapist, standing by his left shoulder, places her left hand over his sternum and her right hand under the occipital area. She then gently flexes his chin towards his chest and directs her right hand so that the heel of her hand is under his occiput and the fingers are spread forwards over the occipital area.

The position of the right hand depends upon the level of the cervical spine being treated. The lower the level being treated, the more the heel of her right hand is extended down his neck (*Figure 10.74a*).

If the high cervical area is being treated, the physiotherapist places the occiput in the palm of her right hand and her left hand is placed over his chin (*Figure 10.74b*).

### Method

The right hand is used to flex the head and neck in a small-amplitude oscillatory fashion while the physiotherapist directs her forearm in whatever direction is required to emphasize the flexion at particular intervertebral levels. For example, if the middle cervical area is being treated her forearm is directed approximately horizontally, whereas if the lower cervical level is being treated her elbow points slightly towards the floor. When the upper cervical area is being mobilized she places her left hand on the patient's chin and raises her right forearm so that her elbow points slightly towards the ceiling. Under these circumstances she works both hands in an equal and opposite direction to emphasize the stretch in the upper cervical area.

### Precautions

This technique is not one selected early in treatment, particularly in the presence of disc pathology, neither is it a technique that should be used very strongly for unstable discogenic disorders.

### Uses

The main indication for this technique is stiffness in forward flexion in the absence of pain or when pain is only minimal. It can also be used as a technique when this movement reproduces the patient's pain in any area associated with the vertebral column. This means that if left buttock pain is reproduced by neck flexion

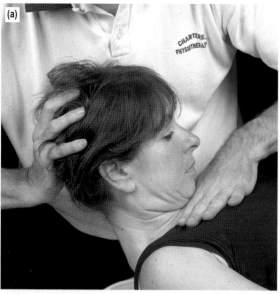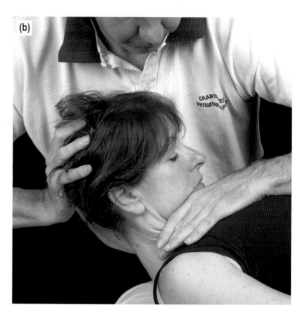

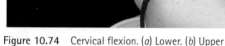

**Figure 10.74** Cervical flexion. (*a*) Lower. (*b*) Upper

in the supine position, then it can be used to mobilize the faulty structures in the lumbar vertebral canal.

### General comment

Techniques can be performed in general or very specific ways. For example, if cervical rotation is being used to treat C4/5, the physiotherapist's 'head' hand can be moved down from the occiput so as to grasp C4. Similarly, if we again take C4/5 as the level, but treatment is by postero-anterior unilateral vertebral pressure on the left side, the technique may be used generally by employing the technique from C3 to C6 or it may be used only on C4 or C5, or on the apophyseal joint line between C4/5. Also, the C4 etc. articular pillar can be held in one hand and the C5 articular pillar in the opposite hand. While C5 is moved posteroanteriorly, C4 can be either moved in the opposite direction to C5 or just stabilized. When transverse pressures are being used, similar accuracy to one level can be achieved by pushing adjacent spinous processes in opposite directions.

## CERVICAL TRACTION

Although cervical traction can be administered by hand it is more efficient if this is done by means of a halter, thus enabling longer periods of traction to be maintained with less effort.

### Halter

There are many types of cervical traction halter in use today, but those that support under the patient's chin and occiput must be adjustable in two of their relationships. When applied to the patient it must be possible to alter the height of the occipital band in relation to the band that supports the chin. It must also be possible to adjust the strap at the side of the patient's head to control the distance between the chin band and the occipital band. Once the adjustments are made they must not be able to slip. Any halter used for different patients that is not adjustable in these two directions must inevitably result in some patients being given traction with too much flexion or extension of the head. Few halters have these two adjustments, and some that do are inadequate because they are not stable when the adjustments are made. For example, one variety has the occipital strap and chin strap constructed out of one piece of material, which is continuous through a metal ring from which the halter is suspended. Though the patient's position may be adjusted with his head in the frontal plane, the position may be lost during treatment because the harness material is able to slide through the rings.

The two adjustments that must be possible are first, the vertical length of the occipital and chin straps; and secondly, the horizontal distance between them. It is necessary to be able to fit the patient who has a long or short jaw as well as the patient who has a small or

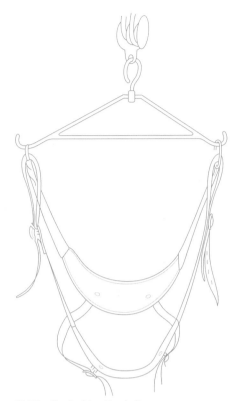

**Figure 10.75** Cervical traction halter

large head. If the head is small it will be necessary to bring the chin strap closer to the occipital strap in its horizontal direction, and if the chin is small it will be necessary to bring the chin strap closer to the occipital strap in its vertical direction. *Figure 10.75* shows the occipital strap and chin strap, each with its own pair of buckles for adjustment in the vertical direction. It is more convenient to have both sections adjustable, although the occipital strap can be of fixed length with a more widely variable length of chin strap, or *vice versa*. The other adjustment is made by the pair of horizontally directed straps from the occipital strap to the chin strap. They pass on each side of the patient's jaw and buckle under the chin to avoid the patient's hair becoming entangled during adjustment.

Discussion surrounding the advisability of giving traction in flexion or in a neutral position is common. However, the amount of flexion or extension of the head on the upper cervical spine during traction treatment should also be considered. This consideration is particularly relevant when the upper cervical spine is treated. It must therefore be possible to adjust the halter, not only to fit the various shapes of head and jaw but also for different 'head–neck' relationships. This is

achieved by vertical adjustment of the occipital strap in relation to the chin strap.

A swivel hook in the spreader bar, as shown in *Figure 10.75*, is not an essential requirement but it makes for convenience. The traction is applied best through double pulley blocks and a rope. With a mechanical advantage of four, small adjustments are possible without losing any feel of the tractive pressure.

## Treatment

Treatment may be administered in three ways:

1. Constant traction requires continuous bed rest for the patient, with the traction applied 24 hours of the day or in cycles of 1 hour of traction followed by a half-hour rest repeated throughout the day. This type of traction is mainly used for patients with severe nerve-root pain.

2. The second method is intermittent traction, administered once or twice a day for short periods. This is the more common variety used in physiotherapy, and is used for patients with less severe nerve root and other intervertebral joint disorders.

3. Thirdly there is the method, also administered only once or twice a day, that comprises a gradual application of traction to a certain weight, which is held momentarily and then gradually released; this is followed by momentary rest before reapplication of the traction. This cycle is repeated for varying periods, and the times for the 'hold' and 'rest' periods, as well as treatment times, can be varied. This 'intermittent variable traction' has a wide application among patients whose joint condition requires movement, and is best performed with an intermittent traction machine. Many brands are available, but the essential qualities it must have are that:
   a) The movement of applying and releasing the traction must be extremely smooth.
   b) Controls must be available to vary the treatment time; the time on 'hold'; the time on 'rest'; the strength when on 'hold'; and the strength when on 'rest'.

4. The speed of the take-up and the speed of releasing the tractive force should be variable.

A gradual stepping up to (and releasing from) the selected tractive force can also be of value.

A patient with severe nerve-root pain, if he is to be treated conservatively, requires cervical traction. A choice needs to be made between cervical traction administered in a hospital or at home on the one hand, and in physiotherapy rooms alone or in conjunction with self-administered traction at home on the other. The former method seriously restricts the patient's daily movements, and this must be borne in mind, but the severity of the pain may demand it as the treatment of choice. If traction is to be given in hospital, the method is as follows.

## Hospital traction

The patient is comfortably supported by pillows in a half-lying position, with a pillow supporting the head and neck in the correct position. If the traction is being administered for a lower cervical nerve-root pain, the neck is flexed slightly on the trunk and the head is supported in a neutral position on the upper neck. If traction is being given for a high cervical nerve-root pain, the neck is supported in a neutral position of comfort for the patient and his head is supported in a position midway between flexion and extension of the upper cervical spine. The halter is then adjusted on the patient's head so that the chosen position will be maintained when the tractive force is applied. The direction of the pulley rope should be in line with the longitudinal axis of the joint to be treated. For the patient with lower cervical nerve-root pain, the rope will form an angle of some 30° with his trunk; for high cervical nerve-root pain, the angle is much shallower. Initial weights used are low, approximately 2–3 kg; these can be increased by 0.5–1 kg per day up to a maximum of 5 kg. The patient's build and general joint mobility on the one hand and the severity of the pain on the other govern the weight. Patient tolerance to the apparatus governs the periods spent on traction, but 1 hour on traction followed by half an hour's rest repeated throughout the waking periods is usually all that is required in the most severe nerve-root pain if it is going to respond to this type of management. Ten days is usually sufficient time for the traction to be maintained, but if there is no improvement over the first few days it is unlikely that the patient will be helped by the constant traction. Traction at home may be used intermittently following the hospital traction.

There are many positions described in the literature for applying traction to the cervical spine, varying from full flexion to full extension. Basically, the position chosen should be one that positions the joint being treated approximately midway between the limits of flexion and extension for that joint. This position may vary from patient to patient because of structural joint changes due to disease, congenital anomalies or trauma. It may also vary in the same patient as treatment effects improvement of a painful restriction (for example, extension). As discussed earlier (*see* p. 172–173), the neck should be positioned in flexion for a

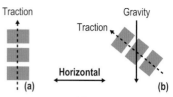

**Figure 10.76** Lines of force. (*a*) Traction in flexion in sitting. (*b*) Traction in flexion in lying

lower cervical intervertebral joint and towards the neutral position for an upper cervical joint.

Whether a patient is treated sitting or lying is governed by factors related to comfort and ease of administering the traction, and not by whether the flexed or neutral position is desired. For example, when traction is being applied in the neutral position the patient is usually more comfortable in the sitting position. If the traction is applied in the supine position, the thoracic spine is more extended and can become uncomfortable during treatment. However, when the supine position is used for traction in flexion the thoracic spine is not extended, so it then becomes the position of choice.

Although the sitting position can be used for traction in flexion, it has the disadvantage that the trunk may be less stable than when supine, and it gives different counter-resistance to stronger tractive forces. Nevertheless, with the patient sitting in a slumped position (supported by a lumbar pillow if necessary) the 'traction-inflexion' position can be achieved, and its line of pull is more direct (no anteroposterior gravity component) than in the lying position (*Figure 10.76*). The following text describes traction in neutral for the upper cervical spine performed in sitting and traction in flexion for the lower cervical spine performed in lying (*Figure 10.77*).

## Traction in neutral (CT ↑)

### Starting position

The patient sits in a comfortable chair with adequate support for his back and, if possible, for his arms, to encourage complete relaxation. This is an important consideration. For this reason, it is advisable to ask the patient to slide his buttocks slightly forwards on the seat to produce slight slumping and therefore better relaxation.

The head halter is applied and the necessary adjustments are made so that when the traction is applied the head, in relation to the neck, will be lifted in the neutral position. The occipital strap must lift under the occiput and must not include suboccipital structures.

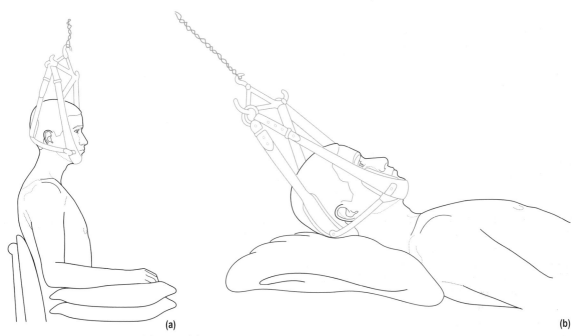

**Figure 10.77**  Cervical traction (*a*) Sitting (*b*) Lying

## Method

Before applying any traction, the physiotherapist should know the area and severity of the patient's symptoms at that moment. The physiotherapist places the tip of her index or middle finger against the side of the interspinous space of the joint to be treated. The traction is then applied and relaxed in an oscillatory movement, very gently at first but gradually increasing until movement can be felt by the finger in the interspinous space. This oscillatory traction should continue until the right pressure is found, which is minimum amount required to produce movement at the intervertebral level being treated. When this pressure has been sustained for approximately 10 seconds, the patient's symptoms are reassessed. The following changes in symptoms will indicate how the pressure should be further altered and how long it should be sustained.

1.  When severe symptoms are completely relieved by this gentle pressure, the pressure must be reduced by half and the traction time kept within 5 minutes because the patient is likely to have a severe exacerbation later unless this reduction is made.

2.  If symptoms have been partly relieved, the traction should be kept at this level and sustained for 5 minutes if the pain was severe before traction, and for 10 minutes if it was moderate.

3.  If the symptoms have not altered, the traction can be increased a little and a further assessment made. The new pressure should be sustained for 10 minutes.

4.  Symptoms made worse by this gentle traction should be given half the pressure and reassessed. If the symptoms are still worse, changes of position of the head–neck relationship by alteration of the harness or sitting position should be carried out and the gentler traction reapplied. If the symptoms are still worse, then one of two courses remains open: if the aggravation is not too great, the gentlest traction can be maintained for 5 minutes or less; if the aggravation is more than minimal, traction should be discontinued. On reassessing the next day, only if the response to the gentle pressure shows improvement can traction be continued.

For the initial treatment, one point must be emphasized. The angle or direction of the pull is not altered during treatment; it is the strength and duration that is modified by changes in the symptoms. The angle of the pull must be as near to the neutral position (midway between the inter-vertebral joint's ranges of flexion, extension, lateral flexion and rotation) as possible so as to achieve the maximum longitudinal movement for that joint with the minimum strength of traction.

## Method of progression

The importance of continually assessing symptoms and signs for changes resulting from treatment was discussed in Chapter 4, and it is by these methods that treatment is guided. As with techniques of mobilization, changes in techniques are guided by checking the patient's movements after the use of a technique and also by the amount of change that is retained from one treatment to the next. When the traction is released the patient's movements should be reassessed, but it is also important to assess the symptoms and the signs on the day following treatment.

Follow-up treatment can be considered in two categories; those patients with severe pain and those with moderate pain. Treatment of a patient who has severe pain should be progressed very slowly, as circumstances allow, until the symptoms become moderate. At first the progression should be by small increases in duration of the traction rather than strength. When there is little or no reaction from treatment, the strength can be increased in small stages also. Progression can be by both strength and duration when symptoms are moderate. With the exception of treatment for severe nerve-root pain, the total time required for traction is not greater than 15 minutes. Results that cannot be obtained with traction of this duration will not be achieved with longer periods, and tractive forces rarely need to be heavy. Traction, as a form of treatment, should be discarded when symptoms and signs remain unchanged after two to four treatments.

No mention has been made regarding strength, and it is assumed that the amount of traction given will be governed by careful assessment of symptoms and signs before, during and following traction. As has been indicated, the application of pressure at first is governed by movement produced at the intervertebral level being treated. Obviously, 4 kg of traction applied to a 102-kg patient will produce less movement than if applied to a 42-kg patient. Therefore, although scales that indicate strength of traction are necessary in research projects and in hospital departments where staff changes occur, it is essential to realize that tractive forces should be governed by assessment and not by the scale.

There is one time when knowledge of the weights that can be considered normal for cervical traction is valuable. People of middle age have some aches that do not worry them and that they class as normal. Examination of their movements frequently exhibits slight pain at the limit of range, but again this is considered normal. However, if this pain increases, these people seek treatment. With these thoughts in mind, a person's cervical spine, even with a degree of symptoms and signs that might be classed as being within normal acceptable limits, should be able to accept traction of up to approximately 10 kg (22 lb) without discomfort or after effects. Similarly, minor discomfort felt with a traction force in excess of 10 kg may, under the circumstances mentioned, be classed as normal. These facts should be borne in mind when treating patients who have discomfort during traction.

## Traction in flexion (CT ⤴ )

### Starting position

The patient lies comfortably on his back with one or two pillows to support his neck in slight flexion in relation to his trunk, so that the joint being treated will be midway between flexion and extension, and so as to support his head neutrally on his upper cervical spine. If he has at any time had any lower back symptoms, it is advisable to have him flex his hips and knees to allow the lower back to rest. The halter is applied and the occipital strap is positioned first. Because the patient rests his head on this strap on the pillows, it will remain in position while the side straps and chin straps are being adjusted. To ensure that the harness is correctly adjusted, the physiotherapist applies some traction via the spreader bar while she watches to see that the head–neck relationship is neutral.

### Method

Knowing the area and the severity of the patient's pain, the operator alternately applies and relaxes pressure through the pulley system while watching and palpating for movement at the intervertebral level being treated. The pressure is sustained at that amount which is the smallest required to produce movement at the joint. After approximately 10 seconds, the patient's symptoms are reassessed. From this point onwards the procedure is identical with that described for traction in neutral.

### Precautions

A frequent problem with strong cervical traction is discomfort or pain in the patient's temporomandibular joints. This pain may be relieved by an alteration of the position of the straps, or by placing a pad between the patient's molars. However, traction of this magnitude is to be avoided unless absolutely essential.

It is surprising how often pre-existing, but possibly dormant, thoracic or lumbar symptoms are irritated by cervical traction. Traction in neutral can irritate either thoracic or lumbar conditions, but traction in flexion only irritates the lumbar spine. Therefore when traction is being used, the patient should be questioned as to the existence of such symptoms, and care should be taken to avoid any aggravation of them.

When traction in neutral is given with the patient sitting, it is as well to be aware of the fact that a patient can experience nausea, but this usually only occurs with prolonged or very strong traction or with excessively apprehensive patients. On releasing traction, patients can experience a feeling of giddiness if the traction has been very strong.

Traction in flexion can cause a burning feeling or pain in the vicinity of the first cervical vertebra. In such a case it is advisable to alter the harness so that the head is extended more on the upper neck, while the lower neck is maintained in flexion.

## Uses

A patient whose neck movements of lateral flexion and rotation towards the painful side are markedly limited by arm pain should be treated by traction only, and it is traction in flexion that should be used. Traction should always be the first choice in treatment when recent neurological changes are present.

Traction is of value in almost any distribution of pain arising from the cervical vertebrae. However, the rapidity with which complete relief of symptoms and signs is obtained is usually slower than with mobilization. When intervertebral joints are stiff, traction may be ineffective if not preceded by manipulation.

Intermittent variable cervical traction (IVCT), referred to on pages 288–289, can be applied in neutral or in flexion for the same reasons as have been given already. Weight and duration are also governed in exactly the same manner. The only factor not already covered is the mode of establishing or progressing the hold and rest periods. When symptoms are severe the amount of movement should be less, which means that the hold and rest periods should be long. As symptoms become less severe, the rest period can be made minimal. When symptoms can be classed as an ache rather than a pain, the hold period should be approximately 3–5 seconds with minimal rest periods.

Examples of treatment include: severe cervical nerve root, pages 414–415; pain simulating cardiac disease, pages 421–422; pain simulating migraine, pages 424–425; acute torticollis, pages 427–428; and shooting occipital pain, pages 429–430.

## GRADE V MANIPULATION

As has been mentioned earlier, there are two kinds of manipulative technique: first, those that are the general techniques; and secondly, those that emphasize the movement, as much as is possible, to a specific intervertebral level.

Of the general manipulations, there are rotation and the direct palpation techniques such as postero-anterior central vertebral pressure. The method is to take up the slack, ease back fractionally, and then add a very fast small-range movement.

It is mandatory that all manipulative (Grade V) techniques must be preceded by testing for vertebrobasilar insufficiency (as described on pp. 242–249).

High cervical rotation manipulations should **not** be the first choice if other manipulative techniques that are generally thought to be less risky in terms of vertebral artery damage can be used with the same effect.

## Cervical rotation (↺)

The symbol indicates the direction of the rotation of the patient's head.

This mobilization can be converted to a manipulation by applying a sudden movement of tiny amplitudes to the neck. Manipulation in this instance presupposes that treatment has progressed through stages from gentle mobilization to the stage when manipulation has become necessary.

The position used to manipulate is the same as that described for the mobilization (*see* pp. 283–284); the head and neck are slowly rotated. Over-pressure is applied, and any indications of vertebrobasilar insufficiency are sought. The over-pressure is then fractionally released, and a quick rotatory movement through 3–4° is given. This movement should never ever be a large movement through a full range from the central position; to do this is to court disaster.

The specific techniques for the different levels of the cervical spine follow, and examples of treatment include acute torticollis, page 427, and shooting occipital pain, page 429.

## Occipito-atlantal joint (rotation lv ↺ 0/1)

### Starting position

The patient lies supine and the physiotherapist stands at the head end towards the patient's left shoulder. By reaching around the right side of the patient's head, the physiotherapist grasps the patient's chin in her right hand. She then places her left hand under the patient's head so that her middle finger is against the posterior margin of the right arch of the atlas, with the pad of the tip of the finger pressed firmly against the posterior margin of the transverse process. A firm grip of this vertebra is then achieved by hooking the thumb round the left transverse process of the atlas to reach its anterior surface. Rotation of the patient's head to the right is then carried out until the occipito-atlantal joint is felt to be stretched (approximately 10° short of

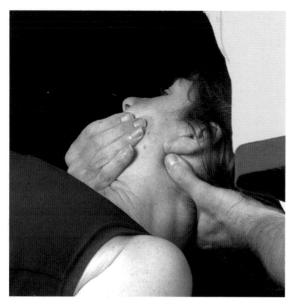

**Figure 10.78**    Occipito-atlantal joint. Rotation (lv ↻ 0/I)

full rotation), from which position the head is rotated back approximately 10°. In this position, the grasp of the atlas is tightened (*Figure 10.78*).

## Method

Sudden rotation of the patient's head to the right through 10–15° should be effected by the physiotherapist's right hand while the left hand attempts to prevent any movement of the atlas. There is no danger attached to this procedure since, although a maximum range of occipito-atlantal movement is achieved, the range of head movement is still short of the patient's full range of active rotation.

## Occipito–atlantal joint (unilateral PA thrust lv ↴ 0/1)

### Starting position

The patient lies supine with his head beyond the end of the couch. If the technique is to be performed on the right side, the physiotherapist stands by the right side of the patient's head. She supports his chin and head in her left arm and holds his right occipital area in her right hand. She places her right hand in such a position that the contact point of her right hand is placed behind the right occipito-atlantal joint. The position she adopts with her right hand is one that is used in many techniques. The contact point is the anterolateral surface at the junction of the proximal and middle thirds of the proximal phalanx of the index finger. If

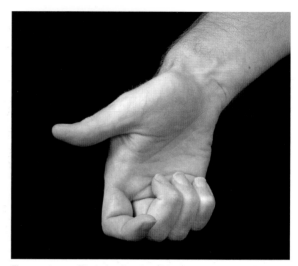

**Figure 10.79**    Thrusting hand position

the contact is made too far laterally, it becomes very painful. The position of the rest of the hand is also important. The fingers are comfortably flexed at the interphalangeal joints while also supporting the patient's head, and the thumb is brought forwards to hold the occiput more laterally. The wrist is ulnar deviated and held in a position midway between flexion and extension. This description of the thrusting hand position (*Figure 10.79*) will be referred to when adopted in other techniques.

The patient's head is now rotated to the left through approximately 30° for convenience, and his head is then firmly stabilized between the physiotherapist's left arm and her shoulder. While the physiotherapist palpates behind the occipito-atlantal joint with the proximal phalanx of her index finger, she adjusts the position of the occipito-atlantal joint with her left arm as follows. First, she adjusts the flexion/extension position of the patient's head on his upper cervical spine until the occipito-atlantal joint is positioned midway between these two movements. Secondly, she adjusts the lateral flexion position for the joint. This she does by tipping his head sideways in an oscillatory fashion on the upper cervical spine. Once this neutral position has been adopted, the head should be held stably so that the position is not lost (*Figure 10.80*).

## Method

The physiotherapist hugs the patient's head firmly in her left arm and tightens her contact against the right occipito-atlantal joint. She then directs her forearm pointing towards his right eye. Small preparatory oscillatory movements are produced by pushing

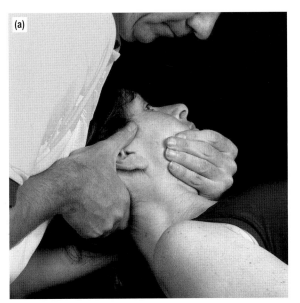 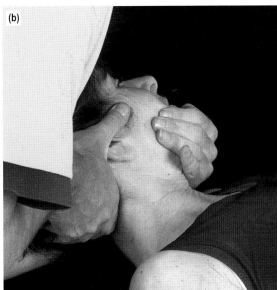

**Figure 10.80**   (*a*) and (*b*) Occipito-atlantal joint. Unilateral postero-anterior thrust (lv ↓ 0/1)

though her right hand, along with very tiny movements of his head with her left arm. These movements allow the head to be tipped by the right-handed push, but do not allow it to move far.

The manipulative thrust is then executed with a short, very fast thrusting-type movement through her right hand and through the right occipito-atlantal joint. This thrust is countered by a controlling and guiding movement with her left arm.

### Upper cervical joints, occiput to C3 (transverse thrust, lv ⟶ opening 0/1, 1/2 or 2/3)

This technique resembles the transverse thrust described on page 298, but a greater range of extension of the head on the neck is incorporated.

### Starting position

To open the joint on the right-hand side, the patient lies supine with his head beyond the end of the couch and his whole body near the left side of the couch. The physiotherapist supports his head in her right arm, holding his chin in her right hand. She then palpates with her left index finger to identify the level she intends to manipulate. The next step is to place the thrusting hand, particularly the proximal phalanx of her index finger, against the posterolateral aspect of the joint. The physiotherapist rotates the patient's head to the right with small oscillatory movements until she can feel that the limit of the range has been reached,

after which she both extends and laterally flexes his head to the left to the limit of their ranges (*Figure 10.81*).

### Method

The technique is the same as with other thrusting-type techniques. When the position has been accurately adopted, the thrust is transmitted as a fast, small-amplitude technique with the physiotherapist's left hand while her body and right arm give a slight increase to the patient's extension, lateral flexion and rotation of his head.

### Upper cervical joints, occiput to C3 (transverse thrust, closing the right lv ⟶)

The technique for closing the intervertebral joints utilizes the same starting position as that described above for opening the opposite side. The difference in the technique is that the thrusting left hand is directed caudally and medially rather than cephalad and medially.

Examples of treatment include cervical joint locking, pages 428–429, and pain simulating migraine, pages 424–425.

### Occipito–atlantal joint (longitudinal movement ⟷)

### Starting position

The starting position for this technique performed on the right side varies in only one aspect from that

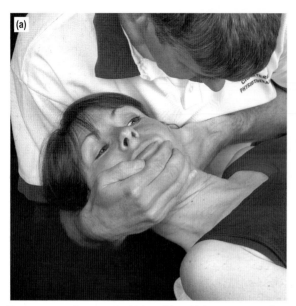 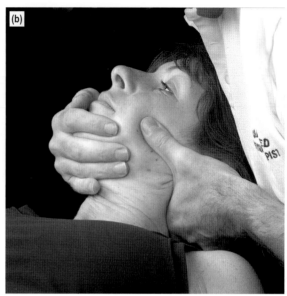

Figure 10.81    Intervertebral joints. (*a*) and (*b*) Upper cervical/transverse thrust opening the right (lv ⟶)

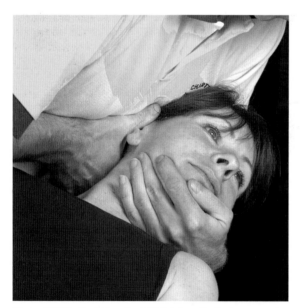

Figure 10.82    Occipito-atlantal joint. Longitudinal movement (⟷ Ⓡ)

described for the postero-anterior thrust. The thrusting hand makes contact with the occiput immediately adjacent to the right occipito-atlantal joint, and the physiotherapist adjusts her right forearm to thrust through the crown of the head. The neutral extension and lateral flexion positions are adopted in the same manner as described above (*Figure 10.82*).

## Method

The physiotherapist hugs the patient's head to hold it firmly, and by pressure directed through the crown of his head with her thrusting hand she takes up the slack of longitudinal movement in his neck. The manipulative thrust is one of very small amplitude performed at maximum speed and without force.

## Atlanto–axial joint (rotation lv C1/2 ↻)

### Starting position

The technique will be described for rotation to the left.

The patient lies supine with his head well clear of the end of the couch. The physiotherapist holds his chin and head in her left arm and rotates his head through 40°. With this degree of rotation there has been no movement of the second cervical vertebra. She palpates for the tip of the spinous process of C2 with her index finger, and then slides her index finger beyond the spinous process keeping firm contact between the spinous process and the index finger's lateral surface. This firm contact must be maintained with the skin and the spinous process throughout so that the tissue can be held tightly. This sliding movement is continued, her arm at right angles to the skin of his neck, until the spinous process of C2 is cradled in the first interosseous space. She is then in a position to hold C2 firmly cradled between the metacarpophalangeal joint of her index finger behind the left articular pillar of C2 and her thumb, which holds the transverse

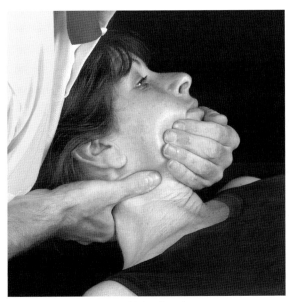

Figure 10.83    Atlanto-axial joint. Rotation

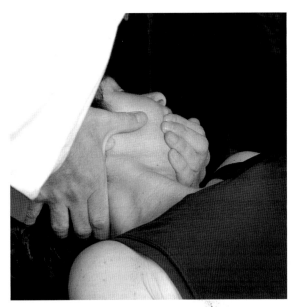

Figure 10.84    Intervertebral joints. C2–7 (lv ↺)

process of C2 on the right-hand side almost from in front. Her forearm is by this time well underneath the patient, with the elbow pointing towards the floor. This hand position is vital if the technique is to be a success. The physiotherapist's hand remains at right angles to the skin throughout the technique, and the fingers of her right hand pass the back of the left hand during the manipulation. The physiotherapist needs to stand behind the patient's head to be in the most efficient position (*Figure 10.83*).

## Method

Before carrying out the manipulation, the position is checked by two movements. First, the physiotherapist rotates the patient's head back and forth through a small amplitude to ensure that all slack has been taken up between the two hands. This is done by rotating the patient's head with the left arm to see if the right hand is forced to follow. This is followed immediately by a derotation movement with her right hand to see if the left hand is forced to return to its original position, because in fact the head is being turned back by the right hand's contact against C2. The second exploratory movement is a counter-clockwise movement with both hands. These movements are done as small jabbing movements with both arms, and are the forerunners of the manipulative thrust. These exploratory movements will give a good guide to the strength of the movement required to manipulate the joint. The manipulation consists of a tiny rotary movement with the left hand and a small-amplitude sharp thrust with the right hand. The

movement of the right hand consists of a unilateral postero-anterior thrust on the left side of C2, while the physiotherapist's whole contact with that vertebra with her right hand effects a rotary movement of C2.

## Intervertebral joints C2–7 (rotation lv ↺)

### Starting position

The technique is described for rotation left of the C3/4 joint.

The patient lies supine with his head beyond the end of the couch. The physiotherapist stands by the right side of his head, supporting his head in the crook of her left arm and holding his chin in her hand. She flexes his neck to place the C3/4 joint midway between flexion and extension. With the tip of her right index finger, the physiotherapist finds the C3/4 interspinous space and then moves her hand laterally to bring the anterolateral surface of the proximal phalanx of the index finger behind the C3/4 apophyseal joint. She places her fingers on the back of his neck and head to provide support, and her thumb lightly on his jaw. While holding this proximal phalanx stationary against the articular pillar of C3/4, she oscillates the head in a rotary movement, starting from the straight head position and gradually turning the head further until rotation is felt by the phalanx at the C3/4 joint. She then tightens her right-hand grip with the fingers and thumb so that if the head is turned further and the right hand follows the turn, C3 also follows the turn. This unifying of the spine above C3 with the head is vital (*Figure 10.84*).

## Method

The manipulation consists of a small-amplitude sharp rotation of the unit, head to C3, with a thrust being exerted behind the articular pillar of C3.

## Intervertebral joints C2–7 (lateral flexion Iv ⌐⌐)

### Starting position

The patient lies supine with his head beyond the end of the couch and the physiotherapist, standing at the head of the couch, grasps the patient's chin in her left hand while her left forearm lies against the left side of the patient's head. With the palm of the right hand at right angles to the neck, and the fingers supporting under the head and neck, the patient's head is laterally flexed to the right through a few degrees while the physiotherapist moves her body and feet until she is standing by the patient's right shoulder facing his head.

To localize the level of the manipulation, the physiotherapist uses the tip of the right index finger to palpate for the desired interspinous space. When the level has been ascertained, the anterolateral surface of the base of the proximal phalanx of the right index finger is placed against the articular pillar on the right at that level. The physiotherapist then combines a push against the articular pillar with the right hand (thus displacing the neck to the left), with a lateral flexion of the patient's head to the right by the left hand and forearm. In this way a position can be reached where the intervertebral joint opposite the base of the physiotherapist's right index finger can be felt to be fully stretched. To complete the tension at this joint, the head must be passively rotated to the left by the physiotherapist's left hand until the stretch can also be felt under this finger. The right wrist is held flexed to the mid-position to keep the heel of the hand away from the patient's right ear, thereby keeping the more lateral aspect of the proximal phalanx to bear against the articular pillar. At the same time the physiotherapist directs her forearm in line with the plane of the apophyseal joint under the base of the index finger. To perform this manipulation with minimum effort, the physiotherapist should crouch over the patient's head to hug it and hold both arms firmly against her sides (*Figure 10.85*).

## Method

When the physiotherapist is sure that she has the joint fully stretched she gives a sudden thrust through the base of the right index finger along the line of the right forearm, at the same time applying an equal counterpressure with her left arm at the head and neck. The aim is to produce a sudden stretch at the apophyseal joint opposite the fulcrum. This stretch may result in a crack-like sound.

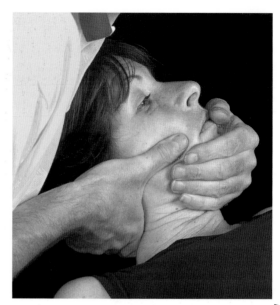

**Figure 10.85** Intervertebral joints. C2–7 (lateral flexion Iv ⌐⌐)

## Intervertebral joints C2–7 (transverse thrust Iv opening ←•–)

### Starting position

This technique will be described to open the joints on the left-hand side.

The patient lies supine with his head extended beyond the head of the couch and his right shoulder near the right-hand edge of the couch. The physiotherapist supports his head in her left arm, holding his chin with her hand, and stands by the right side of his head. With her right index finger, she finds the interspinous space between the two vertebrae that she plans to manipulate. She then places the anterolateral border of her thrusting proximal index finger phalanx against the articular pillar at that level on the right-hand side. She then rotates his head to the left in a series of small-amplitude oscillations, increasing the range until the movement can be felt to take place at the joint to be manipulated. This rotation will vary between 45 and 55°, depending on the level being manipulated; the higher the level the smaller the rotation. The right palm is at all times kept at right angles to the skin surface. The physiotherapist, with firm contact held against the articular pillar, tilts the patient's head back towards his right shoulder with her left arm. This movement is a combination of slight extension with lateral flexion. The movement is continued until the joint can be felt to be tight under the physiotherapist's right hand. At the same time that she tilts back the patient's head and neck, the physiotherapist displaces the mid-cervical area away from her towards his left shoulder (*Figure 10.86*).

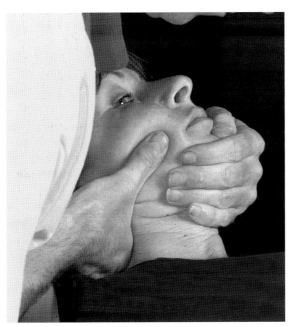

**Figure 10.86**    Intervertebral joints. C2–7 (transverse thrust lv ←•← opening)

### Intervertebral joints C2–7 (transverse thrust closing the right side lv ←•←)

As with the transverse thrust for the upper cervical joints, the technique can be adapted to either open (wider) or close the joints. The description of the technique here is the same as that described on page 296 with *Figure 10.81*.

#### Method

Small oscillatory thrusting movements are employed by the physiotherapist through her right hand to ensure that the right degree of slack has been taken up. These small-amplitude thrusting movements are countered by tiny tipping movements of the patient's head, which is held in her left arm. A small-amplitude manipulative thrust with the body transmitted through the right hand directed towards the left and caudad effects the technique.

#### Extension–acceleration injuries

In contrast to the vigorous techniques described, mobilization must at times be extremely gentle to be effective. One such example is extension–acceleration ('whiplash') injuries in the minor category. To learn more, especially in the area of injuries, Jeffreys (1991, pp. 26–29) gives excellent detail.

Whiplash injury typically occurs when the injured person's car is hit directly from behind, especially if the injured person is looking straight ahead and is totally unaware of the impending blow. It is encouraging to see that flexion and lateral flexion acceleration injuries do cause less damage (Jeffreys, 1991). At the moment of impact, the movement of the head and neck is a totally unguarded movement. Such unguarded movements can occur in a myriad of different ways, but they ALL occur in a manner that flicks the vertebral system into and beyond a normal range of active extension at a speed and suddenness that prevents the protecting muscles from saving the structures from injury. The speed of the colliding car may be as low as 4 kmh, and the gap between the patient's head and the headrest need only be approximately 10 cm to cause a damaging acceleration injury. Obviously, faster speeds and the lack of an effective headrest leads to greater damage.

When a moderate injury occurs there is damage to anterior and posterior structures; posterior damage occurs in bony and ligamentous tissues as well as in 'rim lesions of the intervertebral disc and zygapophyseal joint' (Taylor and Twomey, 1993). Anterior damage occurs in two phases, the first being when the head is hurled backwards and the second soon afterwards when the anterior flexor muscles try to stop the head going backwards and then endeavour to pull the head and neck forwards.

Treatment will not be discussed other than to state two principles:

1.  A soft soothing collar (not one aimed to prevent *all* movement) should be used when the patient feels that this gives some relief (day or night).

2.  Active movement should be encouraged, but should be under the instruction and guidance of a physiotherapist. The initial movement should be a rotary-type movement while supported on a down-filled pillow, and with the soft collar on if this provides greater comfort. The movement is of minimal range, and should cause NO discomfort whatsoever. The words 'rotary-*type* movement' are used here to differentiate the movement from a 'chicken on a spit' rotation, which is to be avoided. The rotary-type movement is a rolling of the head in rotation with a functional ipsilateral lateral flexion. The range may, in the beginning, need to be only 2–3° each side. Also, it is often more comfortably and successfully performed with the patient's head and neck fully supported in neutral on a soft pillow while the therapist's hands, *underneath the pillow*, assist and guide the rolling motion of the head and neck.

# Thoracic spine

## INTRODUCTION

Fascinating facts about the thoracic spine:

- The potential visceral origin of symptoms in and around the thoracic spine
- The costal joints as a source of breathing-related symptoms
- The influence on the thoracic spine of dynamic postural stabilization around the shoulder girdle
- The potential for mechanical irritation of the sympathetic chains to produce symptoms
- The effects of open-heart and thoracic surgery on the neuromusculoskeletal structures

For the manipulative physiotherapist there are several fascinating facts regarding the thoracic spine. The first is that the palpation findings are easy to identify and interpret. However, the patient is often surprised to find that his thoracic spine is 'sore' and 'tender' on palpation. He is even more surprised to find that the source of his aching shoulder and arm, for example, may well be his thoracic spine. The second is that it is an area of the spine that produces symptoms that can mimic many of the pains of visceral disorders. Frequently the endeavour to prove that a patient's abdominal pain is or is not vertebral in origin is extremely challenging. Patience and care with assessment is of the utmost importance, particularly when the symptoms have both vertebral and visceral components. It is important to take great care in determining the area of the patient's symptoms and their behaviour, particularly in relation to the effect of rest on the pain. A patient with visceral pain rarely seeks lying down as a position to adopt to gain relief.

Patients who have intermittent difficulty with breathing are far more likely to have an inter-costal, costovertebral or intervertebral problem than a pleural disorder.

There are many manipulators of the vertebral column who confidently believe that the spine can be the original source of visceral disorders. However, although the cervical spine can cause shoulder joint PAIN, it has yet to be proven that the thoracic spine can cause visceral PAIN. Nevertheless, the shoulder, when disordered, can cause cervical pain, thus forming a double component to the shoulder symptoms. Visceral disorders accompanied by pain can do the same thing, and thereby produce a situation where there is a mixture of vertebral and visceral components, which adds to the difficulty of assessing the differential diagnosis and thus prognosis. Even so, the cervical spine can cause shoulder pain but not pathological change, and it would seem reasonable to assume that the same applies to visceral pathology – that is, it cannot arise from the thoracic spine.

Three further factors to note about the thoracic spine are that:

1. The upper/mid-thoracic spine, the ribs and their attachments can influence the scapulothoracic and shoulder regions. This can be by directly referring symptoms or by influencing the dynamic postural stabilization and relative mobility of the shoulder and shoulder girdle. The lower thoracic spine and the transitional thoracolumbar region may influence disorders of the lumbo-pelvic region in a similar way.

2. The sympathetic chains are in close proximity to the costovertebral joints. Evans (1997) has suggested that arthritic costovertebral joints can cause mechanical irritation of the sympathetic chains. Subtle autonomic symptoms, especially in the limbs, may well be a consequence of such mechanical irritation.

3. Mobilization or manipulation of the thoracic spine and ribs may be necessary after thoracic or open heart surgery. In fact, trauma to the ribcage during surgery may well result in postoperative musculoskeletal pain and stiffness.

## SUBJECTIVE EXAMINATION

*Table 11.1* outlines the subjective examination for the thoracic spine. One item that is peculiar to this area is the effect of breathing on the patient's symptoms.

Inspiration frequently causes pain, expiration does so far less commonly, and if a patient answers that breathing is unaffected he should be asked to take in a deep breath, gradually sniffing more and more into the lungs to prove the point. This is because, if his symptoms are mild or intermittent, his normal expansion does not reach the range of movement that provokes pain.

When listening to the patient's story of his pain problem, one must bear in mind the costochondral articulations and the scapulothoracic movement as well as the obvious costovertebral and intervertebral joints.

## 'KIND' OF DISORDER

> More often than not the patient does not associate his symptoms with the thoracic spine, even though they may well be generated from this spinal region

Often it is not so obvious that the thoracic spine is involved from the patient's initial complaints. The main problem may be 'pressure' headaches, or aching at the back of the shoulder or over the pelvis. Heaviness and tiredness of the arms or legs may well be the only clue. Understandably the patient does not associate the thoracic spine with symptoms in these seemingly unrelated areas, unless there has been an obvious trauma to the thoracic spine or a predisposing activity such as heavy or unusual work which has strained the thoracic structures.

Consequently, if a patient complains of neck pain or shoulder pain or low backache in the absence of movement restriction in the neck or low back, it is worth examining the thoracic spine.

Examination of the thoracic spine may also be crucial in the differential diagnosis of the patient's chest, abdominal or kidney pains, or 'indigestion' in cases where medical investigation has proved unremarkable.

## ASSOCIATED SYMPTOMS

> Disorders of the thoracic spine are often accompanied by symptoms originating from the autonomic nervous system

**Table 11.1**    Thoracic spine. Subjective examination

---

**'Kind' of disorder**
Establish why patient has been referred for or sought treatment:
   (i)    Pain, stiffness, weakness, instability, etc.
   (ii)   Acute onset.
   (iii)  Post-surgical, trauma, MUA, support, traction, etc.

**History**
Recent and previous (see 'History' below)
Sequence of questioning about history can be varied.

**Area**
Is the disorder one of pain, stiffness, recurrence, weakness, etc.?
Record on the 'body chart':
1. Area and depth of symptoms indicating main areas and stating types of symptoms.
2. Paraesthesia and anaesthesia.
3. Check for symptoms all other associated areas, i.e.:
   (i)    other vertebral areas;
   (ii)   joints above and below the disorder;
   (iii)  other relevant joints.

**Behaviour of symptoms**
**General**
1. When are they present or when do they fluctuate and why (associate/dissociate with day's activities, bed/pillow, inflammation).
2. Effect of rest on the local and referred symptoms (associate/dissociate with day's activities, bed/pillow, size/content, inflammation). (Compare symptoms on rising in the morning with end of day.)
3. Pain and stiffness on rising: duration of.
4. Effect of activities. (Beginning of day compared with end of day.)

**Particular**
1. What provokes symptoms – what relieves (severity – irritability)?
2. Any sustained positions provoke symptoms?
3. Are quick movements painless?
4. Where is pain felt on full inspiration, expiration, coughing or sneezing?

**Special questions**
1. Does the patient have bilateral tingling in the feet, or any disturbance of gait (cord signs).
2. General health and relevant weight loss. (Medical history.)
3. Have recent X-rays been taken?
4. What tablets are being taken for this and other conditions (osteoporosis from extensive steroid therapy)?

**History**
1. Of this attack.
2. Of previous attacks, or of associated symptoms.
3. Are the symptoms worsening or improving?
4. Prior treatment and its effect.
5. Socio-economic history as applicable.

HIGHLIGHT MAIN FINDINGS WITH ASTERISKS

---

Disorders of the thoracic spine are often accompanied by associated symptoms other than those generally accepted as being of neuromusculoskeletal origin. The reason for this may lie in the presence of overlapping visceral disease or mechanical irritation of the sympathetic chains in the thoracic spine. A relevant question to ask at this stage may be, 'If the pain between your shoulder blades disappeared, would you be cured?'. Further spontaneous information about associated symptoms may then be revealed. Symptoms commonly associated with thoracic disorders include pressure-type headaches, lightheadedness, nausea, tiredness, 'heavy' arms and legs, swelling of the extremities, excessive sweating, temperature changes of the extremities, depression and anxiety.

Because of the autonomic nervous system supply to the limbs, trunk and head, thoracic spine disorders can manifest as symptoms anywhere in the body. Therefore, when patients complain of generalized, non-segmental, vague heaviness or paraesthesia in the limbs, trunk or head, the thoracic spine should be considered as an area worthy of further investigation. It is very important therefore to define the area of pain. Suggestions as to the distributions were made on page 115, but there are two other important matters. The first is that the thoracic spine quite frequently causes symptoms and signs of irritation and conduction faults of the posterior primary ramus. Three posterior primary rami in the thoracic spine of interest to the manipulative physiotherapist are T2, T7 and T12. These rami are long loops, and therefore supply areas well away from their origin. *Figure 11.1a* shows the areas supplied by these rami. Secondly, there are far fewer occurrences of nerve-root compression. Nevertheless, assessment for sensory changes must be kept in mind, particularly if the patient's pain is distributed in an area that inclines parallel to the anatomical position of the ribs.

Also, the first rib can be singled out for its typical pattern of presentation when stiff or sore (*Figure 11.1b*).

## BEHAVIOUR OF SYMPTOMS

Due to the vagueness of some symptoms originating in the thoracic spine (e.g. limb heaviness/tiredness), the patient often has difficulty establishing a pattern of behaviour of these symptoms. There may be vague relationships to position, posture or activity, but these are often inconsistent and do not necessarily occur on a daily basis. For example, the patient may report that 'Sometimes my arms become very HEAVY and tire easily when I am working with them above my head. But sometimes they can start aching when I'm sitting down'. In such cases there is little value in pursuing the symptoms behaviour to the *n*th degree, as the patient just does not know what consistently aggravates and eases his symptoms. More value may be gained by noting, in detail, the behaviour of less obvious but consistent 'comparable' signs and symptoms emanating from the thoracic spine. The behaviour of 'stiffness' between the shoulder blades may be a more consistent means of evaluating treatment effects. The patient may admit, 'Ah yes, my upper back always feels stiff in the morning, but I thought that this was because I'm getting

(a)

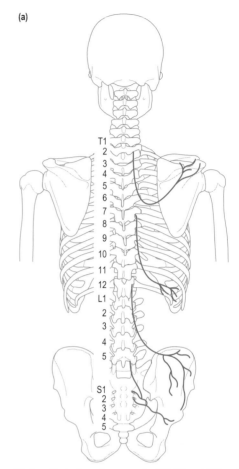

**Figure 11.1a**  Posterior primary rami of T2, T7 and T12 and the areas they supply

older'. Such associated symptoms are part of an acceptable level of aches and pains to the patient, rather than part of the wider spectrum of his disorder.

Likewise, the patient will recognize his limitations in retrospect. He may admit, 'Thinking about it, I've noticed that when I play golf my swing has gradually deteriorated because my upper back is getting stiffer'.

Detailed questioning about the behaviour of the symptoms in the thoracic spine may be a means of helping to **differentiate** the source of the symptoms. For example, a patient may complain about experiencing pain in the scapula whilst reversing his car and twisting his head and body to do so. This pain may be cervical in origin (Cloward, 1959), and specific questioning can help to determine this. Ask whether the patient feels the scapula pain when turning his body or his neck itself. Once an activity that reproduces the symptoms has been established, the potential source of these symptoms can be clarified with specifically detailed questions.

(b)

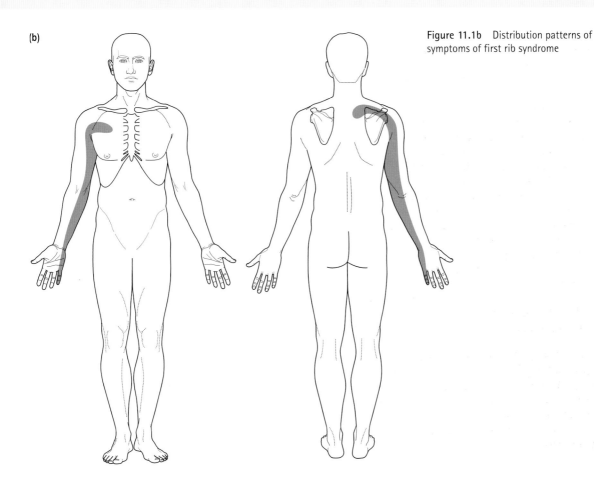

**Figure 11.1b**   Distribution patterns of symptoms of first rib syndrome

## SPECIAL QUESTIONS

> Special questions need to be covered thoroughly; potential visceral, respiratory and cardiac disease should be considered, and spinal tumours occur more readily in the thoracic spine. Furthermore, developmental abnormalities and juvenile disease should not be overlooked when children and adolescents present with thoracic pain

In the presence of thoracic symptoms, the manipulative physiotherapist should always be aware of non-neuromusculoskeletal sources. Medical history and relevant medical symptoms should be detailed. In this way, the manipulative physiotherapist is constantly questioning and stretching the boundaries of her own diagnostic abilities. Potential visceral, respiratory or cardiac involvement should always be considered, as should the propensity for spinal tumours and metastases to occur in the thoracic spine. The thoracic spine may be a site for developmental abnormalities such as scoliosis, juvenile disease such as Scheuermann's disease and inflammatory arthritis such as ankylosing spondylitis. The manipulative physiotherapist must look more deeply at the problem when the given diagnosis is 'growing pains' in adolescence. Communication is especially important with children and adolescents. The manipulative physiotherapist must gain the trust of the child, thus giving them the confidence to express themselves. The child or adolescent often instinctively 'knows' what the problem is, and therapists need to be skilled at gaining the appropriate information (*see* Chapter 3, p. 28).

## HISTORY

Involvement of the thoracic spine and rib cage may be established if there is a clear incident, trauma or predisposing activity. Examples of this mode of onset include a direct blow to the ribcage or thoracic spine during a fall, rib fractures, a 'whiplash' injury, or following thoracic surgery.

Insidious onset of symptoms may be related to a change of job, or to unusual or heavy work. For example, the patient may say 'I've started working more on my computer recently', or 'I've started aerobics and I find some of the exercises difficult because I am not mobile enough'.

> Disorders with thoracic spine components often do not recover at the rate that would be expected. In such cases, it is likely that maintained sympathetic outflow is influencing the stability and progression of the disorder

In some cases thoracic symptoms may vary from day to day, suggesting an element of disorder instability. Expected recovery may not occur at the rate it should. The patient thinks his symptoms are resolving, but then they come back as strong as ever for no apparent reason. In such cases a strong involvement of the autonomic nervous system is evident. 'Desensitization' of excessive sympathetic outflow by mobilizing the thoracic spine, ribs and related neural tissue is often required before the disorder stabilizes and the recovery commences (Wright, 1995).

## PHYSICAL EXAMINATION

*Table 11.2* lists the examination tests that are used, although not every listed movement is required for every patient.

## OBSERVATION

Observation of the thoracic spine is often unremarkable. Postural adaptations such as rounded shoulders, pseudowinging of the scapulae, poking chin, flat thorax, kyphosis and scoliosis of the thoracic spine may be evident. However, these observations need to be related to the patient's signs and symptoms to be of significance.

## PRESENT PAIN

Before starting examination of active functional movements of the thoracic spine the patient should always be asked whether he has any symptoms at present, and if so what and where they are. It is important that the assessment of the pain (symptoms) responsive to movement starts here.

## FUNCTIONAL DEMONSTRATION (AND DIFFERENTIATION WHERE APPROPRIATE)

Although the patient may not be able to perform a specific functional demonstration reproducing his symptoms, there may be a few cases when a functional demonstration or an 'injuring movement' will be useful to the manipulative physiotherapist.

One example is the patient who is able to reproduce his chest pain by taking a deep breath as mentioned earlier. In other cases it may be possible to differentiate the vertebral level responsible for the patient's symptoms using the functional demonstration. For example, when a patient has symptoms in the upper thorax area posteriorly, it is often difficult to determine whether the symptoms are arising from the cervicothoracic junction (or even C5/6 or C6/7) or the upper thoracic intervertebral joints. The procedure to differentiate between them if pain is reproduced by rotation is as follows:

1. With the patient seated and facing straight ahead towards the physiotherapist, he is asked whether he has any symptoms or not (*Figure 11.1c(A)*).

2. Assuming that his symptoms can only be provoked at the end of the range of rotation, he is asked to turn his head fully to the right with his trunk still facing straight ahead. If he feels no change in symptoms, the physiotherapist applies over-pressure to the cervical rotation by pressing her right forearm behind his right shoulder and her right hand behind the back of his head on the right side, while also placing her left hand against his left zygomatic arch. In this position she is able to apply over-pressure to the cervical area without movement of his shoulders. This test is not testing cervical rotation to the exclusion of any thoracic rotation, as the upper thoracic spine does also rotate somewhat. Nevertheless, it is a useful attempt at differentiating (*Figure 11.1c(B)*).

3. Once the pain response with over-pressure to cervical rotation is assessed, the patient is asked to rotate his thorax to the right without there being any rotation of the head to the right. The physiotherapist applies over-pressure to the thoracic rotation by applying further rotary pressure through his shoulders (*Figure 11.1c(C)*).

4. With the pain response noted when over-pressure is applied to the thoracic rotation, the patient is then asked to turn his head fully to the right and any further change in symptoms is noted. If there is a change of symptoms when the cervical spine is rotated to the right, then movement of the cervical

Table 11.2   Thoracic spine. Physical examination

---

### Observation
Posture, willingness to move.

### Brief appraisal

### Movements
*Movements to pain or move to limit*
F, E; LF Ⓛ and Ⓡ in F and E, Rot$^n$ Ⓛ and Ⓡ in F and E, pain and behaviour, range, countering protective deformity, localizing, over-pressure, intervertebral movement (repeated movement and increased speed).

### When applicable, sitting
Neck movements should be tested for upper thoracic pain. Cervical rotation may need to be superimposed onto thoracic rotation for testing upper thoracic joints.
Sustained E, LF towards pain, Rot$^n$ towards pain (when necessary to reproduce referred pain).
Tap test (when F, E, LF and Rot$^n$ & tap are negative).
Compression and distraction (when F, E, LF & Rot$^n$ & tap are negative).
Combined movement tests.
Active peripheral joint tests.
First rib.
Intercostal, costovertebral.
PPIVM $T_4$–$T_{12}$ F, E, LF, Rot$^n$.
Canal (slump sitting) tests.

### Supine
Passive neck F; range, pain (back and/or referred).
SIJ (ankylosing spondylitis).
First rib.
Neurological examination (sensation).
Passive peripheral joint tests.

### Side lying
PPIVM $C_7$–$T_4$ F, F, LF, Rot$^n$. $T_4$–$T_{12}$ Rot$^n$.

### Prone
'Palpation'
   Temperature and sweating.
   Soft-tissue palpation (muscle & interspinous space).
   Position of vertebrae and ribs especially 1st rib.
   Passive accessory intervertebral movement, costovertebral and intercostal movement (↕ ⇢ ⇠ ⌐ ⌐↓ spine and ribs).
   Combined PAIVM tests with physiological movement positions.
   Isometric tests for muscle pain.

### Examination of other relevant factors

### OTHER TESTS
Check 'case notes' for reports of relevant tests (X-rays, blood tests).

HIGHLIGHT IMPORTANT FINDINGS WITH ASTERISKS.

### INSTRUCTIONS TO PATIENT
(i)    Warning of possible exacerbation.
(ii)   Request to report details.
(iii)  Instructions in 'back care' if required.

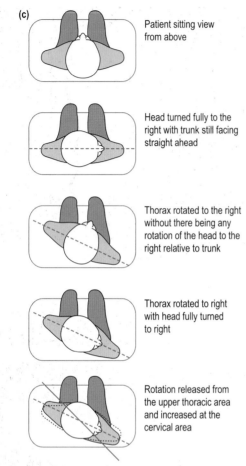

**(c)**

Patient sitting view from above

Head turned fully to the right with trunk still facing straight ahead

Thorax rotated to the right without there being any rotation of the head to the right relative to trunk

Thorax rotated to right with head fully turned to right

Rotation released from the upper thoracic area and increased at the cervical area

**Figure 11.1c**   (A) Patient sitting, view from above. (B)–(E) Various rotation positions

spine must be involved in the patient's symptoms (*Figure 11.1c(D)*).

5. While in the position described above, the physiotherapist changes her application of over-pressure from the upper thoracic area to cervical rotation to the right while at the same time allowing the patient to release the upper thoracic rotation slightly, and the change in symptoms is assessed. With this change of over-pressure, the emphasis of the rotation is released from the upper thoracic area and increased at the cervical area (*see Figure 11.1c(E)*).

## BRIEF APPRAISAL

When the functional demonstration provides valuable information about the sources of the patient's symptoms, the manipulative physiotherapist should briefly appraise the areas involved to give clues to further examination. From the example above, if the thoracic spine appears

to be involved more, detailed examination of this area can commence. The cervical spine should also be tested quickly so that it can be excluded or cleared of involvement.

## THORACIC ROTATION

Thoracic rotation can be assessed in many different positions, but the first position chosen should be that indicated by the patient in response to the question, 'Is there any turning or twisting movement which *you* find provokes your symptoms?'. It may be that he responds with demonstrating his golf swing as the example. Under these circumstances it is necessary to determine at what point in the movement the pain is provoked, so that the passive movement can be assessed more specifically.

Rotation can also be assessed in the standing position, with or without the help of outstretched arms or folded arms. Such rotation is more likely to detect movement of the lower thoracic spine.

With the patient in the sitting position and with his arms folded, ask him to 'hug' himself; rotation can be tested in the erect or extended position of the thoracic spine, and this can be compared with the same rotation but performed in the flexed position. Over-pressure to the movement can be performed by continuing the rotation via pressure against the scapula and pectoral areas (*Figure 11.2a*).

Upper thoracic rotation can be performed in the sitting position, with the patient clasping his hands behind his occiput and the physiotherapist stabilizing his lower thoracic area. In this position, if the patient turns his head and shoulders to the left, with his head kept in a static position in relation to his shoulders, the main movement will occur in the upper and middle thoracic spine.

## THORACIC FLEXION, EXTENSION

Upper thoracic flexion and extension are included in the examination of neck movements, and lower thoracic flexion and extension are included in the examination of lumbar spine movements. Midthoracic flexion and extension are examined by asking the patient to clasp his hands behind his head whilst in the sitting position, and point his elbows forwards so that they come together.

### Flexion

Having adopted the above position, the patient is then instructed to curl his elbows into his groin to produce thoracic flexion. The therapist notes the range of

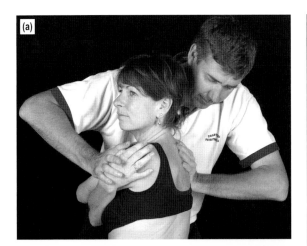

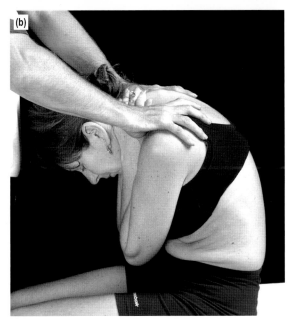

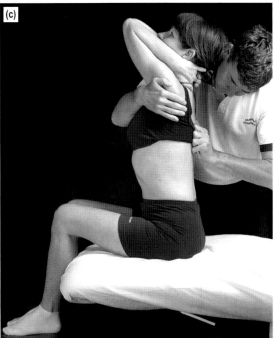

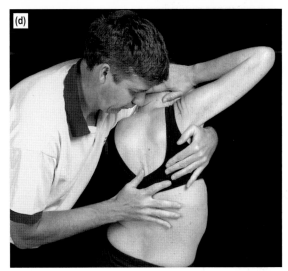

**Figure 11.2**    Examples of adding over-pressure: (*a*) adding over-pressure to thoracic rotation; (*b*) adding over-pressure to thoracic flexion; (*c*) adding localized over-pressure to thoracic extension; (*d*) adding localized over-pressure to thoracic lateral flexion

movement, symptom response and quality of movement. If necessary, over-pressure can be added via the supraclavicular and suprascapular areas. The therapist stands in front of the patient and places her hands over the top of his shoulders with her fingers posteriorly and her thumbs anteriorly. Over-pressure is applied in the direction of the continuing arc of flexion. Over-pressure directed cranially, horizontally or caudally can put emphasis on the upper, middle and lower parts of the thoracic spine respectively (*Figure 11.2b*).

### Extension

The same starting position as for flexion is adopted, with one exception: the patient places one or both feet on a chair in order to flex the lumbar spine. The patient is instructed to direct his elbows upwards. The therapist notes the range, symptom response and quality of movement. If necessary, over-pressure can be added by the therapist, who stands by the side of the patient and places an arm under both his axillae and across his sternum. She places the other hand on his thoracic spine to localize the over-pressure, at the same time side-flexing her trunk in the direction of the thoracic extension (*Figure 11.2c*).

## THORACIC LATERAL FLEXION

Lateral flexion of the upper and lower thoracic spine is incuded in the examination of the cervical and lumbar spines respectively. To localize lateral flexion to the mid-thoracic spine in sitting, the patient is asked to place his hands behind his head and direct his elbows away from his body. He is then instructed to curl his elbows into his side. The range, symptom response and quality of movement is noted. Over-pressure can be applied locally at each intervertebral level by the manipulative physiotherapist standing by the right side of the patient. Taking right lateral flexion as an example, she places her right axilla on his right shoulder and holds under his left axilla with her right hand. Her left thumb is then placed against the side of each spinous process of the thoracic spine in turn, and she bends her knees to increase the thoracic lateral flexion (*Figure 11.2d*).

## WHEN APPLICABLE TESTS

### Combined movement tests

If, at this stage of examination, the patient's symptoms have not been reproduced or comparable signs have not been found, when applicable tests such as combined movements can be used. The sequence of combined movements should reflect the patient's functional limitations.

The following example is but one of many sequences of combined movements that can be used in the examination of the thoracic spine. In the example, thoracic rotation to the left is the starting position, to which is added in turn lateral flexion to the left, lateral flexion to the right, extension and flexion.

1.  With the patient sitting he is asked to turn fully to the left, and when the physiotherapist has added over-pressure to this movement his symptoms are assessed (*Figure 11.3*).

2.  While over-pressure is maintained for rotation to the left, the physiotherapist laterally flexes the patient's trunk to the left while at the same time assessing changes in symptoms. It is important, *during* the movement of lateral flexion to the left, that the same strength of pressure to the rotation is maintained. This is not as easy as it may seem; with her right axilla stabilizing his right shoulder she must follow his lateral flexion (*Figure 11.4*).

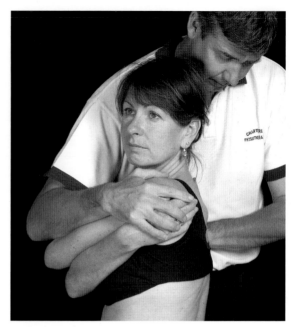

**Figure 11.3**    Over-pressure added to thoracic rotation to the left

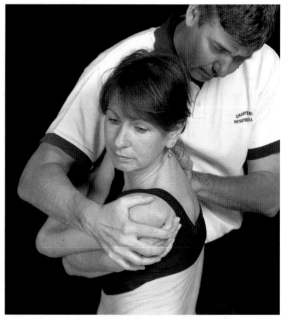

**Figure 11.4**    Adding lateral flexion to the left to the rotation to the left

3.  The physiotherapist then laterally flexes his trunk to the right, again using her right axilla to stabilize and control the lateral flexion, while noting changes in symptoms. Once more, it is necessary to retain

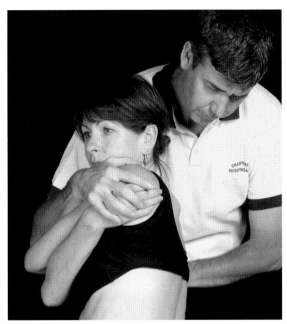

**Figure 11.5** Adding lateral flexion to the right to the rotation to the left

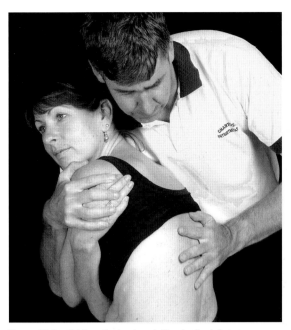

**Figure 11.6** Adding flexion to rotation to the left

the same strength to the rotary over-pressure (*Figure 11.5*).

4. To the sustained over-pressure of the thoracic rotation to the left, the physiotherapist then adds flexing at the appropriate level of the thoracic spine and assesses the changes in symptoms (*Figure 11.6*).
5. To the sustained over-pressure to the thoracic rotation to the left, the physiotherapist then adds thoracic extension at the appropriate level while noting changes in symptoms. To produce the extension, the physiotherapist uses her right forearm as a fulcrum while using her two hands to extend the patient's thoracic spine (*Figure 11.7*).

## COMPRESSION MOVEMENT TESTS

All of the physiological movements can be performed both with and without compression. The patient sits with his arms folded, and the physiotherapist stands behind him and stabilizes his thorax with her body, applying the compression by putting her forearms around in front of his shoulders and grasping over his supraspinous fossa area with her hands. She then uses her hands in conjunction with her upper sternum (at approximately his T3 level) to increase her body weight gradually, thus pushing through his thoracic spine towards the floor.

Localized oscillatory movements of flexion, extension, lateral flexion and rotation can then be performed

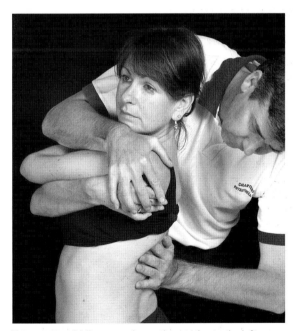

**Figure 11.7** Adding extension to the rotation to the left

while the compression is maintained. It is uncommon in the thoracic spine that the addition of compression makes any difference to the pain response found when the same movement or movements were performed without compression.

## TAP TEST

If active movements are full and symptom free, the patient sits on the plinth with the spine flexed and each spinous process of the thoracic spine and the rib angle are tapped with a reflex hammer. One spinous process or rib angle may exhibit exquisite tenderness over and above any of the others. In some cases, this resonance effect may be a way of detecting bone demineralization, stress fracture or bone tumour.

## SLUMP TEST

This test should form part of the examination of the thoracic spine. However, it is essential to remember that this test causes pain at approximately the T8/T9 area in at least 90 per cent of all subjects. If the patient does experience pain at T8 or T9 and it is for this pain that he seeks treatment, and if the pain is increased during the slump test, then the only way in which a decision implicating the canal structures as a component of the cause of his disorder can be made is to balance it against the physiotherapist's knowledge and experience of what is within the considered norms for this test.

The long sitting slump can be used as an adaptation of the slump test to emphasize the testing of the mobility of the canal structures of the thoracic spine. In this position and with the addition of trunk side flexion to the left, for example, the ribs can be examined and treated on the right. This is a means of influencing the sympathetic chains via the slump position and movement of the costovertebral joints.

Other neurodynamic tests such as the upper limb neural tests (ULNTs), the straight leg raise (SLR), prone knee bend (PKB) and passive neck flexion (PNF) may also be considered as part of the thoracic spine examination.

## PALPATION

The patient lies prone with his arms by his side or over the edge of the couch to widen the interscapular space.

### Areas of sweating and temperature changes

It is not uncommon to find areas of increased temperature situated centrally in the thoracic spine. These areas do not indicate information of either mechanical or pathological origin

The presence of any localized areas of sweating is determined first. Temperature changes are assessed by wiping the backs of the fingers or hands over the thoracic area, particularly in the area between the angles of the ribs or the left and right sides. It is not uncommon to find 9 cm areas situated centrally which do not indicate inflammation of either mechanical or pathological disorders.

### Soft-tissue changes

Thickening of the interspinous tissue and the tissues in the interlaminar trough area is extremely informative. The thickening can be totally lateral, and can be expected to be found on the same side and at the appropriate intervertebral level as unilateral pain. The thickening can extend over more than one level on the same side, or it can be on the left side of, say, T5/6 and the right side of T4/5 and T6/7. The texture of the thickenings can clearly sort them into new and old changes. This sorting is far more difficult in the low lumbar area.

Quite often thoracic physiological, combined movements and movements under compression are pain free. However, palpation anomalies can always be found

At a first consultation, if a patient has upper abdominal pain of skeletal origin it is common for all physiological movements to be pain free even when combined movements and movements under compression are tested. However, palpation anomalies can always be found, provided the examination is perceptively performed and related to the history of progression of the disorder. This reliability makes palpation a skill that should be learned by all general surgeons.

### Bony changes and position tests

The two most common findings when examining the position of the spinous processes in relation to each other in the thoracic spine are:

1. A spinous process that feels to be more deeply set than its abnormally prominent adjacent spinous process above. This is the most informative finding, indicating either that it is the source of a patient's symptoms or that it is a disadvantaged intervertebral area which has the potential to cause symptoms if placed under excessive stress.
2. One spinous process displaced to one side in relation to the spinous process above and below.

This only indicates rotation of the vertebra when it is confirmed by being able to tell that one transverse process is more posteriorly positioned in comparison with the vertebra's transverse process on the opposite side. That is to say, if the spinous process of T6 is displaced to the right, this displacement only indicates rotation of the vertebra if the transverse process of T6 on the left is more prominent (or posteriorly positioned) than the transverse process of T6 on the right. This is rarely the case, and it is surprising to find how often a patient's symptoms, when related to this malalignment, are found to be on the same side as that to which the spinous process is deviated.

When one spinous process is deeply set and the adjacent spinous process above is prominent, pressure over the prominent spinous process usually provokes a superficial sharp pain while pressure over the sore deeply-set spinous process, if firm and sustained, produces a very deeply felt pain. These findings indicate that the joint between them is abnormal and is the possible site of origin of symptoms.

## PASSIVE ACCESSORY INTERVERTEBRAL MOVEMENTS (PAIVMs)

> The two main movements to be tested in the thoracic spine are central postero-anterior and transverse vertebral pressure

The two main movements to be tested in the thoracic spine are postero-anterior central vertebral pressure and transverse vertebral pressure, and these are described on pages 310–311 and 320. As has been stated before, these movements can be varied both in the point of contact that produces them and in the inclination of movement. The other movement that is important for examination purposes by palpation is postero-anterior unilateral vertebral pressure, which is described on pages 321–323. It is also essential that costovertebral and intercostal movements be assessed for their range and pain response. These are described respectively on pages 323 and 323–324.

In earlier editions of this book, in the chapter regarding selection of techniques, the suggestion was made that the direction of transverse pressures should be performed initially towards the side of pain. This statement is based on the fact that the technique opens the intervertebral space on the side of pain, thus avoiding provoking pain. This is not to say that the technique should never be performed in the opposite

direction, and nor should provoking the pain be the aim, as will now be explained.

The usefulness of a 'D-plus-I' response was described in Chapter 6, and use of it should be made in chronic disorders when other test movements are uninformative. Therefore, when a patient with a chronic skeletal disorder causing unilateral referred pain is examined at the first consultation, part of the palpation examination that should be emphasized is the use of transverse pressure from the side of the referred pain against the spinous process of three or four adjacent vertebrae at the appropriate level. The aim is to endeavour to provoke the referred pain. If this is not achieved at the first consultation, its repetition may sensitize the joint at fault and thus make the same transverse pressure provoke the referred pain at the second consultation – i.e. on 'D-plus- I' (D + I).

## DIFFERENTIATION TEST BY PALPATION

When transverse pressure on, say, T7 to the right provokes the patient's pain, it may be necessary to determine whether the symptoms are arising from the T7/8 intervertebral joint or the T7/6 intervertebral joint. The technique for doing this has been described fully on page 162.

## PASSIVE RANGE OF PHYSIOLOGICAL MOVEMENTS OF SINGLE VERTEBRAL JOINTS (PPIVMs)

As has been stated before, the oscillatory testing movement is performed more slowly (as a general rule) than it is when used as a treatment technique. This is only so because sometimes the through-range quality of movement is less easily appreciated with quicker movements. The end-of-range feel can sometimes be determined by applying an over-pressure component to the testing oscillatory movement.

The movements are described below for the selected intervertebral levels.

### C7–T4 (flexion)

*Starting position*

With the patient sitting, the physiotherapist stands in front of him and slightly to the patient's right. She rests her left hand over his right shoulder with the middle finger positioned between two spinous processes, while the index finger palpates the upper margin of the spinous process of the upper vertebra and the ring finger palpates the lower margin of the lower spinous

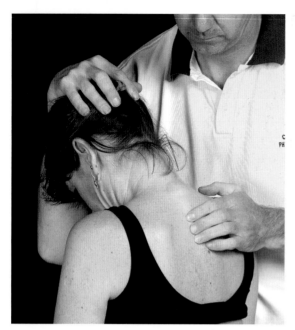

**Figure 11.8**   Intervertebral movement. C7–T4 (flexion)

process. To produce a firm yet comfortable grasp with the left hand, the pad of the thumb is placed in the supraclavicular fossa. The right hand and forearm are placed over the top of the patient's head so that they lie in the sagittal plane. The fingers and thumb grasp the occiput near the nuchal lines, and the wrist is flexed to permit firm pressure on the front of the head by the forearm (*Figure 11.8*).

### Method

Movement of the patient's head is controlled by the physiotherapist's right hand and forearm. All scalp looseness must be taken up by the grasp between the fingers and forearm to permit complete control of the patient's head and make him feel that support of his head can be left to the physiotherapist.

As the amount of movement that can be felt at this level is much less than elsewhere in the vertebral column, two complementary actions are necessary to produce the maximum intervertebral movement. First, the oscillation of the head and neck needs to be through a range at least of 30° performed near the limit of forward flexion. Secondly, because the lever producing movement is long, pressure by the three palpating fingers over the spine will help to localize movement as the head is moved back through a range of 30°.

The intervertebral movement is felt by the ring, middle and index fingers as the spinous processes move

away from and towards each other during the back and forth movements of the head and neck.

### C7–T4 (flexion/extension)

An alternative method for testing flexion, which is more convenient if rotation and lateral flexion are also to be tested, is performed with the patient lying on his side.

#### Starting position

The patient lies comfortably on his right side, near the forward edge of the couch, with his head resting on pillows. The physiotherapist stands in front of the patient, cradling his head in her left arm with her fingers covering the posterior surface of his neck, her little finger reaching down to the vertebral level being examined. She stabilizes his head between her left forearm and the front of her left shoulder. Next she leans across the patient, placing her right forearm along his back to stabilize his thorax, and palpates the undersurface of the interspinous space with the pad of her index or middle finger facing upwards (*Figure 11.9*).

#### Method

With her left arm, the physiotherapist flexes and extends the patient's lower neck as much as possible. The spine above C6 and the head are not flexed or extended, because movement in this area makes movement in the test area less controlled and less isolated. The patient's head and neck are moved only until the particular joint tested has come to the limit of its range.

### C7–T4 (lateral flexion)

#### Method

The starting position is identical with that described for flexion/extension. The purpose of this method is to achieve lateral flexion at the particular joint being tested, and therefore the head does not laterally flex but rather is displaced upwards. Lateral flexion is produced by the physiotherapist lifting the patient's head with a hugging grip of his head, the majority of the lift being achieved by the ulnar border of her left hand against the underside of his cervicothoracic junction (*Figure 11.10*). To test lateral flexion in the opposite direction, the patient must lie on his other side. The palpating finger feels for movement between the two adjacent spinous processes. The upper process moves first, and when the lower process starts to move this will signal the extent of the lateral flexion at this particular intervertebral level.

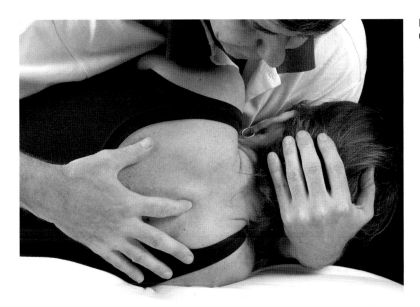

**Figure 11.9**    Intervertebral movement. C7–T4 (flexion/extension)

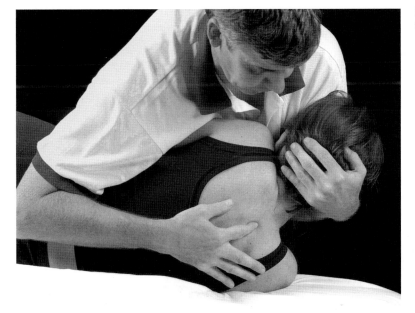

**Figure 11.10**    Intervertebral movement. C7–T4 (lateral flexion)

## C7–T4 (rotation)

### Method

The starting position is again the same as for flexion/extension. To produce the rotation properly, it is necessary to concentrate on moving the joint being examined without causing any tilting or flexing of the head and neck. Movement of the upper spinous process in relation to its distal neighbour is palpated through the pad of the physiotherapist's index or middle finger, which is facing upwards against the underside of the interspinous space.

With the patient's head cradled between the physiotherapist's left forearm and shoulder, and his lower neck firmly gripped in the ulnar border of her hand between the little finger and the hypothenar eminence, she rotates his lower cervical spine towards her. This is achieved by elevating her scapula to its highest point while maintaining a stable thorax (*Figure 11.11*). As the movement is difficult to achieve accurately, more

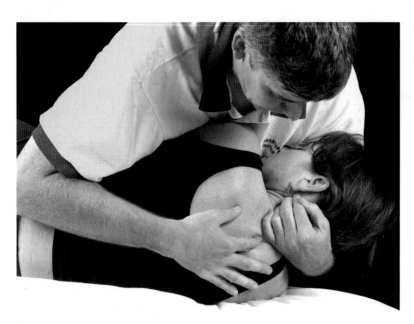

**Figure 11.11** Intervertebral movement. C7–T4 (rotation)

care is needed than with the other movements tested in this area.

## T4–11 (flexion/extension)

### Starting position

The patient sits with his hands clasped behind his neck while the physiotherapist, standing by his left side, places her left arm under his left upper arm and grasps his right upper arm in her supinated hand. She places her right hand across his spine just below the level being tested, and the pad of the tip of the middle finger in the far side of the interspinous space to feel adjacent spinous processes.

### Method

While the patient relaxes to allow his thorax to be flexed and extended, the physiotherapist takes the weight of his upper trunk on her left arm.

To test flexion, she lowers his trunk from the neutral position until movement can be felt to have taken place at her right middle finger; the patient is then returned to the neutral position by lifting under his arms. The oscillatory movement through an arc of approximately 20° of trunk movement is facilitated if the patient is held firmly and if the physiotherapist laterally flexes her trunk to the left as she lowers the trunk into flexion. This makes the return movement one of laterally flexing her trunk to the right rather than lifting with her left arm.

The extension part of the test is carried out in much the same way, except that the physiotherapist assists the trunk extension with the heel and ulnar border of her right hand. In doing this she must be careful to keep the pad of her middle finger in a constant position between the adjacent spinous processes. Movement of the patient's trunk is from the neutral position into extension. It is important to remember that it is movement at only one joint that is being examined, and therefore large trunk movements are not necessary; in fact they detract from the examination.

## T4–11 (lateral flexion)

### Starting position

The patient sits and holds his hands behind his neck or crosses his arms across his chest while the physiotherapist stands side-on behind his right side reaching with her right arm to hold high around and behind his left shoulder. She grips his trunk firmly between her right arm and her right side in her left axilla. This high grasp with the right hand is necessary for examination of the higher levels; as the examination extends below T8, so the grasp needs to be taken down to the lower scapular area. She places the heel of her left hand on the right side of his back at the level being examined, spreads her fingers for stability, and places the tip of the pad of her flexed middle finger in the far side of the interspinous space of the joint to be tested (*Figure 11.12*).

### Method

The physiotherapist laterally flexes the patient's trunk towards her by displacing his trunk away from her

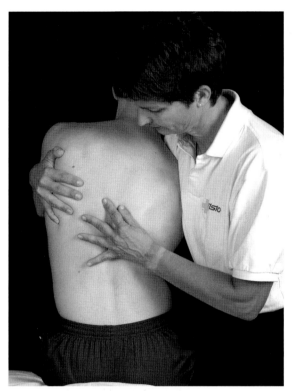

Figure 11.12   Intervertebral movement. T4–11 (lateral extension)

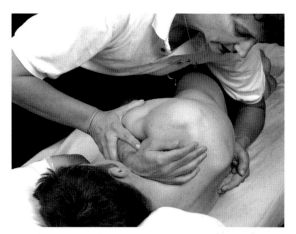

Figure 11.13   Intervertebral movement. T4–11 (rotation)

with the heel of her left hand and her costal margin, and laterally flexing his upper trunk by lifting her right arm and pressing downwards with her right axilla. She palpates for the interspinous movement through the pad of her middle finger, ensuring that during the lateral flexion her finger moves with the spine, maintaining even contact against the spinous processes. The palpating finger feels the space between the spinous processes open and close as the patient's trunk is laterally flexed and returned to the neutral position.

Lateral flexion in the opposite direction can be palpated without a change of position simply by laterally flexing the patient's trunk the other way. However, it is more accurate to change sides and reproduce the technique on the opposite side.

## T4–11 (rotation)

### Starting position

Although rotation can be tested in the sitting position, it is more easily and more successfully tested when the patient is lying down. The patient lies on his left side with his hips and knees comfortably flexed while the

physiotherapist, standing in front of the patient, leans over his trunk to cradle his pelvis between her left side and her left upper arm. This position stabilizes the patient's pelvis. The physiotherapist's forearm is then in line with the patient's spine, and her hand reaches the level where movement is to be examined. She then places her left hand on his spine with the pad of her middle finger facing upwards against the under-surface of the interspinous space to feel the bony margins of the adjacent spinous processes. With her right hand, she grasps as far medially as possible over the patient's suprascapular area and places her forearm over his sternum or grasps the patients elbow over his sternum (*Figure 11.13*).

### Method

The patient's trunk is repeatedly rotated back and forth by the physiotherapist's right forearm and hand through an arc of approximately 25°. Care must be taken to ensure that the movement does not include scapulothoracic movement. To examine movement in the upper thoracic intervertebral joints, the arc of movement should be performed just behind the frontal plane. As lower intervertebral joints are examined, the arc of rotation used to assess movement moves backwards until an arc of rotation between 40 and 60° from the frontal plane is used to examine the movement between T10 and T11. The palpating finger must follow the patient's trunk movement, and when movement occurs at the joint being examined, the upper spinous process will be felt to press into the pad of the middle finger, which is facing upwards. When the lower spinous process starts to move, this is the extent of rotation at the intervertebral level.

## EXAMINATION AND TREATMENT TECHNIQUES

## MOBILIZATION

### Postero–anterior central vertebral pressure (↕)

#### Starting position

The patient lies prone, either with his forehead resting on the backs of his hands or with his head comfortably turned to one side and his arms lying by his sides on the couch. The position depends on the amount of chest tightness created by the 'arms up' position, which is usually reserved for upper thoracic mobilization.

If the patient is on a low couch, the physiotherapist's position for mobilizing the upper thoracic spine (approximately T1–5) needs to be at the head of the patient with her shoulders over the area to be mobilized to enable the direction of the pressure to be at right angles to the surface of the body. The pads of the thumbs are placed on the spinous process, pointing transversely across the vertebral column, and the fingers of each hand are spread out over the posterior chest wall to give stability to the thumbs. As the spinous processes are large, the thumbs may be positioned tip to tip or with the tips side by side in contact with the upper and lower margins of the same spinous process. To gain the best control and feel of movement with the least discomfort to the patient, the pressure should be transmitted through the thumbs so that the interphalangeal joints are hyperextended. This enables the softest part of the pad to be flat over the spinous processes, with a slight degree of flexion in the metacarpophalangeal joints. Not only is this more comfortable for the patient, but it hinders the physiotherapist's intrinsic muscles from producing the pressure.

To mobilize the mid-thoracic spine (T5–9), the physiotherapist should stand at the patient's side with her thumbs placed longitudinally along the vertebral column so that they point towards each other. The fingers can then spread out over the posterior chest wall, to each side of the vertebral column above and below the thumbs.

It may be more comfortable (and this is far easier to do if the patient is lying on a low couch) for the physiotherapist to stand to one side of the patient, approximately at waist level and facing his head, and place the pads of the thumbs on the spinous process pointing across the vertebral column. The fingers of each hand can then spread over opposite sides of the posterior chest wall for stability.

For the lower thoracic spine (T10–12), the physiotherapist's position depends upon the shape of the patient's chest. Either of the latter two positions described

above may be used, but the essential factor is that the direction of the pressure must be at right angles to the body surface at the level. This means that the shoulders may need to be anywhere between vertically above the lower thoracic spine and vertically above the sacrum (*Figure 11.14*). If the patient has difficulty lying prone because extension is painful, a small pillow under the chest will assist. The physiotherapist's position must also allow pressure to be applied to the spinous process using the anteromedial aspect of the fifth metacarpal, similar to that described on pages 370–371 for the lumbar spine. However, it may be essential to avoid direct contact between the pisiform and the spinous process for the sake of comfort (*Figure 11.14*).

#### Method

The mobilizing is carried out by an oscillating pressure on the spinous processes, produced by the body and transmitted through the arms to the thumbs. It is important that this pressure is applied by the body weight over the hands and not by a squeezing action with the thumbs themselves. The fingers, which are spread out over the patient's back, should not exert any pressure but act only as stabilizers for the thumbs. It is easy to dissipate the pressure and lose the effectiveness of the thumbs by faulty use of the fingers.

If the physiotherapist's elbows are kept slightly flexed and the thumbs maintained in the position of hyperextension of interphalangeal joints and slight flexion of metacarpophalangeal joints, the pressure can be transmitted to the pads of the thumbs through this series of strong springs. This springing action at the joints can readily be seen as the body weight is applied during the mobilizing.

#### Local variations

The degree of pressure required in the upper thoracic spine to produce movement is far greater than that required in the cervical spine, and slightly stronger than that required for the remainder of the thoracic spine.

The degree of movement possible in the middle and lower thoracic spine is considerable, and it is here that it is easiest to learn a feeling of movement. The degree of movement possible in the upper thoracic spine is considerably limited, and this is particularly so between T1 and T2.

#### Uses

Postero-anterior central vertebral pressure is as useful for the thoracic spine as rotation is for the cervical

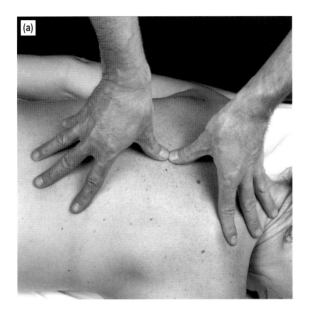

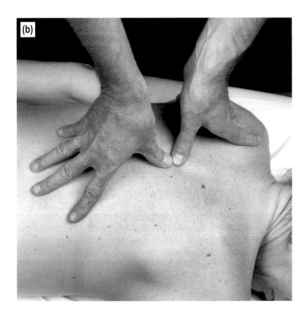

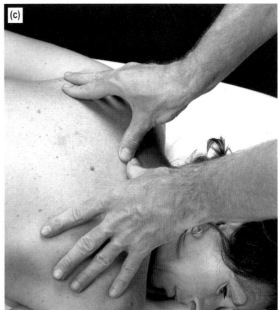

**Figure 11.14**    (*a*), (*b*) and (*c*) Thoracic region. Postero-anterior central vertebral pressure (↕)

spine. In all symptoms arising from the thoracic vertebrae, it is worth trying this procedure first.

'Central pressure' is more likely to be successful with symptoms that are situated in the midline or evenly distributed to each side of the body, but it should also be tried for unilateral symptoms, particularly if they are ill-defined or widespread in their distribution.

Examples of treatment include: glove distribution symptoms, page 438; thoracic backache, page 440; and traumatic girdle pain, pages 441–443.

## Rotary postero–anterior intervertebral pressures

### Starting position

The patient lies prone with his arms by his side while the manipulative physiotherapist stands alongside the patient (in this case by his right side). She places her right hand between the spine and his right scapula, and her left hand between the spine and his left scapula, and transmits pressure through the lateral surface of the hypothenar eminence near the pisiform bone.

To reach the final position, the first step is to place the ulnar border of each hand in a line across the patient's back in parallel lines, the right hand being slightly caudad to the joint to be mobilized and the left hand slightly distal to the joint to be mobilized. At this preliminary stage the physiotherapist's forearms are also directed across the patient's back at right angles to the vertebral column, and her pisiform bone is tucked into the space between the paravertebral muscles and the spinous processes. The next step entails taking up the slack in the soft tissues. This is achieved by applying both postero-anterior and rotary pressures; the rotary pressure is achieved by changing the direction of the forearms, in a swinging or twisting fashion, from across the body to somewhat caudad (the right arm) and cephalad (the left arm) as well as laterally. The final stage is that of being certain that all of the slack has been taken up and that the pisiform bones are now opposite each other at the same intervertebral level (T6/7; *Figure 11.15a*).

## Method

When used as a mobilization, the technique consists of an oscillatory movement with three directions; postero-anterior, cephalad and caudad, and lateral. It can be performed as a very localized movement by using the pisiform as the main contact point through which the pressure is transmitted, or it can be performed much more comfortably over a wider area by utilizing the base of the palm of the hand together with the thenar and hypothenar eminences.

The technique can be performed rhythmically with increasing and decreasing postero-anterior pressure in time with the patient's breathing rhythm.

It can also be used as a manipulative thrust, usually at the end of the patient's expiration. There are times when the technique can be usefully employed in the lumbar spine.

## Uses

The technique can be selected when movement is desired in a postero-anterior direction but the spinous processes are too tender for direct contact.

The ranges of movement of single costovertebral, costotransverse and intervertebral joints are quite small, and yet if this technique is performed through the palm of the hand as described above, quite considerable movement between three or four contiguous levels can be achieved. This can produce immediate comfort and improvement in movement (*Figure 11.15b*).

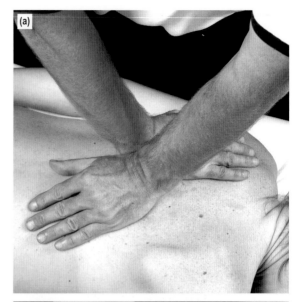

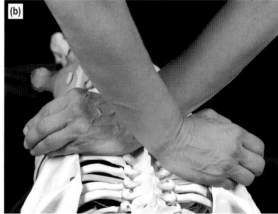

**Figure 11.15**   (*a*) Intervertebral movement, rotary postero-anterior movement mid thoracic–clockwise. (*b*) Movements shown on a skeleton mid thoracic–anticlockwise

## Transverse vertebral pressure (↔)

### Starting position

When the middle and lower thoracic vertebrae are to be mobilized with transverse pressures, the patient lies prone with his arms hanging over the sides of the couch or by his side to aid relaxation of the vertebral column. The head should be allowed to rest comfortably by being turned to one side, preferably towards the side where the physiotherapist stands. However, as this head position tends to produce some degree of rotation in the upper thoracic vertebrae, it is better for the patient to adopt the 'forehead rest' position when these vertebrae are to be mobilized in order to eliminate any rotation. Alternatively, some couches have a hole to allow the head to remain centrally placed. In some cases it may be useful to rotate or derotate the spine using the head position to produce the movement. If the mobilization technique needs to be performed strongly as a Grade IV+, it may help to ask the patient to face towards the manipulative physiotherapist.

The physiotherapist stands at the patient's right side at the level of the vertebrae to be mobilized, and places her hands on the patient's back so that the pads of the thumbs are adjacent to the right side of the spinous processes while the fingers are spread over the patient's left ribs. The left thumb acts as the point of contact and is fitted down into the groove between the spinous process and the paravertebral muscles, so that part of the pad of the thumb is pressed against the lateral aspect of the spinous process on its right-hand side. It is essential to have as much of the pad in contact with the spinous process as is possible. To prevent the thumb sliding off the spinous process, the palmar surface of the metacarpophalangeal joint of the index finger must be firmly brought down on top of the interphalangeal joint of the thumb. This is a valuable position to learn to adopt, as its stability is of value in other techniques. The right thumb, acting as reinforcement, is placed so that its pad lies over the nail of the left thumb. This thumb relationship is chosen because considerable effort is required to keep a single thumb comfortably against the spinous process.

The fingers of both hands should be well spread out over the chest wall to stabilize the thumbs, and the wrists need to be slightly extended to permit the pressure to be transmitted through the thumbs in the horizontal plane. Because of the slightly different functions required of the left and right thumbs, the left forearm is not as horizontal as the right forearm (*Figure 11.16*).

### Method

The pressure is applied to the spinous process through the thumbs by the movement of the trunk; alternate pressure and relaxation is repeated continuously to produce an oscillating type of movement of the intervertebral joint. For the gentler grades of mobilizing, very little pressure is needed. When stronger mobilizing is used, movement of the patient's trunk is involved and timing of pressures should coincide either with the patient's rolling or, in order to make the technique stronger, to go against the rolling.

### Local variations

The upper thoracic spinous processes (T1–3/4) are readily accessible but have a limited amount of movement,

T1 being almost immovable. The lower thoracic vertebrae (T8/9–12) are more easily moved and do not require great pressure. Local tenderness in these two areas is comparatively negligible. Mobilization of the mid-thoracic spine is made difficult by the relative inaccessibility of the spinous processes and natural tenderness, and when a painful condition is superimposed on this natural tenderness, adequate mobilization may be very difficult. Where stronger techniques are required to be performed for longer periods, better effect may be gained by reinforcing the contact thumb with the pisiform of the opposite hand rather than with the opposite thumb pad. In this way, the fingers can be spread over the chest wall and the movement can be produced through the thumb and hand via the therapist's trunk.

### Uses

This technique is particularly useful for pain of unilateral distribution in the thoracic area. In such cases the pressure is best applied against the side of the spinous process that is away from the pain, applying the pressure towards the patient's painful side. When using this technique it is frequently necessary to mobilize the ribcage by a postero-anterior pressure directed through the angle of the rib. If progression is needed, the manipulative physiotherapist may need to clear the joint signs by using pressure on the spinous process on the painful side and towards the pain-free side.

Examples of treatment include pain simulating cardiac disease, page 421; scapula pain, page 426; thoracic backache, page 440; traumatic girdle pain, pages 441–442; and abdominal pain and vague pains, page 443.

### Postero–anterior unilateral vertebral pressure ($\downarrow^{•}$)

#### Starting position

The patient lies prone with his head turned to the left and his arms hanging loosely over the sides of the couch or by his side.

To mobilize the left side of the middle or lower thoracic spine (approximately T5–12), the physiotherapist stands on the left side of the patient and places her hands on the patient's back so that the pads of the thumbs, pointing towards each other, lie over the transverse processes. The fingers of the left hand spread over the chest wall pointing towards the patient's head, while the fingers of the right hand point towards his feet and the thumbs are held in opposition. By applying a little pressure through the pads of the thumbs, they will sink into the muscle tissue adjacent to the

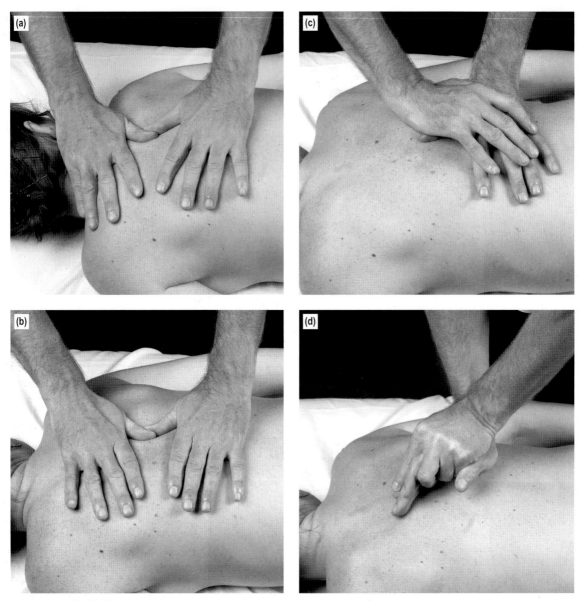

**Figure 11.16**    (a), (b), (c) and (d) Thoracic region. Transverse vertebral pressure (↔)

spinous processes until the transverse process is reached. The metacarpophalangeal joint of the thumb needs to be slightly flexed and the interphalangeal joint must be hyperextended to enable the pad of the thumb to transmit the pressure comfortably. When a much finer degree of localization of the pressure is required, the thumbnails should be brought together so that the tips of the thumbs make a very small but comfortable point of contact. In this position, the metacarpophalangeal joints of the thumbs are brought much closer together to lie directly above the thumb tips. The

physiotherapist's shoulders and arms, with slightly flexed elbows, should be in the direct line through which the pressure is to be applied, and this is at right angles to the plane of the body surface.

Because of the curve of the thoracic spine, it is necessary when mobilizing the upper levels (T1–4) to stand either at the patient's head or towards the shoulder of the side being mobilized to accommodate the necessarily altered angle of the physiotherapist's arms. It is advisable to use the largest amount of the pad of the thumb that can be brought into contact with the

factor of considerable importance. When the hands are used, the technique is frequently more vigorous than is required.

## Uses

Postero-anterior unilateral vertebral pressure is used, almost entirely, for unilateral distributed pain arising from the thoracic spine, and the technique is done on the painful side. Unless the patient's pain is severe, it is less likely to produce a favourable change in the patient's signs and symptoms if it is done on the side away from the pain. When this technique is used in the presence of spasm the pressure must be steadily applied and not hurried, in order to allow time for the spasm to relax.

## Postero–anterior unilateral costovertebral pressure ( ↓ )

### Starting position

The patient lies prone with his arms by his side or hanging over the sides of the couch, and the physiotherapist stands at the side of the patient where the mobilization is to be effected. The physiotherapist's thumbs are placed along the line of the rib at its angle so that the maximum area of contact can be made between the thumbs and the rib (*Figure 11.18a*). Alternatively, the whole ulnar border of the hand and little finger may be used to produce the movement (*Figure 11.18b*).

### Method

An oscillatory movement is transmitted to the rib by the thumbs or hands, and the range of movement produced at one rib angle is compared with that produced at the rib angles above and below. The pain produced by the movement of the faulty rib is also compared with the pain (if any) produced at the rib above and the rib below. Similarly, both the range of the movement and the pain should also be compared with the ribs on the opposite side of the body.

### Local variations

*First rib.* Examination of the first rib is somewhat different from that of the other ribs as the technique can be applied in three ways due to a greater area of the rib being palpable:

1.  The pressure can be applied against the rib posteriorly through the trapezius muscle, and the direction of the pressure is not only postero-anteriorly but is also inclined towards the feet (*Figure 11.19*).

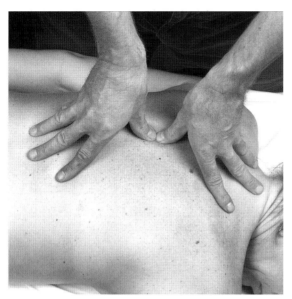

**Figure 11.17**   Thoracic region. Postero-anterior unilateral vertebral pressure ( ↓ )

transverse process, to enable the pressure to be administered as comfortably as possible (*Figure 11.17*).

## Method

A very steady application of pressure is necessary to be able to move some of the muscle belly out of the way and make bone-to-bone contact. As this procedure can be quite uncomfortable for the patient, care must be given to the position of the arms and hands to enable a spring-like action to take place at the elbows and the thumbs. This reduces the feeling of hardness and soreness between the physiotherapist's thumbs and the patient's transverse process that is present if the pressure is applied by intrinsic muscle action.

   Once the required depth has been reached, the oscillating movement at the intervertebral joint is produced by increasing and then decreasing the pressure produced by trunk movement.

## Local variations

Because of the structure and attachments of the ribcage, it is not possible to produce very much movement with this mobilization.

   Some people may find it easier to carry out the mobilization using the hands (as described for the lumbar spine) instead of the thumbs, but this should be discouraged as the thumbs have a greater degree of 'feel' and can localize the mobilization more accurately. They also cause much less discomfort to the patient – a

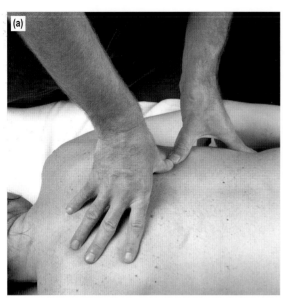

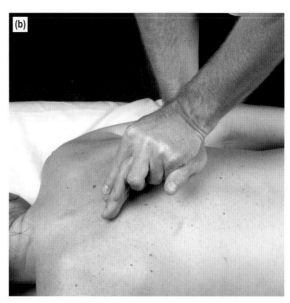

**Figure 11.18** (*a*) Postero-anterior unilateral costovertebral pressure using thumb. (*b*) Postero-anterior unilateral costovertebral pressure using hands ( )

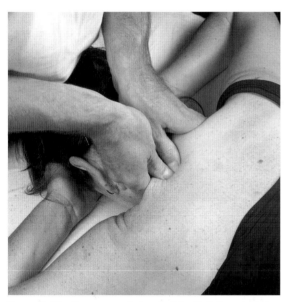

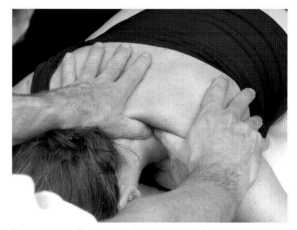

**Figure 11.20** Pressure applied against the first rib posteriorly under the trapezius

**Figure 11.19** Pressure applied against the first rib posteriorly through the trapezius

2. Alternatively, the physiotherapist can place her thumbs underneath (anterior to) the muscle belly of the trapezius and the direction of the pressure can be inclined a little more towards the feet as well as being postero-anteriorly directed (*Figure 11.20*).

3. For this next technique that mobilizes the first rib, the patient lies supine while the physiotherapist,

standing at the patient's shoulder level of the side to be treated, applies the pressure to produce the oscillatory anteroposterior and caudad movement on all parts of the first rib that are palpable (*Figure 11.21*). The symbol for this technique is ⌐ R1.

*Other ribs.* All of the ribs can be examined throughout their entire length by thumb palpation, including the costochondral junctions and the junction with the sternum. The freedom of movement between adjacent ribs can also be tested, but as these are not part of the vertebral column they are not described in this book. They

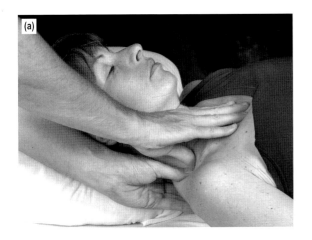

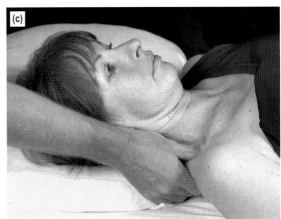

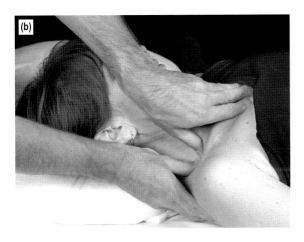

Figure 11.21   (a), (b) and (c) Pressure applied to the first rib anteriorly

are, however, described in *Peripheral Manipulation* (Maitland, 1970a).

A technique performed with the patient supine is described below.

### Uses

Whenever treatment is applied to the thoracic intervertebral joints, the inclusion of mobilization of the ribs should be considered for two reasons:

1. It is frequently difficult to assess whether a patient's pain arises from the intervertebral joint, the costovertebral joint or the costotransverse joint. Therefore, if mobilization of the thoracic intervertebral joint is not producing adequate improvement when used on a patient, mobilization of the rib at its angle should be added to the intervertebral mobilization.

2. If the rib is moved as a treatment technique, it must also create some movement at the intervertebral

joint. This combination may hasten the rate of progress.

If pain is in a referred area of the ribcage, the symptoms may be arising from some abnormality between adjacent ribs. Palpation will reveal abnormalities of position and of movement between adjacent ribs. This aspect of treating costal pain is described in *Peripheral Manipulation* (Maitland, 1970a).

### Thoracic spine: rotation to the right (T2–12)

#### Starting position

The patient lies supine with his arms folded across his chest, resting his hands on the opposite shoulders (*Figure 11.22*). The physiotherapist stands on the right-hand side of the patient, taking hold of the left shoulder with the left hand and the left iliac crest with the right hand (*Figure 11.23*). The trunk is then rolled towards the therapist so that the left shoulder comes off the couch, exposing the thoracic spine. The right hand is then placed so that the flexed interphalangeal joint of the thumb is placed over the transverse process of the thoracic vertebrae to be rotated, allowing the fingers to lie across the thoracic spinous process.

The contact hand is positioned in such a way as to allow the thumb to be flexed at the interphalangeal joint and adducted and slightly opposed at the metacarpo-interphalangeal joint so that it lies in contact with the palm of the hand, the proximal phalanx being in line with the index finger.

The index finger of the right hand is placed over the spinous process of the vertebrae being rotated

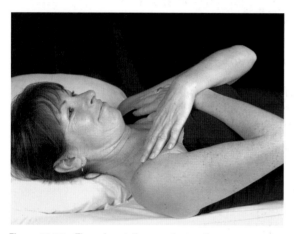

**Figure 11.22**    Thoracic rotation – patient supine

(*Figure 11.24*). The patient's trunk is then rolled backwards over the right hand, and the therapist leans over the patient so that the patient's flexed forearms are tucked into the physiotherapist's chest (*Figure 11.25*).

### Method

The mobilization is then carried out by the physiotherapist rolling the patient's trunk over the right hand. This is done in an oscillating manner.

## Mobilization of the ribs (R2–12)

The same position is adopted as above, with the exception that the right hand is placed so that the right flexed thumb is over the angle of the rib, allowing the fingers to be directed towards the thoracic spinous processes. The index finger is in contact with the spinous process of the vertebrae, to whose transverse process the rib is attached (*Figure 11.26*).

## THORACIC TRACTION

An example of treatment is thoracic backache, page 440.

Traction can be administered to the thoracic spine just as readily as it can to the cervical and lumbar areas, and the guiding principles are exactly the same. However, it is true to say that it is less frequently successful than it is in either of the other two areas, and

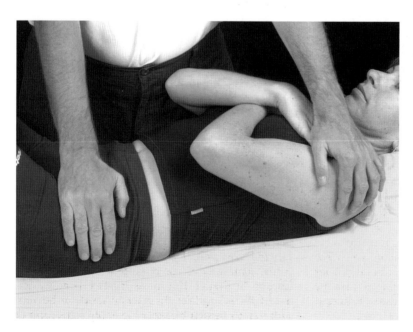

**Figure 11.23**    Thoracic rotation – reaching across to hold the patient

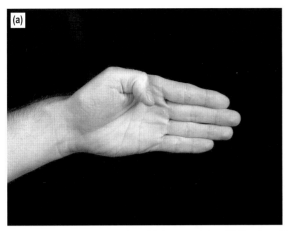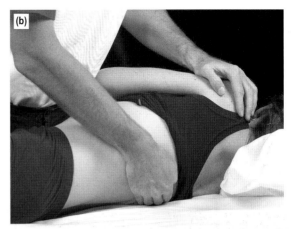

Figure 11.24    Thoracic rotation. (*a*) Hand position. (*b*) Hand position on spine

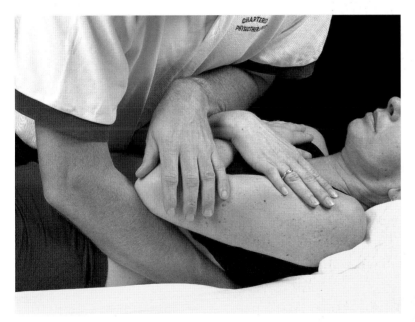

**Figure 11.25**    Thoracic rotation. Final starting position

this may be due, at least in part, to the presence of the thoracic cage.

The principle is to position the vertebral column so that the particular joint to be treated is in a relaxed position midway between all ranges. The amount of pressure to be used is guided first by movement of the joint, with further changes in tension made in response to changes in the patient's symptoms as outlined for cervical traction. Further treatments are guided by changes in symptoms and signs, as already discussed with cervical traction (*see* p. 288).

## Upper thoracic spine (T T ↗)

### Starting position

The patient lies on his back with one or two pillows under his head to flex the neck until the intervertebral level to the treated is positioned midway between flexion and extension. A cervical halter is then applied in the same way as has been described for cervical traction in flexion. If a lower level is to be treated and if the strength of the traction needs to be very firm, it may become necessary to apply some form of

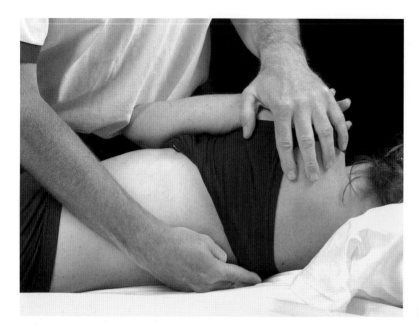

**Figure 11.26**   Costovertebral mobilization

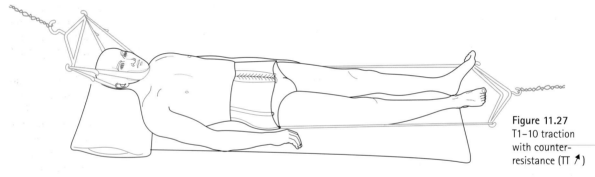

**Figure 11.27**
T1–10 traction
with counter-
resistance (TT ↗)

counter-traction. A belt is fitted around the pelvis and is attached to the foot end of the couch to stabilize the distal end of the vertebral column. The halter is then attached to its fixed point so that the angle of the pull on the neck will be approximately 45° to the horizontal. The actual angle used varies with the amount of kyphosis present in the upper thoracic spine, and it should be an angle that will allow the thoracic intervertebral joint to be moved longitudinally while in a position midway between its limits of flexion and extension. To relieve strain on the patient's lower back during the period when the traction is being applied, his hips and knees may be flexed (*Figure 11.27*).

## Method

The traction can be adjusted from either end or from both ends, but whichever method is used, care must be taken to ensure that friction between the patient's trunk and the couch is reduced to a minimum. This can be done while the traction is being applied by gently lifting

the weight of the patient's thorax or pelvis off the couch and allowing it to relax back into a new position. Friction is almost completely eliminated by a couch whose surface is in two halves that are free to roll longitudinally (*see* pp. 389–394). Releasing the traction does not present any problem, but it is advisable to release slowly.

## Lower thoracic spine (TT ↗)

### Starting position

For the lower thoracic spine, a thoracic belt similar to that used for lumbar traction is used in place of the cervical halter. Traction is usually more effective if it is carried out with the patient supine, but it can be done with him prone.

   The thoracic belt is applied to hold the chest above the level of the spine to be treated, and it is then attached to its fixed point. After this the pelvic belt is applied and attached to its fixed point. The direction of the pull is then longitudinal in the line of the patient's trunk, but pillows may be needed to adjust the

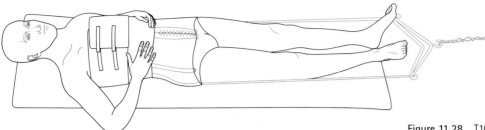

**Figure 11.28** T10–12 traction (TT →)

position of the spine so that the joint being moved is relaxed midway between flexion and extension (*Figure 11.28*).

## Method

Traction is applied from either end or from both ends, but again care is required to reduce friction to a minimum both at thoracic and at pelvic levels. As mentioned previously, a roll-top couch eliminates friction. A simple, cheap and extremely effective roll-top couch is described below (*see* p. 391).

Releasing the traction should be done steadily, and the patient should rest for a short time before standing.

Intermittent variable traction can also be used in this area of the spine, and the details of times for 'rest' and 'hold' periods are the same as have been discussed for the cervical spine.

## Local variations

The thoracic kyphosis varies considerably from person to person, and the positioning of the patient is controlled by this curve. Theoretically, the direction of the pull may be thought of as being at right angles to the upper and lower surfaces of the intervertebral disc at the level that is being moved. The kyphosis usually influences the position for upper thoracic traction more than for the lower thoracic spine.

## Precautions

A check must be kept on the patient to ensure that the traction does not cause any low-back pain.

As with the cervical traction in flexion, it is possible for the head halter in upper thoracic traction to cause occipital headache, but this can be eliminated by the means already described (*see* p. 290).

## Uses

Traction is of greatest value in patients who have widely distributed areas of thoracic pain, particularly if they are associated with radiological degenerative changes in the thoracic spine. It is also of value for patients whose thoracic symptoms do not appear to be aggravated by active movements of the spine or when neurological changes are present. Similarly, it is the treatment of choice for patients with severe nerve-root pain. Whenever mobilizing techniques have been used in treatment without achieving the desired result, traction should be tried.

Sometimes a patient is able to guide the therapist as to what to do because his body tells him what it wants (and what it doesn't want). *Figure 11.29* is a perfect example of such a case. The patient's disorder had been very difficult to help in that progress gained at a treatment session was not retained well enough. The disorder was at the level of T6/7, and had been responding to extremely gentle traction. One day the patient said that he needed the traction, but he also needed to have the vertebra pushed backwards and towards the left while having the levels above twisted to the right. *Figure 11.29* shows how the position was obtained while the mobilizing was produced through the patient's sternum. He claimed that he was 60 per cent better after the first of these treatments, and 80 per cent better after the second. At his suggestion, treatment was discontinued, and on review 12 months later he showed no signs of recurrence.

## GRADE V MANIPULATION

As in other areas of the spine, the mobilization techniques described can be performed as very rapid small-amplitude thrusts. These may be general in distribution, covering more than one intervertebral level (as in rotary PAs described on p. 319), or they can be performed in a much more localized manner so that the emphasis of the movement is focused, as much as is possible, on a single intervertebral level. These more localized manipulative techniques are now described for the thoracic spine.

### Intervertebral joints C7–T3 (lateral flexion ($\curvearrowright$))

#### Starting position

The patient sits well back on a medium-height couch while the physiotherapist stands behind. To provide

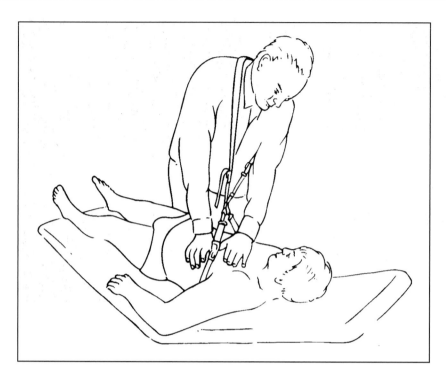

**Figure 11.29** Traction of the mid-thoracic spine combined with localized T6/7 mobilization via the sternum

the patient with comfortable support, the physiotherapist places her left foot on the couch next to the patient's left buttock, rests the patient's left arm over her left thigh, and asks the patient to relax back against her. Localization of the manipulation is achieved by firmly placing the tip of the right thumb against the right side of the spinous process of the lower vertebra of the intervertebral joint. Pressure is applied horizontally in the frontal plane by this thumb, while the fingers spread forward over the patient's right clavicular area. These fingers also stabilize the vertebra. The next step is to flex laterally the patient's head to the right until the tension can be felt at the thumb. While maintaining the lateral flexion tension, the middle position between flexion and extension is found by rocking the neck back and forth on the trunk. After determining this position, rotation (face upwards) is added in small oscillatory movements until the limit of the rotary range is found. The therapist then positions both forearms to work opposite each other (*Figure 11.30*).

## Method

The manipulation consists of a sudden short-range thrust through the right thumb transversely across the body, while a counter-thrust is given by the operator's left hand against the left side of the patient's head.

## Intervertebral joints T3–10 (PAs $\updownarrow$ )

### Starting position

The patient lies supine without a pillow and links his hands behind his neck while the physiotherapist stands by his right side. By grasping the patient's left shoulder in her right hand and both elbows in her left hand, the physiotherapist holds the patient in this position; she releases her hold on the shoulder and leans over the patient to palpate for the spinous process of the lower vertebra forming the intervertebral joint being manipulated. Still holding the patient in this position, the physiotherapist makes a fist with the right hand by flexing the middle, ring and little fingers into the palm but leaving the thumb and index finger extended. A small pad of material grasped in the fingers will give added support. This fist is then applied to the patient's spine (the thumb points towards the head) so that the lower spinous process is grasped between the terminal phalanx of the middle finger and the palmar surface of the head of the opposed first metacarpal. The patient is then lowered back until the physiotherapist's right hand is wedged between patient and the couch. The weight of the patient's trunk is taken on the flat of the dorsum of the hand (not on the knuckles), and the forearm should project laterally to avoid interference with movement of the

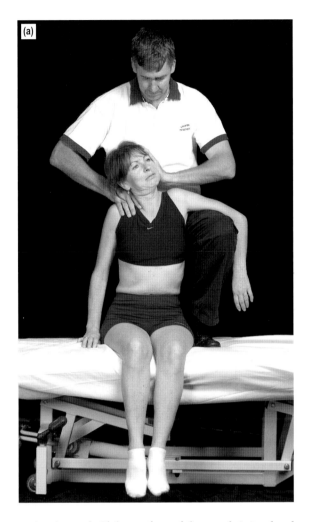

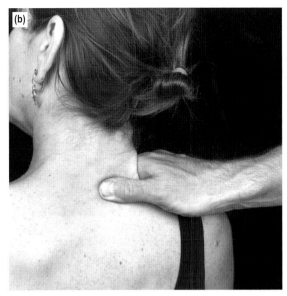

Figure 11.30    (*a*) and (*b*) Intervertebral joints C7–T3

patient's trunk. If the surface of the couch is too hard, it will be difficult for the physiotherapist to maintain her grip on the spinous process. To achieve firm control of the patient's trunk, his elbows should be held firmly and pressed against the physiotherapist's sternum. However, when a patient has excessively mobile joints it may be necessary for him to grasp his shoulders with opposite hands while keeping the elbows in close apposition rather than clasping the hands behind the neck. The patient's upper trunk is then gently moved back and forth from flexion to extension in decreasing ranges until the stage is reached where the only movement taking place is felt by the underneath hand to be at the intervertebral joint to be manipulated (*Figure 11.31*).

### Method

Pressure is increased through the patient's elbows, causing stretch at the intervertebral joint, and the

manipulation is then carried out by a downward thrust through his elbows in the direction of his upper arms. This thrust is transmitted to the patient's trunk above the underneath hand. The thrust may be given as the patient fully exhales.

### Intervertebral joints T3–10 (longitudinal movement ←••→)

#### Starting position

The patient sits well back on the couch and grasps his hands behind his neck, allowing his elbows to drop forwards. The physiotherapist stands behind the patient and threads her arms in front of his axillae to grasp over the dorsum of his wrists. When grasping his wrists, she encourages his elbows to drop forwards while at the same time holding his ribs firmly from each side with her forearms. She then turns her trunk slightly to one side to place her lower ribs against his

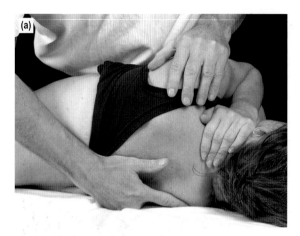

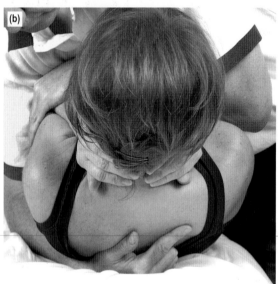

**Figure 11.31** (*a*) and (*b*) Intervertebral joints T3–10 (PAs ↕)

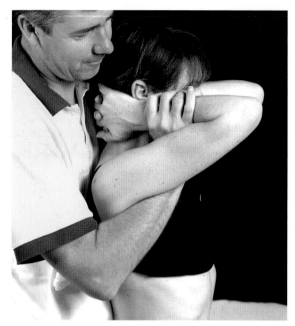

**Figure 11.32** Intervertebral joints. T3–T10 (longitudinal movement)

spine at the level requiring manipulation. While feeling for movement with her ribcage, she flexes and extends his thoracic spine above the level to be manipulated until the neutral position between flexion and extension is found for the joint to be treated (*Figure 11.32*).

### Method

The physiotherapist lifts the patient's trunk in the direction of the long axis of the joint being treated, and makes a final adjustment of the flexion/extension position to ensure that the mid-position has been retained. The manipulation then consists of a short-amplitude sharp lift.

Some degree of extension may be added into this technique. This extra movement is achieved by a very

small movement with the therapist's ribs against the patient's spine, performed at the same time as the lift is executed through the arms.

### Intervertebral joints T3–10 (rotation ↻)

#### Starting position

If rotation to the left is to be performed, the patient sits on the edge of the couch near the right-hand end while the physiotherapist stands behind his right side. The patient hugs his chest with his arms and turns his trunk to the left. For the mid-thoracic area, the physiotherapist reaches with her left arm around his arms to grasp his right shoulder while placing the heel of her right hand along the line of the right rib above the joint to be manipulated. She cradles his left shoulder in her left axilla (*Figure 11.33a*). For the lower thoracic levels, she grasps around his chest under his arms to reach his scapula. This time she places the ulnar border of her right hand along the line of the ribs (*Figure 11.33b*). With both techniques she then takes the movement to the limit of the range, taking up all slack.

### Method

The manipulation consists of a synchronous movement of the physiotherapist's trunk and an extra pressure through her right hand. With her trunk she carries

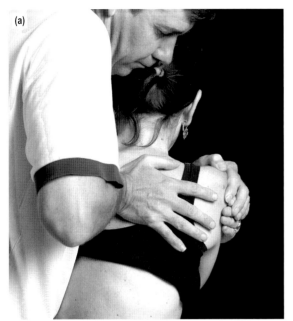 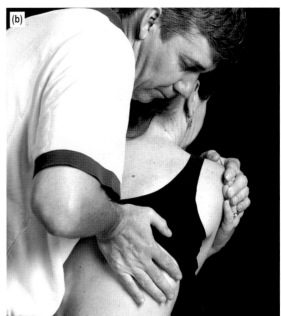

**Figure 11.33**   Intervertebral joints. T3–10 (rotation). (*a*) Mid-thoracic area. (*b*) Lower thoracic area

out an oscillatory rotation back and forth at the limit of the rotary range. At the same time she maintains constant pressure with either the heel of her right hand or its ulnar border exerting an extra rotary push at the limit of the rotation. The manipulation consists of an over-pressure at the limit of the range, being done in a very small amplitude and very sharply.

## CASE HISTORY

The example of treatment given below is included at the end of this chapter for a very specific purpose. It is well known among manipulators (both lay and medical) that many patients have undergone abdominal surgery for symptoms thought to have come from such structures as the gall bladder, the appendix, ovaries, etc. When the patient has not been relieved of the symptoms by the surgeon, the patients often find their way to the manipulators who, under the appropriate circumstances of course, have been able to treat the appropriate level of the vertebral column and relieve the patient of his symptoms. Surgeons who are aware of this possibility are concerned that the examination of such a patient should include a musculoskeletal examination to determine the possibility, when there is doubt with a patient's symptoms, that the symptoms may, in fact, arise from the vertebral column.

### Mrs R
A summary of the report from the physician and gastroenterologist follows.

### Social
This 40-year-old patient was seen 4 weeks ago. She is married with one daughter. She is a housewife and her husband runs a motoring school, which has been poorly attended, causing major financial problems.

### Past history
Her past history revealed asthma, and she was diagnosed by her local medical officer 7 years ago as having acute cholecystitis. She did not have a gall bladder investigation; nor has she had one since that time. She has had an appendectomy and hysterectomy and tubal ligation. She has also been diagnosed as having a hiatus hernia, which was confirmed by barium meal in 1978 when she presented with chest pains. Three years ago she was seen by a cardiologist for a full cardiac assessment because of these chest pains. Finally, she had had a transient right hemiplegia 4 years ago, the cause of which was not known, despite it occurring in a young woman. She had, however, been on the contraceptive pill for some considerable time. There was some possible suggestion that the symptoms were functional.

**Right upper quadrant pain**

The patient was noted to have had backache 14 years ago and again more recently, especially over the past 5 years. She had suffered a constant burning pain in the right upper thorax beneath the right scapula, and she noticed that she developed pain in the right upper quadrant at the same time. The patient herself noted that the pain in the right upper quadrant of her abdomen and her backache tended to occur together consistently. The pain was worse when coughing and deep breathing, and it tended to be worse with walking. She had undergone both an ultrasound of the gall bladder and an oral cholecystogram, both of which were normal, raising the strong suggestion that she probably never did have acute cholecystitis 7 years ago and that this diagnosis was probably incorrect. The patient described episodes of severe gripping pain, which was so severe that she was unable to walk. These pains tended to be worse in bed or early in the morning when she had been lying in bed overnight. She was unable to sleep on her right-hand side because of the discomfort, but had some relief when rolling onto her back or her left-hand side.

Close questioning revealed some abnormality of her bowel habit with small soft stools, and she often noted herself to be bloated with abdominal distension, as if she were pregnant, and she noted that she had relief of many of these symptoms following defecation. If she became a little constipated, she developed pain in the right lower quadrant, passing into the leg, and she noted that this pain tended to be worse if her bowel or bladder were full.

The patient also had fat intolerance in that she described abdominal discomfort after eating an excessively fatty meal. Examination of the patient revealed her to have a blood pressure of 140/190, and examination by the naked eye revealed her to have quite an abnormal posture with a considerable dropped right shoulder; one could quite simply reproduce much of her pain and symptoms by examination of the spine with forced rotation to the right.

Sigmoidoscopy was normal, as was full blood screen, ESR and haemoglobin and WBC. With an MBA-20, and when I first saw the patient, I thought she had colonic symptoms, that the diagnosis made some 7 years previously of cholecystitis was probably incorrect and that her pain in the right upper quadrant was almost entirely musculoskeletal in origin. I considered there was no evidence of biliary disease or any dyspeptic disease, that she did not need endoscopy, and I thought that she should have a barium enema and some treatment for colonic symptoms and be referred for assessment to a manipulative physiotherapist to see if she agreed that the patient's pain was musculoskeletal in origin.

**Neuromusculoskeletal examination and treatment**

The patient's symptoms were as shown in *Figure 11.34*. The examination findings were as follows.

**Flexion**

The patient was only able to reach 5 cm below her knees, and this provoked low back pain. Recovery from that flexed position was difficult and provoked more back pain. After completing the test movement, she developed pain in her right abdomen.

In the flexed position, rotation of the thorax to the right provoked right leg pain.

**Extension**

There was no low lumbar movement at all, but the small amount of low thoracic extension that she could perform provoked what she described as 'shocking pain' in the right buttock and abdomen.

**Lateral flexion right**

This movement provoked her low back pain.

**Rotation left**

This movement was restricted to 50 per cent of her rotation to the right, and it provoked low thoracic pain that extended into the abdomen and also included the whole of her right leg.

**Slump**

Knee extension was limited, reproducing her leg and abdominal pain; there was almost no range of dorsiflexion of the ankle because of markedly increased abdominal pain.

**Right hip**

The movement of flexion adduction was limited by pain. This pain began first in the right buttock, then it spread to the abdomen.

**Palpation**

There was marked thickening in the interspinous spaces on the right side, particularly at the levels between the spinous processes of L2–4. This was greatest at the L2/3 space, which was completely obliterated with both old and new thickened tissue.

**Treatment**

By the seventh treatment, which included very gentle lumbar traction, transverse pressures towards the right

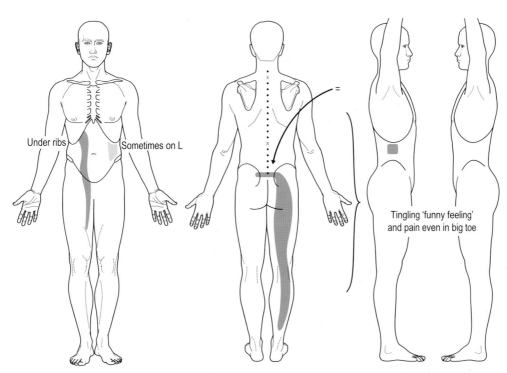

**Figure 11.34**  Patient's distribution of symptoms

from L1–5 as grade II movements, and small-amplitude smooth grade II rotary movements of the hip with it in a neutral position, it became obvious that she had two separate problems, each of which aggravated the other when painful. She had a definite hip disorder and a definite spinal disorder.

The next four treatments consisted of extremely gentle lumbar traction. To perform this, no thoracic or pelvic harness was used; the two movable parts of the lumbar traction couch were separated and blocked in the separated position, and the patient was instructed that the only two things she could do while she was on this traction were to breathe and to blink. The traction was only administered for 12 minutes. She felt that it eased her back symptoms as well as her abdominal symptoms. At the next treatment session treatment for her hip, extremely gentle slow and smoothly executed grade II rotations were used, and this relieved her buttock pain.

Continuing this treatment and adding in accessory movements to her right hip (the accessory movements were longitudinal caudad while she lay on her left side and had pillows between her legs to make the hip position more neutral) improved her further.

These treatments were continued over an interval of 6 weeks on an alternate day basis. As she improved, the techniques could be progressed by making them larger in amplitude and by being prepared to take the techniques into a small degree of reproduced pain. At the end of the 6 weeks her movements were almost normal, and she considered she was not having any real problem.

An interval of 3 weeks was left between her last treatment and the time when she was reviewed by the doctor. This was done deliberately so as to be able to assess the long-term effects of the treatment more clearly. She was again reviewed in 12 months, and she considered herself to be 'cured'.

# Chapter 12

# Lumbar spine

## INTRODUCTION

Symptoms arising from disorders of the lumbar spine are more difficult and complicated to diagnose specifically than at almost any other spinal level. The patterns of presentation of low back pain and associated symptoms give the manipulative physiotherapist little clue as to their precise source. However, Bogduk (1997) suggests that, through clinical trials and with present knowledge, the most important sources of low back pain are the intervertebral disc (40 per cent), the zygapophysical joints (15 per cent) and the sacroiliac joint (15 per cent). There is little evidence available as to how disorders of these structures can be identified from predictable clinical presentations.

The lumbar spine is also the section of the spine that receives the most attention from manipulative physiotherapists and orthopaedic surgeons, and it is the area of the spine that causes the greatest loss of work time. It demands therefore that we should be prepared to put our energies into determining the most successful forms of treatment and also into attempting to understand more clearly the anatomy, physiology, biomechanics and pathologies so that both diagnosis and prognosis can become more accurate.

## GENERAL

For the sake of convenience alone, the manipulative therapist can think of the lumbar spine in two basic groups.

### FIRST GROUP

> The L4/5 and L5/S1 intervertebral discs are frequently a source of symptoms in patients referred to manipulative physiotherapy with low back pain

This group consists of patients whose symptoms arise from the lower two intervertebral levels, with the main emphasis being placed on the intervertebral disc and the structures it can affect when it is at fault. This is not to say that the intervertebral discs at other levels never degenerate, cause symptoms or prolapse. However, it is meant to point to the frequency with which the discs at the L4/5 and L5/S1 levels cause symptoms and are referred to manipulative physiotherapists. It is also necessary to state that these two discs alone are not the greatest cause of low back pain. Nevertheless, there has seemingly been an increase in the number of low lumbar disorders occurring in modern Western society over the last 20 years. This increase may have been brought about by the length of time modern man spends sitting, particularly in the motor vehicles of all kinds, and even more particularly when this position is insulted by the addition of vibration (Troup, 1978).

As well as having hydrodynamic and biomechanical properties, the intervertebral disc may have a proprioceptive role. Note that patients with discogenic problems often lose their position sense and exhibit poor quality and control of movement; proprioceptive dysfunction as well as pain inhibition may contribute to this. The patient may say, 'I feel as though my back is like glass, it just doesn't support me'. Passive mobilization may also influence the recovery of proprioceptive functioning of the disc (Zusman, 1985).

There is now strong evidence that the lumbar intervertebral discs are supplied by dense and microscopic nerve plexuses originating from the sympathetic trunk and the grey rami communicantes (Green *et al.*, 1990). There are strong indications that these nerves have a sensory role. Therefore, the generally accepted sensory supply to the disc, that is, the sinuvertebral nerves, are only a part of the annular innervation.

Nakamura *et al.* (1996) have hypothesized that the lower intervertebral discs have sensory pathways via the sympathetic chain. This may explain why patients with discogenic low back pain have 'visceral' type symptoms amongst their somatic sensory pains. The patient often describes his discogenic pain as 'sickly' or 'nauseous'.

There is now strong evidence from MRI studies that the intervertebral disc can be damaged internally without causing pain, and only when the damage affects the outer part of the annulus is somatic pain more likely. This corresponds to the density of the disc innervation by the sinuvertebral nerve (Bogduk, 1994b). However, patients often complain of experiencing periods of 'stiffness' in the low back prior to an overt disc disorder, and this may well be the warning sign that internal disc damage has already occurred.

### SECOND GROUP

> Posture, muscle balance, muscle weakness, spondylitic and arthritic changes, mechanical movement disorders, etc. can all be a source or cause of symptoms in patients with low back pain

Within this group can be included patients having symptoms from other kinds of disorders such as those caused by posture, muscle imbalance, muscle weakness, spondylitic and arthritic changes, mechanical disorders etc. Most of the disorders considered in this section have been dealt with in Chapter 8.

## SUBJECTIVE EXAMINATION

*Table 12.1* sets out the examination pattern, but certain points require expansion.

### 'KIND' OF DISORDER

In the majority of cases the patient's main complaint is *pain*, either in the back, buttocks, lower abdomen, groin or legs. Any functional limitation will give clues

Table 12.1    Lumbar spine. Subjective examination

---

**'Kind' of disorder**

Establish why the patient has been referred for or sought treatment:

(i)   Pain, stiffness, weakness, instability, etc.

(ii)  Acute onset.

(iii) Post-surgical, trauma, MUA, support, traction, etc.

**History**

Recent and previous (see 'History' below).

Sequence of questioning about history can be varied.

**Area**

Is the disorder one of pain, stiffness, recurrence, weakness, etc?

Record on the 'body chart':

1. Area and depth of symptoms indicating main areas and stating types of symptoms.

2. Paraesthesia and anaesthesia.

3. Check for symptoms all other associated areas, i.e.:

(i)   other vertebral areas;

(ii)  joints above and below the disorder;

(iii) other relevant joints.

**Behaviour of symptoms**

**General**

1. When are they present or when do they fluctuate and why (local and referred).

2. Effect of rest on the local and referred symptoms (associate/dissociate with day's activities, bed, inflammation). (Compare symptoms on rising in the morning with end of day.)

3. Pain and stiffness on rising; duration of.

4. Effect of activities. (Beginning of day compared with end of day.)

**Particular**

1. What provokes symptoms – what relieves (severity, irritability)?

2. What is the pain like with activities that involve the lower back (particularly flexion)?

3. What effect does sitting have on the back pain and the leg pain (or other sustained positions)?

4. Any difficulty rising from sitting or first few steps?

5. What effect does coughing or sneezing have on the symptoms (back and/or leg pain)?

**Special questions**

1. Does the patient have any bladder retention, or anaesthesia in this area? (Cauda equina compression) [initial frequency may indicate cauda equina irritation].

2. General health and relevant weight loss. (Medical history.)

3. Have recent X-rays been taken?

4. What tablets are being taken for this and other conditions (osteoporosis from extensive steroid therapy)?

**History**

1. Of this attack.

2. Of previous attacks, or of associated symptoms.

3. Are the symptoms worsening or improving?

4. Prior treatment and its effect.

5. Socio-economic history as applicable.

HIGHLIGHT MAIN FINDINGS WITH ASTERISKS

to the likely findings on physical examination – for example, 'I cannot put my socks on in the morning'; 'When I lie on my front or arch my back a pain shoots down my leg'.

> Lower limb sporting injuries such as hamstring tears, medial ligament sprains of the knee, achilles tendonitis, ankle sprains, etc. may well have a spinal contributing factor. The history (onset, progression) is vitally important

The manipulative physiotherapist should pay attention to patients referred with lower limb 'joint' problems or lower limb sporting injuries. To pick up on a spinal contributing factor in such cases can be very rewarding.

For example, a patient referred with a chronic sprained ankle revealed: 'I fell and twisted my ankle 10 months ago, but the pain on the outside of my ankle is still making me limp even though the swelling and bruising has gone. I rub cream on it but it doesn't make any difference. The doctor even gave me a cortisone injection and it's still the same. I've got no confidence in it'. On further questioning the patient said that he had an ongoing back problem, which he had learned to live with. He did remember twisting his back when he fell, resulting in stiffness for a few days.

Physical examination revealed tenderness over the lateral ligament of the ankle, but no increase in the pain with movement. SLR was slightly restricted, and his lumbar quadrant revealed local back pain and stiffness on the side of the ankle pain. A unilateral postero-anterior pressure on L5 on the same side as his ankle pain was very 'tender' and stiff, and also made his ankle ache more. Two treatments later, by mobilizing his lumbar spine, his ankle pain had gone.

## AREA OF SYMPTOMS

### Research

Many attempts have been made to carry out research programmes to determine the efficacy of specific treatments (commonly manipulative treatment) for low back pain.

As yet, there is no 'gold standard' research on the efficacy of specific treatments for low back pain. However, in the United Kingdom, encouragement has been given to manipulative physiotherapists by a National Clinical Standards Advisory Group document (CSAG, 1996). All available research on the efficacy of manipulation for low back pain was reviewed, and the advisory group concluded that:

> *Within the first 6 weeks of onset of acute low back pain, manipulation provides better short-term improvement in pain and activity levels and higher patient satisfaction than the treatments to which it has been compared . . .*

> Most research programmes on low back pain fail to take into account the wide variety of clinical problems the patients present with. Grouping of patients needs to be more specific if the effect of manipulative physiotherapy is to be determined usefully

Yet with all the programmes that have been published (and there are many), none of the authors seem to realize that a patient who feels pain as a very localized spot, for example between the spinous processes of L4 and L5, does not have the same problem as the patient who has pain spreading in a line across his back at the L4/5 interspinous space. Nor do they seem to realize that a patient who has a band of pain across his back, which may extend superiorly to L3 or L4 and inferiorly to S1, is different again, as is the patient who has a band of pain spreading across his back at the middle or lower sacral level. These areas of pain that have been mentioned do not take into account the differences that exist if the patient has pain that spreads across his back but is greater on one side than on the other, or if his pain is only felt on one side of his back. Similarly, these are all different from the patient who feels his pain in the area of the sacroiliac joint or in his gluteal area, yet these are still frequently classed in the back pain grouping for survey purposes. It is the author's belief that for any project to determine usefully the effect of manipulative treatment, the groupings of patients must be made much more specific. And this is relating the problems to 'site-of-pain' only. The behaviour of the pains then needs to be classified into separate groups.

### Site

The site of the patient's pain is as important to determine specifically as has been described for the high cervical area (*see* p. 231). This is particularly so when a patient has pain in the region of the iliac crest. It is essential to determine whether the patient's pain is in fact immediately above the crest, on the crest, or immediately below the lip of the crest. Similarly, when a patient has gluteal area pain it is necessary to determine whether this pain is felt medially, centrally, or more laterally; it is also essential to determine whether the patient is able to dig a finger into the gluteal area to define the spot of pain or whether he is unable to do this and can only describe the pain as being vaguely deep-seated in the buttock.

When a patient has symptoms that radiate into the leg it is essential to determine the site and depth of the symptoms, while at the same time differentiating between the kinds of symptoms that a patient can feel. For example, the symptoms may be those of a deep ache, a sharp pain, a burning feeling, a heavy feeling, a feeling of numbness that is in fact not an actual diminution of sensation, or a feeling of tingling or 'pins and needles'. The patient may also comment about cramp (and it is then necessary for us to determine whether he is a person who frequently has cramp or not), a warm feeling or a coldness. It is also necessary to determine whether pains in different areas increase and decrease at the same times as each other and for the same reasons, or whether they behave separately, and whether one area of the symptoms is greater than another. In fact, it is absolutely essential that the manipulative physiotherapist should be able to 'live' a specific patient's symptoms in her own mind.

Three things in particular should be remembered when considering area of symptoms:

1. A patient can feel symptoms centrally in the lower back, yet the origin may be in the upper lumbar, even thoracolumbar, area.

2. A patient can have an area of generalized lower abdominal symptoms that arise from a low lumbar disorder. Occasionally (but far less frequently) symptoms may be felt unilaterally in the lower abdomen, in the groin, or even in the testicular area from the lower lumbar disorder.

3. Some patients with disorders involving the low lumbar nerve roots can have symptoms that they describe as being 'in' the knee or 'in' the ankle. When attempting to differentiate as to whether these symptoms are arising from the back or from the local joint, the possibility of their being related to an old injury to the particular joint must not be forgotten.

## BEHAVIOUR OF SYMPTOMS

When a patient has symptoms in his back, buttock and leg, the symptoms may vary in intensity at the same time as each other. However, it is not uncommon for the back or buttock symptoms to fluctuate at quite different times and for quite different reasons from those in his leg.

Determining the different behaviours helps the manipulative physiotherapist to be aware that during the physical examination she may need to look for test movements that provide different parts of the symptoms, if there is any likelihood that they may be coming from different structures or different aspects of the same structure.

Pain felt on coughing, sneezing or straining can provide useful information. For example, a patient who has back pain that radiates into his leg may, on coughing, provoke back pain. However, it may be that it is the leg pain that is reproduced by the coughing, in which case his symptoms will be much more difficult to relieve than would have been the case if the coughing had provoked pain in his back only.

Again, a patient with pain radiating into his leg, who on getting out of a chair after prolonged sitting or getting out of bed first thing in the morning has difficulty in straightening into the normal erect position because of back pain, has quite a different problem to the patient who is able to stand immediately but has difficulty with his first few steps because of severe leg pain. The latter patient has a disorder that is far more difficult to help than the former. Other aspects of the behaviour of the patient's symptoms are listed in the 'General' and 'Particular' sections of *Table 12.1*.

## SPECIAL QUESTIONS

As well as asking the obvious questions related to general medical conditions, etc., it is particularly important to determine whether there is any indication of cauda equina involvement (*see* p. 18). Naturally, such a patient would not be referred for manipulative treatment, but there is the possibility that the first signs of involvement may not become evident until after the doctor's referral and before the manipulative physiotherapist's first consultation.

## HISTORY

All other aspects of the subjective examination table are straightforward and obvious, but some comments should be made about history for lumbar disorders.

An accurate history is most important if the manipulative physiotherapist is to have any idea of:

1. The structure or structures involved.
2. The state of the structures involved.
3. The rate of progression of the disorder, especially if it is one that tends to have a natural progression.
4. The degree of stability of the disorder at the time of the initial consultation.
5. The likelihood of being able to help the patient's disorder with specific kinds of treatment.

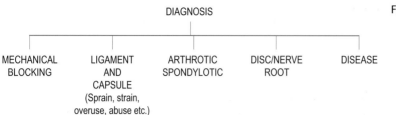

Figure 12.1   Diagnostic groups

6. The likely prognosis for the patient's disorder, and the future 'management of the disorder' in terms of self help and the role of manipulative physiotherapy.

At the beginning of this book it was suggested that patients could be divided into groups (*Figure 12.1*). The history for the group of patients with symptoms arising from sprain, strain, posture, misuse or abuse is obvious and easily determined by appropriate logical questioning, with which all readers are familiar.

> Lumbar discogenic disorders follow fairly common patterns in terms of episodic progression and behaviour of symptoms

The histories of patients with low lumbar discogenic disorders also follow fairly common patterns, both in the episodic progression of the disorder and in the behaviour of the symptoms. There is an element of the history that is indicative of a low lumbar discogenic disorder, which also helps to guide the appreciation of both the severity of the disorder and the stage of development of the progression of the disorder. This element is that the patient may be aware, frequently at the end of the day, of a slight twinge in his back, usually associated with a trivial lifting or twisting incident. He is able to continue working, but when either he cools down later, or when he tries to get out of bed the next morning, he is very much aware that he has a 'bad back'. The degree of the provoking incident is the comparison that provides the information regarding the state of the disc disorder.

Symptomatically, the patient having a discogenic disorder could expect to have stiffness of his lower back on first getting out of bed in the morning, which would last for between 10 and 30 minutes. It would also be likely that after prolonged sitting he would have difficulty in standing straight on first getting out of a chair. He would probably comment on having difficulty getting out of a motor vehicle, it again being difficult for him to stand straight. If he has difficulty getting in and out of the car, it may be the neck flexion (a neural sign) component of the movement that is the problem rather than the straightening process of the

lumbar spine. Coughing and/or sneezing would also probably provoke back pain.

As the disc disorder progressively deteriorates from episode to episode, it will follow one of two paths. The first is that each episode results in back pain only. The second path is that, with each increasingly progressing episode, the pain spreads from the back into the limb in variously increasing degrees and may, in the later stages, include neurological changes.

There are many variations of *referred* pain and radicular pain, and it is not the intention to discuss these in differential diagnostic terms, as it is not the aim of this book. Rather, the information given in this chapter and in Chapter 8 is to give the newcomer to the field of manipulative physiotherapy an outline of the commonly seen disorders.

The mechanical blocking or locking type disorder has the sudden severe onset history, and totally prevents the patient returning to the upright position. This was discussed earlier (*see* p. 232). With regard to the arthritic spondylotic type of disorder, there is one important point to be mentioned. The history is the same as the same kind of disorder it presents when in the limb joints. In the spine, however, if the onset indicates involvement of a single intervertebral level and this level is only one of several levels showing the same radiological changes, it can be clearly said that it will be very difficult to relieve the patient of his symptoms. Conversely, if the symptoms are diffuse aching arising from several adjacent levels, the chances of making a valuable reduction in the symptoms are predictably very good.

Obviously, the foregoing does not provide coverage of the history of all disorders the manipulative physiotherapist may be asked to treat. However, it is hoped that it opens her mind to the kind of questions she should ask to elicit the kind of problem the patient may have. There are many reference texts regarding the subject, including *Practical Orthopaedic Medicine* (Corrigan and Maitland, 1983).

## PHYSICAL EXAMINATION

*Table 12.2* summarizes the physical examination for disorders of the lumbar spine.

**Table 12.2**   Lumbar spine. Physical examination

**Observation**
  Getting out of the chair, willingness to move, gait, posture.

**Movements standing**
  Other joints (quick tests).
  *Move to pain or move to limit* F, E, LF, Ⓛ and Ⓡ and Rotⁿ Ⓛ and Ⓡ and in F and E; pain and behaviour, range, countering protective deformity, localizing over-pressure, intervertebral movement (repeated movement, increased speed and/or under load).
  For lowest lumbar joints do F, E, LF all in standing from below upwards by using pelvic movement when applicable. Also combined movement tests.
  Lateral displacement shift.

**When applicable**
  Sustained E and LF towards pain (when necessary to reproduce pain).
  Quadrants (if F, E, LF, and Rotⁿ are negative).
  Tap test (if F, E, LF, Rotⁿ and Q are negative).
  Compression and distraction (if F, E, LF, Rotⁿ and Q and Tap are negative).
  Neurological (calf).
  Active peripheral joint tests.
  Canal tests (slump sitting).

**Supine**
  Passive neck F; range, pain (back and/or leg pain).
  (May require combining with slump-sitting & SLR.)
  Passive SLR (straight leg raising); range, pain.
  (Compare supine with standing.)
  SIJ.
  Neurological examination.
  Resisted static tests for muscular pain.
  (When applicable compare F and/or SLR in standing with supine.)
  Passive peripheral joint tests.
  Instability test.
  Passive rotation from below upwards, and 'coupling' by using femur–pelvis.
  Lateral flexion from below upwards by using pelvis.

**Prone**
  Passive PKB (prone knee bend).
  Neurological examination.
  Resisted static tests for muscular pain.
  'Palpation'
    Soft-tissue palpation (muscle, interspinous space).
    Position of vertebrae.
    Intervertebral accessory movement.
    Combined PAIVM tests with physiological movement positions.
  Passive peripheral joint tests.

**Side lying**
  PPIVM: F, E, LF, Rotⁿ and F/E instability tests.

**Examination of other relevant factors**

**OTHER TESTS**
Check 'case notes' for reports of relevant tests (X-rays, blood tests).

HIGHLIGHT IMPORTANT FINDINGS WITH ASTERISKS

## OBSERVATION

When watching the patient's lumbar movements of flexion, extension, lateral flexion and rotation, notice should initially be taken of the gross spinal range and the pain response to the movement. This may well be the first asterisk used for assessment purposes. The second aspect is to note (during the movements) the appearance of local intervertebral movement, so that if lateral flexion, for example, is limited, the statement may be recorded that the limitation occurs mainly from L3 downwards. Watching the movements from these two aspects (i.e. the gross movements and the local movements) can be likened to taking a photograph with a wide-angle lens for the gross movement, and a second movement using a telephoto lens to highlight the localized limited movement.

Any sign of a protective deformity in standing must be noted and corrected (*cf.* lateral shift correction, p. 350). The patient should be asked if this is a normal stance for him. If it is indeed protective and only associated with episodes of pain, he may still say, 'What do you mean?' or 'This is usual for me'. Sometimes when it is mentioned to the patient's spouse or partner, they recall having noticed it coming and going with the episodes of pain. To make the picture clear, the deformity must be countered. If by passively correcting (countering the stance or movement) or overcorrecting the deformity the patient's symptoms (associated with this episode) are changed or reproduced, then the antalgic posture is related to this painful episode. This may then serve as another important asterisk to use during reassessment.

## FUNCTIONAL DEMONSTRATION/INJURING MOVEMENT

The patient will often be able to demonstrate a movement or activity, involving the lumbar spine, which reproduces his symptoms. This may be a daily activity that he knows hurts his back, such as bending forwards to tie his shoelaces. He may also be able to demonstrate the movement he was doing when his back was injured – for instance, a backhand at tennis. By asking the patient to demonstrate such an activity or injuring movement to $P_1$, or to the limit, the therapist can analyse the range of movement, symptom response and quality of movement. Thus she has her first asterisks for reassessment.

Differentiation at this stage may help to confirm the structures at fault if there is any doubt. For example, the patient may be able to reproduce his left buttock pain by demonstrating the backhand tennis shot that injured him. This movement principally involves rotation of the spine and hip. By using the lumbar spine/hip differentiation test described on pages 162–163, involvement of the spine rather than the hip may be revealed (or *vice versa*).

Further brief appraisal of the spine and hip will confirm the need to examine the spine or hip in more detail. Treatment should then reinforce the initial hypothesis.

Further differentiation of the functional demonstration or injuring movement may be of value when improvement has slowed or stopped. After several sessions of treatment, the patient may have to stretch a lot further into the backhand shot to reproduce his pain. Further differentiation may reveal that lumbar extension and lateral flexion to the painful side adds to the buttock pain being reproduced by rotation of the spine during the backhand shot. Therefore a lumbar rotation treatment technique in lumbar extension and ipsilateral lateral flexion will be a valuable technique as a progression of treatment.

## LUMBAR FLEXION

> Examination of lumbar flexion can include:
>
> - Forward flexion (FF) with over-pressure and return to the upright position
> - Clearing test of lumbar extension *from* full flexion at speed
> - Clearing test of sustained over-pressure in flexion, flexion rotation then rapidly into full extension
> - Forward flexion with cervical flexion added
> - Forward flexion with rotation to the left and right added
> - Half flexion plus rotation left and right
> - Flexion from below upwards
> - Flexion with any protective deformity countered

Forward flexion is a very important movement in the lumbar spine, and should be examined in depth and with intimacy. Smooth, even unrolling from above downwards occurs during the normal movement. Recovery from flexion to the standing position should also be a smooth movement. However, a patient may have what appears to be a normal movement during flexion but difficulty in dropping into the normal lumbar lordosis when returning to the upright position. This is an important abnormality to be noted, and it must be eliminated if treatment is to be successful.

Taking the considerations surrounding lumbar flexion one step further, it may be necessary to prove that the patient's disorder has not been completely resolved. The following clearing test of forward flexion should be performed. First, the patient is asked to extend backwards as far as he can and the physiotherapist sustains him in this position by giving him gentle support while sustaining gentle over-pressure. Before the patient moves from this position, and while the position is being sustained, she explains to him that when she says 'bend forwards NOW', he is to bend forwards from the fully extended position to the limit of his range of forward flexion at maximum speed; and then immediately and as quickly as possible come up from the fully flexed position to the normal upright standing position. Any disturbance to the normal rhythm of intervertebral movement indicates that the disorder has not been completely resolved. The normal spine will roll and unroll without any distortion of the rhythm of intervertebral movement.

While still considering flexion, and needing to prove that the disorder has not completely resolved, a further variation should be examined. Such tests as this and the one described above should not be performed if, on the normal examination of movements and palpation, it is obvious that the disorder has not been resolved. These special tests should only be used as clearing tests. To perform this test the patient is asked to flex fully and sustain the position (it must be painless). Over-pressure is added to the flexion and sustained (say for 5–10 seconds). The patient then turns his head, thorax and lumbar spine fully to the left, and this position is sustained with over-pressure. The same procedure is performed with rotation to the opposite side, and the patient then returns to the straight position, still sustaining his full flexion. It is then explained to him that he is, as rapidly as possible, to return to the upright position and pass beyond that

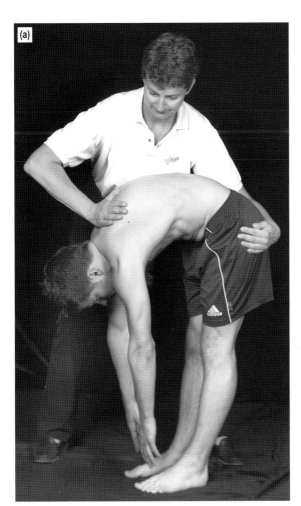 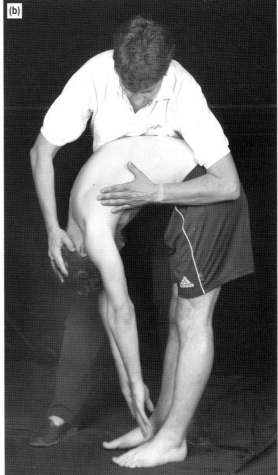

**Figure 12.2**   Lumbar flexion (*a*) with over-pressure at upper thorax; (*b*) superimposed over-pressure to neck flexion

to a fully extended position. The normal spine will show no tendency to a lumbar kyphosis at any stage of this recovery (or extension) movement, and the movement should be smoothly executed.

During the normal examination of lumbar flexion, time can often be saved and information quickly discovered by adding two tests. The first test is adding cervical flexion once the pain response to the normal over-pressure (or to $P_1$.) to flexion is known. Any change in the pain response (in the lumbar spine, buttock or leg) once the neck flexion is added can be attributed to movement of the pain-sensitive structures in the vertebral canal rather than to any change of the movement of the lumbar intervertebral joints (*Figure 12.2*).

The second addition to the flexion test is to ask the patient to fold his arms, turn his head to the left, and then turn his shoulders and trunk to the left. This is a combined movement of flexion and rotation to the left. Over-pressure can be applied to this movement, and its pain response must be noted. This is different from the clearing test described above, because there is no 'sustain' component to this test movement. To add rotation to the left, the physiotherapist stands on the patient's left side to stabilize his pelvis between her pelvis and her right hand, which grasps around the patient's left iliac crest. She then reaches under his thorax to grasp his right shoulder posteriorly.

Over-pressure to the rotation is achieved by the physiotherapist pulling downwards towards the floor with her left hand and assisting the backward rotation of the patient's left thorax by the use of her left arm anterior to his left shoulder. The rotation is then performed to the right (*Figure 12.3*).

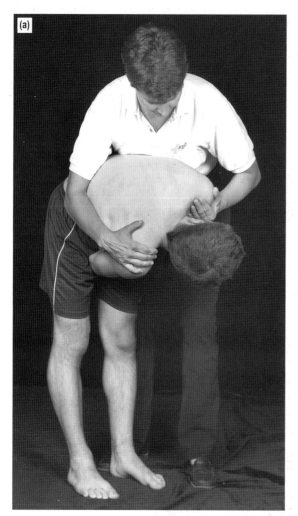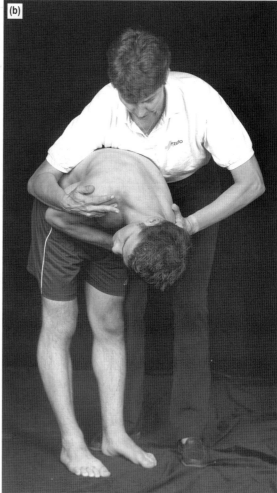

Figure 12.3    Lumbar flexion over-pressure adding rotation with over-pressure. (*a*) Rotation left. (*b*) Rotation right

If there is any sign of a protective deformity (erroneously called 'sciatic scoliosis'; Maitland, 1961) during any test movement, the test movement should be repeated with the physiotherapist countering (preventing the deformity taking place) the protective deformity and assessing the change in pain response. If the pain response increases dramatically, the deformity on movement is directly related to the disorder causing the patient's symptoms, as discussed earlier.

De Seze (1955) describes and illustrates the common varieties of protective deformity very clearly. He states that the L5 sciaticas caused by the L4/5 disc are accompanied most commonly by a contralateral list, while the ipsilateral list occurs more frequently with S1 sciaticas caused by the lumbosacral disc. Lumbar kyphosis occurs with equal frequency at the L4/5 and lumbosacral levels. Sometimes the patient's inability to extend his lumbar spine or laterally flex it towards the painful side is expressed in a one-legged stance, with the leg on the painful side resting on the ball of the foot with the hip and knee slightly flexed. Although De Seze discusses the alternating list, he does not mention the arc of list that can occur during forward flexion. This may be seen as a deviation of the patient's thorax to one side during the middle third of the flexion movement, or alternatively the patient's

pelvis may displace backwards on the opposite side. Nor does he mention that these lists may be present only on extension. In addition they may be present in conjunction with a protective spasm of either the flexor or extensor muscles, or the flexor or extensor spasm can also be present without any list. When spasm is present in the extensor muscles, response to treatment is slow whether this spasm is bilateral, causing a marked lordosis localized to two vertebrae, or unilateral.

Movement in the lumbar spine in particular has one fascinating feature: its movements can produce entirely different pain responses depending upon whether the movement is performed from the top downwards or from the bottom upwards.

All of the basic lumbar physiological movements tested in the standing position can be performed by the patient from above downwards (which is what most examiners would do, and be content with the pain response answers obtained) and also from below upwards. *Figures 12.4–12.7* explain the examples. Rotation from below upwards is of particular value when the lower two intervertebral discs are suspected of being a source of symptoms. It may also be helpful in deciding the direction of rotation as a treatment technique based on the desired effect. For example, if

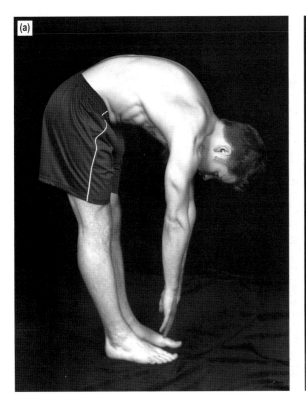
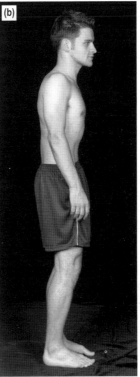

**Figure 12.4** Lumbar spine flexion. (*a*) From above downwards. (*b*) From below upwards

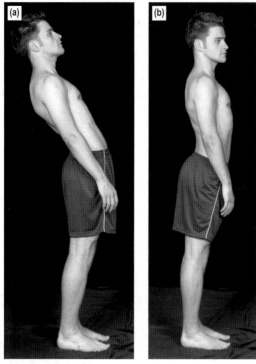

**Figure 12.5** Lumbar spine extension. (*a*) From above downwards. (*b*) From below upwards

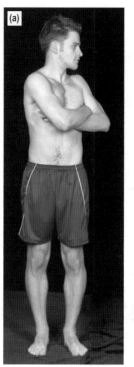
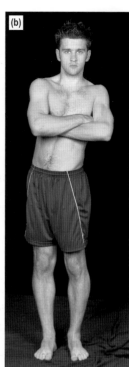

**Figure 12.7** Lumbar spine rotation, commonly referred to as rotation to the left. (*a*) From above downwards. (*b*) From below upwards

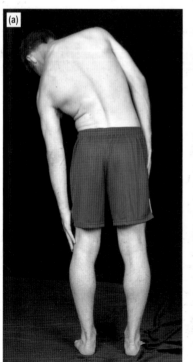
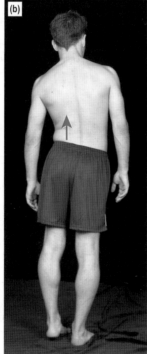
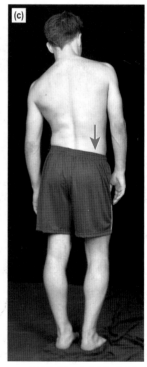

**Figure 12.6** Lumbar spine lateral flexion left. (*a*) From above downwards. (*b*) From below upwards, hitching left hip. (*c*) Dropping the right hip

rotation from below upwards to the right reproduces severe right calf pain and numbness of the right big toe, but rotation from below upwards to the left only reproduces backache, rotation of the pelvis to the LEFT would be the direction of first choice. This would be more likely to influence the intervertebral discs without provoking the nerve-root symptoms.

## LUMBAR EXTENSION

A patient with low lumbar pain may appear to have a full painless range of extension in standing. If it is thought that the pain may be coming from the lumbosacral level, it is advisable to include the following test: the standing patient should be asked to flex his pelvis (i.e. tuck his tail between his legs as a cat or dog can) and then extend his pelvis. This movement, particularly extension, may reproduce back pain in comparison with a pain-free arching backwards of his trunk. This response is accentuated if spinal extension is then added to the pelvic extension. When arching backwards, the movement starts from the top and gradually the lower joints take part in the movement, and it is possible that the low lumbar area is so protected by muscle spasm that the movement is pain free. If the extension movement is done in reverse by moving the pelvis, the intervertebral movement starts from the lowest moving joint and then it extends upwards. If pelvic movement reproduces the patient's back pain, the cause will almost certainly lie in the lumbosacral joint.

When, on examination, a patient appears to have a painless full range of extension, or when he is aware of minimal lumbar discomfort, the technique for applying the over-pressure needs to be performed in a specific manner if important information is not to be missed.

The same technique can be used to differentiate between whether a stiff-looking section of the spine is

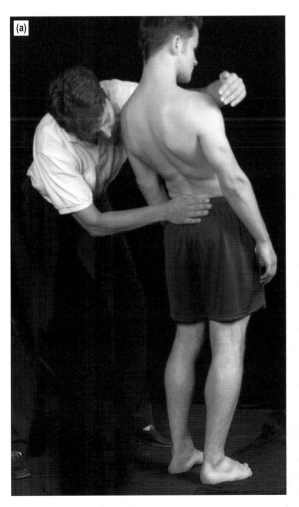 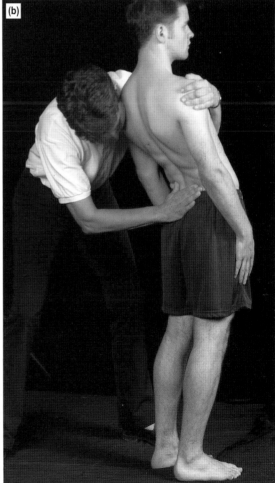

Figure 12.8 Assessing lumbar extension by over-pressure. (*a*) Preparatory positioning. (*b*) Over-pressure applied

painful on extension or whether it is the intervertebral level immediately above or below the stiff section. The differentiation is made by changing the position of the pivoting index finger and thumb (*Figure 12.8a*). There are two stages. The physiotherapist encourages the patient to arch further by intermittently touching his shoulders and chest with her left arm. This is done as light touches combined with a verbal command; constant contact with her hand and arm must be avoided. At the same time she uses her right index finger and thumb in the same manner. It is essential for the physiotherapist that the patient maintains *his own balance*, but she can provide the patient with a degree of security by allowing his hair to touch her neck and left suprascapular area without her taking the weight of his head and neck (*Figure 12.8b*). When she knows he is at the limit of his range of extension, she then applies the over-pressure by carrying his thorax backwards with her left arm, pivoting the further extension over the postero-anterior pressure of her right index finger and thumb, with her neck increasing the support of his head and neck.

## LATERAL FLEXION (IN STANDING)

Examination of lumbar lateral flexion is most valuable when comparing the quality and range of movement from one side to another. The range of lateral flexion is best measured in terms of the curve of segmental mobility. Over-pressure can be added by standing behind the patient and placing both hands over the respective supraspinous supraclavicular areas of each shoulder, and following the arc of lateral flexion beyond the active range. Over-pressure can be applied more locally by the therapist standing at the right side of the patient (for example) and placing her left thumb against the right side of each lumbar spinous process in turn. She adds over-pressure by holding the patient's left shoulder with her right hand and resting her right axilla on top of his right shoulder. She then bends her knees to take the lateral flexion beyond the active range, and her left thumb localizes the over-pressure. Alternatively, if there is height incompatibility between the therapist and patient, the therapist can grasp round the patient's trunk with her right arm.

## ROTATION

Lumbar rotation can be examined either in standing or sitting. However, lumbar rotation as an active movement is often more valuable when performed in combined movements, as described below.

## LATERAL SHIFT

Testing lateral displacement of the thorax on the pelvis is a very important test movement, especially for the lower lumbar spine. McKenzie (1981) described the technique very clearly and its application very fully. His text is extremely valuable and provides a totally original concept, which must be known and understood by every manipulative physiotherapist. In the context of this text, it would be impossible to cover his field adequately; however, it needs to be understood in the depth that McKenzie's book provides. A method of testing lateral shift with the patient in the standing position is described below.

The physiotherapist stands on the patient's left side and places her right hand around his right lateral iliac crest. She then places her left hand on top of his left shoulder in such a manner that she can stabilize his left upper thoracic area between her thorax posteriorly and her left arm anteriorly, and asks the patient to relax and allow his hips and shoulders to slide. She applies an equal and opposite pressure with each hand making sure that, as the movement of the patient's lumbar spine takes place, the lower lumbar spine moves horizontally laterally and does not go into a right lateral flexion movement. The rhythm and range of the lateral movement, together with any pain response, is noted. To test the movement in the opposite direction while still standing on the patient's left side, she changes her hand positions. She now places her left hand over his right shoulder and her right hand cupped around his left lateral iliac crest area. The lateral shift movement from this position moves the thorax laterally to the left over his pelvis (*Figure 12.9*).

To apply strong over-pressure to, say, a shift to the right, she stands by his left side, placing his left elbow between her upper sternum–clavicular– shoulder area, and clasps her hands around his right iliac crest. The over-pressure is produced by a horizontal push to the patient's lower ribs to his right while firmly applying an equal horizontal pull with her hands on his iliac crest towards his left (*Figure 12.9d*).

## WHEN APPLICABLE TESTS

Assessing the quality, range and pain response, particularly as they relate to combinations of flexion and rotation in the low lumbar spine, provides powerful information on which to base the selection of treatment techniques, and for assessment purposes. To read a text that describes all of the details regarding the techniques would be tedious to say the least. Therefore, the drawings with minimal text (and using the

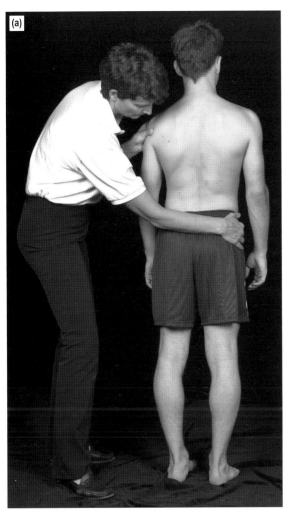

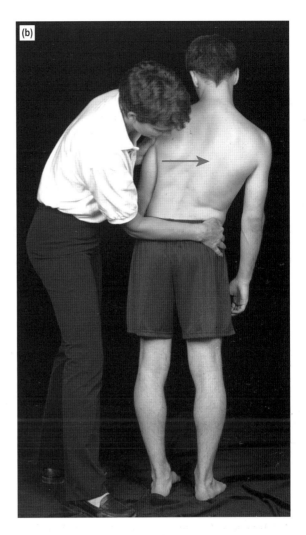

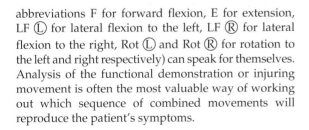

Figure 12.9 (a) Lateral shift. (b) Lateral shift of the trunk right

abbreviations F for forward flexion, E for extension, LF Ⓛ for lateral flexion to the left, LF Ⓡ for lateral flexion to the right, Rot Ⓛ and Rot Ⓡ for rotation to the left and right respectively) can speak for themselves. Analysis of the functional demonstration or injuring movement is often the most valuable way of working out which sequence of combined movements will reproduce the patient's symptoms.

## Combined movements in flexion

*Figure 12.10a* – F. The patient's pelvis is securely stabilized between the physiotherapist's left inguinal fossa with her right hand gripping around his iliac crest to the anterior superior iliac spine.

*Figure 12.10b* – F + LF Ⓛ. While maintaining the flexed position and the stabilized pelvis, the patient laterally flexes to the left and the physiotherapist pulls with her left hand to apply over-pressure.

*Figure 12.10c* – F + LF Ⓛ + Rot Ⓛ. The physiotherapist uses the whole of her left arm and hand to twist the thoracic and lumbar spine into the rotated position. A very strong grasp of the patient's pelvis is needed; in fact she pulls strongly backward with her right hand around the anterior superior iliac spine, and pushes forward strongly with her right anterior superior iliac spine against his mid-to-lateral left buttock.

*Figure 12.10d* – F + LF Ⓛ + Rot Ⓡ. The physiotherapist uses the full length of her left forearm to fingers to produce the thoracic rotation to the right. She also needs to work hard with her left arm to avoid losing the lateral flexion component. Hopefully, it is obvious from the text of this book that the movements of lateral flexion and rotation can be performed in a different

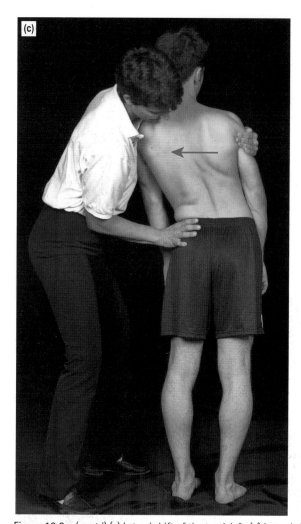

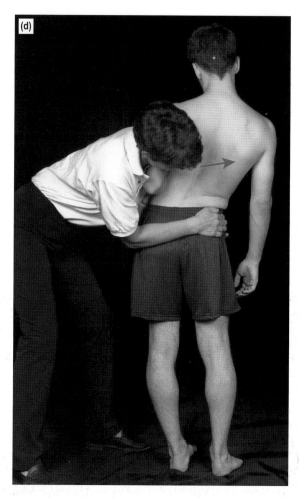

**Figure 12.9** *(contd)* (c) Lateral shift of the trunk left. (d) Lateral shift right of the pelvis left with over-pressure

sequence and that the test can also be performed to the other side.

## Combined movements in extension

*Figure 12.11* – E. The care and sequence of adopting the extension position is described on page 349.

*Figure 12.12* – E + Rot Ⓛ. The physiotherapist pulls with her left fingers, and pushes with her left upper arm/axillary hold. Counter-pressure is needed through her right thumb. If lateral flexion to the left is added to this position the patient is then in the 'quadrant' test position.

When using the quadrant test for the lumbar spine, the physiotherapist should stand behind the patient on the side away from which she intends turning the patient. She encourages him to extend to the limit of his range and then places her hands over his shoulders

for control. Then, and only then, should she apply through her hands some pressure to the extension while ensuring that her nearside shoulder is near his occiput to take the weight of his head if required. By using her hands on his shoulders, she then guides his trunk into the corner by laterally flexing and rotating his trunk away from her. Movement is continued until the limit of the range is reached (*Figure 12.13*).

*Figure 12.14* – E + Rot Ⓡ. The therapist pushes the patient's left shoulder forwards with her shoulder area, and his right shoulder backwards with her left hand. In this direction it is her right index finger that supplies the counter-pressure.

## Combined movements in lateral flexion left

*Figure 12.15* – LF Ⓛ . The localizing (or emphasizing) of the intervertebral level is achieved by the therapist's

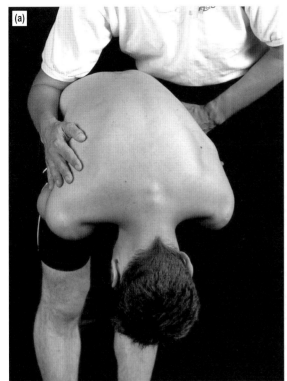

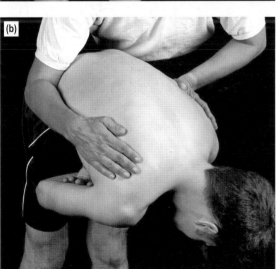

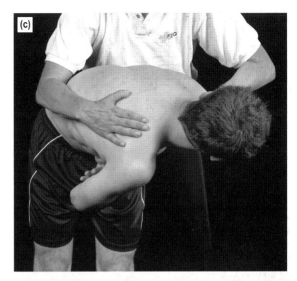

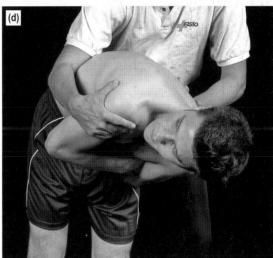

**Figure 12.10**   Combined movements in flexion. (*a*) F.
(*b*) F + LF Ⓛ. (*c*) F + LF Ⓛ + Rot Ⓛ. (*d*) F + LF Ⓛ + Rot Ⓡ

thumb anteriorly and the web of her hand between the thumb and index finger laterally, and her index finger is reinforced by her middle finger posteriorly. She uses her left axilla, her upper thorax and her left upper arm to keep control of the stability and apply the over-pressure.

*Figure 12.16* – LF Ⓛ + E. By careful position of her grasp around his upper thorax, that is by using her clavicular–axillary–arm and hand grasp, the physio-therapist can keep the patient's thorax in the coronal plane during the extension movement. Also, she can emphasize the intervertebral level of extension with

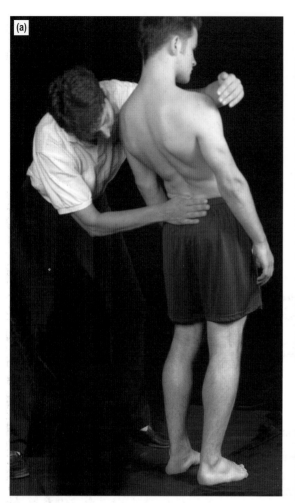
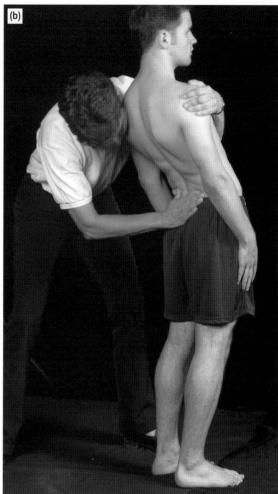

**Figure 12.11**    Combined movements in extension. (*a*) Prepartion position. (*b*) Over-pressure

counter-pressures between her left elbow and her right fingers.

*Figure 12.17* – LF Ⓛ + F. The thorax must still be maintained in the coronal plane. The flexion can be emphasized to various intervertebral levels by appropriate pressures with the physiotherapist's left elbow and right thumb in conjunction with counter-pressure from her all-surrounding grasp of his upper thorax.

*Figure 12.18* – LF Ⓛ + Rot Ⓛ. For this technique, the physiotherapist's grasp of the patient's upper thorax, making maximum use of her left axilla and left hand, is imperative if the rotation is to be totally in her control.

*Figure 12.19* – LF Ⓛ + Rot Ⓡ. As with Rot Ⓛ, the physiotherapist has to have a firm grasp of the patient's upper thorax to maintain the control necessary to produce rotation to the right of the patient's thorax and thus his lumbar spine.

## Combined movements in rotation left

*Figure 12.20* – Rot Ⓛ. After taking the patient into the fully rotated position (*Figure 12.20a*) the therapist changes her grasp so that she can hold the full range of rotation with her left axilla and hand, thus leaving her right hand free.

*Figure 12.21* – Rot Ⓛ + E. The intervertebral level to be tested with this extension has its level emphasized by the physiotherapist's thoracic grasp and her left upper arm/forearm/elbow countering the postero-anterior pressure exerted at the appropriate intervertebral level with her right index finger and thumb.

*Figure 12.22* – Rot Ⓛ + F. While adding the flexion to the rotation, the tension of the rotation needs to be increased; without its being increased, the flexion has a loose feel about it and thus becomes valueless as a combined-movement test.

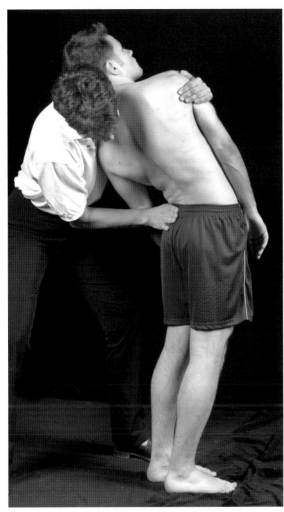

**Figure 12.12**   Combined movement in extension

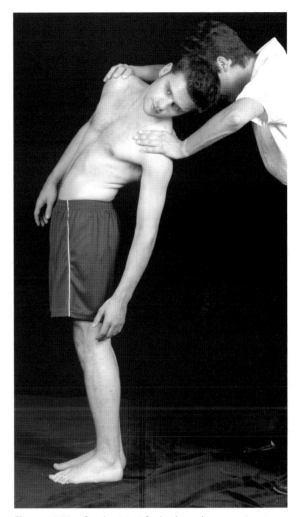

**Figure 12.13**   Quadrant test for lumbar spine

*Figure 12.23* – Rot Ⓛ + LF Ⓛ. The physiotherapist's right thumb localizes or emphasizes the intervertebral level desired, while the patient is guided into the lateral flexion movement towards his left shoulder. This lateral flexion movement can have added to it:

1.  A left-sided compression component by the physiotherapist applying a pressure on the patient's left shoulder with her axilla.
2.  A displacement component towards the patient's right by directing her left axillary pressure on the patient's left shoulder towards his right hip.

*Figure 12.24* – Rot Ⓛ + LF Ⓡ. The direction of the lateral flexion component is towards his right shoulder, and during this movement she needs to lift her body upwards to keep the same grasp of his left shoulder area with her left axilla.

*Figure 12.25* – Rot Ⓛ + F + LFⓇ. Obviously, there are many combinations that can be used, but this is just one combination that uses movement in the three planes.

## PALPATION

Phillips and Twomey (1993) have produced the best evidence yet that manual diagnosis, including palpation examination and passive intervertebral movement testing, can be a reliable means of identifying symptomatic lumbar segmental levels. This is the case when manual diagnosis is compared with the most reliable diagnostic method available, namely segmental spinal anaesthetic block procedures.

As has been stated earlier, the first steps in this palpation examination are to determine sweating and temperature.

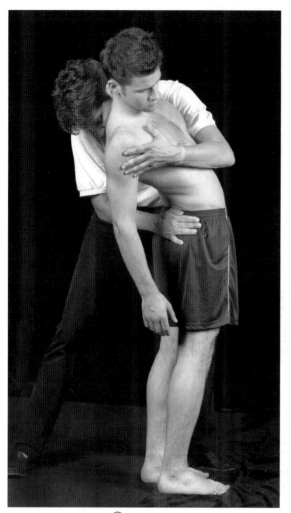

Figure 12.14    E + Rot Ⓡ

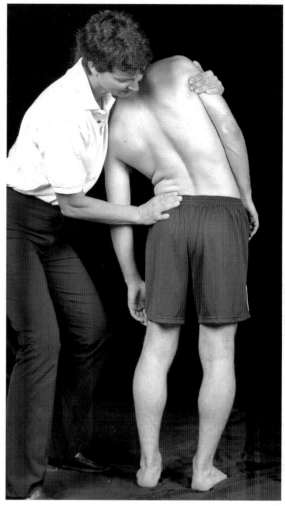

Figure 12.15    Combined movement in lateral flexion left. LF Ⓛ

## Sweating

This is not an uncommon finding at an initial consultation, and it is also a phenomenon that can occur as a result of mobilizing an intervertebral area that is the cause of pain. Its significance to the manipulative physiotherapist is little more than indicating the intervertebral level at fault and, as is quite often important, proof that something abnormal must be present; that is, it is not possible to bring about sweating by mobilizing a normal spine.

## Temperature

In the lumbar spine there is a fusiform area, which is nearly always warmer than surrounding areas. It has its horizontal central level at the iliac crests, and its midline is the line of the spinous processes (*Figure 6.31*). There are times when a patient will mention that his back feels hot, and on examination this statement will be confirmed.

There is a very definite quality to the warmth; it feels as though it is coming from within and working its way out to the surface. When this is present in the patients who are selectively referred for manipulative physiotherapy, it is not likely to be inflammatory due to a disease process but rather from a mechanical disorder. When the temperature change is very definite, treatment strength and progression should be gentler and slower, but the speed with which the increased temperature disappears is quite astounding. On examination the temperature should be assessed using the back of the hand and the palm, with sweeping large

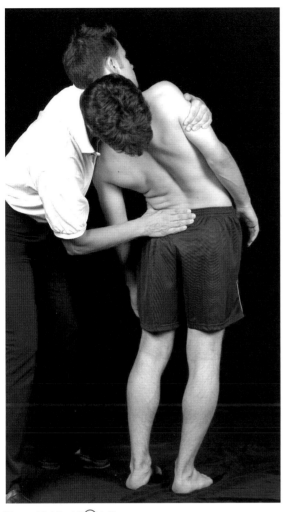

**Figure 12.16**   LF Ⓛ + E

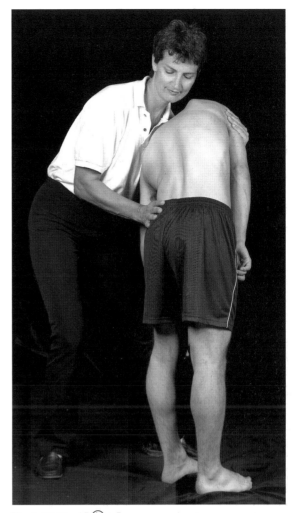

**Figure 12.17**   LF Ⓛ + F

movements at first, gradually reducing the size of the sweep to localized areas when indicated. It is often useful to assess temperature after treatment, especially when it is thought possible that a disorder may have been disturbed unfavourably by treatment.

## Soft tissue, bony tissue and position

> All lumbar interspinous spaces should be palpated *deeply*, as should the lateral surfaces of the spinous processes

This aspect has been covered in depth in Chapters 6 (*see* pp. 149–165) and 10 (*see* pp. 190–192). However,

there are some aspects that are special to the thoracic and lumbar spines.

All lumbar interspinous spaces should be palpated deeply with discernment, as should the lateral surface of the spinous processes. Thickening can occur on one or both sides of the process or in the space, even to the extent where the interspinous space on one (or both) side(s) can be completely obliterated by thickened hard tissue. *Figure 12.26* shows how this can be performed without the examiner having to move her position. She stands alongside the patient facing his feet, and uses her middle fingertip to probe into the right space and her index finger to dig medially into the left space. She can change rapidly from side to side, and equally rapidly from one level to the next, upwards or downwards.

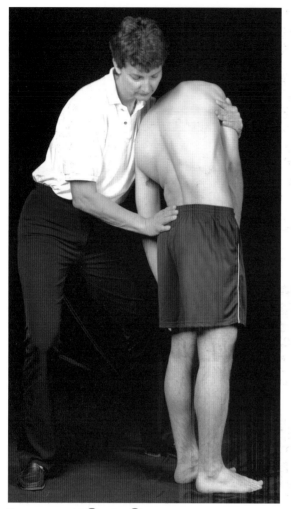

**Figure 12.18** LF Ⓛ + Rot Ⓛ

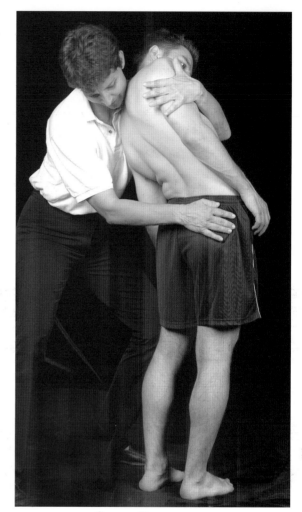

**Figure 12.19** LF Ⓛ + Rot Ⓡ

It is also necessary to use the index and middle fingers to palpate into the interspinous space. When doing so, the fingers are held tightly together and oscillated back and forth sideways in an attempt to sink deeply into the space. This can be achieved in normals but not in abnormals (*Figure 12.27*).

*Figure 12.28* – Deeper palpations of the interspinous area. By using the tip of the thumb a greater depth, even as deep as the lamina, can be reached. An assessment of this depth should be carried out if the more superficial area is normal.

*Figure 12.29* – Palpation of the paravertebral soft-tissue structures. Both thumb tips are utilized, and the probing deep palpation should be carried out in many different directions – medially, lateral, caudally and cephalad. Also, the palpation should not be limited to

the interlaminar area but should be extended to the adjacent upper and lower borders of the lamina and over the lamina itself.

## PASSIVE ACCESSORY INTERVERTEBRAL MOVEMENTS (PAIVMs)

These are fully described in this chapter under the heading of 'techniques', but relate to those techniques that involve direct contact on superficial parts of the vertebra. As described in Chapter 6, it is necessary to vary the point of contact through which the movement is produced, and to vary the inclination of the manipulative physiotherapist's arm and thereby the direction of the movement.

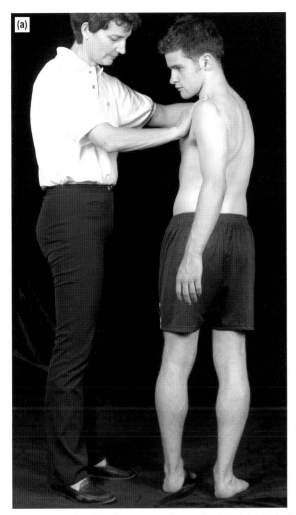

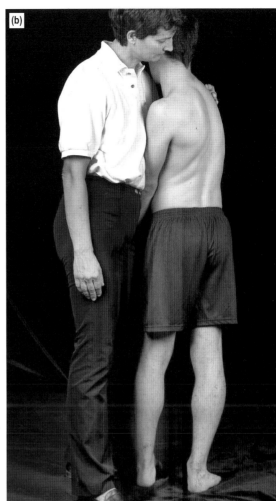

Figure 12.20    Combined movements in rotation left. (*a*) Initial adopting position. (*b*) End-position before adding other movements

The techniques used to assess the quality and range of movements are described in detail on pages 368–372 (*Figures 12.37–12.41*).

## Pain response

Having come to a decision as to where there is any hypomobility, hypermobility or protective muscle spasm, the movement produced by palpation is assessed for pain response with the movement. As a joint may be hypermobile yet painless or hypomobile yet painless, the relationship between pain and movement can only be identified by the patient. An important example of this is the examination of a patient who has an inactive Scheuermann's disease in the upper lumbar spine. His pain may be arising from the stiff diseased joints or, more commonly, from the joint above the diseased section because it has had to take over mobility functions from the stiff area below. For example, while carrying out postero-anterior pressures, the patient should be asked two particular questions:

1. 'Does the pain feel superficial or deep?' Superficial pain felt directly under the physiotherapist's hand or thumb may be unassociated with the disorder, or may be a referred tenderness and therefore an abnormal response. A deep pain is always an abnormal response.

2. 'Is the pain felt under my hand ONLY, or does it spread at all?' Any spread of pain is classed as abnormal.

*During examination for low lumbar pain even the upper lumbar area must be subjected, if necessary, to firm*

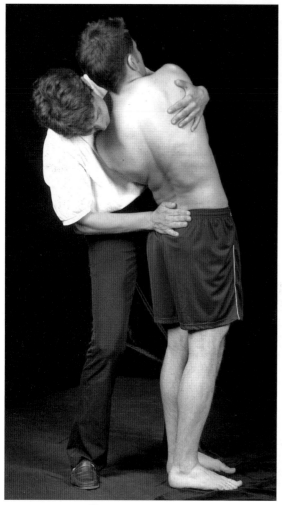

**Figure 12.21**  Rot Ⓛ + E

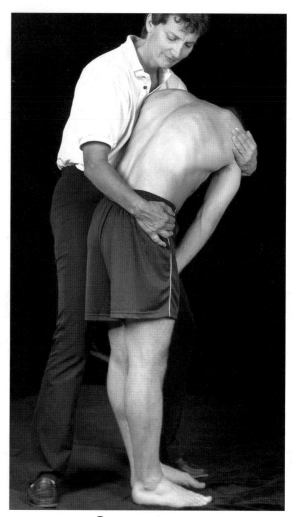

**Figure 12.22**  Rot Ⓛ + F

*sustained over-pressure in the postero-anterior direction because this level quite frequently reproduces the low lumbar pain.*

There is one palpation technique that is performed for its pain response rather than to enable the assessment of movement, and is of particular value in the examination of spondylolisthetic-type pain. The technique is anteroposterior pressure on the body of the vertebra. When performing the procedure it should be done slowly, gradually sinking through the abdomen to reach the promontory of the sacrum. The contact position can then be moved to wherever it is needed to make the examination complete. Abdominal discomfort is lessened by using all the fingers of both hands (*Figure 12.30*). This technique is of value for the lower lumbar vertebral bodies only, thus avoiding compromise of the descending aorta.

## PASSIVE RANGE OF PHYSIOLOGICAL MOVEMENTS OF SINGLE INTERVERTEBRAL JOINTS (PPIVMs)

These passive test movements are described in detail below. It must be remembered that the examining movements are usually performed at a slower speed than when they are used as treatment techniques. Also, the examination movement should be taken to the end of the available range and then over-pressure applied so as to assess the end-feel of the movement.

### T11–S1 (lateral flexion)

*Starting position*

The patient lies on his right side with his hips and knees flexed to allow his lumbar spine to lie relaxed

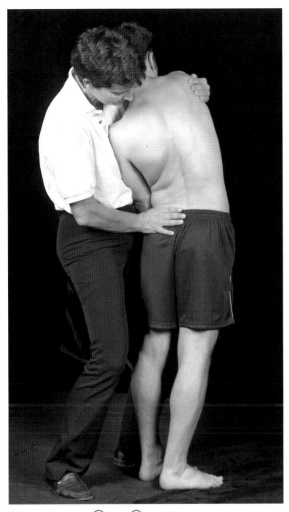

Figure 12.23   Rot Ⓛ + LF Ⓛ

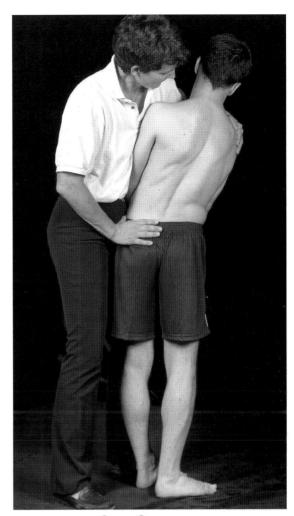

Figure 12.24   Rot Ⓛ + LF Ⓡ

midway between flexion and extension. If the patient has unusually large hips compared with the size of the thorax, a pillow should be placed under the lumbar spine to prevent it sagging into lateral flexion. The physiotherapist, standing in front of the patient and facing his feet, reaches across his left side while resting her lower ribs against his side with her left forearm pointing caudad along his spine and her right forearm grasping around his pelvis under the ischial tuberosity. She places the pad of her left middle finger facing upwards in the underside of the interspinous space to feel the bony margin of the adjacent vertebrae (*Figure 12.31*).

### Method

With the physiotherapist grasping the patient's pelvis and upper thigh with her right forearm and her right

side, she laterally flexes his lumbar spine from below upwards by rocking his pelvis. She tips his pelvis cephalad on the left by pulling with her right forearm, and returns it by pushing against his thigh with her right side. An oscillatory movement produced in this way rocks the pelvis, with the underside hip and femur acting as the pivot. The movement is easy to produce and easy to palpate (*Figure 12.32*).

To test lateral flexion to the opposite side the patient should be asked to turn over.

### T11–S1 (rotation)

#### Starting position

This starting position is similar to that described for lateral flexion, but it is necessary to ensure that the patient's top knee will slide freely forwards over the

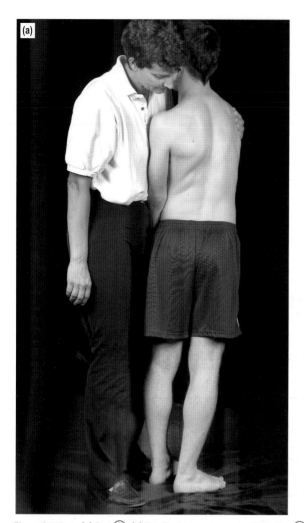

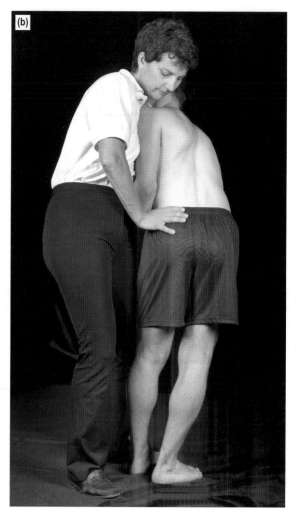

**Figure 12.25** (a) Rot Ⓛ. (b) The flexion component added. Rot Ⓛ + F

underneath knee. The physiotherapist leans across the patient, placing her left forearm along his back to palpate the interspinous space from underneath, whilst twisting her trunk slightly to face his hips. She holds over his left hip with her right hand, her fingers spreading out behind his trochanter and the heel of her hand anterior to the trochanter. Her right forearm holds along his left femur (*Figure 12.33*).

## Method

While the physiotherapist stabilizes the patient's thorax with her left arm and side, she rotates his pelvis towards her by pulling with her right hand. As his top knee slides forwards over his right knee, the pelvis and lumbar spine rotate forwards on the left side. Ensuring that her palpating finger keeps pace with this movement, she will feel the displacement of the distal

spinous process in relation to the proximal one. She effects the return movement of the pelvis with the heel of her right hand and her right forearm.

Rotation in the opposite direction can be tested without changing the patient to the other side. However, uniformity of 'feel' is best achieved by repeating the technique on the other side.

## T11–S1 (flexion/extension)

### Starting position

The patient lies on his right side with hips and knees flexed. The physiotherapist, standing in front of the patient, reaches behind and under the patient's flexed knees to grasp anteriorly around the right knee. She then lifts his knees and rests the lower legs against her own upper thighs, placing the knees just beyond her

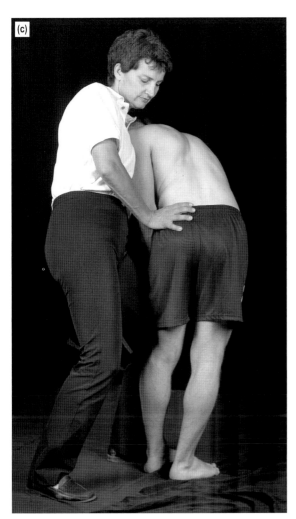

Figure 12.25 (*contd*) (c) Lateral flexion right added.
Rot Ⓛ + F + LF Ⓡ

left thigh. With her left arm stretched over the patient's lower scapular area to prevent any backward rotation of the thorax, the physiotherapist places the tip of the pad of the index or middle finger in the interspinous space to be tested, where it can feel the adjacent margins of two spinous processes. To help palpate more deeply without losing sensibility, this finger can be reinforced over the nail by the middle finger (*Figure 12.34*).

### Method

Passive movement of the spine is produced by rocking the patient's knees back and forth towards his chest through an arc of 30°. Over-pressure should be applied at the limit of extension to assess any backward sliding of a vertebra, which may indicate instability. The test movement is produced by a side-to-side movement of

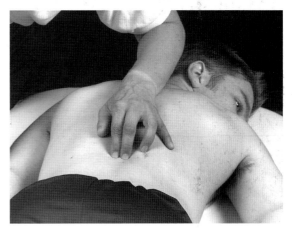

Figure 12.27 Palpating postero-anteriorly in depth

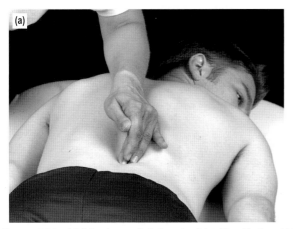

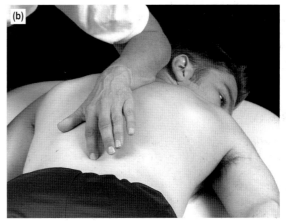

Figure 12.26 (*a*) Palpating medially into the right side with the middle finger. (*b*) Palpating medially into the left side with the index finger

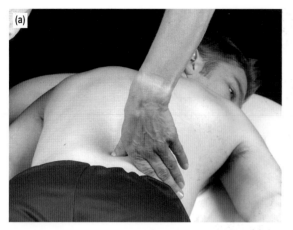

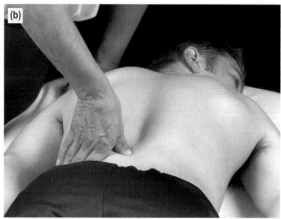

**Figure 12.28**  Deeper palpation of the interspinous area. (*a*) Right side. (*b*) Left side

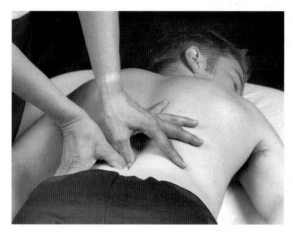

**Figure 12.29**  Palpation of the paravertebral soft-tissue structures

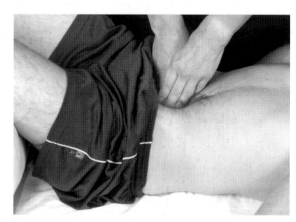

**Figure 12.30**  Anteroposterior pressure

the physiotherapist's pelvis, carrying the patient's legs with her. The palpating hand can help to increase the intervertebral range by pressing against the spine when the patient's legs are released from their flexed position. An opening and closing of the interspinous gap can be felt with the rocking of the patient's pelvis and legs. The arc of 30° will be with the legs in relatively less flexion when palpating movement in the upper lumbar spine, and relatively more flexion when palpating for movement in the lower lumbar spine.

### Instability

Particularly in the lower lumbar spine, excessive mobility or instability in the sagittal plane can be assessed by varying the above technique slightly. During the testing of extension, the manipulative physiotherapist pushes along the direction of the femoral shaft so as to push a lower vertebra backwards beneath the neighbouring vertebra above it. When instability exists, the excessive movement backwards of the lower spine can be appreciated by her palpating finger. Similarly, during the assessment of flexion the manipulative physiotherapist, by pulling in line with the shaft of the femur, will produce excessive interspinous movement if instability in flexion is present.

### T11–S1 (flexion/extension) – single-leg technique

As some physiotherapists find the technique using both of the patient's legs to produce the movement awkward, a single-leg technique is described. However, accurate positioning of the underneath leg becomes important.

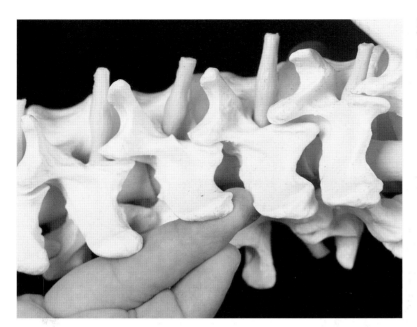

Figure 12.31    Intervertebral movement. T11–S1 (lateral flexion). Position of palpating finger for lumbar spine

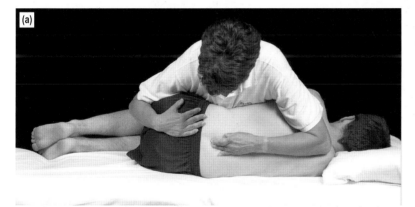

Figure 12.32    (*a*) and (*b*) Intervertebral movement. T11–S1 (lateral flexion)

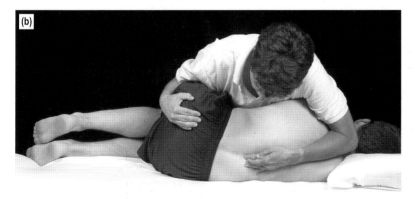

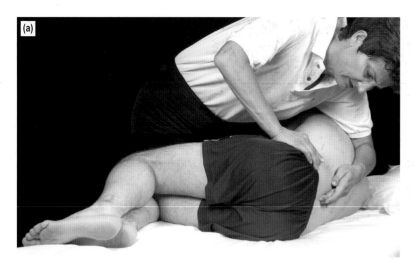

**Figure 12.33** (*a*) and (*b*) Intervertebral movement. T11–S1 (rotation)

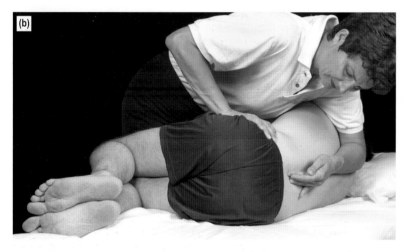

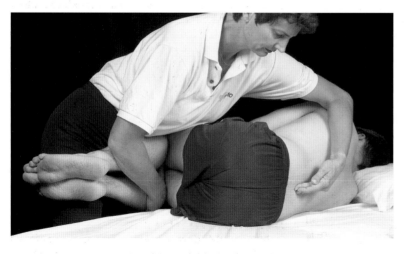

**Figure 12.34** Intervertebral movement. T11–S1 (flexion/extension)

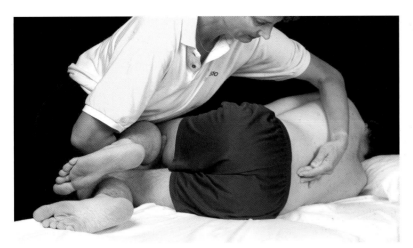

**Figure 12.35** Intervertebral movement. T11–S1 (flexion/extension). Single leg technique

### Starting position

The patient lies on his right side and the physiotherapist stands in front of his upper chest facing towards his hips. She places her left forearm along his back to palpate between adjacent spinous processes from underneath with her middle finger while stabilizing his thorax between her left arm and left side. With her right hand she grasps his left upper tibia from in front (*Figure 12.35*).

### Method

The physiotherapist produces flexion and extension of the patient's lumbar spine by flexing and releasing the flexion of his left hip while she assists extension by pressure with the heel of her left hand against the lumbar spine.

*Disturbances of spinal movements*. These can be evaluated more clearly by study of the physiological and pathological changes that occur in the disc and apophyseal joints (Harris and Macnab, 1954). Similarly, it is important to be familiar with the radiological appearance of the normal spine; for example, the contour and position of vertebrae, the size and appearance of disc spaces and the intervertebral foraminae. This knowledge helps in the correlation of congenital and developmental abnormalities with physical findings.

### Slump test

Testing for movement of pain-sensitive structures in the vertebral canal, as distinct from movements of the lumbar intervertebral joints, is the most important test that should be included in the examination of all patients so that it can be determined whether there is normal movement or not.

The slump test, so called because of its agreement with the term as used by engineers and architects, is described fully with diagrams on pages 144–149. The description of this test was placed in Chapter 6 because it is a test that should be used for cervical and thoracic disorders as well as lumbar disorders. However, its most useful applications are in the lumbar spine and secondly in the cervical spine.

As well as performing the test in the sagittal plane, it can also be performed by applying over-pressure to lateral flexion or rotation in sitting, before incorporating the initial slumping of the thoracic and lumbar spines.

The information being sought is a relationship between the range of movement and reproduction of the patient's symptoms. Added to this is the change of range/pain response that can occur when one aspect of the tensioned section is released. For example, extending the left knee may be limited by 30° compared with extending the right knee, and it may reproduce buttock pain. On releasing neck flexion, the buttock pain may disappear and the patient may be able to extend his knee a further 15°. This is the most common kind of response.

There are many ways in which the test can be carried out to reveal abnormalities in the movement of the pain-sensitive structures in the spinal and vertebral canals and along relevant peripheral nerves. The thing that is important is that, when signs are present, the treatment should initially be aimed at improving intervertebral movement while watching to see if there are parallel changes in canal movement. If the improvements are not parallel, then the canal movement that reproduces the lumbar symptoms should be substituted or added as treatment.

Because the dura mater is structurally different from ligamentous-type tissue, it can accept very strong mobilization. Its pain response, when produced by strong mobilization, is usually greater than that which is predictable when mobilizing ligaments, and the pain takes longer to settle than does ligamentous pain.

The slump test can be adapted to investigate all parts of the lumbar and lumbrosacral plexuses. For instance, if a patient has back pain and anterior thigh pain, the extent to which the canal structure and the femoral nerve are contributing may need to be tested. The patient can be 'slumped' in side lying. The addition of knee flexion and hip extension may reproduce his anterior thigh pain. Further addition of cervical flexion may increase the thigh pain and tighten the leg so that less hip extension or knee flexion is possible. Such a response would strongly implicate the neural structures as part of the mechanism of symptom production (Butler, 1991).

## EXAMINATION AND TREATMENT TECHNIQUES

As has been stated repeatedly, there is no limit to the treatment techniques that can be used. *There are no such things as 'Maitland techniques'.* However, a basis needs to be formulated to cover the 'teaching situation', but it must be remembered that all need to be tailored to the patient's symptoms, signs and pathology. The techniques described in the following pages form that basis.

## MOBILIZATION

### Postero–anterior central vertebral pressure (↕)

#### Starting position

The patient lies face downwards with his arms by his side or hanging over the sides of the couch and his head turned comfortably to one side.

When extremely gentle mobilizing is being performed the starting position and method is identical with that described for postero-anterior central vertebral pressure for the middle and lower thoracic area (*see* p. 318). However, as the need for stronger pressure arises the thumbs are inadequate, because the technique becomes uncomfortable for the patient and the physiotherapist loses the degree of feel that she should have. It is better to change to using the hands as the means for transmitting the pressure.

The physiotherapist stands at the left side of the patient and places her left hand (this one is chosen for convenience) on the patient's back so that that part of the ulnar border of the hand between the pisiform and the hook of the hamate is in contact with the spinous process of the vertebra to be mobilized. For this bone to be the major point of contact while the physiotherapist's shoulders are positioned directly above the vertebra, it is necessary to extend the left wrist fully and hold the forearm midway between full supination and full pronation. If complete wrist extension is not maintained the whole of the ulnar border of the hand will become the contact area and accurate localization will be lost. This left hand is then reinforced by the right by fitting the carpus of the right hand, cupped by the approximation of the thenar and hypothenar eminences, over the radial aspect of the left carpus at the base of the left index finger (*Figure 12.36*). Then, by allowing the right middle, ring and little fingers to lie between the left index finger and thumb, and by allowing the right index finger and thumb to lie over the back of the left hand, stability is gained by grasping the palm of the left hand between the thenar eminence and the middle, ring and little fingers of the right hand.

To hold this right-hand position with the physiotherapist's body weight over the hands, the right wrist must be extended.

The physiotherapist's shoulders are balanced over the top of the patient, and the elbows are allowed to flex slightly (*Figure 12.37*).

#### Method

The position is taken up by gradually moving the therapist's body weight forwards more directly over the patient's vertebral column, and the oscillating movement of the vertebra is obtained by a rocking movement of the upper trunk up and down in her vertical axis. The pressure is transmitted through the arms and shoulders, which act as strong springs.

#### Local variations

There is no natural tenderness to be felt when mobilizing the lumbar spine. Movement can be felt readily, but is noticeably less at the level of the fifth lumbar vertebra than it is above this level.

When a patient has an excessive lordosis, a small firm pillow placed under the abdomen may be necessary for joint positioning. Whether a pillow is used or not, the physiotherapist often needs to alter the direction of her arms to enable the push to be at right angles to the surface of the body.

#### Uses

Postero-anterior central vertebral pressure is best used in conditions of the lumbar spine that cause a

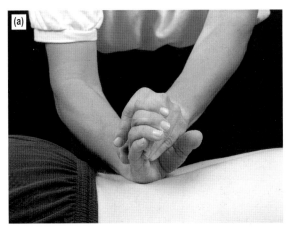
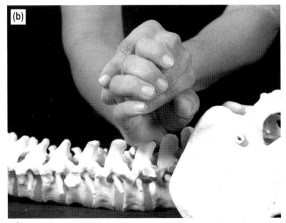

Figure 12.36    (a) and (b) Postero-anterior central vertebral pressure ($\updownarrow$)

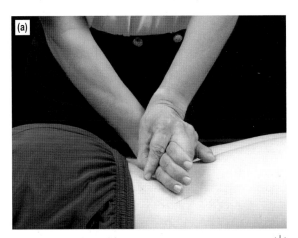
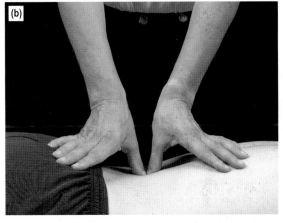

Figure 12.37    (a) and (b) Postero-anterior vertebral pressure ($\updownarrow$)

pain which is evenly distributed to both sides of the body.

As in the cervical spine, this technique is of value in patients whose symptoms arise from an area of the lumbar spine that has marked bony changes, whether these changes arise from degeneration or an old injury, or are structural changes associated with faulty posture.

This technique is indicated when pain or protective muscle spasm is felt with movement in this direction, but under these circumstances it is performed in such a way that the pain or spasm is not provoked.

Examples of treatment include chronic lumbar nerve root ache, pages 414–415; low back pain, page 430; buttock pain, page 432; spondylitic spine with localized lesion, page 433; coccygodynia, page 434; juvenile disc lesion, page 436; and abdominal pain and vague pains, page 443.

## Postero–anterior central vertebral pressure as combined movement, in lateral flexion right (in LF ® do $\updownarrow$)

### Starting position

The patient lies prone and the manipulative physiotherapist positions his lumbar spine in lateral flexion to the right. She does this by moving his trunk nearer to her, his pelvis away from her and his legs towards her. In fact his right hip should be abducted and his left hip adducted so that they stabilize his pelvis in the position, which laterally flexes his lumbar spine to the right.

Once the patient has been positioned correctly, the therapist places her hands on the level to be mobilized and then ensures that her shoulders are vertically above her hands (*Figure 12.38*).

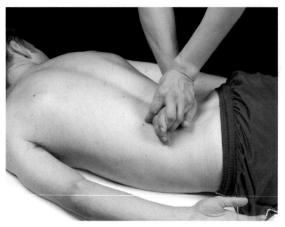

Figure 12.38   Postero-anterior central vertebral pressure as a combined movement, in lateral flexion right (in LF (R) do ↕)

### Method

The technique is the same as that described above without the lateral flexion positioning.

### Uses

This technique is used as a grade IV (nudging at the start of pain), or as a grade IV+ if stiffness is the main component.

## Anteroposterior central vertebral pressure (↕)

### Starting position

The patient lies supine with his hips and knees flexed and his feet resting on the couch. He relaxes his abdominal wall as the therapist very gradually sinks her fingers into his abdomen until she reaches the sacral prominence.

The manipulative physiotherapist overlaps the middle three fingers of each hand and places as much of their pads as possible on the patient's abdomen centrally and midway between his umbilicus and symphysis pubis. She slowly and carefully, so as to avoid abdominal discomfort as far as possible, sinks her fingers to reach the sacral prominence (*Figure 12.39*).

### Method

In producing the anteroposterior movement, the therapist needs to allow the distal interphalangeal joints to hyperextend fully so that the broadest contact possible of the pads of her fingers is made on the sacrum. During the oscillatory pressure, all of the flexors of her fingers and wrists must work eccentrically, not concentrically.

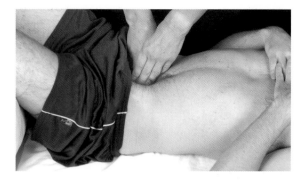

Figure 12.39   Anteroposterior central vertebral pressure (↕)

### Uses

This technique can be used for any low lumbar disorder, but has a special value for those patients experiencing pain from a spondylolisthesis or intradiscal disorder.

## Postero–anterior unilateral vertebral pressure (↓⟋)

### Starting position

The patient lies prone with his arms by his side, and his head can be turned to the side. If the technique is to be performed on the left side of the spine, the physiotherapist stands by the patient's left side and places her thumbs on his back, pointing towards each other, immediately adjacent to the spinous process on the left. It is wise not to reinforce one thumb with the other, as this destroys the feel that can be obtained through the pad of the thumb. The fingers are spread around the thumbs to provide stability. The base of the thumb is brought as near directly above the tip of the thumb as possible. This position is governed by the ability to hyperextend the thumbs (*Figure 12.40*).

Because the muscle bulk in this area is large, it is difficult to feel the transverse process clearly. However, if the points of the pads of the thumbs are used and the pressure is applied slowly, the majority of the muscle bulk can be penetrated to reach a firm bony base.

### Method

The physiotherapist positions her shoulders above her hands, and transmits the pressure of her trunk through her arms to her thumbs. The thumbs act as springs as the pressure is applied, and in no way do the thumb flexors act as prime movers.

The hands can be used to perform this technique, and when using this method the position of the hands

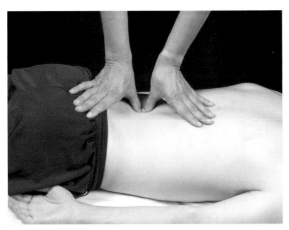

**Figure 12.40**  Postero-anterior unilateral vertebral pressure ( )

is the same as that described for postero-anterior central vertebral pressure (*see* p. 369). However, the disadvantage of using the hands is that the pressure cannot be localized as well, nor can there be as much feel for the very localized abnormalities of movement that can be palpated with the thumbs.

### Local variations

In the upper and middle lumbar areas it is easy to palpate the lateral margin of the transverse processes, as they are quite long. In the lower lumbar spine, however, the technique must be performed near the spinous process and time must be taken over penetrating the muscle bulk to reach the bony base.

### Uses

This technique is extremely valuable when muscle spasm of the deep intrasegmental muscles can be felt. The technique is carried out on the side of the muscle spasm or the pain, and its angle can be varied as indicated by the response to the technique.

### Transverse vertebral pressure ( ←•— )

#### Starting position

The patient lies prone with his arms by his side or hanging over the sides of the couch and his head comfortably turned to the side.

The physiotherapist stands by the patient's right side and places her hands on the patient's back so that the thumbs are against the right side of the spinous process of the vertebra to be mobilized. As much as possible of the pad of the left thumb is placed against the right lateral surface of the spinous process. The

right thumb is used as reinforcement by placing the pad of the right thumb over the nail of the left thumb. It is necessary to hyperextend the interphalangeal joint of the thumb and hold the metacarpophalangeal joint in a position of slight flexion. The left thumb is then wedged into position by the palmar surface of the base of the index finger to prevent the thumb sliding up and over the spinous process. The fingers of both hands are then spread out over the patient's back to help stabilize the position of the thumbs, and pressure is applied to the thumbs through the forearms held near the horizontal plane (*Figure 12.41a*).

### Method

When applying body pressure through the thumbs against the one spinous process, a certain amount of care is necessary to differentiate between the intervertebral joint movement and the rolling movement of the patient's trunk. The pressure is applied and relaxed repeatedly to produce an oscillating type of movement, small movement being produced by small pressures and larger movement by stronger pressures.

### Local variations

Movement is much greater at L1 than it is at L4, and in fact is felt readily at L1. The spinous process is far more accessible at L1 and L2 than it is at the lower levels. When stronger pressure is required, it may be easier to reinforce the left thumb with the ulnar border of the right hand in the area of the pisiform and hook of hamate as described on pages 320–321 (thoracic spine transverse vertebral pressure).

### Uses

This technique is of greatest value when used with symptoms that have a unilateral distribution. Under these circumstances it is more likely to produce an improvement in the patient's symptoms and signs if it is done from the painless side, pushing the spinous process towards the painful side. In this way the joint of the painful side is opened.

When used in the lower lumbar spine this mobilization is less valuable than either rotation or postero-anterior central vertebral pressure. It is useful, however, when used for conditions of the upper lumbar spine, and the higher the lumbar level causing the symptoms the more likely this technique is to succeed.

If a strong technique is required for the purpose of stretching the joint, which is not painful, the following technique may be adopted.

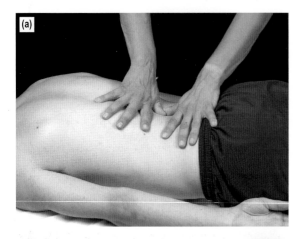

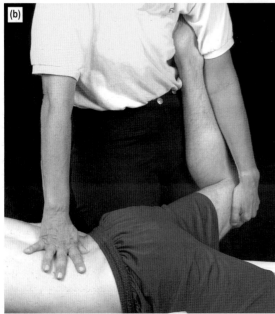

**Figure 12.41** (*a*) Transverse vertebral pressure (◄—►), starting position. (*b*) Transverse vertebral pressure (◄—►), strong technique

### Starting position

A position similar to the above is adopted, but with the right thumb pad placed against the spinous process of the vertebra being mobilized. The patient's right knee, flexed to a right angle, is then cradled in the physiotherapist's left hand so that the grasp is around the medial aspect of the knee (*Figure 12.41b*).

### Method

When the leg is used as a lever, care is needed in taking up the slack because of the movement that takes place at the hip joint. With the right thumb against the spinous process, the left arm abducts the patient's right leg until movement is felt to take place at the vertebra under the right thumb. The oscillating movement is then produced by a combined action of the right thumb against the spinous process and the left arm acting on the patient's leg. The range through which the femur is moved to assist with mobilizing after the slack has been taken up is quite small.

Examples of treatment include spondylitis and a spondylitic spine with a localized lesion, pages 433–434.

## ROTATION

Rotation, as a technique, is almost the most important technique. The manipulative physiotherapist needs to:

1. Master the rotary movement.
2. Know where the centre of the axis of the movement is.
3. Know how to vary the technique to alter the central axis of the movement.
4. Know how to combine the technique with different starting positions for the lumbar spine.
5. Know how to perform the rotation from the bottom upwards and the top downwards.

If these concepts have not been consciously considered, most people would think that when performing the rotation movement as described on pages 374, 375 (*Figure 12.44*), the centre of the rotation would be somewhere in the middle of the vertebra. This would be quite wrong, the centre is somewhere between the under-surface of the treatment couch and the floor. Imagine the rotation grade III (*Figure 12.44*) being performed – as the patient's left iliac crest is rolled forwards, the right iliac crest's contact with the couch is, at first, the lateral or posterolateral margin, and at the end of the movement the contact point has moved forward towards the anterior superior iliac spine. Therefore, the centre of the arc of the circle described by the left iliac crest must be below the top of the treatment couch.

It may be more easily understood if an analogy with the old-style wagon wheel is used (*Figure 12.42*). Imagine that the rim of the wheel represents the crest of the ilia (plus the sacrum and abdominal wall). Although the lumbar vertebrae are nearer to the back than the abdominal wall, the analogy is just as pertinent if the hub of the wheel represents the vertebra. We tend to imagine that when we perform the simplest of lumbar rotation techniques, the centre of the movement is the axle of the wagon wheel. However, if the pelvis at its highest superior surface is pushed forward, as occurs in performing lumbar rotation, it is the same as pushing the

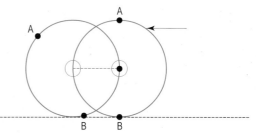

**Figure 12.43**    Changed positions of points A and B during rotation

2.  What effect do I think I am having on any pathological disorder?

Variations of lumbar rotation techniques are now described.

### Rotation (↻)

#### Starting position

For this mobilization, the patient should be lying on his right side with pillows supporting his head. While the patient remains relaxed, the physiotherapist moves the patient around to adopt the position required. The patient's left arm is adjusted so that his hand rests on the left side of the abdomen with the shoulder extended and the elbow flexed. When the gentlest rotation is being used, the patient's thorax is kept in the side-lying position while both hips and knees are flexed, the top one slightly more than the right. The physiotherapist then stands behind the patient and, with her hands, grasps the patient's pelvis. Positioning of the intervertebral joint being treated so that it is midway between flexion and extension is achieved by the degree of hip flexion and the therapist's grasp of the pelvis. This grasp enables the physiotherapist to tilt the pelvis towards flexion or extension; the pelvis carries the lumbar spine with it.

If the rotation is to be performed further into the range, the physiotherapist rotates the patient's thorax to the left by lifting the patient's right arm towards the ceiling so that the chest faces upwards. This range of rotation is governed by the flexibility of the patient. His underneath leg (right leg) is slightly flexed in relation to his trunk. However, this leg can be extended slightly or flexed more depending upon whether the rotation is to be applied with the lumbar spine towards extension or flexion. The left leg is positioned so that the hip and knee are flexed with the medial tibial condyle resting just beyond the edge of the couch. When additional pressure is required during mobilization, this top leg can hang over the side of the couch.

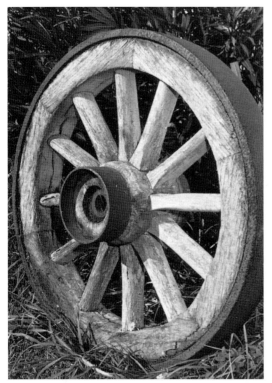

**Figure 12.42**    A waggon wheel – an analogy for lumbar rotation

top of the wagon wheel forwards. Simultaneously, the lowest point of the wagon wheel moves forwards, albeit a far shorter distance, and the axle moves forwards in a line parallel to the surface along which it is being moved (*Figure 12.43*).

If we want to apply maximum rotational torsion to the intervertebral joint, we would have to pull point B on the wagon wheel backwards as far, and at the same time, as we move point A forwards. If we do this, the axle of the wheel remains at one point and the rim of the wheel spins around this axle. It is quite possible to do this, and the technique is shown and described on page 371 and in *Figure 12.50*. And this is not taking into account the 'instantaneous centre of axial rotation' (Farfan, 1973), which is a separate consideration altogether.

When thinking of performing the rotation in different coronal axes, as would be the case when performing the rotation with the patient's lumbar spine in flexion or extension; or in different sagittal axes, as in lateral flexion left or right, there are endless things on which to ponder. The aspects that are primary in the clinical application of the rotation technique are:

1.  Am I performing the rotation to provoke or ease the symptoms:
    a) When performing it; or
    b) After having performed it?

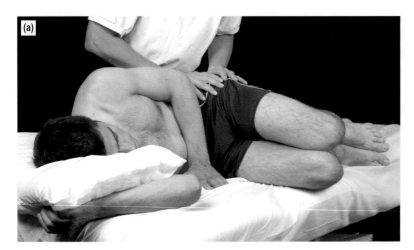

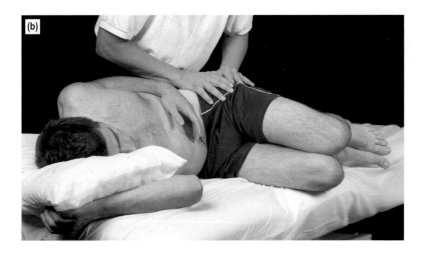

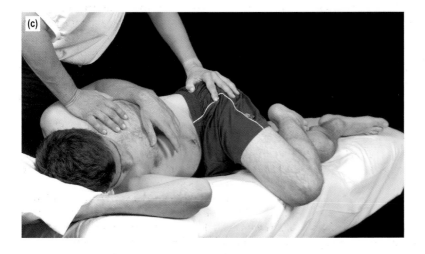

Figure 12.44 Rotation. (*a*) Grades I and II. (*b*) and (*c*) Grade III

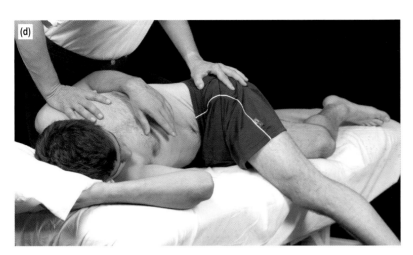

Figure 12.44    (*contd*) (*d*) Grade IV, with neural emphasis

The physiotherapist then stands behind the patient and places the palms of her hands over the patient's pelvis and left shoulder with the fingers pointing forwards. The hand on the shoulder is cupped over the head of the humerus, with the fingers spreading forward over the pectoral muscles. In some cases where the shoulder itself is painful it is necessary for the patient's shoulder to be in a lesser degree of extension and for the physiotherapist's hand to be moved further towards the pectoral area to apply the pressure. The hand over the pelvis is placed near the crest if the rotation is to be carried out with the lumbar spine towards extension, or over the greater trochanter if the rotation is to be carried out towards flexion.

When the technique is being carried out as a general rotation with the patient's lumbar spine midway between flexion and extension, the physiotherapist's shoulders are placed over the patient's body midway between the hand positions. The elbows should be minimally flexed. If the rotation is to be performed with the lumbar spine tending towards extension, the physiotherapist should move slightly towards the patient's shoulder to enable the line of the left arm operating on the patient's pelvis to encourage extension by its altered position. Similarly, if the rotation is to be done in some degree of flexion, it is necessary for the physiotherapist to move towards the patient's pelvis to enable the left arm operating on the pelvis to encourage flexion with the rotation.

When a stronger mobilization is required, the patient's position remains unchanged but the physiotherapist kneels on the couch behind the patient. The physiotherapist can then carry her weight directly over the patient and use her knee under the patient's buttock to assist the rotation (*Figure 12.44*).

## Method

Because the leverage is long, the physiotherapist must at all times be in a position to see the patient's back to watch the movement taking place.

With the gentle techniques the small oscillatory movements are produced through the physiotherapist's left hand, which has a double function. First, by its grasp of the pelvis the intervertebral joint is positioned midway between flexion and extension. Secondly, while the pelvis is held in this position, the left hand imparts the rotary movement to the pelvis. No counter-pressure to prevent thoracic movement is required, but great care is necessary to be sure that the movement is purely rotary.

Even with the change of starting position required for stronger techniques, the rotary movement is still a movement of the pelvis (not the thorax) about a central axis. There is a need for the thorax to be stabilized by the hand on the shoulder, but this counter-pressure is not one that pushes the shoulder and thorax backwards; it is rather a holding action, which allows the thorax to follow the direction of the pelvic movement but only to a limited degree.

During the oscillation it is often desirable from time to time to roll the patient's trunk back and forth, without attempting any increase in the amount of rotation, to be sure that maximum relaxation is being obtained and that all slack has still been taken up.

With these techniques the axis of the rotation is beneath the surface of the couch, as explained on page 372 (*Figure 12.43*). The same comment applies to the descriptions of the local variations, which follow. However, if they are compared with the lumbar rotation technique described on page 378 it will be seen that the centre of the rotation is much nearer the vertebra than the hub of the wagon wheel.

### Local variations

The sense of movement than can be obtained here is quite marked, and a noticeable degree of feel can be acquired despite the fact that the leverage is so great. This is aided by watching the patient's lumbar area of movement throughout the procedure.

Rotation with the lumbar spine towards extension is better used when mobilizing the middle or upper lumbar spine, and rotation towards flexion is best reserved for the lowest joints.

### Precautions

Occasionally a patient will develop cervical discomfort following treatment by lumbar rotation. It is preferable, therefore, not to alter the head position from that which he feels is comfortable unless this is necessary to improve the starting position. This cervical irritation usually settles without any difficulty, but it is better avoided if possible.

The possibility of irritating the lower thoracic spine or of creating a thoracic condition can become a very real problem with strong mobilization, and requires watching. Particular care is required with those patients who have (or have had) lower thoracic symptoms as well as the lumbar condition for which they are being treated.

If the rotation is done too vigorously while rotating the pelvis towards the painful side, symptoms of referred pain can be produced in the pain-free leg.

### Uses

Rotation is one of the most useful procedures in treating painful conditions arising from the lumbar spine. It is most valuable when used for symptoms that are unilateral in their distribution, whether they are referred to the leg or localized to the lumbar area. In examples where the symptoms are central but the signs are unilateral, these signs can be taken as the guide to the painful side. In such cases the technique is more likely to succeed in relieving the patient's symptoms and signs if it is done with the patient lying on the painless side; that is, with the painful side uppermost so that the pelvis can be rotated away from the painful side.

One further aspect regarding the application of mobilization techniques for distally referred pain requires emphasizing. Frequently a technique performed early in the range results in an exacerbation, even when symptoms are not created during the performance of a technique. In this event the cause of the pain is being excited and nothing is being done to alter the pathology. Under these circumstances the same technique performed at the limit of the available range, in very small amplitudes, will often effect improvement. For example, if lumbar rotation used as grade I does not produce pain yet causes an exacerbation, the same rotation performed as a very gentle and very small amplitude grade IV may well effect improvement.

### Alternative method of rotation (↺)

When the physiotherapist has difficulty in obtaining sufficient patient relaxation to produce good movement, the following alternative method may give the patient more feeling of security, thus enabling him to relax better.

### Starting position

The patient lies on his left side, well forwards on the couch, with his underneath hip and knee flexed slightly and comfortably. He rests his right upper arm on his side and places both forearms, parallel to each other, in front of his abdomen, with his left forearm nearer his chin. The physiotherapist leans across his trunk, facing his pelvis, to place her right forearm along his back. She then holds behind his right femur distally to grasp his inner knee with her left hand. She supports his right leg in approximately 90° knee and hip flexion (*Figure 12.45*).

### Method

With her trunk and right arm, the physiotherapist stabilizes the patient's trunk while rotating his pelvis forwards on the right side through the medium of his

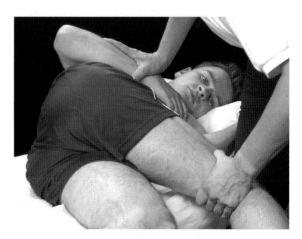

**Figure 12.45**    Alternative rotation method (↺)

right leg. It is important that the technique does not involve any abduction or adduction of the patient's hip; the leg is used merely as a lever to produce the pelvic, and therefore lumbar, rotation.

To assist the movement, the physiotherapist can use her right hand on his back:

1. To feel the rotation between adjacent spinous processes.
2. To encourage the rotation at a particular level by lifting the lower spinous process in rhythm with the rotation.
3. To hold back against the spinous process of the upper vertebra, so localizing the movement more to the single appropriate joint.

## ROTATION WITH COMBINED MOVEMENT POSITIONS

There are many ways in which the same direction of a lumbar rotation can be performed, and obviously the combined positions can also be varied both in combination and sequences.

1. The first technique described demonstrates that the rotary movement can be performed from the top downwards (that is, the rotary movement is performed by rotating the thorax backwards) (*Figure 12.46*).
2. The next four techniques are examples of exactly the same direction of intervertebral rotation (that is, rotation of L5 clockwise (viewed from on top in the standing position) under L4, or rotation of L4 anticlockwise on L5), and in the same combined movement position.

3. The first three of these four techniques have the axis of the rotation below the surface of the couch, the first two with the axis below the patient's right ilium and the third with the axis below the left ilium. In the fourth technique, the axis is in or near the vertebra.

## Rotation in extension from above downwards (in E do Th ↺)

### Starting position

The patient lies on his right side with his left hand resting on his abdomen at the level of the upper vertebra of the joint to be mobilized. The manipulative physiotherapist sits behind the patient, facing his head, and uses her left pelvis to stabilize his pelvis in a position that encourages a lumbar extension position (*Figure 12.46*).

### Method

With her right hand holding his elbow and her left hand pushing his left hand into his upper abdominal quadrant, the therapist oscillates the rotation through her two arms. Her stabilization of his pelvis is not one that is equal and opposite to the direction of movement being produced by her arms but is rather a holding, which prevents his pelvis rolling backwards as far as his lower thorax.

### Uses

All lumbar rotation combined movements are performed in a manner, determined from the examination combined movement tests, aimed at reproducing or avoiding reproduction of the patient's symptoms.

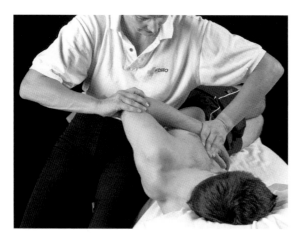

**Figure 12.46** Rotation in extension from above downwards (in E do Lx ↺)

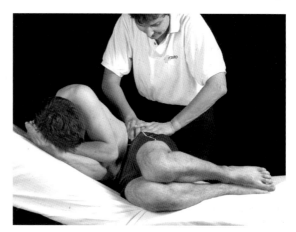

**Figure 12.47** Rotation in flexion and lateral flexion left from below upwards (in F + LF Ⓛ, do ↑ Lx ↻)

## Rotation in flexion and lateral flexion left from below upwards (lie on Ⓡ in F + LF Ⓛ, do Lx ↻)

### Starting position

With the head end of the couch raised, the patient is positioned in lateral flexion and flexion for the lumbar spine. The manipulative physiotherapist firmly grasps his left pelvis with the fingers of her right hand around the anterior superior iliac spine and her left hand grasping around his left buttock. Her grasp should be such that the patient's left pelvis and her two arms become a single unit and will move as one (*Figure 12.47*).

### Method

With her grasp of his pelvis, the therapist directs her rotary pressure towards his arms. No counter-pressure is required for the patient's thorax. The direction of her rotary movement must encourage or maintain the lumbar flexion and the lateral flexion left.

## Rotation in flexion, and lateral flexion left, from above downwards (lie on Ⓡ in F + LF Ⓛ, do Th ↺)

### Starting position

The patient's starting position is the same as that described for the technique above. However, this time the manipulative physiotherapist stabilizes his pelvis with her pelvis to prevent it from rolling backwards during the technique. She holds his left elbow with her right hand, and makes a solid unit of his lower thorax by pressing against his left hand with her left hand (*Figure 12.48*).

### Method

The rotary movement is produced through the therapist's arms so as to roll the patient's thorax backwards (i.e. to the left) while maintaining the flexion and the lateral flexion left to his lumbar spine.

## Rotation in flexion, and lateral flexion left, from below upwards (lie on Ⓛ in F + LF Ⓛ, do Lx ↻)

### Starting position

This time the patient lies on his left side with the couch arched upwards at his waist angle (pillows or blankets rolled up on a flat couch can produce the same position) to produce the lateral flexion left in the lumbar spine. He is also positioned in lumbar flexion. The manipulative physiotherapist kneels on the couch just distal to his buttocks and grasps around his iliac crest in such a way that she can make a stable single unit of his right ilium and her two hands (*Figure 12.49*).

### Method

The therapist produces the rotation by using her body weight through her arms. No counter-resistance is needed during the technique, but she should watch the patient's lumbar spine to see that she is producing the rotary movement and is not losing the positioning of lumbar flexion and lateral flexion left.

## Rotation in flexion, and lateral flexion left, from below upwards with a vertebral axis

With this technique, the aim is to raise the axis of the pelvic/lumbar rotation from below the surface of the couch to the vertebrae themselves.

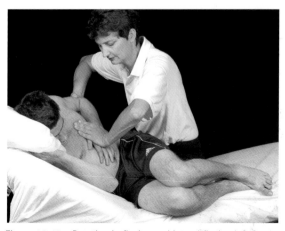

**Figure 12.48** Rotation in flexion and lateral flexion left from above downwards (in F + LF Ⓛ, do Th ↺)

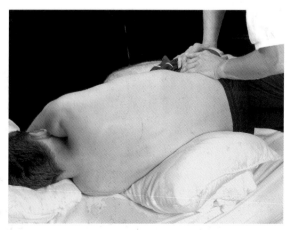

**Figure 12.49** Rotation in flexion and lateral flexion, and lateral flexion left, from below upwards (in F + LF Ⓛ, do ↺)

## Starting position

The patient lies on his right side, positioned in lumbar flexion and lateral flexion. This time the manipulative physiotherapist grasps his left iliac crest with her left hand so that she can push it forwards, while at the same time grasping under his left iliac crest, reaching as far anteriorly as his anterior iliac spine so that she can pull his right ilium backwards (*Figure 12.50*).

## Method

The rotary movement is produced by a synchronous movement of the therapist's left and right hands in opposite directions. Her right hand under his pelvis needs to slide backwards and forwards on the couch so that both of her hands move equal distances, thus centring the rotation near the vertebrae.

### Rotation with straight leg raising (↻)

Lumbar rotation and straight leg raising have been described as separate techniques. However, it is sometimes useful to allow the patient's leg to hang over the side of the couch during a lumbar rotation technique. One advantage of this is that the weight of the leg assists the rotation being performed by the physiotherapist. However, another important use is that sometimes the effect of the leg hanging over the side acts almost like a straight leg raising technique. Under circumstances when a firm straight leg raising technique is desired, the lumbar rotation needs to be done slightly differently so that the physiotherapist can stand in front and use her legs to strengthen the straight leg raising stretch.

## Starting position

The patient lies on his right side and the physiotherapist positions him for lumbar rotation as described previously. She allows his leg to hang over the side of the couch with his knee projecting beyond its edge.

She stands in front of the patient and places her right lower leg behind his calf and her left knee in front of his left knee. She leans over the patient to place her left hand cupped over the front of his left shoulder and her right hand cupped over his left hip. She leans far enough across to be able to direct her right forearm back towards herself (*Figure 12.51*).

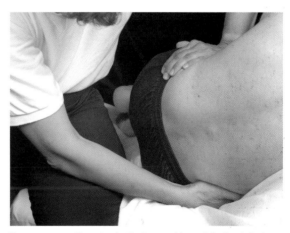

**Figure 12.50** Rotation in flexion, and lateral flexion left, from below upwards with vertebral axis (in F + LF Ⓛ, do Lₓ axis)

**Figure 12.51** Rotation with straight leg raising (↻)

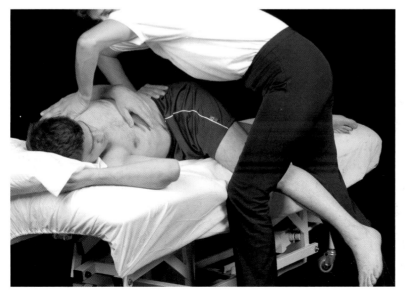

## Method

The physiotherapist provides a holding action with her left hand against the patient's shoulder and performs the rotation with her right hand against his femur. At the same time as she applies rotation to his lumbar spine, she also increases the tension in the straight leg raising by pivoting on her feet to both maintain knee extension and increase the angle of hip flexion.

## Precautions

This technique should not be used until other techniques have been tried and it is known that straight leg raising is a necessary part of treatment. It should not be done when radicular pain is reproduced in the lower leg, unless the pain is longstanding and the disorder stable.

Examples of treatment include: severe lumbar nerve root pain, page 414; chronic lumbar nerve root pain, page 418; insidious onset of leg pain, page 419; low back pain, page 430; acute back pain, page 431; spondylitic spine with localized lesion, page 433; coccygodynia, page 434; juvenile disc lesion, page 436; and bilateral leg pain, page 437.

## LONGITUDINAL MOVEMENT (↔)

There are two methods for producing this movement. The operator may use either one or both of the patient's legs.

### Using two legs (↔ 2)

#### Starting position

The patient lies on his back on a low couch with pillows placed under his head, while the physiotherapist stands at the foot end of the couch facing the patient and grasps the patient's heels and ankles from the outside. The patient's legs are lifted, while maintaining some traction, to a height that will allow the lumbar spine to relax in a position midway between flexion and extension. To do this, the legs need to be raised approximately 25° from the horizontal plane.

It is advisable for the physiotherapist to stand with one foot in front of the other and crouch forwards over the patient's feet. The physiotherapist's body and arms are then in the position where maximum pull can be given with minimum effort (*Figure 12.52*).

## Method

All looseness of contact between the patient and the couch is taken up by gently pulling on the

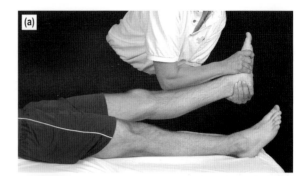

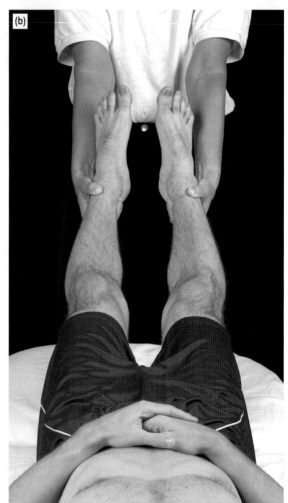

Figure 12.52    (*a*) and (*b*) Longitudinal movement

patient's ankles. Longitudinal movement is then produced by the physiotherapist flexing her elbows and extending her shoulders while in the crouched position. With gentle mobilizing there is no movement of the patient along the couch, but with stronger grades only three to six tugs can be transmitted because the patient slides a little along the couch. The patient should not make any effort to prevent this movement.

## Using one leg (↔ Ⓛ)

### Starting position

The patient lies on his back on a low couch with pillows under his head. To mobilize, using the patient's left leg, the physiotherapist stands by the left side of the couch towards the foot end.

The important part of the technique is executed when the patient's leg is straight. It is better, therefore, to take up this position first, so that the physiotherapist can stand comfortably in an efficient position. The physiotherapist grasps the patient's left ankle so that the left hand is placed under the heel, grasping it from the outside in the area of the Achilles tendon, while the right hand is placed in front of the ankle with the thumb lying over the outer aspect of the foot in front of the lateral malleolus with the fingers spreading over the inner aspect of the foot and the medial malleolus. This should give a comfortable encircling grasp of the ankle. The physiotherapist places her feet in a 'walk-standing' position opposite the patient's lower leg, with the feet pointing towards the foot end of the couch, and crouches forwards over the patient's left foot. The angle at which the patient's leg is held should allow the lower lumbar spine to lie comfortably in a neutral position midway between extension and flexion while traction is maintained on the leg, and the knee should be relaxed in extension.

To move from the position described to the true starting position, the physiotherapist flexes the patient's hip and knee without moving her own feet. The amount of hip and knee flexion employed is governed by the gentleness of the mobilization desired. If the technique is to be done strongly, a rather full hip and knee flexion position is adopted. If the mobilization starts from a lower position of hip and knee flexion, it becomes correspondingly more gentle. As it is necessary for the patient's leg to be relaxed, it may be necessary to prevent any abduction of the hip by supporting the lateral aspect of the lower leg with the physiotherapist's right forearm (*Figure 12.52*).

### Method

From the flexed position the physiotherapist guides the leg and allows it to drop, but should be sufficiently ahead of the movement to be in control of the leg position. As the knee drops into the relaxed, fully extended position, the physiotherapist applies a gentle, sharp

pressure to the patient's ankle so as to continue the elongating action of the leg. The line traversed by the patient's heel must be a straight line from the starting position to the point where the traction is applied, and the line is the position of the straight leg chosen at the outset to place the intervertebral joint being mobilized in its mid-position. *The timing of the physiotherapist's action to coincide with the final dropping of the patient's knee into extension is vital.* The physiotherapist's arms and the patient's foot must at all times be held close to the thorax.

If the patient is unable to allow his knee to drop freely into extension, this action can be assisted by asking him to kick gently through his heel. Dorsiflexion of the ankle may assist further.

Once the physiotherapist's action is completed, the patient's leg is returned to the flexed hip and knee position ready for the next movement. A series of three to six movements should be done before reassessing progress. The patient must not hold on to the sides of the couch to prevent sliding, as this may hinder adequate relaxation. As the patient slides along the couch, the physiotherapist must move her feet to remain in control of the procedure.

### Precautions

When using the single-leg procedure, the state of the patient's hip and knee must be checked before and during treatment to avoid injury. If back pain or muscle spasm is produced when the double-leg procedure is being used, the technique should be done gently and changes accurately assessed afterwards.

### Uses

The double-leg method is used for evenly distributed painful conditions, and the single-leg method (using the painful leg) for symptoms that are unilateral when these symptoms have a lumbar origin below the fourth lumbar vertebra.

This is a very useful technique, particularly when applied as a gentle double-leg procedure for acute pain that is localized to the lumbar spine.

Examples of treatment include: acute back pain, page 431; abdominal pains and vague pains, page 443.

## FLEXION (F)

Flexion is often considered a movement to be avoided, but there are times when it is a necessary part of treatment, both with the very gentle and the stronger techniques. Four techniques showing varying strengths are described below.

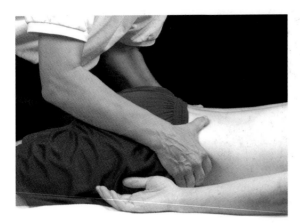

**Figure 12.53** Flexion: first starting position (F)

## First starting position

The patient lies prone, arms by his side and with his head turned comfortably to one side. The physiotherapist stands to his left side at the level of his thigh, facing his pelvis. She leans across the patient to grasp his right anterosuperior iliac spine in her right hand while holding the left anterosuperior iliac spine in her left hand. She places her right forearm against his lower right buttock (*Figure 12.53*).

### Method

Using a very gentle pulling action with her hands, the physiotherapist raises and lowers the patient's upper pelvis slightly. The movement is facilitated by pivoting her right forearm against his buttock.

## Second starting position

The patient lies supine with his hips and knees flexed and his feet resting on the table. The physiotherapist stands alongside his trunk, facing across his body, and passes her right arm behind his knees. She reaches across with her left arm in front of his thighs to link her hands together on the outside of the farthest knee. By lifting and pulling with her arms, she flexes his knees towards his chest (*Figure 12.54*).

### Method

The physiotherapist uses both arms to flex and return the patient's legs; this gently flexes his lumbar spine and then allows it to unroll. Most of the action is carried out by her right arm, but her left arm assists the flexing action. By virtue of the position of her right arm behind his knees, she is able to exert a certain amount of traction along the line of his femur, assisting

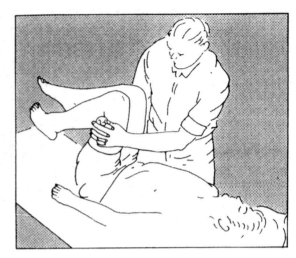

**Figure 12.54** Flexion: second starting position (F)

the flexion action on the lumbar spine by raising the pelvis. The oscillatory flexion action can be performed in any part of the flexion range.

## Third starting position

The patient sits with his legs extended in front of him and his hands on his shins. The physiotherapist stands closely by his left side, with her left hand over his knees and her right hand positioned approximately over his thoracolumbar spine. Her legs are positioned in walk-standing. She crouches forward towards his feet (*Figure 12.55*).

### Method

The technique has four phases, the first two of which are identical. For the first phase, the patient takes his hands off his knees and gently stretches his hands towards or beyond his toes and then returns to the hands on knees position. The second phase involves repeating this gentle stretch and return. During both these movements the physiotherapist follows his two gentle stretches, maintaining light pressure with her right hand against his thoracolumbar spine while following his trunk movement with her trunk flexion. The third phase is the actual mobilization, which is an exaggeration of the first two phases. In this third phase the patient stretches as far beyond his feet as he can while the physiotherapist, holding his knees down, pushes against the thoracolumbar spine with her hand, using her body weight to produce an efficient stretch. The fourth phase involves returning to the original starting position where the patient's hands rest on his knees.

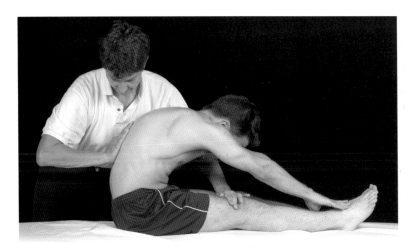

Figure 12.55   Flexion: third starting position (F)

## Fourth starting position

The patient stands with his feet 10 cm (4 in) apart. The physiotherapist, standing behind the patient, places her right foot between his feet. She places her right forearm across his middle or lower abdomen and grasps her hands firmly together in the region of his left iliac crest. The patient then flexes forward, and the physiotherapist controls the range to which she allows him to flex by the position of her right forearm through which she exerts pressure (*Figure 12.56*).

### Method

The patient repeatedly but gently bounces down into flexion. The physiotherapist allows him to go as far as she chooses, then returns him some short distance by pulling with her forearm. While pulling with her forearm she leans backwards, levering her right pelvis against his sacrum.

### Precautions

The last two methods are not used in the presence of a herniating disc. Flexion is not a technique to use until others that effect movement at the intervertebral joint have been tried without success.

When it is first used it should be performed gently so that its effect can be assessed before progressing to stronger techniques.

### Uses

The very gentle technique, described first, is extremely valuable when the patient, on forward flexion, exhibits considerable lordotic muscle spasm. The two stronger

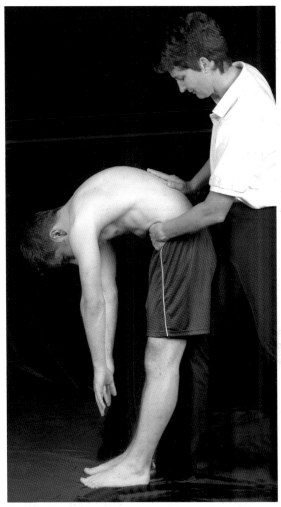

Figure 12.56   Flexion: fourth starting position (F)

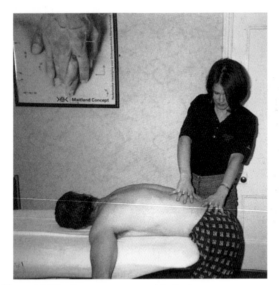

**Figure 12.57** Accessory movement in flexion

techniques cannot be used under these circumstances, but are valuable when flexion is limited by stiffness and is not hindered by muscle spasm or pain.

### Accessory movement in flexion (e.g. IN Lx FF 20° do ↰↓ L4)

#### Starting position

The patient rests on the end of the plinth with the end just proximal to his anterior superior iliac spine, and lies down over the plinth. He then bends his knees under the plinth to allow the lumbar spine to flex via the pelvis. The physiotherapist stands by the right side of the patient and places her thumbs on his back, pointing towards each other and immediately adjacent to the spinous process on the right as described on pages 370–371.

The method is identical to that described on pages 370–371 for the postero-anterior unilateral vertebra pressure (*Figure 12.57*).

#### Uses

This technique may be useful as an end-of-range mobilization if flexion is stiff. On the other hand, it may be valuable to use as a pain-relieving technique if the patient is most comfortable in this position.

## DEBILITATING LOW BACK PAIN CONFINING PATIENT TO BED

There are many ways in which extremely gentle mobilizing techniques can be administered advantageously.

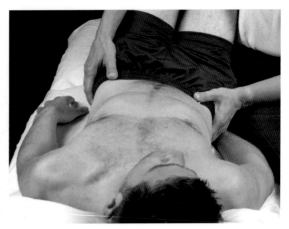

**Figure 12.58** Rotation

The first technique that may be considered is bilateral longitudinal movement (*see Figure 12.52*) caudad as a grade I movement.

The following techniques can be performed in a very localized and smooth manner.

### Rotation

#### Starting position

The patient lies supine with his hips and knees comfortably flexed. The manipulative physiotherapist stabilizes his knees with her axilla, and places her hands comfortably on his lateral iliac crests. For rotation of the pelvis to the right she places her left thumb in front of his anterior-superior iliac spine (*Figure 12.58*).

#### Method

Both of the therapist's hands work simultaneously, the right hand lifting and rolling its crest anteriorly and to the right while the left hand encourages a backwards and rotary movement of his right ilium. The technique must be smooth and slow, and must avoid provoking pain and spasm.

### Extension

#### Starting position

Again, the patient is supine with his hips and knees comfortably flexed while being supported by the therapist's right axilla. She places the full palmar surface of all fingers on the posterior lateral iliac crests (*Figure 12.59*).

#### Method

A very gentle, smooth and slow oscillatory movement is transmitted through her hands to his iliac crests, lifting

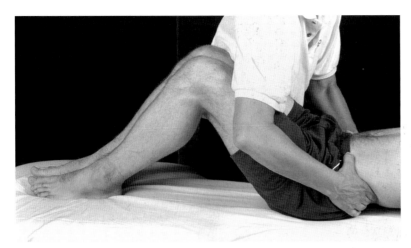

**Figure 12.59**    Extension

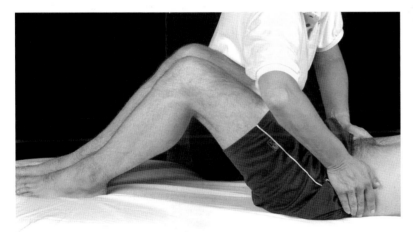

**Figure 12.60**    Flexion

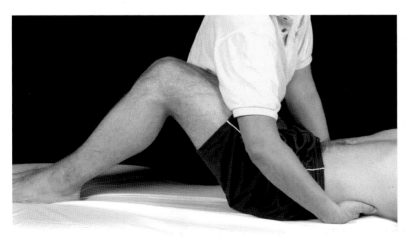

**Figure 12.61**    Postero-anterior movement

them towards the ceiling and thus producing an extension of the low lumbar spine.

## Flexion

The same starting position is used, but the manipulative physiotherapist's hands are placed near the greater trochanter of the femur. The oscillatory flexion of the pelvis, through her arms, produces a flexion of the lumbar spine. Again, the technique must not cause pain or provoke spasm (*Figure 12.60*).

## POSTERO-ANTERIOR MOVEMENT

### Starting position

This is the same as for the preceding techniques, except that this time the manipulative physiotherapist places the palmar surfaces of her fingers as close to the vertebral column as she can comfortably reach (*Figure 12.61*).

### Method

It requires great care to apply the lifting movement in the loin area without producing a poking feeling with the fingertips. However, a very satisfactory movement, slowly, gently and smoothly, can be produced. The level at which the movement is emphasized can also be varied. It is wise in the stages of severe pain to avoid direct contact with the spinous processes, but as movement improves some of the pressure can be transmitted to the area of the transverse processes.

## FLEXION, EXTENSION, LATERAL FLEXION, ROTATION FROM BELOW UPWARDS AND 'COUPLED' BY USING THE FEMUR AND PELVIS

### Starting position

The patient lies supine with his hips and knees flexed to 90°. The manipulative physiotherapist stands by the left side of the plinth, for example, facing across the patient. She then places her right foot on the plinth so that her thigh is placed under the patient's knees and calves. Her right hand holds his knees together from above, and her left hand holds under both his heels (*Figure 12.62*).

### Method

Flexion, extension, lateral flexion and rotation are produced using the legs and pelvis of the patient as lever-

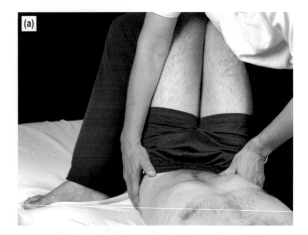

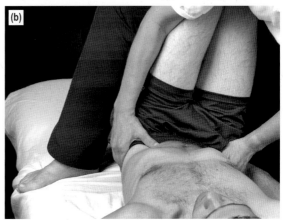

**Figure 12.62**    (*a*), (*b*) Starting position for flexion, extension, lateral flexion, rotation from below upwards and 'coupled' by using the femur and pelvis

age. For flexion, the therapist lifts her heel in order to lift his femur and pelvis, thus producing lumbar flexion. Lowering of his hips and knees will produce extension. Lateral flexion is produced by swinging his feet horizontally in an arc from left to right or *vice versa*. Rotation of the lumbar spine is produced by moving his knees and feet in a parallel arc from left to right and *vice versa*.

When gentle mobilization of the lumbar spine is required and direct contact with the vertebrae is not possible due to tenderness and sensitivity, this technique may be of value (*Figure 12.62*).

## STRAIGHT LEG RAISING (SLR, Ⓛ)

This is not a technique to mobilize an intervertebral joint, but it is a mobilizing procedure frequently essential in the treatment of lower lumbar conditions.

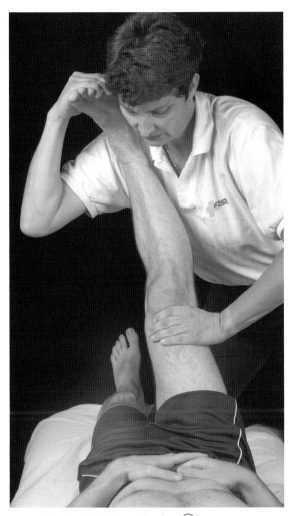

**Figure 12.63**    Straight leg raising (SLR Ⓛ)

### Starting position

The patient lies supine and rests his left leg on the physiotherapist's left shoulder, which is kept as low as is required by the limited range of the patient's straight leg raising. While the physiotherapist kneels alongside the patient, she endeav-ours to keep the patient's right knee extended by resting her left knee lightly just above the patient's knee. The patient's left knee must be kept extended and slightly medially rotated by the physiotherapist's left hand (*Figure 12.63*). To this position, inversion and eversion in dor-siflexion and plantarflexion can be added.

### Method

Tension is applied, usually as a single fairly rapid stretching movement or as a series of small oscillatory movements, by the physiotherapist raising and lower-ing her trunk from the squatting position.

As tension is applied, the patient may lift his pelvis on the painful side. If this does occur it can be pre-vented by thumb pressure in the iliac fossa. Similarly, he may abduct and laterally rotate his left leg. This action can be prevented by the physiotherapist's left hand holding the patient's leg medially rotated, and by directing her stretch into flexion and slight adduc-tion of the hip.

### Precautions

When lower leg pain is severe or paraesthesias are present, this technique should not be used or should be used extremely gently with careful assessment. Care must also be exercised when neurological changes are present. However, such changes are not necessarily contraindications.

### Uses

Straight leg raising can be used when the symptoms or signs indicate pain is arising from the nerve root or its associated investments, whether this is due to nerve-root compression or otherwise. The most common indication is unilateral limitation of straight leg raising with minimal pain, and when over-pressure produces a pelvic lifting. This sign may be present when the patient has back pain or limb pain. Under some cir-cumstances the range of straight leg raising may be full; the technique then merely mobilizes and tensions the nerve.

It is not the method of choice when the limitation is muscular, and it is not a technique that should be used until other techniques that do not move the nerve root so much have been found ineffective. SLR is also a valuable method of improving neuro-dynamic mobility following lower limb peripheral nerve entrapment.

### SLUMP

Any of the positions of the slump test (*see* pp. 144–149) can be used as a treatment mobilizing technique. The circumstances when it would most be used are:

1.  When the knee extension is limited and reproduces the patient's pain.
2.  When the dorsiflexion of the ankle reproduces his pain.

The one qualification is that mobilizing for the inter-vertebral joints at the appropriate level has not produced any improvement, or enough improvement, in the canal signs.

### Precautions

These are the same as those referred to in relation to straight leg raising.

## LUMBAR TRACTION

Examples of treatment include: severe lumbar nerve-root pain, page 416; chronic lumbar nerve root pain, page 418; insidious onset leg pain, page 419; low back pain, page 430; spondylitic spine with localized lesion, page 433; and juvenile disc lesion, page 436.

There exists quite commonly a false impression of traction. One false impression is that traction is different to mobilization. This is quite wrong and it is unfortunate – particularly when a patient does not improve because gentle movement in this direction (the traction direction; long-axis extension; longitudinal movement caudad) has not been utilized. Joints have the capacity to flex, extend, rotate, laterally flex *and to be both distracted and compressed* as well as being moved in accessory movement directions. When a manipulative physiotherapist does this, it is seen that she is mobilizing. However, when she is seen to use a longitudinal direction (by means of harness and a machine of some kind), it is seen to be traction and not mobilization. The second false impression related to traction is that it is thought by many that the strength of the pull must be great enough to distract the vertebrae by a measurable amount. Many surveys have been carried out to prove that a force of 136 kg (300 lb) is required to separate the vertebrae. Other writers go as far as to say that even with that force there is no separation. These attitudes are indeed unfortunate. Earlier in this book, the text referred to grade I movements. Also, reference has been made to the rhythms of mobilizing techniques – these references relate first to extremely gentle techniques, and secondly to a sustained pressure, the latter being used, for example, in overcoming muscle spasm. Traction IS just another direction of movement, and the very important intersegmental intervertebral muscles are capable of protecting this direction of movement in just the same way as they can for any other direction of movement. Traction is a mobilization in the sense that that word is used in this book. Therefore there is no clinical reason why a very gentle grade I traction (3–4 kg) cannot be used as effectively as mobilizations.

Traction for the lumbar spine has been described in a variety of ways and using many different types of harness. Some writers have described it with the patient standing (Lehmann and Brunner, 1958) while others have the patient lying; some use a thoracic belt as the means of fixing the upper end of the spine, while others use padded pillars against the axillae (Crisp, 1960); some have described it with the patient in the straight position, while others insist on lumbar flexion (Mennell, 1960); some give traction on canvas-top couches (Scott, 1955) while others use roller-top couches (Judovich and Nobel, 1957); some administer it as constant traction (Cyriax, 1975) and others as intermittent traction (Judovich and Nobel, 1957). Even the application of manual lumbar traction has been described (Crisp, 1960). A useful summary of these and other authors in relation to all forms of traction is given by Licht (1960).

A patient with severe nerve-root pain, if he is to be treated conservatively, should be treated with lumbar traction. However, a choice needs to be made between constant traction administered on a 24-hour basis in hospital and traction administered in physiotherapy rooms on a 30-minute per day basis. Provided traction in rooms stands a reasonable chance of success it is the treatment of choice, as it leaves the patient freer than does traction in hospital. When pain is severe it is not easy to make the correct decision from the outset. If constant traction in hospital is to be used, the method is as follows.

### Hospital traction

The patient lies supine either on a horizontal bed or with the foot of the bed raised 25 cm (10 in). A comfortable soft pelvic belt is placed on the patient, to which ropes are attached and fitted to a spreader. From the spreader a single rope passes over a pulley at the foot of the bed to the weights attached at its end (*Figure 12.64*). It is wisest for the patient to remain supine at all times, but a change of position may sometimes be permitted. The patient should be allowed commode facilities, as the use of a bedpan is too traumatic to the back of a patient with severe pain. Fowler's position (*Figure 12.64*) is only required if the patient has a marked lumbar kyphosis that is not largely reduced when recumbent. If Fowler's position is required, as soon as the kyphosis improves the normal traction position described first should be adopted. Initially the tractive force should be approximately 5 kg. This weight can be increased on a basis of approximately 1 kg per day up to a maximum of 9–11 kg. Ten days is usually long enough for the traction to be maintained, after which the patient should become fully ambulant over the next 3 days. If there is no improvement after

1 week on constant traction, persistence with the traction will not produce any change.

Fundamentally, the two essentials for lumbar traction administered in treatment rooms are a comfortable, adjustable harness for attaching the thorax and pelvis to fixed points, and a comfortable position for the patient, to assist relaxation. With these two factors in mind, the following method is given as a basis for traction therapy.

### Starting position

A belt is firmly fixed around the patient's thorax while he is standing and a second belt around the pelvis while he is lying, making sure that no single garment is caught under both belts.

The patient then lies face upwards on the traction couch. In the supine position it may be necessary for the patient's hips and knees to be flexed. The position of choice is the one that places the intervertebral joint midway between flexion and extension to permit the greatest longitudinal movement.

By means of straps, the thoracic belt is then attached to some fixed point beyond the head of the couch and the pelvic belt is attached to a fixed point beyond the foot of the couch. Before the patient is ready for the traction to be applied, these straps must be tightened to remove all looseness from the harness (*Figure 12.65*).

### Method

It is necessary to assess accurately the patient's area and degree of pain, while he is lying ready for the traction to be applied.

The traction is then applied from either the head end or the foot end of the apparatus, or from both ends, but care must be taken to eliminate friction between the patient and the couch if a roll-top traction couch is not being used. The physiotherapist does this by raising and lowering the patient's thorax and pelvis alternately to ensure that the stretch is being applied between the belts and that it is not lost in friction between the patient's body and the couch.

Although a friction-free couch is not essential, it is such a tremendous advantage that if it is possible to make up a simple one cheaply the effort is more than rewarded. Most patient roll-top couches consist of a fixed thoracic section and a rolling lumbar section, but this arrangement has little to recommend it. An efficient friction-free couch has both sections on rollers. It is also essential to be able to lock the sections together, not only to make it stable for the patient to climb onto but also to make it usable for purposes other than traction.

### A friction-free traction couch

A friction-free couch is not an essential requirement for traction therapy, but the advantages to both patient and physiotherapist are considerable. These advantages can only be appreciated fully by the comparative use of traction with and without the friction-free top. The time saved in eliminating friction when applying traction on a friction-free couch is valuable, but probably the most important factor is the ease and accuracy with which small increases and decreases in the tractive force can be made, knowing that they are immediately

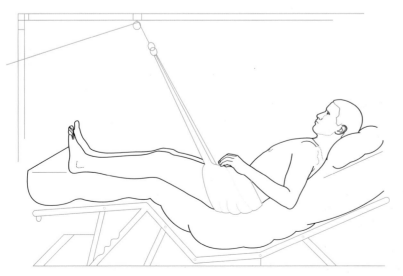

**Figure 12.64** Traction in flexion (Fowler's position)

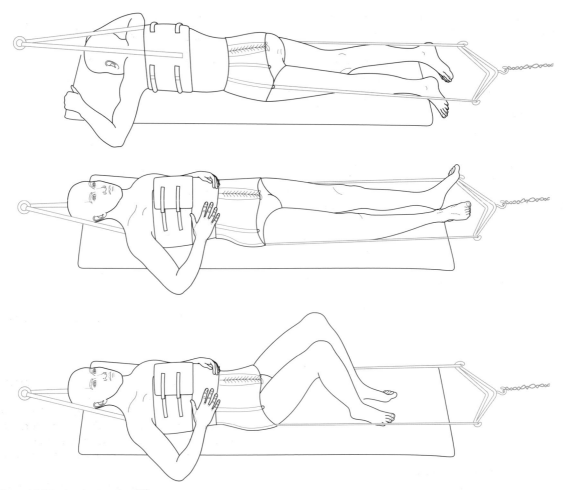

**Figure 12.65** Lumbar traction (LT)

effective in the spine. Another important factor is that a scale used during traction provides a more true measure of the tractive force between the thoracic and pelvic belts.

Many varieties of patented friction-free couches are available, but mostly they have a mobile lumbar section and a fixed thoracic section. This is not satisfactory because the thorax moves when traction is applied, even though the movement may sometimes be small. If the thoracic part of the couch is not free to move, some of the tractive force will be taken up by friction between the patient's thorax and the couch. Therefore, both lumbar and thoracic sections must be free to move. It must also be possible to fix the friction-free roll top in a stable position to allow the patient to get on and off the couch, and to enable it to be used for other treatments. These requirements are met in the

couch described, and the modifications can be adapted for any couch that has a wooden top, or wooden edges to its top.

The friction-free top is formed by placing two sections of 1.85 cm (¾-in) plywood end to end on top of a normal couch, with dowelling to act as rollers between the plywood and the top of the couch. The thoracic plywood section is 76 cm (30 in) long and the lumbar section 107 cm (42 in) long, and their widths equal the width of the couch. If the top of the couch measures 1.98 m (6.5 ft) in length, and both plywood sections are placed end to end with the head end of the thoracic section level with the head end of the couch, there will be 15 cm (6 in) of the couch uncovered by plywood beyond the foot end of the lumbar plywood section. Four pieces of dowelling 1.85 cm (¾ in) in diameter and equal in length to the width of the couch are placed across the couch under the plywood. Two dowels are used to support each plywood section.

To prevent the sections of plywood from rolling off the head end of the couch, a piece of timber is nailed to the end of the couch so that the top of the timber is level with the top of the plywood when it is in position on top of the dowels (*Figure 12.66a*). To prevent the plywood from rolling off the foot end of the couch, a U-piece is made to fit into an L-shaped hole cut out of the table top immediately below the foot end of the lumbar section of plywood (*Figure 12.66b*). To lock the friction-free top in a stable position against the piece of timber nailed to the head of the couch, the U-piece is lowered into the largest part of the cut-out section of the couch, pushing forwards to clamp over the top of the plywood and under the top of the couch, and then pushed sideways to lock the U-piece into the smaller part of the hole. In this position the U-piece also prevents the foot end of the lumbar section of plywood from lifting when a patient sits in the middle of the couch. This lifting must be prevented if the couch is to be used for treatments other than traction. When the U-piece is removed, both plywood sections are free to roll independently towards the foot end of the couch.

The four dowels must be carefully positioned to enable each plywood section to roll far enough for traction treatments, and for the friction-free top to be made stable enough for use with other forms of physiotherapy. One dowel should be positioned under each plywood section 12.7 cm (5 in) from the head end, and the other should be level with the foot end. Each plywood section can then roll 27.5 cm (12 in) before each head-end dowel reaches the end of its plywood section. The position of the dowel under the foot end of the thoracic section also allows the patient to sit in the middle of the couch where the two plywood sections meet, without the head end of the thoracic section lifting. The foot end of the lumbar section is prevented from lifting, as would be the case if the patient sat on the lumbar section nearer its head end than the dowel, by the locking effect of the U-piece.

The total cost of material for converting a normal treatment couch into a stable and efficient friction-free couch is minimal, and the labour costs are very small.

Because many physiotherapists are deterred from acquiring friction-free lumbar traction equipment by high prices and by equipment which is too cumbersome to be used for routine physiotherapy, a cheap and simple method for providing the two fixed points required for traction on a normal treatment couch is described. The tractive force is effected by a system of ropes and pulleys. The ropes and pulleys are attached to one end, usually the foot end, and a scale is inserted

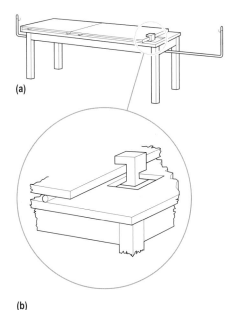

(a)

(b)

**Figure 12.66**  (*a*) Roll-top traction table. (*b*) Enlargement of the end

at the opposite end. This method is preferable to wheel-operated traction on a screw thread because of its quicker action. Also, the rope and pulley system gives the operator some feel of the tractive force during application. Accommodating for the stretch of the harness during the first few moments of treatment is also far easier with the pulley system.

If a tube having an internal diameter of 3.17 cm (1.25 in) is fixed under a normal treatment couch by metal straps at each end, two tubes having a slightly smaller external diameter than 3.17 cm can slide inside the fixed tube from each end. Each inner sliding tube should be half the length of the outer fixed tube. A strut should be welded at right angles to one end of each inner tube, and a length of the end strut should be such that when it is positioned vertically, with the inner tube within the fixed outer tube, its top is approximately 13 cm (5 in) above the level of the top of the couch. When the couch is not being used for lumbar traction, these sliding tubes can be slid out of the way inside the fixed tube. When they are in use, they should be extended a distance of approximately 36 cm (14 in) at the head end and 81 cm (32 in) at the foot end, and are held with the end struts upright by a pin inserted through holes appropriately placed through the outer and inner tubes at each end of the couch. These distances allow the ropes and pulleys to be fitted to the foot end, and the scale at the head end.

While on the subject of couches, there are many different brands and varieties of couch available and they are all expensive. A good manipulative physiotherapist should be able to improvise using a normal examination couch, without purchasing special ones. Having said this, a special couch can be an enormous advantage both in conserving strength and in being able to apply smooth rhythmical movements to heavy patients.

For those patients with low thoracic pain or lumbar pain, when a large-amplitude through-range technique is needed, the axis of the mobilizing couch for lateral flexion and rotation techniques must be in the right place. Akron Therapy Products supplied the drawings of their couch in *Figure 12.67*, showing the different axes. It is the only couch the author knows of at this time that has the correct axis for lateral flexion. The caption for each of the drawings should be interpreted as the direction of movement that would take place if the patient were lying supine.

It should be stated here that the surveys that have been performed to show how small is the intervertebral movement produced by firm traction forces show a lack of clinical appreciation of the relief of a patient's symptoms and improvement of his signs with minimal weights. Quite frequently, traction produced by merely wedging the thoracic and lumbar sections of the friction-free couch apart is all that is needed. Under such circumstances, the patient must not move – other than to breathe and blink his eyes. It is not the intention of traction to pull the vertebrae apart and produce negative intradiscal pressure; this is only one other direction of mobilizing technique, as are all the others mentioned in this chapter.

When a patient is given lumbar traction for the first time, a very low weight (not greater than 13 kg) should be used and this should be maintained for a period not exceeding 10 minutes. The patient should not be permitted to have his arms above his head, and if he wants to read while on traction this is permissible if, and only if, his elbows are rested on the couch. A careful watch should be kept for low back symptoms caused by the traction, even if these are only felt with movement of the lumbar spine or coughing. If low back pain is experienced by the patient, the duration and pressure of this first treatment should be reduced. If 13 kg can be applied, the patient's symptoms, both local back pain and referred limb pain, should be assessed after a waiting period of 10 seconds. One of the following courses of action should then be taken.

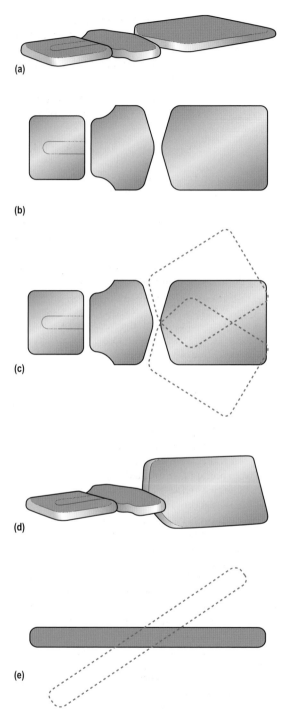

**Figure 12.67** Examples of a mobilizing couch. (*a*) Floor plan. (*b*) Rotation. (*c*) Extension. (*d*) Lateral flexion. (*e*) Rotation

1. When severe symptoms are completely relieved (particularly symptoms in the leg), the weight should be reduced by at least half and the duration should not exceed 5 minutes. If this action is not taken, the patient will almost certainly suffer a marked exacerbation of symptoms.

2. The symptoms may be relieved minimally by 13 kg of traction, and under these circumstances the

strength may be increased to approximately 20 kg and the duration can be 10 minutes. However, if 20 kg completely relieves symptoms (especially if they are severe), this strength should be reduced to something less than 18 kg.

3. If the symptoms remain unchanged, the traction should be increased to 20 kg and sustained for 10 minutes.

4. If the symptoms are worse, the traction should be reduced to a weight where the patient is the same as before the traction was applied, and the duration should be reduced to 5 minutes.

While the traction is being released slowly, the patient should move his pelvis gently by rolling from side to side and tilting it. If pain is experienced with this pelvic movement, the traction should be held at that point until the pain disappears. When the traction has been removed, the patient should rest for a few minutes before standing. This is not always necessary, but should be insisted upon at the first treatment. The patient should be warned that it is normal for his back to feel strange for approximately 2 hours.

### Method of progression

On the day following the first 'stretch', the patient's symptoms and signs are assessed and compared with those present before traction. From these facts it is possible to determine whether traction should be repeated and how it should be graduated. Signs can be assessed immediately following the traction, but flexion frequently does not provide any useful information, and certainly it is not the main criterion on which to base further treatment because it is frequently more limited immediately after traction. Reassess the asterisk signs, leaving flexion to the last. If the initial attempt at flexion looks difficult, 'stiffish' and slow, stop the patient and ask what he felt, then explain that this is a frequent finding following traction but does not mean that traction isn't helpful. The reassessment of lateral flexion and extension can provide helpful information. Sometimes lateral flexion may not be painful, even with over-pressure, but when comparing right to left there is definite restriction or stiffness. Following traction, this difference between the sides may be lessened. In a similar way extension may exhibit more movement, albeit small.

In the absence of other signs, one factor that will show whether traction is being successful is if it is known that at a certain weight pain is produced, and this weight can be increased at a subsequent treatment without producing the discomfort. In this case, the patient's condition must be improving.

If, during the first treatment, the symptoms were made worse initially and the weight had to be reduced considerably, and if the symptoms remain increased and the signs have also deteriorated, traction must be discontinued. If, however, the symptoms do not remain worse and the signs do not deteriorate, the traction can be repeated. During the second treatment, an assessment should be made of the weight that can be applied without increase of symptoms, to be able to compare this with the previous treatment. If a higher weight is possible, then favourable progress has been made.

When the strength on the first day was reduced because symptoms were completely relieved while the patient was on traction, the progression is guided as much by changes in the severity of any temporary exacerbation that followed the treatment as by the changes in signs. Over the period of the first three or four stretches, the improvement in signs will probably be small. When signs indicate that traction should continue, any increase in the treatment should be in the length of time and not in the weight. When there is no exacerbation following treatment or after the duration of 15 minutes, the weight can be gradually increased.

Under circumstances other than the two just discussed, weight and time can be increased together. Generally, the average weight is reached between 30 and 45 kg. However, occasionally when the rate of progress seems too slow with lower strengths, stretches of up to 65 kg are necessary. Duration does not need to exceed 15 minutes, as longer periods do not produce any further progress except when treating disc pathology causing nerve-root symptoms.

Although strengths have been suggested, the scale should not be the controlling guide during treatment. In fact it should only be referred to when traction has been applied to the level required by the patient's symptoms and signs. The main value of a scale measurement is for recording purposes.

As in other areas of the vertebral column, intermittent variable traction can be used for the lumbar spine. The duration and strength of such treatment falls within the same limitations as set out above. Timing for the hold and rest periods varies as discussed on page 289.

Unfortunately, there is still no intermittent traction machine that can be varied in its speed of pulling up or letting down. For the patient who has generalized aching in an area of the spine where marked degenerative changes are evident on X-rays, intermittent traction with no rest or hold time is very useful. It would be better still if the speed of pulling up and letting down could be doubled compared with that which exists in the better machines. Similarly, if pain is severe yet it seems the joint needs movement in this longitudinal direction, it would be nice if the speed could be halved.

## Precautions

With the exception of discomfort from the harness used, there is no natural soreness to be felt with low weights of traction. With this in mind, great care should be taken when any low back discomfort is felt while the traction is being given. It is advisable, once the traction has been applied, to ask the patient to attempt alternate flattening and lordosing of the lumbar spine as well as coughing to see if this causes any back discomfort.

It is wise to consider the first session of traction as a 'dummy run' so that the embarrassing but harmless situation of a patient having difficulty getting onto his feet is avoided. Following carelessly strong traction, particularly the first time, a patient may be unable to get to his feet because of sharp pains in the lower back. This is unpredictable, but can be avoided if care is exercised with every first treatment.

## Uses

Traction has three primary uses in the treatment of pain arising from the lumbar spine:

1. Any symptoms, whether they are localized to the lumbar area or referred into the leg, which have gradually appeared over a period of days or longer, and which have not been preceded by any known trauma, may be treated successfully by traction.

2. An ache arising from the lumbar spine in the presence of marked bony changes, whether this has been brought about by excessive degeneration, old trauma or postural deformities, usually responds well to gentle traction or intermittent variable traction.

3. Pain arising from the lumbar spine in the absence of any obvious loss of active range of movement in the lumbar spine usually responds better to traction than to manipulation.

Traction should always be tried when no further progress can be obtained by mobilization. When treatment is primarily for stiffness, traction can be added to the mobilization, usually after the effect of mobilization has been reassessed. Intermittent traction is commonly chosen for its mobilizing effects.

It is often necessary for traction to be preceded by manipulation, particularly when traction is given in the presence of painless limitation of movement at an intervertebral joint. When traction of a particular patient has reached a stage when it is not producing any further progress it is advisable to return to mobilization, as this is then often successful where it had not been before traction.

## GRADE V MANIPULATION

Most of the mobilizations can be performed as manipulations by merely increasing the speed of the technique at or near the limit of the available range. Of the two types of manipulations (general or localized), in the general group the main one is rotation.

## Lumbar rotation (↻) generalised V

The symbol indicates the direction of the rotation of the pelvis.

Although the mobilization described on pages 379–300 can be converted to a manipulation by a sudden increase of the operator's effort, the starting position described below is easier to perform.

### Starting position

The patient lies on his back with his head supported on a pillow, while the physiotherapist stands by the right side of the couch facing the patient and abducts the patient's right arm out of the way. The physiotherapist cups her left hand over the patient's left shoulder, grasps behind the patient's left knee from the outside with her right hand, and flexes the hip and knee to a right angle. Then, by adducting the patient's left hip to pull the knee across the body and downwards towards the floor, the pelvis will be rotated to the right. Careful positioning of the patient at the beginning will prevent squeezing his left leg against the edge of the couch (*Figure 12.68*).

### Method

When the position of full rotation has been reached, the physiotherapist changes her right hand to grasp the posterolateral aspect of the upper calf; the heel of the hand lies behind the head of the fibula and the fingers extend down the calf. Rotation is stretched further by increasing the pressure against the patient's shoulder and leg, then a sudden downward and rotary thrust is applied to the leg and strong counter-pressure at the shoulder. The all-important factor is that the direction of movement of the patient's left leg must produce rotation of the pelvis and not adduction of the hip. This rotation can be done with the lumbar spine in flexion or extension by positioning the underneath leg and altering the angle of hip flexion used for the leg, which acts as the lever.

The more localized manipulations, which are merely mobilization techniques performed at greater speed, are mentioned below.

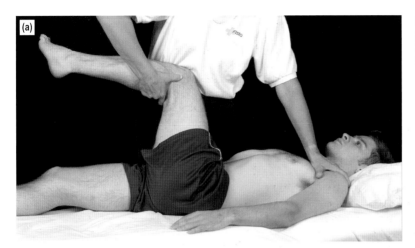

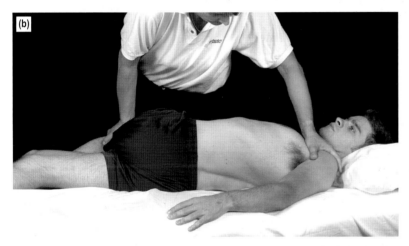

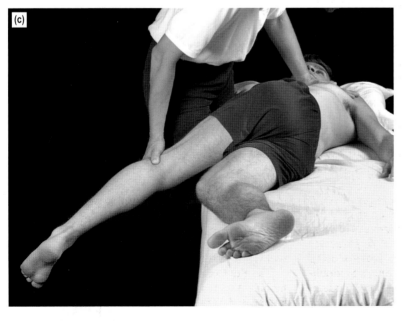

Figure 12.68 Lumbar rotation, generalised manipulation (*a*) Bent knee upwards; (*b*) bent knee to side on back; (*c*) bent knee across body

## Postero–anterior central vertebral pressure, postero–anterior unilateral vertebral pressure and transverse vertebral pressure

Conversion of these mobilizations to manipulations necessitates a sudden tiny amplitude increase of pressure, given from the position where the joint is stretched to its limit, to produce a sudden movement of very small range. The pressure required to produce this small movement is considerably greater for the lumbar region than for the remainder of the spine. To increase the effectiveness of the manipulation in the lumbar spine the patient's trunk or legs can be supported in extension, thereby increasing the lumbar lordosis (*Figure 12.69*).

## Intervertebral joints T10–S1 (rotation ↻) localised manipulation

### Starting position

The patient is asked to lie on his right side while the physiotherapist stands at the side of the couch facing the front of the patient. From this position it is advisable to tell the patient to relax, explaining that he will be put into the required position. The first step is to flex the patient's left hip and knee until the dorsum of the foot can lie behind his right knee, and then the straight right leg is put into slight hip flexion sufficient to place the particular intervertebral joint midway between flexion and extension. The patient's left arm is extended at the shoulder and flexed at the elbow to allow the forearm to rest on his side. To achieve the next step, involving rotation at the intervertebral joint, the patient's right arm is pulled towards the ceiling to twist his thorax until his left knee lifts from the table. Care must be exercised to see that the joint is still in the mid-flexion–extension position. The arm is then allowed to relax in an abducted and laterally rotated position out of the way. The physiotherapist leans over the patient, threads her left forearm through the triangle made by the patient's left arm and trunk, and places her left upper forearm against the patient's left shoulder. At the same time, she places her right upper forearm

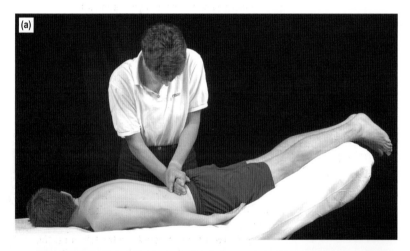

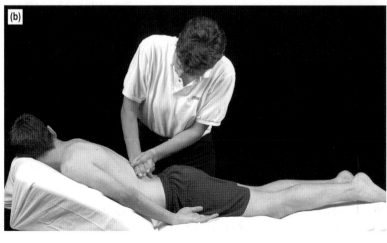

**Figure 12.69**    Postero-anterior central vertebral pressure (lumbar) localised manipulation. (*a*) Distal end raised. (*b*) Proximal end raised

behind the patient's left hip. This position leaves both hands free to add to the rotation at the intervertebral joint. The left thumb presses downwards against the left side of the spinous process of the upper vertebra, and the right middle finger (usually the strongest) pulls upwards against the right side of the spinous process of the lower vertebra (*Figure 12.70*).

## Method

Maximum rotary stretch is applied by rocking the patient back and forth with the forearms, altering the position of the right forearm on the buttock if the lumbar spine position needs to be adjusted. Gradually, as more and more stretch is achieved, the pressure against the spinous process is increased until the joint is tight. The manipulation then consists of increasing the push through both forearms and sharply increasing the pressure against the adjacent spinous processes.

## CASE HISTORIES

Even though there are case histories at the end of the book, it seems useful to include here an example of how the manipulative physiotherapist thinks her way through a patient's difficulty and atypical spinal problem. This particular example demonstrates how to link the theory with the clinical presentation. It also demonstrates the different components a patient's problem may have, and how one component may improve and another not. This patient's disorder demonstrates how the therapist must adapt her techniques to the expected and unexpected changes in the symptoms and signs. The example also demonstrates how open-minded she must be, and how detailed and inquiring her mind must be in making assessments of changes and interpreting them.

### Mr L

Eighteen months ago, a 34-year-old fit, well-built man (Mr L) with no history of previous back problems wakened with pain in his left buttock area. Over the previous 2 days he had suffered very bad low lumbar backache, which his doctor had diagnosed as being viral because he also had general aching in other parts of his body. Mr L did say that, although he had 'flu-like aches all over', his lower back was the worst area. He had been on holiday during the previous week and had done a lot of lifting and been wind-surfing (a new experience for him). Two days after the onset of his buttock pain it spread, overnight, down the left leg with tingling into the big toe area of his left foot (? L5 radicular symptom). Some days later, the big toe tingling alternated with tingling along the lateral border of his foot and into the lateral two toes (? S1 radicular symptom). At no time prior to 18 months ago had he ever had any back symptoms, and there was no familial component. He had undergone numerous forms of treatment (orthodox and unorthodox) over 6 months, but without success. Over a period of time the symptoms eased, but he did not become symptom free.

Following a fall 3 weeks ago, which exacerbated his disorder, he had a lumbar puncture (which proved negative) and hospital traction for a week. Following this, his low back pain increased. When he first went for physiotherapy his symptoms were as follows (*Figure 12.71*):

1. He would waken in the morning with back pain and back stiffness, and the stiffness would last for a few hours. (Unusual for a non-inflammatory musculoskeletal disorder.)
2. Coughing caused both back pain and left calf pain.
3. He was using indomethacin (Indocid) suppositories every night, and he felt that these were essential to lessen the level of his pain. (Perhaps this means there must be an inflammatory component.)
4. Bending caused him severe back and leg pain, both of which eased immediately on standing upright. (This latter fact indicates that a treatment technique that provokes leg pain may not be a contraindication to its use; the technique, to be effective, may in fact need to provoke leg pain.)
5. On standing for 1 minute, the pain would increase in his back and would spread down his leg. (This indicates that a sustained technique may be required.)
6. The only neurological change present was calf weakness.

The initial physiotherapy treatment, which he had undergone elsewhere, had improved all of his symptoms marginally. The first three of these treatments consisted of PAs on L5 and unilateral PAs to the left of L4. The latter, he said, provoked calf pain in rhythm with the technique. On the third treatment intermittent traction had been introduced, but this did not help him.

### Assessment
I saw him for the first time 5 days later.

1. On more positive questioning to determine his area of pain, it was interesting to note that, although his main lower leg pain was posterior, he had what he described as 'a different pain' in the upper posterolateral calf. These two pains were sometimes present at the same time, but were more frequently felt separately. (This tends to indicate that they may arise from two different sources – two components.)

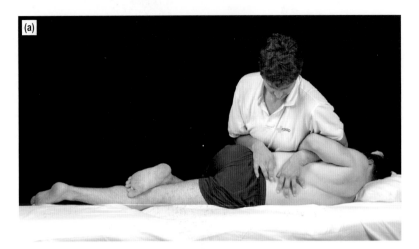

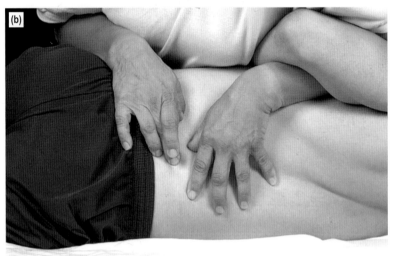

Figure 12.70    (a) Intervertebral joints, T10–S1 (rotation) localised manipulation; (b) close up on hands

2.  Standing (and he could not stand erect, in fact he had a lumbar kyphosis) provoked pain in his left leg, and he was unable to bend backwards because of increased leg pain.

3.  He had an ipsilateral list on flexion. (Items (2) and (3) seem to indicate that he has a disc disorder, which is provoking possible radicular pain. The offending part of the disc is probably medial to the nerve root and its sleeve, and will therefore be harder to help by passive movement techniques.) Neck flexion while he was flexed was limited by increased leg pain. (There must be a canal component in his disorder.) It did not increase his back pain. (The cause of his back pain is probably not causing his leg pain. Two aspects of the one structure perhaps? The disc?)

4.  While still in the flexed position, rotation to the left increased his leg pain by about 100 per cent.

Rotation to the right in flexion decreased the leg symptoms, slightly but definitely. (It is very helpful from a treatment point of view to have different responses with the different directions of rotation.) In this man's circumstances it is wise, when considering the selection of technique, to choose the relieving position while performing the relieving direction for the rotation.

5.  In the upright position, performing a lateral shift of his trunk towards the left decreased his pain; shift to the right slightly increased the symptoms. (Because of this pain response, the list must be directly related to his disorder.)

6.  Straight leg raise on the left was 35°, causing posterior leg pain. On the *right* it was 70°, and he said it caused an uncomfortable tight feeling, plus tingling, in the *left* foot laterally. (Crossed SLR

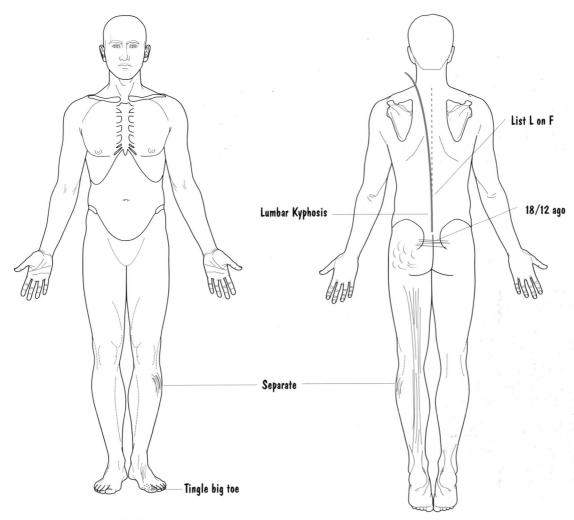

List L on F

Lumbar Kyphosis

18/12 ago

Separate

Tingle big toe

Figure 12.71    Body chart, Mr L

response – treatment may need to include mobilizing the right SLR.)

7. Testing the power of his calf in standing demonstrated some weakness, which may have been a neurological weakness but may also have been a pain inhibition reaction.

8. Attempting to stand, from sitting only a short time (half a minute), he had back pain and a severe lumbar kyphosis, which took some 15 seconds or more (a long time) to dissipate. (Because the kyphosis developed so quickly, this meant that the disorder causing his back pain was *very mobile*.)

9. His leg pain was minimal on first standing but then gradually increased in intensity and also in the length of the pain referral down his leg. (This meant that the disorder causing his leg pain had a *latent component*.)

10. His leg pain and his back pain could be provoked separately. (This meant that there were *at least two components to his disorder*. With the added information in number (1) above, he has at least three components. Number (4) above makes it four components.)

11. Tingling was felt either in the big toe or the lateral border of his foot. (This indicated the *possibility* of two nerve roots being involved. This could mean that two intervertebral discs may be involved, or the patient may have an anatomically abnormal formation of the nerve roots; *see Figure 8.2*.)

**12.** He also had canal movement abnormalities as well as intervertebral joint movement abnormalities.

Mr L's disorder was obviously atypical. The disc component seemed to be causing him more disability than the radicular aspect, but obviously the radicular aspect took higher priority. Being atypical means that one has to be very quick to notice the changes in the examination signs of the separate components, and to react with appropriate technique changes.

### Treatment

Because it seemed to be discogenic (getting up from sitting) with a nerve-root irritation:

1. The choice of technique would be rotation, as the symptoms and signs are clearly unilateral.

2. The rotation would be performed in the 'symptom-relieving' position and direction to avoid provoking pain.

3. Thinking ahead to further treatment techniques, it seemed possible that the canal signs would not improve in parallel with the joint signs, and that therefore SLR stretching may be required later.

Mr L was positioned lying on his left side with a support (folded towel) under his iliac crest to gain a lateral shift to the left position (his comfortable shift position, *see* item (5) above). He was also positioned in a degree of flexion to keep his lumbar spine away from the painful and markedly limited extension position. A rotation of this thorax to the right in relation to the pelvis was also adopted, and his right leg was kept up on the couch to avoid any canal tensioning (which would occur if his right leg were allowed to hang over the edge). The technique was to rotate his pelvis to the left (that is, the same direction as thoracic rotation to the right, but performed from below upwards) as a sustained (sustained because of the latent component) grade IV.

- During the performing of the technique he felt an easing of his leg symptoms, which was a favourable indication.

- On reassessing his movements after the technique, the joint movements were improved but SLR was unchanged.

The technique was repeated, but more firmly and for a longer sustained period. During the performing of this technique all tingling in his foot disappeared.

Following the technique:

- Movements had further improved, but

- SLR was still unchanged.

- Symptomatically, he felt more comfortable and felt he could stand straighter.

After four such treatments Mr L was greatly improved, but SLR, although improved, was nowhere near as much improved as were the joint movements. Sitting was also improved. His calf power was normal. During this stage of treatment, a scan revealed posterior disc protrusions slightly lateral to the left of the posterior longitudinal ligament at both the L4/5 and L5/S1 levels.

Because the, ?discogenic?, component was improved, and also the radicular symptoms were less (plus calf power improvement), left SLR was used as a technique and after four treatment sessions of this his left SLR became full range and pain free. However, the right SLR still felt tight and did provoke minimal left leg symptoms. It was decided to do right SLR as the treatment technique. The tightness cleared and remained clear for 4 hours.

The next treatment session consisted of performing SLR on each leg and ending off the session with a repeat of the previous positioning and rotation technique. It was decided to stop treatment (unless he had an exacerbation) and review all aspects in a month.

The assessment after a month revealed that he had not only retained all of the improvement from treatment but also found he could sit, stand and be much more active. His movements were full and almost free of any discomfort. He was reviewed again after 2 months and discharged. Aspects of 'back care', especially in relation to the 'weak link', the capacity for harm to accumulate painlessly and the need to be aware of predisposing factors (*see* Appendix 4) were forcibly emphasized.

This presentation emphasizes that the manipulative physiotherapist must understand the pathology that may be involved in such a patient's disorder, yet she must take most notice of the changes in symptoms and signs. For example, the fact that his disorder may have been progressing towards a nerve-root compression did not prevent SLR being used as treatment, because the possible nerve condition signs were improving and the possible radicular symptoms were also improving. Nevertheless, the first SLR mobilization had to be done only once, and that once was a mild stretch. The 24-hour assessment indicated that it should be continued with care.

# Chapter 13

# Sacroiliac region: sacroiliac joint, symphysis pubis

## INTRODUCTION

> In reality, the true incidence of sacroiliac pain and disorders is unknown

The sacroiliac joint, as a joint that can cause local and referred pain, has had periods of favour and periods of disfavour. There was a time when all low back pain was considered to have its origin in the sacroiliac joint. The mood changed, and people then considered that there was so little movement in the joint that it could hardly be the source of pain. In reality, the true incidence of sacroiliac pain and disorders is unknown.

Probably the main reason for confusion lies in the fact that many of the physical examination tests used by those who favour the sacroiliac joint in fact move many other joints at the same time.

The sacroiliac joint has a diverse and extensive innervation from L2 to S4. This may partly account for the inconsistency and variability in suggested sacroiliac joint pain patterns. The joint also possesses a relatively small amount of movement, which is difficult to measure. This is what makes testing indiscriminate, and the differential diagnosis may then lead to a wrong conclusion.

Furthermore, the inaccessibility of parts of the joints make manual evaluation of clinical signs difficult. The insensitivity of passive testing of the sacroiliac joint, therefore, always leaves the manipulative physiotherapist wondering whether, in fact, she has located relevant clinical signs that correspond to a sacroiliac disorder.

> The manipulative physiotherapist should seek to establish a series of relevant findings that build into a case implicating the sacroiliac joint

However, by encountering subtle clinical clues, the manipulative physiotherapist may build a case to implicate the sacroiliac joint. More often than not, retrospective assessment will be the final determinant, and even then she is never entirely sure that her intervention has influenced the sacroiliac joint alone. Therefore, she should seek to establish a series of relevant findings that build into a case implicating the joint.

Although the statement that follows is only a relative statement, and therefore hard to evaluate, the author's view is that this joint is not the most common mechanical source of pain, even when the pain is in the sacroiliac area.

> Most patients with pain in the sacroiliac area do not have sacroiliac disorders. The pain is usually referred from the lumbosacral spine

Most patients with pain in the sacroiliac joint area who are selectively referred for manipulative physiotherapy do not have sacroiliac joint disorders. Rather, their pain is usually referred from the lumbosacral area. Because of this, it is essential to examine this area and be able to declare it 'clear' before stating that the pain is probably coming from the sacroiliac joint (assuming, of course, that the sacroiliac joint tests are positive). In some cases the symphysis pubis should also be examined as part of testing of the pelvic region. The manipulative physiotherapist should also be aware of the contribution that altered neurodynamics makes to disorders of the pelvic region.

## SUBJECTIVE EXAMINATION

Sacroiliac disorders present most frequently in the second and third decades. Pain in the sacroiliac region in the elderly is more likely to originate from a spinal source, or from a pathological process such as Paget's disease or metastases from a prostate cancer.

However, if the patient complains of a very localized deep, often 'sickly' ache in the sacroiliac area accompanied by 'jabs' of pain with certain activities, the sacroiliac joint should be one of the structures considered.

## AREAS OF SYMPTOMS

> True sacroiliac joint strains or sprains are unlikely to produce symptoms that cross the midline. The hip may feel 'out of place', and the whole leg may feel heavy

A true sacroiliac joint strain or sprain is unlikely to produce symptoms that cross the midline. If the sacroiliac region is bilaterally painful in the absence of pregnancy or inflammatory disease, the symptoms are more likely to be referred from the spine. Schwartzer *et al.* (1995) found that groin pain was consistently associated with sacroiliac disorders identified by anaesthetic block and MRI techniques. However, the authors did not specify whether the pain was below, above or in the groin.

Referred pain and associated symptoms related to sacroiliac joint problems are not always consistent. There may be pain and aching down the inside of the leg or under the testicles in men. The hip joint may feel 'out of place', and the whole of the leg may feel heavy. Symptoms often overlap with those from neural tissue, the spine and the hip.

The symphysis pubis normally presents with pain or aching locally over the joint with referral into the groin or down the inside of the legs. Associated symptoms such as crepitus or a feeling of the joint 'shearing' with walking may be present.

## BEHAVIOUR OF SYMPTOMS

Local sacroiliac strains often result in difficulties with weight transference in standing and during walking.

It is difficult to distinguish sacroiliac problems functionally from those of the spine, hip and neural structures. However, there may be consistent clues that make the manipulative physiotherapist suspect the sacroiliac joint. Local 'jabs' of pain felt 'in the sacroiliac joint' with weight transference to the offending side, as in walking or stepping off a kerb, is such a clue.

In the acute stage, the patient 'cannot get away from the pain'. This can be very wearing and disabling. Night pain and prolonged morning stiffness may be a red flag sign for inflammatory disease. Patients with sacroiliac pain on weight bearing will often flex their hips or flatten their back against a wall for relief.

## SPECIAL QUESTIONS

Where pelvic symptoms are concerned, it is relevant to ask about genito-urinary and bowel function as well as saddle anaesthesia.

## HISTORY

Sacroiliac pain is common: during pregnancy; when an inflammatory disorder exists; as a result of repeated vigorous sporting activity (such as fast bowling at cricket); and as a result of overuse strain. Pelvic postural alignment faults or disorders elsewhere, such as a stiff hip or lumbar spine, may contribute to strain of the sacroiliac joint. If there has been a history of pelvic trauma, such as fracture or a fall on the base of the spine, involvement of the sacroiliac joint should be suspected.

## PHYSICAL EXAMINATION

### OBSERVATION

'Zoom lens' observation of the pelvic region should include orientation of the sacrum about the horizontal and sagittal axes, and the sacrum's relationship to the lumbar lordosis. Visual differences may be seen in the relative prominence and position of the posterior and anterior superior iliac spines and the greater trochanter. Any subtle changes in the gluteal and abdominal musculature should be noted. Any pelvic tilt or shift may also be contributing factors to a sacroiliac or pubic symphysis disorder (*Table 13.1*).

## MOVEMENTS

The sacroiliac joint should be examined functionally along with the lumbar spine and hip. The quality of pelvic movement compared with spinal or hip movement may be useful to note. Generally speaking, there is little value in trying to differentiate the sacroiliac joint in functionally demonstrated movements. Any attempt at sacroiliac joint differentiation would be indiscriminatory and invalid.

**Table 13.1**   Sacroiliac joint. Physical examination

| | |
|---|---|
| **Observation**<br>Getting out of the chair, willingness to move, gait, posture.<br>**FUNCTIONAL DEMONSTRATION/TESTS**<br>1. Their demonstration of their Functional movements affected by their disorder.<br>2. Differentiation of their demonstrated Functional movement(s).<br>**Brief appraisal**<br>**Active movements**<br>  Routinely<br>    As for lumbar spine.<br>  As applicable<br>    Flexing each knee onto chest in standing and lying.<br>**Isometric tests**<br>**Other structures in 'plan'**<br>**Passive movements**<br>  Routinely<br>    Supine, spread and compress ilia.<br>    Prone, ↕ S1 to 5<br>      ↙ ↘ S1–5 and on adjacent ilium.<br>      ⟶ laterally on ilium.<br>  As applicable<br>    Rotation in side lying.<br>    Bilateral isometric contraction of hip abductors and adductors in 90° hip F.<br>    ULNT<br>**Palpation**<br>+ Ligamentous thickening.<br>**Check case records etc.**<br>**HIGHLIGHT MAIN FINDINGS WITH ASTERISKS**<br>**Instructions to patient.** | **Symphysis pubis. Physical examination**<br>**Observation**<br>  Getting out of the chair, willingness to move, gait, posture<br><br>**FUNCTIONAL DEMONSTRATION/TESTS**<br>As applicable<br>1. Their demonstration of their Functional movements affected by their disorder.<br>2. Differentiation of their demonstrated Functional movement(s).<br>**Brief appraisal**<br>**Active movements** (move to pain or move to limit)<br>  Routinely<br>    As for lumbar spine<br>  As applicable<br>    Folding each knee onto chest in standing and lying.<br>**Isometric tests**<br>**Passive movements**<br>  Routinely<br>    Supine<br>    1. Spread and compress ilia, + angling these movements.<br>    2. Ⓛ ASIS caudad + Ⓡ ASIS ceph. and vice versa.<br>    3. F Ⓛ hip (OP) while E Ⓡ hip (OP), and vice versa.<br>    4. 2 hips abducted.<br>    5. With 2 hips and knee F'd 90° do 2 hips HE.<br>  As applicable<br>    Lying alternate sides.<br>    Pelvic rotation (top ilium) forward and backward.<br>**Palpation**<br>**Check case records etc.**<br>**HIGHLIGHT MAIN FINDINGS WITH ASTERISKS**<br>**Instructions to patient.** |

## WHEN APPLICABLE TESTS

When pain is reproduced in the sacroiliac joint during vigorous sporting activity, it may be necessary to perform the movement at speed as in throwing a javelin. Alternatively, it may be necessary to repeat an aggravating activity such as heel strike during fast bowling at cricket, or it may be necessary to sustain a provoking position such as extension of the back as in a butterfly swimmer.

In such cases, the speed of the movement, the number of repetitions or the sustained time can act as a measure of symptom reproduction and therefore as a measure for reassessment.

Neurodynamic tests such as the slump, SLR and prone knee bend will also be useful in order to determine whether the neural structures are contributing to pelvic symptoms, notably groin pain or buttock pain.

Exclusion of the hip and spine also plays an integral part of the examination of the pelvic region.

Of all the physical tests that can be used to implicate the sacroiliac joint, only two, if performed properly, involve this joint without involving the lower spine (Grieve, 1980). The first test involves moving the ilia synchronously so as to produce an opening effect of the anterior surface of the two sacroiliac joints and then opening the posterior surfaces; the second test involves direct pressure over the sacrum and adjacent ilium in an endeavour to reproduce the patient's symptoms.

## EXAMINATION AND TREATMENT TECHNIQUES

### OPENING THE ANTERIOR AND POSTERIOR SURFACES

#### Opening anterior surfaces

*Starting position*

The patient lies supine. A small pillow under his knees will help to position the low lumbar spine for most people in a neutral position, thus lessening any movement there as the sacroiliac joint is stressed. The physiotherapist, standing by the patient's right side at thigh level and facing his head, places the palmar surface of her right hand against the medial surface of his right anterior superior iliac spine. This necessitates her leaning across his pelvis so that she can direct her right forearm in the coronal plane from his left side to the iliac spine. She places the palmar surface of her left hand against his left anterior superior iliac spine, directing her left forearm from right to left across his

pelvis. Both of her forearms should now be touching each other and be flat on his lower abdominal wall. To achieve the best mechanical advantage, her sternum should be close to her forearms.

*Method*

To produce an opening stress on the anterior surface of both sacroiliac joints, the physiotherapist uses her pectoral muscles quite gently at first but gradually builds up to a firm oscillatory action, which pushes her hands from each other. This pushes the anterior superior iliac spines away from each other, which thereby stresses the sacroiliac joints anteriorly (and compresses them posteriorly).

For the test to be considered positive, local sacroiliac pain should be reproduced in rhythm with the oscillatory testing movement.

#### Opening posterior surfaces

*Starting position*

The patient lies supine and the physiotherapist stands by his right side, as described above. For this technique she places the palmar surface of her right hand against the patient's left iliac crest laterally, and leans across his lower abdominal area to enable her to direct her right forearm coronally from his left towards his right. The palmar surface of her left hand is placed on the lateral surface of his right iliac crest; this forearm also in the coronal plane. The fingers of both hands should be pointing anteriorly around the anterior superior iliac spines, and to produce the best movement her sternum must lie against his abdomen to enable her elbows to be closer to the floor than her palms.

*Method*

This again needs strong pectoral muscle work, but the oscillatory movement for stressing the joint posteriorly (and compressing it anteriorly) is achieved if the line of the forearms has an anterior inclination.

#### Direct pressure over the sacrum and the ilium

*Starting position*

The patient lies prone and the physiotherapist places her hands centrally at first over the upper sacrum. The hand position is the same as that described on page 368.

*Method*

At first the oscillatory pressure is applied to the S1 level (*Figure 13.1a*), but it should be applied to all

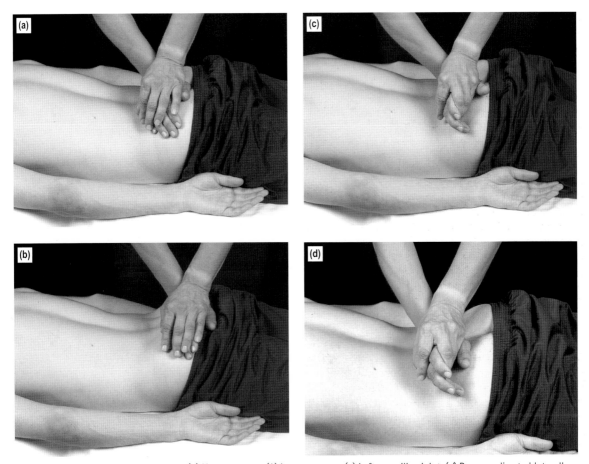

**Figure 13.1**    Postero-anterior pressures. (*a*) Upper sacrum. (*b*) Lower sacrum. (*c*) Left sacroiliac joint. (*d*) Pressure directed laterally

levels until reaching the distal end of the sacrum (*Figure 13.1b*).

The point of contact is then elongated to the posterior superior iliac spine area, and the pressure directed postero-anteriorly (*Figure 13.1c*). With all of the above techniques, varying angles should be used to complete the tests; for example *Figure 13.1d* shows the postero-anterior pressure being directed laterally on the left posterior superior iliac spine.

The sacroiliac test should be performed as part of the examination of every patient with back pain, whether there is any likelihood of the symptoms arising from these joints or not, as pain with this movement can be the first sign of ankylosing spondylitis.

Two further tests that examine the rotary movements of the pelvis about the sacrum through a transverse axis should be used when the sacroiliac joint is thought to be the source of pain. The first test tilts the upper pelvis backwards and the second tilts it forwards. Tilting the upper pelvis backwards is commonly associated with

spinal flexion related activity or extension of the hip, and tilting the upper pelvis forwards is commonly associated with spinal extension activities or flexion of the hip.

## FURTHER TESTS

### Backward tilt of the upper pelvis

#### Starting position

To test the left sacroiliac joint, the patient lies on his right side with his hips and knees comfortably flexed less than 90°. The physiotherapist stands in front of his hips, facing his shoulders, and leans across his hips to place the heel of her right hand over the posterior surface of his left ischial tuberosity, with the fingers and forearm pointing over his hip towards her face. She places the heel of her left hand over his anterior iliac spine, with her fingers and forearm pointing over his pelvis towards her other hand. She then stretches over

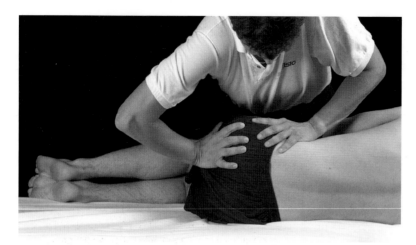

**Figure 13.2** Sacroiliac joint movement in the direction of lumbar flexion

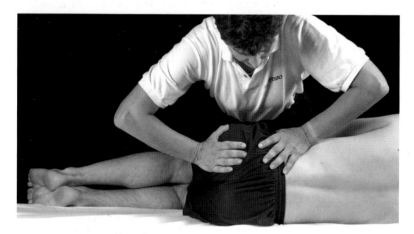

**Figure 13.3** Sacroiliac joint movement in the direction of lumbar extension

the patient's hip to be able to direct her forearms towards each other (*Figure 13.2*).

### Method

By squeezing both arms towards each other and simultaneously displacing her pelvis to the left, the physiotherapist exerts a rotary strain on the sacroiliac joint by pushing the anterior iliac spine upwards and backwards and the ischial tuberosity forwards. Rotary movement in the opposite direction is similarly effected. This test can be repeated with the left hip and knee retained at 90° but the right hip and knee straightened out. This has the effect of putting the spine into relatively more extension and hence, as the upper pelvis is tilted backwards, there is relatively less flexion strain on the lumbar spine and the movement is biased more to the rotary strain on the sacroiliac joint.

## Forward tilt of the upper pelvis

### Starting position

The patient adopts the same starting position, but this time the physiotherapist stands in front of the patient's waist facing towards his hips, and leans forwards across the patient to place the heel of her left hand against the posterolateral margin of the iliac crest. Her fingers point upwards, continuing around the ilium. She cups the palm of her right hand over the left ischial tuberosity so that the heel of her hand, pressed into the patient's upper thigh, reaches as deeply as possible. Her fingers point backwards over the patient's buttock (*Figure 13.3*).

### Method

Using the same alternating pressure method mentioned above, a rotary strain is placed on the sacroiliac joint.

Similarly to the backward tilt test, if the left leg is allowed to straighten and the right leg is fully flexed, this will have the effect of flexing the lumbar spine and hence, as the upper pelvis is tilted forwards, there will be relatively less extension strain on the lumbar spine and the movement is biased more to the rotary strain on the sacroiliac joint.

## PALPATION

> It is vital to palpate for soft-tissue changes around the sacrum, the sacroiliac sulcus, and other relevant sites around the pelvis

When a sacroiliac joint disorder is suspected, palpation around the sacrum and the sacroiliac sulcus, especially for soft-tissue changes, is vital. However, because the sacroiliac joint has effects on tissue around the pelvis as a whole, it is important to palpate beyond the sacrum and sacroiliac sulcus. Relevant sites for extended palpation are: the various layers of tissue in the buttock, including the sciatic nerve; the sacrotuberous ligament and the sacrospinous ligament regions; the symphysis pubis and the pubic rami; the anterior superior iliac spine; and the groin, including palpation of the femoral nerve and lateral cutaneous nerve of the thigh. In this way, tissue changes associated with sacroiliac joint strain or alignment faults of the pelvis can be detected.

Palpation in this region may also have a valuable role to play in reassessment and retrospective assessment. For example, the sacroiliac sulcus may be tender to touch but the lumbar spine is also stiff and painful. If the tenderness in the sulcus is referred from the spine, treatment of the spine should produce a marked reduction of the tenderness in the sulcus on re-palpation.

## TREATMENT TECHNIQUES

When the test movement gives a positive pain response and adjacent joints are implicated, the technique that reproduced the pain should be used first. At the outset it should be performed at such a grade that only minimal discomfort is produced. The assessment 24 hours later will indicate whether it can be performed more strongly or whether it should be gentler.

Wells (1986) also describes a comprehensive series of techniques that may be relevant to the treatment of sacroiliac joint and pelvis problems.

## CASE HISTORY

### Mrs P

#### Subjective examination
Two weeks ago, 34-year-old Mrs P picked her 3-month-old baby son out of his cot. She felt a sharp, deep, sickly pain immediately, in the area of her left posterior superior iliac spine. She felt as though 'something had slipped out of place'. The pain was accompanied by a 'grinding' feeling. She had previously felt this area to be sore, with occasional jabbing pains whilst walking. This had started about 8 months into her pregnancy.

She felt the sharp sickly pain (*Figure 13.4*), which seemed to be coming through just above her groin, every time she put weight on her left leg. She could not stand with her weight on the left leg. She could only gain relief from the sickly pain by sitting and pulling her left knee to her chest, or by lying on her side and curling up in a ball. When she aggravated the pain it could linger for a few hours, and her whole leg would feel heavy and achy.

Apart from a bit of high blood pressure, her general health was fine. She was tired because the baby wasn't sleeping. Her doctor gave her some Brufen, but that only helped to ease her pain slightly.

#### Physical examination
Observing Mrs P in standing revealed that she had a lordotic lumbar spine with laxity of the lower abdominals and a pelvis tilted anteriorly. Her hip was in slight flexion, and she was only partially weight bearing through her left leg. A few centimetres of weight transference onto the left leg increased her left-sided pain deep to her L PSIS.

#### Forward flexion
Mrs P was able to forward flex so that her fingertips touched her ankles. At this point, the pain deep to her L PSIS became 'sore'. The addition of head and neck flexion did not change this soreness.

#### Extension
Almost immediately she was asked to extend her spine 5°, the pain deep to her PSIS became severe.

#### Lateral flexion
When asked to laterally flex her spine to the left, the pain deep to her L PSIS was only felt as a discomfort at the end of the movement.

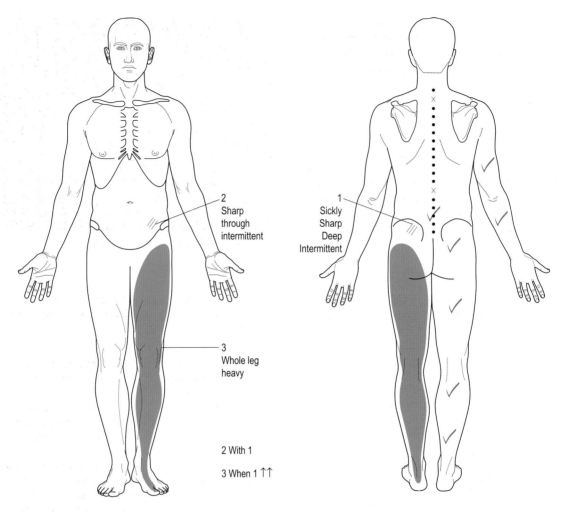

**Figure 13.4** Body chart for case history

(On squatting, there was no extra pain, no discomfort, no restriction and good quality of movement.)

### Slump
In the slump position, the pain deep to her L PSIS came on more when her left knee was 20° short of full extension. Head and neck flexion and extension did not change this.

### SLR
At 70° of L SLR she felt her pain deep to the PSIS, but this did not change when the ankle was dorsiflexed or plantarflexed.

### Hip F/ADD
When left hip flexion was performed passively at 100° of flexion, the pain deep to her PSIS on the left was reproduced early in the movement; the addition of hip medial rotation did not change the pain.

### Iliac approximation and separation
Almost immediately, approximation of the ilia made her pain deep to the L PSIS worse.

### Rotation backwards of the left side of the pelvis
When performed, this movement gave her the feeling of relief from the deep pain in the L PSIS area.

### Palpation
L3–5 were stiff and locally tender pain when postero-anterior and unilateral postero-anterior pressures were

applied. The sacroiliac sulcus was thickened and tender to palpate. The deep pain was reproduced by a unilateral postero-anterior pressure on the L PSIS, and even more so by a transverse pressure to the left on the PSIS.

### Treatment

The first three treatment sessions involved mobilization using the technique of posterior rotation of the upper part of the pelvis on the left (p. 405), as this was the main direction that relieved the sickly, deep pain in the L PSIS area. After three treatments her walking was still as bad, although her leg aching was reduced and when aggravated her pain settled in minutes rather than hours. Her hip flexion adduction was a little better, but her spinal extension was unchanged.

Once there was no more improvement using the backward pelvic rotation technique, a more direct technique was chosen to try to influence the deep, sickly pain. This had been reproduced using the transverse pressure on the PSIS. A grade III was chosen in order to respect the pain. Almost immediately, her extension improved and she was able to put more weight through her left leg when walking. On her next visit she said that she had had a few days of being able to walk easier, then her pain had returned to its pre-treatment level. This happened on a further three occasions.

It appeared that, although relief was being obtained by treating the PSIS locally, there was some reason for her symptoms returning. As the lumbar spine was stiff, it was decided to mobilize L345 on the left using a unilateral postero-anterior technique. After three sessions using this technique her back felt a lot looser and her spinal extension had improved, but her pain deep to the PSIS remained the same. On returning to local palpation around the PSIS, the unilateral postero-anterior technique was now most painful. After three sessions of using this technique as a grade III, her walking and pain deep to the PSIS improved by 50 per cent.

She then could not attend for 2 weeks due to personal reasons. In that time her pain had settled to a slight ache, and the only sign remaining was with hip flexion adduction. Two treatments of mobilizing hip flexion adduction settled the last bit of aching.

A programme of transverse abdominal and pelvic stabilization exercises was also instigated as part of a home programme.

## THE SYMPHYSIS PUBIS

If the patient's symptoms suggest a symphysis pubis disorder, pain is likely to occur in the area of the

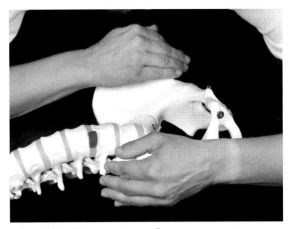

**Figure 13.5**   Ⓡ ASIS cephalad, Ⓛ ASIS caudal

joint, especially when weight bearing on one leg. The relevant testing of the symphysis pubis should include:

- Spreading an approximation of the ilia (p. 404).
- Forward and backward rotation of the upper pelvis (pp. 405–407).
- Supine lying on the edge of the plinth so that the right leg is allowed to fall into full extension; the left hip is then fully flexed with the right hip held in full extension.
- In supine lying, both the patient's hips and knees are flexed to 90° and the hips are allowed to fall into horizontal extension. Over-pressure can be applied by pushing outwards on the insides of both knees simultaneously.

## TREATMENT

### Left anterior superior iliac spine caudad, right anterior superior iliac spine cephalad

#### Starting position

With the patient in supine lying, the therapist stands on the patient's left side, for example, the heel of her right hand is placed against the left anterior superior iliac spine (ASIS) from above. Her right elbow is pointed towards the patient's left shoulder so that the direction of movement of her right hand is caudad on the ASIS.

The heel of her left hand is placed against the underside of the right ASIS. Her left elbow points along the femoral line so that the direction of movement of her left hand is cephalad on the ASIS.

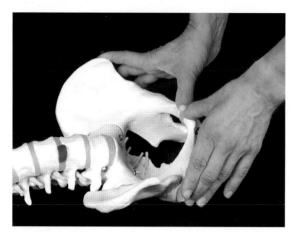

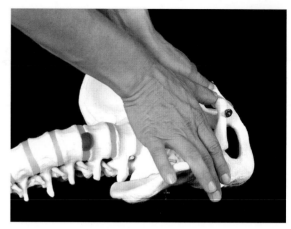

**Figure 13.6**   Joint line symphysis pubis. This technique can be modified so that pressure is applied to the pubic ramus on the Ⓡ➚or on the Ⓛ ➚.

**Figure 13.7**   ←•→ caudad joint line symphysis pubis. This technique can be modified so that pressure is applied to the pubis ramus on the Ⓡ or Ⓛ or from the lower border of the joint line or pubic ramus ( ←•→ cephalad)

## Method

The movement of the symphysis pubis via the ASISs is produced by the therapist using her pectoral muscle to simultaneously move the ASISs in opposite caudad and cephalad directions (*Figure 13.5*).

## Other accessory movements

More localized accessory movements can be performed on the symphasis pubis using thumb pressure:
Joint line (↑)
Pubic rami (➚, ➚) (*Figure 13.6*)

Caud ( ←•→ ) (*Figure 13.7*)
Ceph – joint line ( ←•→ )

# Chapter 14

# Sacrococcygeal and intercoccygeal regions

## INTRODUCTION

This area is quite commonly the site of pain, and it is not always easy to determine whether the pain is a referred phenomenon from the lumbosacral area or whether it is a local pain from a joint disorder. Palpation in either case will be painful. If pain is present on pelvic movement in the sitting position, a differentiation test is used to determine its source. The pain response while moving the pelvis in sitting in a firm chair is compared with the pain response with the same pelvic movements and in the same chair but with two padded blocks, one under each ischial tuberosity. In this position there is no pressure on the coccyx. In cases of chronic coccydynia, where mobilization has had little effect, it is important to examine the slump test or SLR as restrictions in neural mobility in this area are readily treatable using neural mobilization techniques (Butler, 1991).

## EXAMINATION

### PALPATION

Palpation is the most important part of the examination. Alignment of the segments is the first essential, and pain response on palpatory movement is the second and most important essential. The first palpatory passive movement test involves a central postero-anterior pressure.

## EXAMINATION AND TREATMENT TECHNIQUES

### POSTERO-ANTERIOR CENTRAL COCCYGEAL PRESSURE

#### Starting position

The patient lies prone and the physiotherapist places as much of the pad of the tip of her thumb as is possible over the mid-coccyx (*Figure 14.1*).

#### *Method*

The technique is the same as that described with similar techniques, but it is important here that pain produced by a bone-to-bone contact is avoided (*Figure 14.1*).

Gentle movements should be used at first, and the depth of the grade should be increased only if the pain response permits it. The important part about the technique is that the greatest use possible should be made of:

1. Varying the point of contact, even to the extent of changing by 1 mm at a time.
2. Varying the angle of the pressure – cephalad, caudad, left, right and combinations of these.

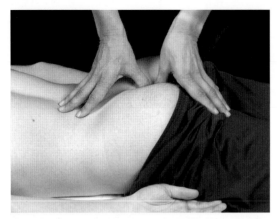

**Figure 14.1**    Postero-anterior central coccygeal pressure

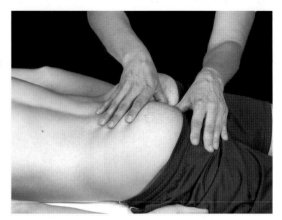

**Figure 14.3**    Anteroposterior coccygeal pressure

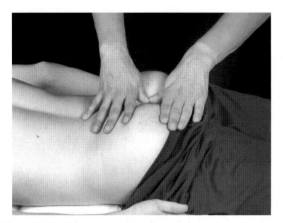

**Figure 14.2**    Transverse coccygeal pressure

Differentiation between the manipulative physiotherapist's technique soreness and the disorder's soreness should be attempted, because the patient can frequently pick the difference. If the patient believes it is the therapist's thumbs and not the disorder causing the soreness, the therapist must change (and keep changing) her thumb contact until all of the bruising feeling has been eradicated.

## TRANSVERSE COCCYGEAL PRESSURE

### Starting position

The only change from the above technique is that the therapist directs the pad of her thumbs to the patient's left side and places them on the right-hand side of the coccyx (*Figure 14.2*).

### Method

The same situation regarding contact soreness and varying the inclinations applies as in the technique above. It is necessary with this technique to maintain a very deep position of the thumbs if the whole lateral border of the coccyx is to be reached.

## ANTEROPOSTERIOR COCCYGEAL PRESSURE

### Starting position

Again, the only change is that of the manipulative physiotherapist's thumbs. This time she must sink her thumbs deeply alongside the coccyx to reach the anterolateral margin of the coccyx (*Figure 14.3*).

### Method

The technique can be performed unilaterally, as in *Figure 14.3*, which gives the direction of movement an angled inclination. However, it can also be performed with each thumb in the same anterolateral point of contact, one on each side. The thumbs then transmit synchronous pressure to the coccyx, and a straight anteroposterior movement is achieved. There is no need for the anal approach to produce an anteroposterior movement.

## TREATMENT TECHNIQUES

Those examination techniques that produce the predicted pain response are used as the treatment techniques. However, it is wise to use the techniques as grade II or III techniques until it is known that there will not be any unfavourable reaction to firmer techniques.

# Chapter 15

# Examples of treatment

## CHAPTER CONTENTS

The appropriate case histories are also referred to at the end of each individually described treatment technique

The foregoing part of this book has been concerned with describing techniques and the principles of their application. Now this knowledge must be put into practice. Supervised treatment of patients is, of course, the best way to do this, but selected case histories have been given in some detail as a guide. These will indicate the reasons for each step taken, and the results that followed.

In the case histories that follow there will be aspects of the examinations that have not been mentioned, but it can be assumed that all relevant abnormalities known at the time of treatment have been included. The case histories have been set out so that they can be readily used for quick reference. With each history there is a quick reference diagram showing the area of pain of which the patient complained, and a title showing the particular reason for its inclusion.

## EXAMINATION

The examination deals with the appropriate aspects of the patient's history and the associated signs, and is divided into the following:

1. Brief statements setting out the history of the condition as it stood at the time of treatment.

2. The relative physical findings on examining the patient at the first visit.

## TREATMENT

> Although diagnosis is important, a clear appreciation of the symptoms and signs present on examination is the vital issue

Treatment is divided into the following:

1. A list of the general principles involved in the manipulative treatment.
2. A record of the treatment given and its effect, and the factors involved in any alteration.

It is hoped that the following section will guide the student through the early stages of making decisions on treatment, and also guide the medical practitioner in assessing the treatment results the physiotherapist should be getting when patients are referred for such treatment. These cases are intended not as reading material, but as references and guides for the student.

The basis for this book has been to relate treatment to the symptoms and signs found on examination. This concept is unacceptable to many medical practitioners, and it is reasonable to consider that manipulation should not be undertaken unless a diagnosis is possible. However, two sets of circumstances apply. Sometimes it is not possible to make a diagnosis, and mobilization cannot be administered diagnostically. Secondly, although a diagnosis may be possible, this does not necessarily give enough indication to guide

the type of treatment necessary. This is so because under one diagnostic title the patient may have any one of a number of related symptoms and signs, each of which may indicate a different approach to treatment. Hence, although diagnosis is important, a clear appreciation of the symptoms and signs present on examination is the vital issue. This also eliminates boundaries in our thinking. Stoddard's *Manual of Osteopathic Practice* (Stoddard, 1969) clearly relates treatment to the diagnosis, but the divisions can be carried even further.

As an example, in the first four case histories the patients all had a diagnosis of 'disc lesion with nerve-root compression'. However, on examination their signs were markedly different, and each was treated in a different manner. It is for these reasons that symptoms and signs play such an important part, and they must be given much consideration.

## CASE HISTORIES

> The case histories which will be dealt with are listed in Table 15.1.

## NERVE ROOT

### SEVERE CERVICAL NERVE-ROOT PAIN

#### Examination

*History*

A man aged 42 years developed aching in his right scapula in November, for no apparent reason. Over a

**Table 15.1**   Case histories dealt with

period of 2 weeks, these symptoms subsided but did not completely go away. In January the symptoms recurred, but they settled over a period of 3 weeks. The symptoms recurred again in April and gradually, over a period of 4 days, spread into his right arm. Treatment began 3 weeks after the April onset. When first seen, he was obviously in distress because of pain. The two main areas of pain were the right scapula and right forearm. He also complained of a general puffy, numb feeling through his whole hand (*Figure 15.1*).

## Physical findings

All cervical and arm movements were full range, while cervical extension, lateral flexion to the right and rotation to the right all produced right scapular pain. If these three movements were sustained at the limit of the range, right forearm symptoms developed and a general tingling appeared in the right hand. Following examination of the patient's cervical movements there was a marked exacerbation of his symptoms, which took 5 minutes to subside. Moderate weakness of the right triceps was the only definite neurological change.

## Treatment

### Guiding factors

1. With the example of severe cervical nerve-root pain, traction is the only form of conservative treatment that should be considered from the physiotherapist's point of view.
2. With an exacerbation so easy to produce, initial treatment must be very gentle.
3. Mobilization of any form is not considered appropriate at this stage.
4. The patient should be advised that he may not notice much improvement in his symptoms for the first 7 days. Despite this, we should be able to assess that progress is forthcoming by the signs.
5. The patient should also be warned of the possibility of some exacerbation following the first treatment.

### First day

Very gentle cervical traction in flexion in lying was administered for 15 minutes. This treatment was continued daily for 5 days, and over the last 2 days the duration of each stretch was increased. By the fifth day the patient was having 25 minutes' traction. At this stage he was unaware of any improvement, although on examination his extension was slightly less painful in the scapula area and the position required sustaining longer before arm symptoms developed.

### Sixth day

By the sixth day the patient was able to say he was feeling better, and traction was then increased to 30 minutes.

### Eleventh day

By the eleventh day the patient was feeling 70 per cent better, and at this stage sustained extension did not produce any symptoms.

On the fifteenth day the patient was able to say the arm was the best it had been, and his movements were then almost symptom free. Treatment was discontinued, and he was reviewed 2 weeks later. His symptoms were then 90 per cent better and were not worrying him. Movements were painless and the triceps muscle power was unchanged.

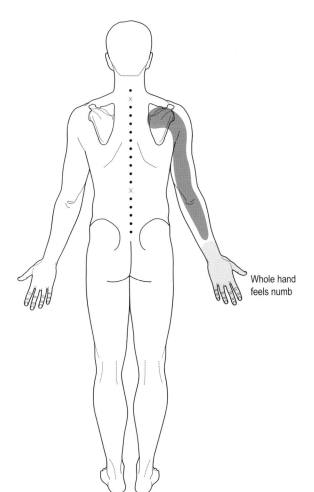

Whole hand feels numb

**Figure 15.1**   Severe cervical nerve-root pain

## SEVERE LUMBAR NERVE-ROOT PAIN

### Examination

#### History

This man aged 45 years had had a sudden onset of back pain 6 weeks previously while lifting. Over a 3-week period he developed lower leg and foot symptoms and muscle weakness. He was admitted to hospital and given constant traction for 12 days. He was then referred for continuing physiotherapy (*Figure 15.2*).

#### Physical findings

In forward flexion the patient was only able to reach his knees, and at this position he had pain only in his back. Extension was full range and painless. Lateral flexion to the left was limited and caused pain in his back at 40°, and at 45° the pain increased in his back and appeared also in his foot. His tibialis anterior was 1, extensor hallucis longus 2, and toe extension 2+.

### Treatment

#### Guiding factors

1. Traction would probably be the first treatment that should be considered. However, as the patient has had traction in hospital and been considerably relieved of his symptoms, the last improvement in his movements may come more rapidly with mobilization.

2. If mobilization is to be used, general rotation would be the treatment of choice because symptoms are unilateral and the cause of the pain is likely to be the disc.

3. In the presence of marked neurological changes treatment must be gentle and cautious, and assessment of the neurological changes made daily.

#### First day

Lumbar rotation, pelvis rotated to right, was performed very gently as a grade IV. Following two uses of this technique, the assessment was as follows. Symptomatically his lower leg felt better, and his left lateral flexion seemed a little improved. Left straight leg raising was unaltered.

#### Second day

On assessment the patient's movements were unchanged, but he thought his leg might have been better at times. The same technique was repeated, this time for three times. The technique improved his flexion and straight leg raising by 5 cm (2 in), but his symptoms were unchanged.

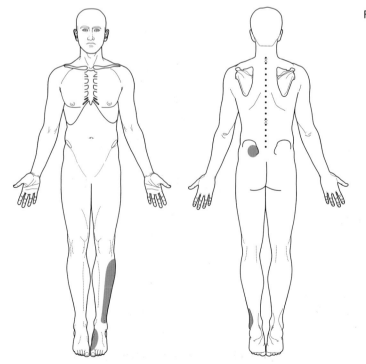

Figure 15.2  Severe lumbar nerve-root pain

### Third day

The patient's symptoms and signs were unchanged, so it was decided to make a change in treatment. Traction was chosen, and it was decided to use intermittent variable traction instead of constant traction because the oscillatory movement of the lumbar rotations did seem to produce some change. A weight of 12 kg was given for 10 minutes, with a 5-second hold and no rest period.

### Fourth day

The patient reported feeling definitely a little better, so the treatment was repeated for a duration of 12 minutes.

### Fifth day

The patient still felt a little improved, and both flexion and straight leg raising had maintained the 5-cm (2-in) improvement in range. It was then decided that perhaps rotation could be added to the traction to see if this would gain a slightly quicker improvement. Therefore, following a period of 15 minutes on 14-kg traction, two periods of rotation were given gently.

### Sixth day

The patient reported feeling worse again, and his flexion had lost some of what had been gained. It was then decided to give the traction and leave out any other treatment. The traction was gradually increased daily in weight until 25 kg was being given for 15 minutes.

### Fourteenth day

By this stage the patient's symptoms were minimal, his forward flexion was 70 per cent recovered and he was able to reach two-thirds of the way down his shin. Straight leg raising on the left was to 70°, and painless. On examining his muscle power, the extensor hallucis longus and toe extensors were normal, and the tibialis anterior was almost fully recovered.

## RESIDUAL INTERMITTENT NERVE-ROOT PAIN

## Examination

### History

Four months previously, this woman aged 35 years had what she said had been diagnosed as a disc lesion with nerve-root compression. She had traction, which relieved her symptoms considerably in the first month. Following this she did not have treatment, but found that she still had intermittent symptoms in her left elbow. Physiotherapy was tried again, but this time it did not help her symptoms. She complained of intermittent symptoms in the left elbow many times a day. They did not last long and were not severe, but were unpleasant (*Figure 15.3*).

### Physical findings

All cervical movements and arm movements were full range and painless. Even a sustained quadrant movement was pain free. There was marked weakness of the patient's left triceps, but the reflex activity appeared normal. On examination by palpation, it was easily determined that there was a loss of at least 50 per cent movement at the left C6/7 intervertebral joint.

## Treatment

### Guiding factors

1. As the symptoms are unilateral, the selection of techniques would be between postero-anterior unilateral vertebral pressure and rotation.
2. Traction would not be required, not only because it has been attempted before without success but also because the symptoms are not severe.

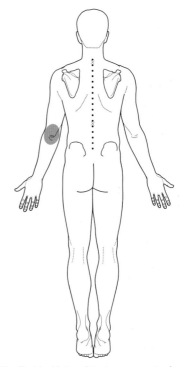

**Figure 15.3**    Residual intermittent nerve-root pain

3. Mobilization would be quicker in its effect than traction, and therefore should be attempted first.
4. As the joint signs were found only with palpation, it would be wise to use this sign as the first treatment movement.

### First day

Postero-anterior unilateral vertebral pressure on the left side of C6/7 was given in three periods of 1 minute. The only assessment that could be made was that this movement appeared to improve slightly as treatment continued. The patient was warned of possible exacerbation as a result of the first treatment, but was asked to note any change in the pattern of symptoms.

### Second day

The patient reported that there had been a reduction of at least 50 per cent in the number of times she had had symptoms. On examination by palpation, the movements seemed to have retained the improvement that had been gained the previous day. The treatment was repeated.

### Third day

The patient reported having had almost no symptoms, but when they had come they were as uncomfortable as previously. The treatment was repeated, and the movement was felt to be almost normal by the end of the third period. It was decided to leave treatment for a week to see whether further treatment was necessary. The patient was advised to come for treatment if the symptoms showed signs of returning.

### One week later

As symptoms had gone, the patient was pleased and treatment was discontinued.

## CHRONIC LUMBAR NERVE-ROOT ACHE

### Examination

#### History

This man aged 35 years had had recurrent back symptoms over a period of 8 years. In the last 18 months he had had some symptoms in his left leg. Previous bouts had been successfully relieved by an osteopath. Two and a half months ago, while weeding in the garden, he noticed minor symptoms in his buttock and throughout his leg. These developed as the day progressed, and over the next 3 days increased to a constant ache. This made sitting difficult and interfered with his work as a clerk. His osteopath had not been able to relieve the pain, so he went to his doctor and was referred for physiotherapy (*Figure 15.4*).

#### Physical findings

Flexion was to within 23 cm (9 in) of the floor, and straight leg raising was limited to 60°. Other than these two signs, the patient's movements were painless. He had slight weakness of his calf and there was some tingling in the lateral border of the sole of his foot, but no sensory change. His reflexes were normal.

### Treatment

#### Guiding factors

1. As this is probably a discogenic nerve-root problem, the choice of technique lies between rotation and traction.
2. As the patient's symptoms are not severe and mobilization is quicker in its effect, it would be wiser to try rotation first.
3. As the nerve root is involved, it may be necessary at a later stage to make use of straight leg raising as a technique.

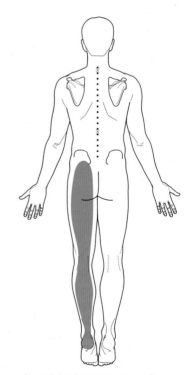

**Figure 15.4**    Chronic lumbar nerve-root pain

### First day

On determining that the patient's symptoms were not irritable, it was decided to use rotation quite strongly and in a sustained manner. The rotation was done, rotating the pelvis to the right, and this was sustained strongly. It was repeated four times. At the end of the treatment the patient said his symptoms felt a little easier, and straight leg raising had improved by 5 cm (2 in). Flexion had also improved.

### Second day

The patient reported feeling much the same, though his movements had maintained their slightly increased range. It was decided to repeat the rotation, but to add postero-anterior central vertebral pressure. This was done, and movements improved by a further 5 cm.

### Third day

There was a slight lessening of pain, and the range of movements had been maintained. The treatment was repeated, after which the patient reported that his calf felt much more comfortable.

### Fifth day

By the fifth day it was decided to add traction, following which the patient felt much better. His movements were improving, but more slowly, and it was thought that these should be progressing more quickly.

### Seventh day

By this stage it was decided to give traction, followed by postero-anterior central vertebral pressure and rotation. To this was added straight leg raising as one strong stretch. Two days later, the patient said he considered he was almost symptom free. His movements seemed almost normal for him, and treatment was discontinued.

## INSIDIOUS ONSET OF LEG PAIN

### Examination

#### History

For 10 years a woman aged 35 years had had many bouts of back pain, each necessitating rest in bed. They had all begun suddenly from minor lifting incidents. Three months ago she noticed an ache superficially in the lateral aspect of the right thigh. Aching was intermittent at first, but became constant over a period of 1 week. A tingling feeling, which also developed in the lateral aspect of the lower leg and foot, later developed to an ache and a feeling of numbness on the dorsum of the foot (*Figure 15.5*). These symptoms developed over a period of 3 weeks. Her doctor put her into a plaster jacket for 6 weeks, but the symptoms did not improve. Three weeks after the plaster was removed, she was sent for a 'trial of manipulation and traction'.

### Physical findings

With forward flexion the patient was able to reach to 40 cm (16 in) from the floor. With this movement the leg pain increased, and a sciatic scoliosis, which caused a tilt of the trunk to the left, became evident. The scoliosis disappeared on resuming the upright position. Lateral flexion to the right performed in that range of forward flexion that caused the scoliosis was very limited, and caused slight back pain. All other spinal movements were stiff, but they were not noticeably painful. Firm pressure over the vertebral column did not cause any pain or muscle spasm, but there was a general feeling of intervertebral tightness in the lumbar spine. Right straight leg raising lacked 20° of movement and was painful at the back of the whole leg. Reflexes, sensation and muscle power were all normal.

### Treatment

#### Guiding factors

1. Slow onsets of this type are more likely to respond to traction than to manipulation.

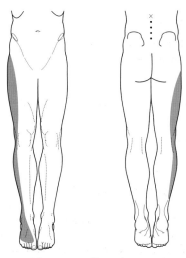

**Figure 15.5**   Insidious onset of leg pain

2. A general limitation of intervertebral movement, if it is contributing to the symptoms, will be improved by mobilization rather than by traction.
3. This patient probably will be helped by a combination of traction and mobilization.
4. If mobilization were attempted, rotation should be the first choice.
5. As there are no neurological changes and straight leg raising is not markedly limited, the possibility of completely relieving symptoms is good.

### First day

It was decided to institute traction first to assess its value before including mobilization. Very gentle traction in supine was applied for 10 minutes. While the traction was on there was a lessening of pain in the leg, and on releasing the traction the symptoms remained eased. After a 5-minute rest the patient's straight leg raising had improved by 10°. The patient went home and was asked to rest.

### Second day

The patient felt that she had improved from the traction. She had not had any back discomfort. Forward flexion had improved by 5 cm (2 in), and straight leg raising had maintained the improvement of 10°.

Traction was repeated, but as there had been no trouble with back pain it was done in prone. A strong pull (35 kg) was given for 15 minutes, and all leg pain disappeared. Some pain returned on releasing the traction. After a short rest, straight leg raising was found to have improved a little further.

### Third day

Further slight improvement was felt by the patient. Forward flexion was 32 cm (13 in) from the floor (an improvement of 2.5 cm), and straight leg raising still lacked 10°.

The same strength of traction was used, and similar relief of symptoms was experienced. Traction was maintained for 30 minutes.

### Fourth day

In comparison with the first day there had been considerable improvement, but the rate of progress appeared to have been less over the last 2 days. Forward flexion now lacked 31 cm (12 in), and straight leg raising lacked 5°.

Stronger traction (70 kg) was given, and the patient was then given a long rest.

### Fifth day

Forward flexion lacked 25 cm (10 in), straight leg raising was full and there was further symptomatic improvement.

As it was felt that progress should have been quicker, mobilization was commenced. Rotation with the patient lying on her left side was given four times. Following each movement there was an improvement in forward flexion consisting of a 5-cm (2-in) improvement after the first and second times, 2 cm (0.8 in) after the third and only 1 cm (0.4 in) after the fourth. Strong traction followed the mobilization.

### Sixth day

The patient felt much better. Her back felt freer and the leg ache was almost gone. Forward flexion had maintained its increased range, and the fingertips were now 11 cm (3 in) from the floor. Straight leg raising was normal.

A repetition of the rotation increased forward flexion to 2 cm (0.8 in) from the floor. Traction was also repeated.

### Seventh–ninth days

The routine of the fifth and sixth days was repeated, and by the tenth day the patient was free of all symptoms. Her straight leg raising was normal and forward flexion was full, with all signs of the sciatic scoliosis gone. She had lost all tingling sensation by the seventh day. All active and passive movements were much freer than when examined on the first day.

## POORLY DEFINED LEG SYMPTOMS

### Examination

#### History

For 2 years a man aged 45 years had noticed intermittent tingling, which began over the dorsum of the left foot and gradually extended to the lateral aspect of the leg, thigh and buttock (*Figure 15.6*).

Two weeks ago he had been hospitalized for a heart condition, and during this period the symptoms had worsened until at the time of treatment he had a constant dull ache in the left lateral buttock, thigh and leg with tingling over the dorsum of the foot.

#### Physical findings

Active movements of the spine were full and painless with the exception of forward flexion, which caused a dragging feeling posteriorly in the left leg when his fingertips were 13 cm (5 in) from the floor. Passive movements of the lumbar spine showed a marked limitation of the flexion–extension movement between the fourth and fifth lumbar vertebrae. Other tests of the spine, sacroiliac joints and hips were normal.

The referring physician asked for 2 days of treatment, as the patient was then returning to his home in the country.

## Treatment

### Guiding factors

1. The only objective sign is the L4/5 stiffness.
2. These is no muscle spasm protecting movement of the L4/5 intervertebral joint.
3. As only 2 days of treatment are possible, and as the L4/5 stiffness (if this is the cause of the symptoms) has probably taken at least 2 years to reach its present stage, it could waste time to begin with mobilizing techniques.
4. From the above three points it would appear best to begin with manipulation of the intervertebral joint between L4 and L5.

### First day

The rotary manipulation localized to the L4/5 joint was done twice to the right and twice to the left. The range of forward flexion improved each time until the patient was able to touch his toes without any dragging feeling in the left leg. The leg ache improved from the beginning, and the foot tingling had gone after four manipulations.

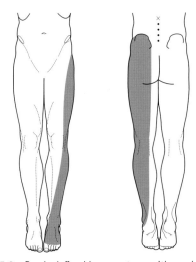

**Figure 15.6**   Poorly defined leg symptoms with good movements

### Second day

The patient was still able to touch his toes, and all limb and buttock pain had gone. Tingling had been intermittent and less severe since the manipulation. The L4/5 joint was sore from the manipulation.

The first day's treatment was repeated, and this cleared the tingling in the foot. On re-testing, the L4/5 movement was greatly improved.

The patient wrote 10 days later to say that he had remained symptom free.

## CERVICAL

## PAIN SIMULATING CARDIAC DISEASE

### Examination

### History

A man aged 54 years was treated 7 years ago for Ménèire's disease and deafness. Three years later he had a very bad bout of left chest and arm pain, which came on during the night. He later recalled that he had been waking with a feeling of slight neck stiffness for a few days before this onset. At that stage his doctor considered that a heart condition was the cause of the pain, and he was treated for this.

Ten days ago he was again wakened by left chest and arm pain, and since then the pain had been unbearable at times (*Figure 15.7*).

His referring specialist said there was little evidence of cardiac disease and, as neck movements were restricted, manipulation and traction should be given as a diagnostic trial.

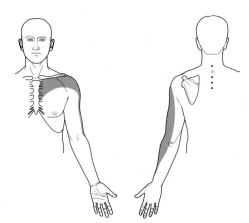

**Figure 15.7**   Severe left chest and arm pain simulating cardiac disease

## Physical findings

Neck movements were markedly restricted. Extension was impossible, forward flexion, left lateral flexion and left rotation lacked 60° of their range, and right lateral flexion and right rotation were limited by approximately 25°. All of these movements caused pain in the arm.

Radiologically the body of C6 was narrowed vertically, and there was marked narrowing of the C6/7 interbody space with over-riding of the apophyseal facets.

## Treatment

### Guiding factors

1. Pain in the left chest and arm, which may simulate cardiac disease, can arise from T4 or C7 levels.
2. With such severe symptoms and with all movements limited by a marked increase in arm pain, traction would be preferable to manipulation.
3. With marked limitation of movement and with a definite painful limitation of forward flexion, the result can be expected to be slow.
4. As pain subsides with traction, and flexion becomes free, mobilization could be used to hasten the result.

### First day

As extension was so limited, cervical traction in flexion (approximately 35°) was given, which almost completely relieved the pain. Treatment comprised two stretches, each of 10 minutes' duration. Pain returned on lowering the traction each time. The patient was warned of the possible flare-up of symptoms following the first treatment. He was attempting to continue his own clerical business throughout treatment.

### Second day

Movements and pain were approximately the same as on the first day. Traction was repeated, but it was given as a stretch of 15 minutes. Some degree of relief remained on releasing the traction.

### Third day

Pain had eased a little, and rotation showed a little improvement. Traction was repeated.

### Fourth–seventh day

Marked progress continued with this daily traction.

### Eighth day

By this stage, pain had been reduced and all movements were less limited. Forward flexion was painless, and pain was in the same areas – namely the chest and the whole of the arm.

As symptoms were less severe and forward flexion was painless, it was decided to commence mobilization as well as continuing with the traction. Cervical rotation to the right carried out three times resulted in freedom from the forearm part of the pain and lessening of the upper arm pain, but the chest pain remained unchanged.

The thoracic spine between T1 and T5 was then mobilized three times, pushing the spinous processes from right to left with transverse vertebral pressure. This relieved the chest pain, but only slightly improved the forearm pain.

The usual traction was given, and this completely relieved the forearm pain.

### Ninth day

The pain had eased its usual amount, but movements had made more progress than previously. As thoracic soreness had increased from the mobilizing of T1–5, only traction was given on this day.

### Tenth day

Local tenderness had improved, so the eighth day's treatment was repeated.

By the thirteenth day, the alternate-day mobilizing plus the daily traction had resulted in freedom of movement and only occasional sensations of ache in the arm.

## PAIN SIMULATING SUPRASPINATUS TENDINITIS

### Examination

Reference of pain from the vertebral column into joints is common, and it is sometimes difficult to determine the origin of, say, shoulder pain, as demonstrated in the example that follows. When pain is referred, the joint signs consist of pain on movement without restriction. Sometimes there is pain in an associated area (such as the scapula) to guide the examiner, but this is not necessarily so. Sometimes there are no vertebral column signs to indicate that the shoulder pain arises in the neck. The only way of finding out is to treat the neck and observe the shoulder pain. The response to treatment when the neck is the cause is always quick which makes assessment easier. This problem of vertebral cause of peripheral joint pain is common in the hip and shoulder, and less common in the elbow or knee. The following case history is given as one example.

### History

A young man aged 25 years was referred for physiotherapy treatment to his right shoulder, which had been painful for 2 months. Cortisone injections into the shoulder 18 days ago had caused a severe reaction.

The patient said the symptoms had come on gradually, and he knew of no previous history of pain or injury. His symptoms consisted of an ache in the shoulder at night, and jabs of pain on top of the shoulder with movements of the arm during the day (*Figure 15.8*).

### Physical findings

There was an arc of pain felt on top of the shoulder during mid-range abduction, and a static contraction of the supraspinatus muscle also caused pain on top of the shoulder. Passive movements of the acromioclavicular joint and glenohumeral joint were painless. All cervical movements were full range and painless. Except for slight tenderness in the region of the insertion of the right supraspinatus tendon, all tissues felt normal.

## Treatment

### Guiding factors

Shoulder treatment with emphasis on the supraspinatus tendon is to be given by electrotherapy and deep-friction massage to the tendon.

### First–tenth days

During the first 10 days of treatment, there were some nights when the shoulder did not ache. However, the arc of pain on abduction remained unchanged. On the eleventh day, the site of the pain had changed to the middle of the supraspinous fossa.

### Eleventh day

With the pain in a new position, cervical movements were rechecked and were found to be full, but rotation

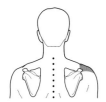

**Figure 15.8** Shoulder symptoms of cervical origin

to the right and extension reproduced this right supraspinous fossa pain. With closer questioning, the patient recalled the pain in this area approximately 2 weeks before his shoulder pain developed. He also mentioned that in recent years he occasionally wakened with a slightly stiff neck, which always disappeared within 1–2 hours of getting up. Mobilization of the cervical spine by left rotation was used as an oscillation for 1 minute and, upon favourable assessment of progress, was repeated twice more. Abduction had then lost its painful arc, and cervical movements were painless. The static test of the supraspinatus had also become painless. Local shoulder treatment was discontinued.

### Twelfth day

The patient reported feeling much better, but cervical rotation to the right still caused supraspinous fossa pain. Cervical extension and shoulder abduction were still painless. Rotation mobilization to the left was repeated three times, and resulted in painless neck movements.

### Thirteenth day

Pain had returned to the top of the shoulder, and the painful arc of abduction had also returned. Cervical rotation to the right again caused pain in the right supraspinous fossa. Treatment mobilizing the cervical spine with a rotation to the left was repeated, and resulted in freedom from all symptoms and signs, including the arc of pain with abduction.

### Fourteenth day

Treatment was cancelled as the patient had no pain, and neck and shoulder movements were painless.

## Treatment of further developments

There was a slight return of supraspinous fossa pain 2 weeks later, which was cleared by mobilizing the cervical spine by rotation to the left on 2 consecutive days. The patient was later known to have remained symptom free for 4 months.

It should not be concluded from this case history that all shoulder conditions that have a painful arc of movement must be treated by mobilization of the cervical spine; rather that such symptoms may have a cervical component. It is useful to treat the cervical component first while assessing changes at the shoulder. Should there be little or no improvement in the shoulder either at the initial treatment session or in the

24-hour assessment period, then treatment must focus on the shoulder.

## PAIN SIMULATING MIGRAINE

### Examination

#### History

A woman aged 40 years had a 21-year history of what the doctor had called migraine. During this time, her longest period without pain had been 2 years. In each bout of pain the symptoms began at the back of the neck, and then spread into the right occipital area and then over the head to the right ear and the right frontal area. The pain, which she described as a vicious throb, lasted from 2–8 days, enforcing bed rest in the early stages. Symptoms of pain were accompanied by nausea and blurring vision. The only prodrome was a 'feeling of well-being' (*Figure 15.9*).

#### Physical findings (at the end of an attack)

Head and neck movements were quite full, but flexion and extension gave general discomfort in the right upper neck area. Right lateral flexion gave moderate pain on both sides of the neck at the level of C1, whereas left lateral flexion hurt only to the right of C1. Rotation to the left was normal, but to the right it caused pain to the right of C1.

### Treatment

#### Guiding factors

1. While the patient's symptoms are severe, gentle and sustained traction in neutral would possibly ease the symptoms considerably.
2. Rotation is usually the best procedure for helping neck conditions, particularly when they are unilateral.
3. It needs to be explained to the patient that, once the pain to the right of C1 (which can be produced by testing movements) has been eliminated, treatment will only be given during attacks, and therefore the end-result may appear slow in coming.

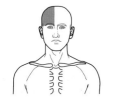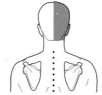

Figure 15.9    Cervical headache

4. The progress should consist of a lessening of the severity of the attacks and an extension of the pain-free period between attacks.
5. Treatment should be instituted as soon as an attack begins, whatever the hour of day.
6. While treating during an attack, the treatment sessions can be expected to be long because extended rests should be given between techniques.
7. The changes that can be anticipated from the various procedures should be the same as would be expected with other vertebral syndromes.
8. The first aim is to make all cervical movements free of the pain at the right of C1 and to note how freedom from this alters the patient's pain cycle.

#### First–third day

Rotation mobilizations (done only to the left) were given as gentle but sustained procedures, twice the first day and four times on the second and third days. This produced a gradual clearing of the pain felt to the right of the first cervical vertebra.

#### Fourth day

The patient reported with all of the disturbances that accompany an attack, but she did not have the usual throbbing head pain. The pain to the right of C1 had reappeared and become more noticeable.

Gentle traction in neutral was given for 10 minutes, and this eased the feeling of nausea and cleared her blurred vision. These symptoms did not return on releasing the traction. After a 5-minute rest, the traction was repeated.

#### Fifth and sixth days

The nausea, although less, was still present, returning 2 and 4 hours respectively after the fourth and fifth day's treatments.

Traction was repeated in two periods (one of 20 minutes and the other of 10 minutes) on each day, but this only produced a slight improvement.

#### Seventh day

Vision was normal and nausea was absent, but the pain to the right of C1 was still in evidence on rotation, especially if this was done to the right, and there was slight right frontal pain.

Rotation mobilization to the left was done four times as a much stronger oscillatory procedure. This resulted in a clearing of all symptoms and signs.

## Eighth day

The patient reported feeling well, and the only remaining sign was pain to the right of C1 when the head was put into full extension and then laterally flexed and rotated to the right.

Rotation mobilization to the left was done twice as a strong full-range procedure, allowing a 10-minute rest between. This made the patient free of pain on testing.

## Treatment of further developments – 1

The patient remained symptom free for 10 days (a much longer period of freedom than usual), and then returned with pain on the right side of the neck radiating over the right side of the head to the frontal area, with blurred vision and a feeling of nausea.

On examination, rotation to the right caused pain in the right side of the neck at the C1 level. This pain increased both in intensity and area, to a right hemi-cranial pain, if the rotation was combined with right lateral flexion and full extension (the upper cervical quadrant).

## First day

The patient was given transverse manipulation to the right at C1–2 three times during a 2-hour period, which allowed for long periods of rest. Symptoms were greatly eased and movements became less painful.

## Second and third days

The patient felt pleased that she had not had to resort to drugs. There were fewer symptoms, and by the third day she only had slight right frontal pain with testing rotation in the position of right lateral flexion and extension.

Transverse manipulations to the right were repeated, with shorter rests between as they became less necessary. By the end of the treatment on the third day she was both symptom free and sign free again.

## Fourth and fifth days

There was a mild overnight recurrence of right hemi-cranial ache (not pain), which indicated that treatment should continue. There was no nausea or blurring of vision. During the treatment on the fourth and fifth days, longitudinal movement, rotation to the right and postero-anterior central vertebral pressure were attempted in turn, but as each was used it caused an increase in symptoms, and rotation to the left had to be reinstituted in order to settle them. It was now known

that rotation manipulation to the left was the effective treatment in this case.

## Sixth and seventh days

Transverse manipulation to the right was the only technique used, and by the end of this period the patient was again symptom free and sign free.

## Treatment of further developments – 2

The patient remained symptom free for 13 days, indicating further improvement, and then developed moderate pain in the right occipital and adjacent neck area with slight right frontal pain. The feeling of nausea was minimal. The usual sign of pain with rotation to the right was present.

## First day

At this stage, rotation left manipulation without traction was the most effective treatment for this patient, and it was known that it could be done as a strong procedure with safety. As nausea was not excessive, long rests between manipulations were unnecessary. Rotation to the left was given four times as a very strong and sustained oscillating movement followed by a manipulative flick. The patient's neck on the left side was then too sore to allow further treatment. Active rotation to the right was almost painless, and all nausea and head pain had gone.

## Second day

There was no nausea and only slight frontal pain. Rotation to the right still caused some pain to the right of C1.

Maximum-range forced rotation to the left was given three times, with complete relief of symptoms and signs.

## Treatment of further developments – 3

The patient remained symptom free for a further 3 weeks; she then developed a mild right frontal pain. Active rotation to the right was painless, even when done in conjunction with right lateral flexion and extension.

## First day

Transverse manipulation to the right was given twice, followed by a 30-minute period of rest. As the symptoms did not return, further manipulation was considered unnecessary.

This treatment was given in 1957, and she is known to have remained free from attacks until her death in 1965.

## SCAPULAR PAIN

### Examination

#### History

One week ago, while yawning and stretching, a woman aged 40 years felt a sharp pain over the left scapula. During the next 2 hours the ache increased slightly in intensity, and spread over a greater area to cover the left side of the lower neck and the left middle and upper scapular area (*Figure 15.10*). After that, the symptoms remained unaltered.

The patient had had a similar episode a year ago, which recovered without treatment in 4 days.

#### Physical findings

The symptoms consisted of a constant nagging scapular ache, which was aggravated by movement and partially relieved by rest. Trunk and shoulder movements were full and painless, but the cervical movements, except for left lateral flexion and right rotation, were all very limited and caused scapular pain. Forward flexion lacked 50 per cent of its movement, and although it was possible to initiate extension, pain then prevented further movement. Rotation of the head to the left was limited by 50 per cent, and pain prevented all but the first few degrees of right lateral flexion. (This combination of limited rotation to one side and lateral flexion to the opposite side is unusual.) With all of these movements, pain in the left scapula was markedly increased. The only tenderness that could be found was over the spinous processes between T2 and T4.

### Treatment

#### Guiding factors

1. Scapular pain can be caused by either a cervical or an upper thoracic condition; therefore both areas may need to be treated.

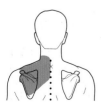

Figure 15.10    Scapular pain

2. As the cervical movements are so limited, it would be wiser to treat this area first.
3. Conditions of sudden onset usually respond more rapidly to manipulation than to traction.
4. Rotation right would probably be the main technique here.

#### First day

Mobilization of the cervical spine by rotation to the right was given very gently for 20 seconds. Following this, cervical extension and right lateral flexion had increased by 20°. The technique was repeated, but as there was no pain or muscle spasm with the oscillation it was done with greater pressure. Following three applications of this rotation, the patient had 50 per cent of her range of extension and right lateral flexion; full flexion and left rotation only lacked 20°. All these movements still caused scapular pain. The patient was warned of the possibility of an increase in symptoms following treatment.

#### Second day

There had been no increase of symptoms, and the patient felt much better. The range of movement had remained the same as had been obtained following the first treatment. The same mobilization was given, but it was done seven times. There was no improvement with the last two applications of the rotation, but overall the movements made further improvement. Flexion and right lateral flexion were full and painless. Rotation to the left increased by 10° and now lacked the last 10° of movement, while extension increased 10° and still lacked 30° of movement. Both these movements caused left scapular pain.

#### Third day

The improved movement was maintained, and it was decided that, as progress had been slower on the second day, the upper thoracic spine should be included in the mobilization. As it was known how much improvement the rotation had produced on the second day, the thoracic mobilizing was done first to assess the comparative values of thoracic and cervical mobilization. Transverse vertebral pressure was directed against the right side of the spinous processes of T2–4. The technique was done firmly for 1 minute. The result was full left rotation and extension of the head, although both movements still caused pain. Following two further applications of transverse vertebral pressure, all pain had gone.

## Fourth day

The patient could feel pain only in the left scapular area on full extension of the head or full rotation to the left. For the final treatment, the patient was given transverse vertebral pressure against the spinous processes of T2–4 followed by rotation to the right for the cervical spine. All movements were painless following the mobilization. No further treatment was required, as the patient was free of symptoms and signs on the following day.

## ACUTE TORTICOLLIS

### Examination

#### History

A boy aged 16 years was wakened two nights ago at 3 am by pain in the right side of his neck. He had never had any trouble with his neck previously, and had not been carrying out any unusual work during the few days immediately prior to the incident; nor had he been unwell (*Figure 15.11*).

#### Physical findings

The head and neck were held in a position of approximately 35° of left lateral flexion and slight forward flexion. The patient said that there had been no improvement following one day of complete rest in bed.

His active range of flexion was full, but gave some right middle neck pain. Both extension and right lateral flexion were grossly limited by the pain. Rotation to the left and right gave pain, but with rotation to the left the range was full, while to the right it was moderately restricted.

### Treatment

#### Guiding factors

1. As there is some flexion deformity of the neck, the result is likely to be slower than if only lateral flexion deformity were present.
2. If a day of rest has not made any difference, the patient is unlikely to respond to treatment as

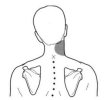

**Figure 15.11** Acute torticollis

quickly or easily as would some patients with symptoms and signs of this type.
3. If manipulation is given it should be done gently, being guided by the patient's comfort.
4. The best result will possibly be obtained by doing a small amount of mobilizing to produce an increase in range of movement, followed by gentle traction to maintain the improvement while allowing soreness to subside. More mobilizing could then follow. This cycle should be repeated until the maximum progress has been gained. The last part of the treatment would need to be a period of traction.
5. As the patient is unable to extend his neck, the traction will need to be given in flexion. This also applies to the mobilization used.
6. Following treatment, the patient will need to rest with pillows supporting the neck.
7. If there is marked improvement during treatment on each of the first 2 days but with an overnight deterioration, a soft collar may be required to help maintain the progress. Under these circumstances, the collar should not be needed for many days.
8. As symptoms are right-sided, the ideal technique will be rotation to the left; however, as there is deformity, care will be needed to ensure that a physiological rotary movement is produced.

#### First day

A rotation mobilization to the left was given first. This was done with the neck comfortably flexed. The rotation was taken gently to the limit of the range allowed by the pain and spasm. Once the limit was reached a gentle oscillation was carried out, attempting all the time to increase the spasm-free range. This was continued for approximately 1 minute. As there was quite a marked improvement from this one mobilization, it was decided to give traction in flexion while lying. This was done for 15 minutes. By doing this, the following mobilizations would possibly be more effective and of less discomfort to the patient than if more mobilization was done at the beginning.

Following the 15 minutes' traction the angle of deformity was reduced, but there was still marked limitation of right lateral flexion. Extension was greatly improved. Rotation mobilizing to the left was repeated three times, producing further improvement. During the mobilizing, the rotation was easier to produce and the muscle spasm was much less. Traction was repeated.

The range of lateral flexion was then 50 per cent of normal, and extension was 75 per cent of normal, but each movement still caused right neck pain. Some indication of the deformity was still present, but the patient was able to adopt the normal head position without pain. Rotation was repeated three times. It was possible to do this much more strongly at this stage. Traction was repeated.

Following this, terminal extension caused pain, right lateral flexion was 75 per cent of full range, and the deformity was almost gone. Rotation mobilization to the left was repeated twice more, and traction reapplied. Movements were then full but were performed cautiously, and the deformity had gone.

The patient was asked to rest, using adequate neck support. As he had been using a rubber pillow, its disadvantage was explained; being rubber it has the tendency to maintain its shape, and during sleep this will result in a constant nudging against the relaxed neck. Although this may seem trivial, it is sufficient to irritate an easily disturbed neck. To give treatment every assistance, the patient was shown how to make an ordinary flock or feather pillow into a butterfly shape by shaking the stuffing to the ends and tying the centre isthmus lightly with ribbon. He was asked to lie with the isthmus under his neck for support, leaving the wings to stabilize the head. Then, whether he lies on his back or side, he has adequate support for the neck and the head. If necessary, a second small pillow can be used temporarily under the 'butterfly' pillow to give the amount of flexion needed to relieve the pain.

### Second day

The deformity was almost gone, and extension was full but caused slight right neck pain at the limit of its movement. Right lateral flexion was limited by approximately 25 per cent of its movement. Rotation to the left was full and painless, but to the right there was pain at the limit of the range. There had been more progress than was anticipated (*see* Treatment, (1) and (2), p. 427), and therefore more could be done without causing the patient discomfort.

Rotation left was repeated as a strong oscillating procedure. This made right lateral flexion almost full range after three mobilizations, but further repetition of the rotation did not produce much further increase. Extension was now full and painless, as was rotation left. Both lateral flexion right and rotation right caused terminal pain. Treatment was changed to mobilizing with left lateral flexion, and after being carried out twice it produced slight improvement. As the patient's neck was sore from the stronger procedures, he was given supine traction in flexion.

Following this, there was no deformity and only pain with rotation to the right. One strong rotation was then given, but this time to the right. Assessment was made difficult by soreness from the mobilization, but the patient was told that he need not rest at home.

### Third day

There was no deformity, and only right neck pain with full right lateral flexion and full right rotation.

The patient was manipulated twice with rotation without traction to the left, after which the movements were painless.

## CERVICAL JOINT LOCKING

### Examination

#### History

A girl aged 15 years had, while playing basketball, suddenly turned her head to the left, and it had become stuck in this position. She felt pain on the right side of her neck. She had had no previous neck injury or symptoms, and was not otherwise unhealthy (*Figure 15.11*).

#### Physical findings

The patient was unable to extend her head or laterally flex or rotate it to the right. Examination by passive intervertebral movement showed the C2/3 joint to be fixed.

### Treatment

#### Guiding factors

1. As it occurred easily, it may clear easily.
2. Gentle longitudinal movement and rotation should be tried first.
3. If mobilization does not help, a localized manipulation should be used to open the C2/3 joint on the right.
4. Complete restoration of range should be achieved on the first day, although the movement may still be sore.

#### First day

Longitudinal movement was tried without success. Rotation to the left was tried next, and this produced slight improvement. Repeating the movement did not help further. A localized diagonal thrust was used next, tipping the patient's head to the left, patiently coaxing the position to relieve spasm first. One manipulation completely restored movement. The test for range by passive intervertebral movement was made following the manipulation, to ensure that range was restored. Heat and massage were then given to relieve soreness.

## Second day

Movement was normal, but soreness was still present. Palliative treatment was given, but further manipulation was considered unnecessary.

## SHOOTING OCCIPITAL PAIN

### Examination

#### History

A man aged 38 years bent over a handbasin 5 weeks ago, and sustained a sharp pain across the neck at the level of C1. Following this, he was unable to move his head without pain.

He complained of 'shooting' pains across his upper neck at the level of C1 when turning his head, and an ache which spread downwards in the midline from C1 to T1 (*Figure 15.12*).

#### Physical findings

Neck flexion caused a pulling feeling in the area of the upper cervical spine, but was full range if carried out cautiously. Extension and lateral flexion were painless. Rotation to each side was full range and caused moderate pain in the sub-occipital area, but all movements had to be done slowly. Quick movements in flexion or rotation produced sharp suboccipital pain.

The referring doctor asked for treatment by traction and manipulation, to be attempted in that order.

### Treatment

#### Guiding factors

1. As the symptoms are predominantly sharp pains with movements, an ineffective procedure should be changed quickly for another.
2. Sudden onsets with immediate limitations that do not become progressively worse over the following 2 or 3 days are more likely to be helped by mobilization than by traction.
3. Upper cervical conditions are usually more difficult to help than mid-cervical conditions.
4. Rotation is usually the most effective procedure for the cervical spine, although postero-anterior

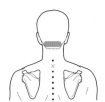

**Figure 15.12**  Shooting occipital pain with movements

central vertebral pressure is usually best for evenly distributed symptoms.
5. If traction is to be used, traction in neutral would be preferred to traction in flexion, as the condition is probably arising from the upper cervical spine.
6. As the patient can only attend for treatment for two consecutive days at a time, it will be reasonable to give a long treatment on the second day despite soreness if progress is being achieved, as the patient will have a week before further treatment can be given.

### First day

Traction in neutral was applied gently at first, but as this produced no improvement in the pain felt with movements while it was on, it was gradually increased until a firm traction was applied for 10 minutes. After the traction there was a feeling of burning suboccipitally and a feeling of general loosening of the neck, but there was no improvement in the sharp pains. It seemed pointless continuing with traction, as there had been no quick progress.

With the patient lying, longitudinal movement as an oscillatory procedure was applied. After 20 seconds of this, rotation to the left was improved, but other movements remained unchanged. This was repeated twice more without further change.

As right rotation now caused more pain than left rotation, it was decided to use left rotation as the next mobilization. This was done firstly as an oscillating procedure, then as a manipulation without traction. As this did not produce any improvement, the same order was tried with rotation to the right, but this also did not produce any improvement. No further treatment was given that day, and the patient was warned of a possible exacerbation of symptoms following the treatment.

### Second day

The patient reported a bad night with a lot of shooting pains, but these symptoms had subsided to their usual level today.

As traction and rotation had failed, postero-anterior central vertebral pressure was used next, localizing it to C1 and C2 and commencing gently, for approximately 15 seconds. There was an immediate improvement in the freedom of rotary movements following this technique.

This mobilization was continued, as it was producing a steady improvement in the freedom from pain with movements. Because the patient could not come in again for a week, the technique was carried out

12 times with gradually increasing pressure. The patient was again warned of the possibility of a temporary flare-up of his symptoms.

### Third day (1 week later)

Thirty minutes after the last treatment the patient had vomited and had a lot of shooting suboccipital pain, but by the following day he felt markedly improved, and had been almost free of pain ever since. Currently his symptoms were 'a feeling of limitation to turning the head but no real jabs of pain'.

The same postero-anterior central vertebral pressure was used for a further five times. This made rotation painless and unrestricted.

### Fourth day (following day)

Except for a slight pain on full, quick, active rotation, the patient felt normal. There was no recurrence of vomiting. The treatment given on the third day was repeated, resulting in full, free rotation.

The patient wrote 1 week later stating that he had lost all his symptoms.

## LUMBAR

### LOW BACK PAIN

### Examination

#### History

A woman aged 43 years was limited in the amount of housework she could do because of backache and pain with movement of the back. Since the age of 20 she had had bouts of back pain, usually following heavy work.

She had had her present bout for 2 weeks, during which time it had not improved (*Figure 15.13*).

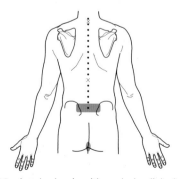

**Figure 15.13**  Low back pain with marked radiological degenerative changes

The ache was relieved by short rests, but a full night's rest in bed caused stiffness of the lower back. This stiffness readily disappeared on moving about, but the backache became much worse by the end of the day. Sitting increased the patient's backache, and she always experienced difficulty rising from a chair. Sneezing caused considerable back pain.

### Physical findings

With forward flexion the patient's lower lumbar spine was lordosed, and she was only able to reach her knees before pain prevented further movement. Backward bending was limited, and lateral flexion to the right was more limited and more painful than to the left. Rotation and straight leg raising were normal. The lumbar spine was generally tender in the area of pain (L4–S1). Radiologically the body of L4 was almost sitting on L5, and they were fused on the left. The lumbosacral disc space was extremely narrow, and this was narrower to the left. This created a scoliosis convex to the right from L4 to S1, and there was a compensating scoliosis about L4 convex to the left together with a slight amount of rotation. Passive intervertebral movements of the lower spine could not be adequately tested for range, because of pain.

### Treatment

#### Guiding factors

1. Painful movements, when associated with marked radiological degenerative changes, are often helped by gentle oscillating mobilization, particularly postero-anterior central vertebral pressure.

2. Even though the symptoms are bilateral, the pain felt with lateral flexion is worse when done to the right. It may therefore be better to use a rotation mobilization using the right side as the dominantly painful side.

3. Symptoms that have a gradual onset usually respond better to traction than to manipulation.

#### First day

Postero-anterior central vertebral pressure was chosen, and was done for a period of 20 seconds as a very gentle oscillating procedure over L4 and L5. Forward flexion became more limited, and the patient was only able to reach to 50 cm (20 in) from the floor.

Mobilization was then changed to a gentle oscillating rotation, with the patient lying on her left side. As this produced improvement in the range of forward flexion, it was repeated three times. Forward flexion improved to 30 cm (13 in) from the floor. The patient was warned of a possible exacerbation.

### Second day

The patient reported feeling easier for a while after treatment, but by the time she reached home the symptoms were very bad and she had a bad night. On examination, forward flexion was still 30 cm (12 in) from the floor. The amount of treatment was possibly the cause of the exacerbation, rather than the technique used, so rotation was repeated three times with the patient lying on her left side. To reduce the possibility of a further exacerbation, it was decided to stop at three times. Forward flexion was improved by only 5 cm (2 in).

### Third day

The patient reported another bad night. Forward flexion remained 25 cm (10 in) from the floor. Traction was considered to be the next step. Because movement was required it was decided to use intermittent variable traction, and 12 kg was given for 10 minutes with a 5-second 'hold' period and no 'rest' period. At this low weight she felt relieved of pain, but said that if it had been any stronger it would have given her back pain.

On releasing the traction there was moderate back soreness. After a short rest, the patient reported feeling better than before the traction. Forward flexion was not tested because this movement is often stiffer for a short period immediately following traction.

### Fourth day

The patient felt greatly improved, and forward flexion was now 20 cm (8 in) from the floor. Traction was repeated.

### Fifth–ninth days

There was steady and marked progress from day to day, and traction was able to be slightly increased in pressure each day until on the ninth day she felt no back discomfort with 30 kg of traction. The duration of traction did not exceed 15 minutes.

After the fifth traction (on the ninth day), all movements were full and painless actively, and the patient had been able to carry out housework without discomfort.

## ACUTE BACK PAIN

### Examination

#### History

During the last 5 years a heavy man aged 62 years had had three comparatively minor bouts of back pain, each of sudden onset from trifling incidents. His present bout commenced with a slight backache following weeding in the garden 1 week ago. The pain improved, but was aggravated by an 8-hour drive in his car 3 days ago. Gradually the symptoms became more severe and changed in nature from an ache to a sharp pain with movement, which eventually prevented walking. After 2 days in bed without any improvement in his symptoms, his doctor requested manipulation. At the time of treatment, the patient was in bed unable to move because of jabs of pain in the centre of the lower back (*Figure 15.14*).

#### Physical findings

It was impossible to examine more than straight leg raising, spreading and compressing the ilia, and neck flexion, as the patient was unable to move. Straight leg raising was almost full on both sides, but more back pain was produced with raising the right leg than with raising the left. Flexion of the neck with the chin on the chest produced slight back pain, and the sacroiliac joint test was negative.

### Treatment

#### Guiding factors

1. Examination is too limited to be conclusive, but at least the symptoms are localized to the back and straight leg raising is good.
2. The fact that the response to straight leg raising varies slightly when comparing the left leg with the right leg may call for a unilateral technique when the patient is more mobile.

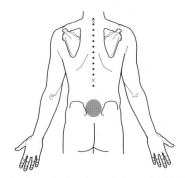

Figure 15.14   Acute back pain confining patient to bed

## First day

The only technique possible with such an immobile patient, and possibly the best choice in view of the nature of the patient's symptoms, is longitudinal movement. The movement was done gently but sharply as three tugs using both legs. It caused marked pain each time at the site of his symptoms. Following this, the pain with neck flexion was less. The tugs were repeated, and neck flexion then became painless. Straight leg raising was then normal on the left, and although full range on the right, it still produced some back pain. The patient was still unwilling to try to move in bed. It was then decided to give the longitudinal movement using the right leg only. This was done in the same way as the two-leg technique, as it was obvious that the patient would not be able to kick. This procedure was done twice, with two tugs each time. Right straight leg raising was then normal. The patient was given adequate warning that some exacerbation might occur during the next few hours.

## Second day

There was only a slight flare-up of symptoms, and the patient was able to walk about but unable to bend. He had lost most of his 'catching' pain. On examination he had a slight protective scoliosis, with the displacement of his shoulders being to his left side. Forward flexion was very limited, and this caused central pain at the level of L5. Right lateral flexion was very limited and painful, but to the left it was full and painless. Backward bending, straight leg raising and neck flexion were all normal.

The protective scoliosis resulting in a tilt to the left and the unilateral straight leg raising of the previous day suggested a unilateral problem (predominantly right-sided), even though symptoms were central.

Rotation mobilizing was given with the patient lying on his left side. After two rotations, the protective scoliosis had gone and lateral flexion right was full and painless. Forward flexion had improved, but was still limited and painful. Rotation was repeated twice without any further improvement. It was suggested that the patient should rest for an hour, after which he should walk about as much as possible, provided that the symptoms were not aggravated.

## Third day

There was no exacerbation, and the patient had been up most of the day. There were also fewer symptoms. The scoliosis had returned, but right lateral flexion was full and painless. Forward flexion was still limited.

Rotation, which was repeated twice, eliminated the scoliosis and partly improved the range of forward flexion. This technique was repeated twice more, but did not produce any change.

Longitudinal movement using the kicking action of the patient's right leg was used four times. With each of the first three there was an increase in the range of forward flexion until it became almost full, but the fourth did not produce any further improvement. The patient was asked to move about normally.

## Fourth day

There was no scoliosis, and only slight limitation of forward flexion. The patient said he felt almost normal.

Rotation was repeated twice and followed by two applications of longitudinal movement using the patient's right leg. Forward flexion was then full range and painless.

Forward flexion remained normal, and treatment was discontinued.

# L1 BUTTOCK PAIN

## Examination

### History

A man aged 55 years gradually developed right buttock pain over a period of 5 days while engaged on heavy shovel work 6 months ago. He was able to continue work, and although the aching did not become any worse it did not improve. After a long period of unsuccessful treatment involving what he called 'adjustments', he went to his local doctor. After a week of bed rest failed to help him, his doctor suggested a further trial of manipulation (*Figure 15.15*).

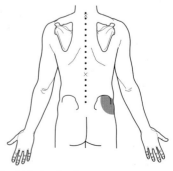

**Figure 15.15**   L1 buttock pain

### Physical findings

The patient's symptoms consisted of a constant ache felt superficially in the right upper gluteal area. The ache did not seem to vary much with moderate activity or rest. With the exception of extension (which reproduced the buttock pain) his spinal movements were painless, although all movements were stiff. His thoracolumbar area was kyphosed, but the patient said that it had always been so. There was no tenderness in the buttock or spine, but with firm pressure over the spinous processes of L1 and L2, a deeply situated protective muscle spasm could be felt. With the application of this pressure, it was possible to feel a limitation of movement in this postero-anterior direction when compared with the areas above and below this level. By questioning the patient, it was noted that his treatment by adjustments had consisted of rotation of the lumbar spine, pressure over the lower lumbar spine, and a whip-cracking action of the back produced by using the patient's leg as the handle of the whip while the patient was lying prone.

### Treatment

#### Guiding factors

1. When a patient has been unsuccessfully treated elsewhere by manipulation, more difficulty can be expected in alleviating the symptoms.
2. The whip-cracking and pressure of the previous treatment would have been effective only on the lower lumbar spine. Rotation is more valuable for treating the lower lumbar spine than the upper lumbar spine.
3. In view of the deep spasm in the upper lumbar area and the limitation of postero-anterior movement, it would be better to direct mobilization at this level using postero-anterior central vertebral pressure.
4. It is possible for buttock pain to arise from the upper lumbar spine.
5. As rotation did not help in the patient's earlier treatment, it would be better to begin with postero-anterior central vertebral pressure or transverse vertebral pressure.
6. Because the symptoms developed slowly and did not respond to adjustments, it may be better to begin treatment with traction.

#### First day

With the presence of muscle spasm and the likelihood of the symptoms having an upper lumbar origin, it was decided to begin by mobilizing between T12 and L2. Postero-anterior central vertebral pressure was given firmly, attempting to give the maximum pressure possible without causing muscle spasm. One minute was spent mobilizing the area at this pressure. The procedure caused no change in the patient's symptoms or signs. This technique was repeated twice more, because it was felt that the muscle spasm was lessening. By the end of the treatment, the ache in the buttock had eased by 50 per cent.

#### Second day

Although there was little change, the patient considered he could feel some improvement for the first time in 6 months. This indicated that treatment was probably being directed at the right level. Postero-anterior central vertebral pressure was repeated, but this technique was interspersed with transverse vertebral pressure pushing the spinous processes from left to right. The result following four applications of each technique was a further noticeable improvement in symptoms.

#### Third–sixth days

The second day's treatment was repeated during these 4 days. Symptoms gradually lessened day by day, until by the sixth day postero-anterior movement felt normal and it was free of muscle spasm.

It may be that if traction had been incorporated into the treatment routine on the third day, the total treatment time might have been shortened by 1 or perhaps 2 days. However, it seemed unwise to change from measures that were obviously proving successful.

## SPONDYLITIC SPINE WITH SUPERIMPOSED LOCALIZED LESION

### Examination

#### History

An elderly man developed sharp pain in his left groin and quadriceps area following rest in bed for a kidney infection. He complained of a constant dull ache with intermittent sharp pains (*Figure 15.16*).

#### Physical findings

Radiologically, the patient had marked spondylitic changes throughout his lumbar spine. Examination of his lumbar movements revealed that extension and left lateral flexion were both markedly limited, causing pain in the left thigh. All other movements were pain free. Palpation in the L2/3 area revealed that transverse

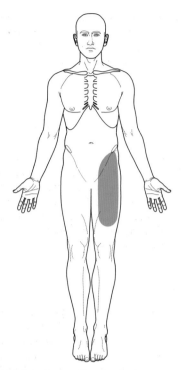

**Figure 15.16**   Superimposed localized pain

pressure at this joint, pushing towards the right, reproduced his right quadriceps pain.

## Treatment

### Guiding factors

1. An elderly patient with a lot of spondylitic change, having a superimposed localized joint lesion, is likely to be very difficult to help.
2. Localized mobilizing techniques are more likely to be helpful than general techniques.
3. Traction, if it is to be used, will need to be of the intermittent variable type rather than the constant type.
4. It is likely that all suitable techniques will need to be used in concert.

### First day

Transverse pressure towards the left at the L2/3 level and above and below this joint was performed three times. There was an improvement in extension and left lateral flexion, but the movement was still very painful.

### Second day

There was no unfavourable reaction from the first treatment, so intermittent variable traction was added

after the transverse pressures. The traction used was gentle and for a short time; 12 kg was given for 10 minutes, with 3-second hold periods and no rest period.

### Fourth day

There appeared to be a gradual but slow improvement in the range of extension and left lateral flexion, so the treatment was continued and postero-anterior central vertebral pressure was added.

### Sixth day

A further technique, that of lumbar rotation, pelvis to the right, was added.

### Subsequent days

This treatment was continued daily for 3 weeks, at the end of which time the patient said he had had no pain in his leg for the previous 3 days and had been able to play 18 holes of golf without trouble. Treatment was discontinued.

## COCCYGODYNIA

### Examination

#### History

Six months ago, after an unusually long ride on a bicycle which had a wide seat, a woman aged 34 years developed pain in the region of the coccyx. This pain gradually increased until it reached a stage when she was unable to sit through a full cinema programme. The area ached for at least an hour after prolonged sitting, but provided she did not sit again she would remain symptom free.

Since the age of 16 years she had had minor low backache following gardening or heavy housework, but this symptom had not altered during the last 6 months (*Figure 15.17*).

The referring doctor felt that the patient's symptoms might be from her lower back rather than of local coccygeal origin, and requested a trial of manipulative treatment directed to the back, to aid in assessing the source of the symptoms.

#### Physical findings

All movements of the lumbar spine were full and painless, but the patient was able to elicit pain in the coccyx by sitting on a hard seat and leaning back 10°. Both the coccyx and lumbosacral joint were tender on pressure.

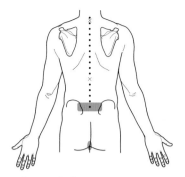

Figure 15.17   Coccygodynia

## Treatment

### Guiding factors

1. During each treatment period, the only guides to progress are tenderness to pressure and the patient's ability to lean backwards while sitting on a hard seat.
2. As the symptoms are not unilaterally distributed, the first choice for mobilizing should be postero-anterior central vertebral pressure.
3. As tenderness is one of the guides, it might be better to begin treatment with rotation to avoid the possibility of causing back soreness, which could make it difficult for the patient to assess coccygeal soreness.
4. If rotation is used as the first mobilization, it may be necessary to perform it to one side only at one treatment, and then assess the patient's ability to sit during the following 24 hours.

### First day

Treatment by mobilizing with postero-anterior central vertebral pressure was given first as a gentle oscillating procedure from L3 to L5. Although there was some tenderness over L5, there was no muscle spasm. On reassessing the patient's ability to sit and lean backwards, the pain was still produced after 10° of movement. The procedure was repeated twice more, after which the degree of leaning backwards had increased to 20°. A further mobilization was given, but this did not produce any further increase and so the treatment was stopped.

### Second day

The patient had not noticed any improvement, but it now required 20° of leaning backwards to produce the coccygeal pain while sitting. As this improvement had been maintained, it was decided to repeat the postero-anterior central vertebral pressure. After the first three times there was an improvement of 5° with the sitting test, but there was no further progress after the fourth.

### Third day

There was a marked increase in lower back discomfort, but no improvement in the ability to sit for prolonged periods. Coccygeal pain was caused by 15° of leaning backwards in sitting. This was almost back to the original range. Rotation with the patient lying on her left side was the next mobilization chosen. This side was chosen merely because only one side should be used on one day. Four applications produced an improvement of 10° (to 25°) in the sitting test.

### Fourth day

As no improvement could be reported and the sitting test had maintained its range of 25° from the previous day, the rotation was applied with the patient lying on her right side. After three applications of this technique there was a further increase of 10° (to 35°) in the sitting test, but a fourth use of the rotation did not produce any further improvement.

### Fifth day

All low back discomfort had gone, and the patient noticed that the coccygeal ache had taken longer than usual to come on with sitting. On examination, the tenderness over the coccyx was approximately the same, but the sitting and leaning back test had maintained its range of 35°. Rotation with the patient lying on her right side was repeated three times, after which she could sit and lean backwards without feeling any discomfort. There was also noticeably less coccygeal tenderness.

### Sixth day

The patient considered that her ability to sit without pain had improved to 80 per cent of normal. There was very little tenderness on palpation, but at the limit of leaning backwards in sitting the patient could feel coccygeal discomfort. The rotation was repeated four times, after which the sitting test was normal and tenderness had gone. It was decided to discontinue treatment for 1 week to assess progress, and suggested that the patient should return earlier if the symptoms became worse.

*One week later*

There were only odd times when pain was present, and the patient had been to the cinema twice during this time. On examination, the sitting test was normal and palpation was painless. The rotation mobilization was repeated four times, and treatment discontinued.

## JUVENILE DISC LESION

### Examination

#### History

Following a boating accident a youth aged 19 years developed pain in his right buttock, extending into the hamstring area. He had no previous history of back injury. Although symptoms were not severe, they were preventing him from his normal work and he could not rest properly at night (*Figure 15.18*).

#### Physical findings

On standing the patient had a contralateral tilt, which increased with the limited range of forward flexion he had. He was unable to reach beyond his knees, but the limitation was due more to tightness than to a feeling of pain in his buttock or leg. Right straight leg raising

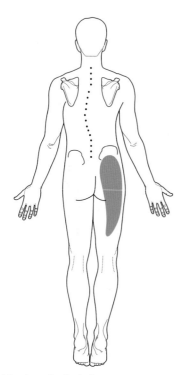

**Figure 15.18**  Juvenile disc lesion

was also limited to 40°, but all other movements were full range and painless. There were no neurological changes.

### Treatment

#### Guiding factors

1. Being young, this patient will be slow in his response to treatment.
2. Because the diagnosis is a disc lesion, rotation and traction are probably the two most important techniques.
3. The techniques will probably need to be used quite firmly.
4. Treatment will probably effect an improvement in symptoms without making as much improvement in the signs.

#### First day

Rotation of the pelvis to the left was performed four times, and although this did not seem to make much difference to his movements, the patient was able to say that his leg felt freer.

#### Second day

The patient had retained the free feeling in his leg for 4 hours, but it then returned to the previous state. The treatment was repeated, and postero-anterior central vertebral pressure was added. The treatment again produced a freeing of his leg.

#### Third day

The patient retained the free feeling in his leg for longer, although by the third day his symptoms were much as they had been. Treatment was repeated, and traction was added. This again produced freedom, which was maintained for a similar period.

#### Subsequent days

The same treatment of rotation, central pressures and traction was repeated for the next 5 days, during which time the symptoms became much easier. The freedom was retained from treatment to treatment, and the scoliosis was reduced by 50 per cent. Straight leg raising and forward flexion were essentially the same, except that the pain felt at the limit of the ranges was decidedly less. Treatment was discontinued, and the patient was reviewed 1 month later. At this stage, his symptoms had remained relieved and his movements were approximately the same. On review 12 months later his scoliosis had gone, and his straight leg raising and forward flexion had both improved by 30 per cent but were not normal. However, at this range they were pain free.

## BILATERAL LEG PAIN

It is perfectly obvious that not all patients will respond to treatment by mobilization or manipulation. However, even when treatment is unsuccessful, if it is administered in a methodical and constructive manner the result can be so conclusive as to be of advantage to the referring doctor. Frequently it is obvious that a patient requires surgery and would not respond to conservative measures. Although this is so, the unexpected occurs sufficiently often to justify a trial of manipulation, because the number of treatments required to reach a conclusive result is usually few.

### Examination

#### History

A woman aged 27 years had a 5-year history of trouble with her lower back and intermittent symptoms radiating into the buttocks and hamstring area. The onset had been insidious, with periods of back pain during the first 18 months before pain spread into her leg. She had been able to continue with her domestic work throughout this time. Two weeks prior to admission to hospital she had been cleaning floor-level cupboards, and after working in the bent position for half an hour was unable to straighten up. She was admitted to hospital and put on constant lumbar traction. After 11 days, there had been no improvement in her symptoms or her signs (*Figure 15.19*).

#### Physical findings

On examination, the patient was only able to reach her knees in flexion and she was unable to flex laterally to the left at all. Right lateral flexion was approximately 50 per cent of full range, and she only had 10° of extension. Straight leg raising on the left was 30°, and on the right was 45°. Movement produced by pressure over the fourth and fifth lumbar spinous processes was limited by 50 per cent in all directions, and at this point was strongly protected by muscle spasm. There were no neurological changes.

### Treatment

#### Guiding factors

1. Symptoms are likely to be discogenic in origin; therefore the treatment techniques most likely to succeed are rotation and traction.

2. The patient has had traction administered on a constant basis without success; therefore further traction is unlikely to succeed.
3. The techniques that can be used in quick succession to give clear-cut information for the lumbar spine are rotation, central pressure, traction and, possibly, straight leg raising.
4. Patients with bilateral leg symptoms are always slow to respond to treatment and difficult to help.
5. As this patient has a lot of pain as well as marked limitation of movement, care will be necessary with techniques to avoid exacerbation.
6. Very careful assessment will need to be made to be sure of the effect of treatment as quickly as possible.
7. If rotation is to be used, then the left side is the dominant side from the point of view of both signs and symptoms.

#### First day

Rotation to the right was administered first as a grade I movement. However, this irritated the symptoms while it was being done, and produced no improvement in straight leg raising or other signs. The same movement was then attempted as a very gentle grade IV. Less pain was provoked during this technique. On examination, the patient's forward flexion had improved

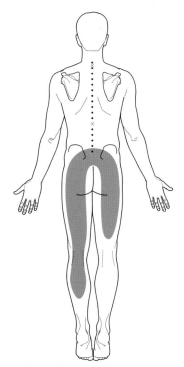

Figure 15.19    Bilateral leg pain

5 cm (2 in), and her left lateral flexion showed the first signs of movement. The technique was repeated, but did not produce any further improvement. The patient commented that the symptoms in her back were much worse.

### Second day

Symptomatically, the patient had been much worse. However, it was her back that was worse, and not her leg symptoms. On examination, her flexion and left lateral flexion had maintained their progress. The same rotation was attempted again, but muscle spasm was present, preventing as good movement as could be achieved previously. On re-examination, her movements had not improved further. It was decided to discontinue with that rotation, and to attempt rotation on the other side. This could be done a little less easily than to the right, and the technique did not produce any improvement in movements. The patient then lay prone and postero-anterior central vertebral pressure was attempted, but this movement was found to be worse than on the day of the initial examination. Following its use as a very gentle grade I technique, movements were reassessed and found to be unchanged.

### Third day

The patient again reported feeling worse in her back. Movements had not changed from those achieved following the first day's treatment. Attempted rotation and postero-anterior central vertebral pressure were both more difficult to achieve this day than on the second day. It seemed fairly obvious that there was no point in continuing treatment further.

A myelogram revealed a massive lumbosacral central protrusion, and decompression surgery produced relief of symptoms.

## THORACIC

### 'GLOVE' DISTRIBUTION OF SYMPTOMS

The T4 syndrome is commonly referred to. This does not mean that T4/5 is the joint always involved – it may refer to T3–7 – but it does imply symptoms of an ill-defined nature probably having their reference via the autonomic nervous system. It can be applied to symptoms in the arm or head. Symptoms are dull in nature, and cover the whole of the head or hand or arm. The following example is one where symptoms were felt locally at the T4 level. However, this is not essential, although signs at the appropriate thoracic

joint can always be found when symptoms arise from it.

## Examination

### History

A woman aged 42 years complained of intermittent 'pins and needles' involving the whole of the right hand. The symptoms appeared at least five times during a day, lasting for as long as an hour each time. There were no symptoms at night. She had had these symptoms to a lesser degree during the last 2 years, but they had recently increased in intensity and duration. As far as she knew, there was no injury or strain that could have caused the onset 2 years ago or the more recent increase of symptoms.

There was an area of extreme sensitivity in the mid-thoracic area, which she had had for many years without change. Although hard rubbing of this area eased the sensitivity, she could not tolerate soft rubbing (*Figure 15.20*).

Treatment by traction and mobilization was requested.

### Physical findings

Forward flexion was the only cervical movement that was painful. This movement lacked 40 per cent of its range, and caused sharp pain along the anterior aspect of the right arm from the shoulder to the wrist. Trunk and upper limb movements were full and painless. There was no tenderness in the cervical spine, but T5 was extremely tender and pressure here caused pain in the region of the right elbow. The patient was able to produce tingling in the hand by going through the actions of combing her hair, and the symptom could be relieved by shaking her hand vigorously.

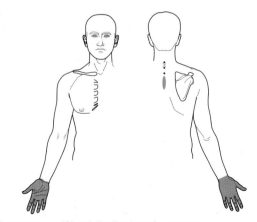

Figure 15.20   'Glove' distribution of symptoms

## Treatment

### Guiding factors

1. As there has not been a sudden or traumatic origin to account for these symptoms, traction may be the technique to try first.
2. Traction in flexion should be used before traction in neutral, as the symptoms could hardly be of upper cervical origin.
3. Of the mobilizing techniques, rotation of the cervical spine should be used before postero-anterior central vertebral pressure because the symptoms are distributed unilaterally.
4. If none of the above techniques relieve the symptoms, mobilization of the T5 area should be included. It must be remembered that the autonomic nerve supply for the arm arises from as low as T8.

### First day

Traction in flexion was applied with firm pressure (approximately 15 kg) for 10 minutes. As there were no symptoms present in the hand at the time of treatment, the pressure of the traction could not be gauged to suit the symptoms. On releasing the traction, neck flexion had improved a little but hand tingling could still be produced by the patient combing her hair. After applying traction in flexion for a further 15 minutes, neck movements and hand tingling were unchanged.

### Second day

The patient felt that there may have been a slight lessening of the intensity of the hand symptoms, but the discomfort felt with combing her hair was unchanged. Neck flexion had maintained the slight improvement from the previous day. Traction in flexion was repeated, but this time it was carried out much more strongly (25 kg) because there had been little change, favourable or otherwise, from the previous traction. It was given for periods of 20 minutes and 15 minutes. Following the treatment, neck flexion had increased by a further 5° (making a total improvement of approximately 10°), but the hair-combing test was still unchanged.

### Third day

Neck flexion had maintained its slight improvement, but there had been no further improvement in the hand symptoms. To enable the traction to be given more strongly, it was changed to traction in neutral and applied at a pressure that almost lifted the patient from the chair. While in this position she attempted the hair-combing test and found that, although she could still bring about a tingling, it was less intense. The patient was only able to tolerate 3 minutes of this traction the first time and 2 minutes the second, because of pain in the mid-thoracic area. Following the second traction, her neck flexion was 5° less than previously and the hair-combing test was unchanged.

### Fourth day

The patient reported feeling about the same as she was before treatment, and on examination there seemed to have been no progress. Treatment was changed from traction to mobilization, and the first technique used was cervical rotation to the left. Remembering that the patient had been given strong traction without any ill effects, the mobilizing was sustained for 1 minute. Following this, the hair-combing test was unchanged and neck flexion had improved by 10°. The rotation was repeated even more strongly, but this did not produce any change in symptoms or signs. As no headway was being made, the next mobilization given was a strongly applied postero-anterior central vertebral pressure, alternating three times with transverse vertebral pressure directed against the left side of the spinous processes between C4 and T1. However, these techniques did not produce enough change to warrant continuing with them. It was therefore decided to mobilize the midthoracic spine before attempting cervical lateral flexion. Postero-anterior central vertebral pressure was applied from T3 to T7, at a pressure that did not cause pain in the patient's elbow. The oscillating was continued for 1.5 minutes. Following this treatment, neck flexion was full and painless and the hair-combing test had improved by approximately 50 per cent. While the mobilizing was being repeated, it was found that the pressure could be markedly increased without causing local pain or referred pain. By the third application of the mobilization, the patient was unable to induce the hand tingling by combing her hair.

### Fifth–seventh days

There was a marked reduction in severity and duration of symptoms following the fourth day's treatment, and neck flexion had remained full in its range although it still caused anterior arm pain. The postero-anterior central vertebral pressure was repeated between T3 and T7 without producing any elbow pain, and again made the patient free of symptoms and signs. After treatment on the sixth day the patient remained symptom free, but as T5 was still tender the mobilizing was repeated on the seventh day.

### Treatment of further developments

One month later there was a mild recurrence of symptoms, which was eliminated by 2 days of mobilizing the mid-thoracic area.

This case history has been included to show that the therapist must be aware that atypical symptoms can and do occur, and that one must be ready to treat the less obvious areas sometimes.

## THORACIC BACKACHE

### Examination

#### History

A woman aged 31 years first noticed thoracic backache 4 years ago. It came on following heavy work of an unusual nature, and took 2 weeks to subside. After this attack she had similar aches following any particularly heavy work, even though there was never any incident of sudden pain with this work. The ache would subside in 2 weeks. More recently the ache had become continuous, but it was always further aggravated by heavy work. On waking each morning there was a marked feeling of stiffness in this area of the thoracic spine (*Figure 15.21*), but the stiffness would disappear after she had been up and about for 30 minutes.

#### Physical findings

Symptoms were evenly distributed to each side of the spine. There were few positive signs. Trunk rotation to each side was limited by 20–25°, and each movement caused pain 2.5 cm (1 in) to the left of the T8/9 area. When the intervertebral joints were tested passively, there was a limitation of rotation between T4 and T5 and between T5 and T6. There was very marked tenderness to pressure over the spinous processes of T4, T5 and T6, and to a lesser extent over T3 and T7. When

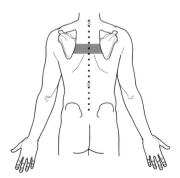

**Figure 15.21**   Thoracic backache

firm pressure was applied over this area of the spine, strong muscular contraction came into play to prevent intervertebral movement.

### Treatment

#### Guiding factors

1. Mobilization will need to be kept within the limits of the spasm.
2. Symptoms are evenly distributed but there is left-sided pain with rotation to left or right, which may therefore require a unilateral technique.
3. The thoracic spine responds best to postero-anterior central vertebral pressure first and transverse vertebral pressure towards the painful side (left side in this case) next.
4. With this patient there are three things to eliminate; the ache, the stiffness on rising, and the tenderness with limitation of movement between T4 and T6. The tenderness and movement will be helped by mobilization, but the ache and stiffness may require traction.
5. As mobilization is quicker in its effect, it should be used first.

#### First day

Postero-anterior central vertebral pressure was given first over the spinous processes from T3 down to T8. There was marked tenderness between T4 and T6, necessitating a gentler pressure. The oscillating was done steadily, taking approximately 1.5 minutes to cover the area. The spasm did not prove to be any obstacle, as localized tenderness prevented the depth of oscillation that would have caused the muscle spasm. There was an increase of 10° in the rotation to each side following this procedure, and pain was still left-sided.

This gently oscillating mobilization was repeated another three times. Rotation, which improved but was not yet full range, caused a feeling of general thoracic soreness rather than a left-sided pain. After a short rest, the patient thought the ache was less than before the treatment.

Adequate warning of a possible increase of symptoms was given, and the patient was asked to refrain from any work that she knew would aggravate her symptoms.

#### Second day

The ache and the stiffness on rising were unchanged. The centre of the patient's back was sore (presumably from the mobilization), and rotation to the left produced left-sided pain but now lacked only 15° of its full range.

The same postero-anterior central vertebral pressure was given, but it was done more firmly. Even though the area was sore, it was possible to increase the pressure to the level of the muscle spasm. This was repeated four times, still maintaining the oscillating and taking 1.5 minutes to complete each time. The range of movement was then full and painless, but the spine felt very sore.

It was decided to leave treatment for 48 hours to allow the soreness to subside and thus make assessment more informative.

### Third day

During the day following treatment the patient's back was sore, but she reported that the ache was less severe. Stiffness on rising had remained unchanged. Rotation was now only slightly limited, but still caused left-sided pain. There was less tenderness than at the beginning of treatment, and there was now no muscle spasm.

Postero-anterior central vertebral pressure was repeated gently as a continuous oscillation four times, and was interspersed with transverse vertebral pressure pushing against the right side of the spinous processes from T3 to T7, pushing them towards the painful left side. This was done three times. Rotation became full and painless, being the best result obtained with treatment of this patient so far.

It was decided to leave assessment for 3 days to allow all soreness to subside again.

### Fourth day

All soreness had gone and backache was almost nil. However, the patient still had stiffness on rising, and although rotation was full, it gave a general feeling of soreness in the thoracic area.

The movements appeared normal but some backache and stiffness remained, so it was decided to give the patient traction.

The passive range of intervertebral rotation was found to have improved and to be almost normal. As some limitation remained, it was decided that the mobilizations should be repeated. Had this movement not improved, it would have been necessary to manipulate these intervertebral joints.

The oscillating techniques of the third day's treatment were repeated. There was no muscle spasm and very little soreness. Following this, the patient was given traction in two periods lasting 15 minutes and 10 minutes. The angle of pull on the cervical halter was approximately 30° from the horizontal, and although the patient had not had any low back pain, the flexed hip and knee position was adopted.

### Fifth day

In the morning the patient reported feeling very much better. There was no ache, and almost no stiffness on rising. Rotation was normal both actively and on passively testing the movement at the intervertebral joint.

No mobilization was given, but traction was repeated for another two periods of 15 minutes and 10 minutes.

The patient reported 1 week later, having had no backache or stiffness since the last treatment.

## TRAUMATIC GIRDLE PAIN

### Examination

#### History

Following a vehicular accident 1 week ago, a man aged 33 years suffered a collapse of the left upper lobe of the lung and girdle pain (left side greater than right side) at the fifth thoracic level. Because of chest pain, breathing was difficult, coughing was impossible, and the man was unable to lift his left arm above his head. He had two nerve blocks, but these gave only temporary relief (*Figure 15.22*).

Figure 15.22    Traumatic girdle pain

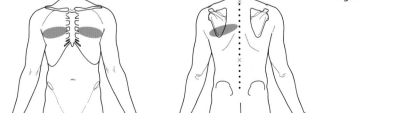

## Physical findings

The trunk was held rigid as if to avoid all movement, as movements of the head caused chest pain. On the left side of the trunk, the constant pain radiated throughout the fifth thoracic level from the vertebra around the thoracic cage to the sternum. The right-sided pain, which was mild and intermittent, would subside with rest. Trunk rotation to the left caused pain throughout the area, but particularly posteriorly on the left after 10° of movement. Rotation to the right caused pain after 40°. With lateral flexion of the trunk, pain was produced at the beginning of the movement to the left and after 20° of the movement to the right. Trunk flexion could be performed more readily than other movements, but it still had to be done slowly. Without any obvious movements of the trunk, 50 per cent of head and neck extension caused the thoracic pain. Cervical rotation to the left, which lacked 20° movement, also caused thoracic pain. Tenderness was most marked over the spinous processes of the third to the sixth thoracic vertebrae.

## Treatment

### Guiding factors

1.  As symptoms are severe and movements grossly limited, mobilizing will need to be done extremely gently.
2.  Traction may be made difficult by the patient's inability to lie on his back without pain, but perhaps it could be done sitting.
3.  Although symptoms and signs have a unilateral dominance, postero-anterior central vertebral pressure will probably be the best procedure because it is the main technique for the thoracic area and because symptoms spread to both sides.

### First day

Postero-anterior central vertebral pressure was given very gently over the spinous processes from the second to the seventh thoracic vertebrae. The mobilizing, which was done so softly that spasm and pain were avoided, was continued over a period of 2 minutes. Trunk rotation to the left improved from 10° to 25°. The procedure was repeated twice more, after which rotation to the left was 45°. All other movements improved, including raising the arm. The patient said that the pain had had the 'sting' taken out of it. To avoid joint soreness, it was decided to stop treatment for that day. Warning was given of the possibility of an increase in symptoms later in the day.

### Second day

The patient reported having felt wonderful for 5 hours, but in the morning he had felt worse. On examination, the arm movement had remained improved and trunk rotation to the left was possible through 30°. This is an example of a patient feeling worse, possibly due to treatment soreness, but whose signs show improvement. Patients may complain of severe pain and continue to feel that they are worse, despite improvement in signs, for as long as 5 days. However, the improvement in signs guides the therapist in the choice of techniques. Postero-anterior central vertebral pressure, repeated as a firmer procedure, was more uncomfortable than on the first day, but it still was not done firmly enough to cause muscle spasm. The procedure was repeated three times, and the result was an increase in trunk rotation to the left to 60°.

### Third day

The patient felt much better, and left trunk rotation was possible through 45°. Transverse vertebral pressure was used against the right side of the spinous processes of the second–seventh thoracic vertebrae, moving them towards the more painful left side. After two applications of this technique, rotation of the trunk to the left was possible through 65°. This technique did not appear to be superior to the previous procedure in the results it produced. Postero-anterior central vertebral pressure was then carried out twice, resulting in a range of painless rotation to the left of 75°. The overall rate of progress was considered to be satisfactory.

### Fourth–sixth days

Treatment was continued as a combination of postero-anterior central vertebral pressure and transverse vertebral pressure, alternating from one to the other four times. These mobilizations were gradually increased in pressure day by day as symptomatic progress was made. Traction was not given for two reasons; the rate of progress was satisfactory, and the patient could afford only the minimum of time necessary for treatment now that he was able to resume the full responsibilities of his job. By the sixth day, his pain was only of nuisance value and movements were full, although left trunk rotation and extension still caused slight left thoracic pain. Arm movements were normal, and there was no discomfort with breathing or coughing.

## Further treatment

Treatment was then continued on alternate days for the next three visits, this break being caused by the pressure of his work. The same routine as had been used previously was repeated strongly, and by the last visit movements were normal and painless and the ache had gone.

## ABDOMINAL PAINS AND VAGUE SIGNS

The following case history is an example of uncertain diagnosis where manipulative physiotherapy was used as a diagnostic trial. It is included in this chapter to show how manipulation, although an empirical form of treatment, can be used methodically and constructively as an active yet safe eliminative treatment.

### Examination

#### History

This patient was a girl aged 12 years who was training for competitive swimming. While swimming 18 months ago she had a severe bout of left-sided abdominal pain, and had to be lifted out of the water. She was able to return to swimming 3 weeks later, and then had only occasional twinges. Two months ago, vague left-sided abdominal symptoms began to return and gradually became more persistent, preventing full swimming training. On questioning, she mentioned mild soreness across the back between the levels of T12 and L2 (*Figure 15.23*) during 'out of pool' training 6 months ago.

The patient's only symptom at the time of treatment was a predominantly left-sided abdominal pain brought on by swimming and, to a lesser extent, by prolonged walking.

Her referring doctor suggested that she should discontinue swimming temporarily, but that after a trial of manipulative physiotherapy she should go back into the water to assess progress.

#### Physical findings

On examination, all active movements were painless but active lateral flexion to the left appeared to be limited between the T12 and L2 spinous processes when compared with the same movements to the right. Passively

testing the range of intervertebral movement revealed a limitation between T12 and L1 and between L1 and L2.

With the patient prone, strong pressure against the left side of the spinous process of T12 pushing it towards the right sometimes caused a pain in the left side of the abdomen.

### Treatment

#### Guiding factors

1. Young people with persistent symptoms of a severity necessitating treatment are often more difficult to help than middle-aged people with similar symptoms.

2. If the symptoms arise from the thoracolumbar junction, the three main mobilizations are postero-anterior central vertebral pressure, transverse vertebral pressure and rotation, as used for the lumbar spine, and the order of preference would be as listed.

3. With a limitation in the active range of movement between T12 and L2 as it exists in this patient, the transverse vertebral pressure mobilization could either be done to restore the movement, or could follow the general principle of pushing the spinous processes towards the painful side. Each of these principles would result in transverse vertebral pressures, but from opposite sides.

4. The intervertebral joints T12–L1 and L1/2 can be manipulated if symptoms do not improve with mobilization.

5. The only two true guides to progress are pain with walking and pain with swimming. If walking can be regulated, and thereby used as a guide, the swimming test can justifiably be tried when walking becomes painless.

#### First day

Postero-anterior central vertebral pressure was chosen to be used in conjunction with transverse vertebral

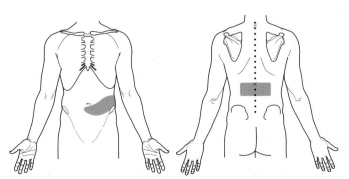

**Figure 15.23**  Abdominal pains and vague signs in a young patient

pressure directed against the left side of the spinous process from T11 down to L2, aiming at reducing the active limitation of left lateral flexion (contrary to the principle 'push towards the pain'). These two mobilizations were carried out three times in each direction. The patient was asked to walk 3.2 km (2 miles) before breakfast to assess the timing and the severity of pain.

### Second day

The patient reported left abdominal pains of short duration after 460 m (500 yd) and again after 830 m (900 yd). Active left lateral flexion looked unchanged, and there was some local vertebral soreness from the previous day's treatment. As no reason could be seen for assuming that the patient was either worse or better, the previous day's treatment was repeated. She was asked to repeat her walking test before breakfast.

### Third day

Pain was less severe with walking this morning. Left-sided twinges were experienced once at 550 m (600 yd) and once at 740 m (800 yd). As this indicated possible progress, the same mobilizing procedure was repeated.

### Fourth day

Twinges of pain experienced with the walking test were approximately the same as on the previous day.

Lateral flexion appeared unaltered. It was felt that this should have improved, and also that the walking test should have shown further progress after the third day's treatment. Treatment was therefore altered to transverse vertebral pressure only, but directed against the right side of the spinous processes of T11 and T12, pushing towards the painful side. This was carried out four times, each time lasting approximately a minute, with an assessment of the patient's active left lateral flexion between. This movement did not appear to change.

### Fifth day

There was no pain with walking this morning, and on examination left lateral flexion showed slight improvement. The fourth day's treatment was repeated, and it was suggested that a 0.8-km (half-a-mile) swim should be attempted.

### Sixth day

Only two momentary twinges were felt with the swim. Lateral flexion had improved a little more. Very strong pressure against the left side of T12 no longer produced abdominal pain. The treatment of the fourth and fifth days was repeated, and a 3.2-km (2-mile) swim was suggested.

### Seventh day

No symptoms resulted from further swimming. Lateral flexion appeared to be unchanged from the sixth day. It was decided to discontinue treatment, as normal swimming training the preceding day did not produce any symptoms.

At the end of the patient's full summer training programme 4 months later, she reported that there had been no further trouble.

# Appendix 1

# Movement diagram theory and compiling a movement diagram

*Geography would be incomprehensible without maps. They've reduced a tremendous muddle of facts into something you can read at a glance. Now I suspect ... economics [read passive movement] is fundamentally no more difficult than geography except it's about things in motion. If only somebody would invent a dynamic map.*   (Snow, 1965)

The movement diagram is a dynamic map representing the quality and quantity of passive movement perceived by the manipulative physiotherapist during her examination of any passive movement direction. This will include the amount, behaviour and relationships of any abnormal physical findings present, i.e. pain, resistance, spasm

## THE MOVEMENT DIAGRAM: A TEACHING AID, A MEANS OF COMMUNICATION AND SELF-LEARNING

The movement diagram is intended solely as a teaching aid and a means of communication. When examining, say, postero-anterior movement of the C3/4 intervertebral joint produced by pressure on the spinous processes (*see Figure 10.59*), newcomers to this method of examination will find it difficult to know what they are feeling. However, the movement diagram makes them analyse the movement in terms of range, pain, resistance and muscle spasm. Also, it makes them analyse the *manner* in which these factors interact to affect the movement.

> Movement diagrams are essential to the understanding of the relationship that the various grades of movement have to abnormal joint signs

The movement diagram (and also the grades of movement) are not necessarily essential to using passive movement as a form of treatment. However, they are essential to understanding the relationship that the various grades of movement have to a patient's abnormal joint signs. Therefore, although they are not essential for a person to be a good manipulator, they are essential if the teaching of the whole concept of manipulative treatment is to be done at the highest level. Movement diagrams are essential when trying to separate the different components that can be felt when a movement is examined. They therefore become essential for either teaching other people, or for teaching one's self and thereby progressing one's own analysis and understanding of treatment techniques and their effect on symptoms and signs.

> The components considered in the diagram are pain, protective involuntary muscle spasm and spasm-free resistance or stiffness

The components considered in the diagram are *pain*, *spasm-free resistance* (i.e. stiffness) and *muscle spasm* found on joint examination, their relative strength and behaviour in all parts of the available range and in relation to each other. Thus the response of the joint to movement is shown in a very detailed way. The theory of the movement diagram is described in this appendix by discussing its components separately at first. The practical compilation of a diagram for one direction of movement of one joint in a particular patient follows on page 460–461.

Each of the above components is an extensive subject in itself, and it should be realized that discussion in this appendix is deliberately limited in the following ways. The spasm referred to is protective muscle spasm secondary to joint disorder; spasticity caused by upper motor neurone disease and the voluntary contraction of muscles is excluded. Frequently this voluntary contraction is out of all proportion to the pain being experienced, yet in very direct proportion to the patient's apprehension about the examiner's handling of the joint. Careless handling will provoke such a reaction, and thereby obscure the real clinical findings. Resistance (stiffness) free of muscle spasm is

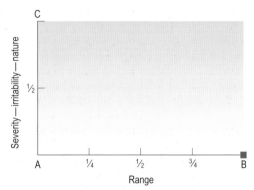

**Figure A1.1**    Beginning a movement diagram

discussed only from the clinical point of view; that is, discussion about the pathology causing the stiffness is excluded.

A movement diagram is compiled by drawing graphs for the behaviour of pain, physical resistance and muscle spasm, depicting the position in the range at which each is felt (this is shown on the horizontal line AB) and the intensity or quality of each (which is shown on the vertical line AC) (*Figure A1.1*).

The base line AB represents any range of movement from a starting position at A to the limit of the average normal passive range at B, remembering that when examining a patient's movement of any joint, it is only considered normal if firm proportionate over-pressure may be applied without pain (*see* p. 127–128). It makes no difference whether the movement depicted is small or large, whether it involves one joint or a group of joints working together, or whether it represents 2 mm of postero-anterior movement on the spinous process of C4 or 90° of cervical rotation to the left from the neutral position.

Because of soft-tissue compliance, the end of range of *any* joint (even 'bone to bone') will have some soft-tissue component, physiological or pathological. Thus the range of the 'end of range' will be a movable point, or have a depth or position on the range line. To locate half way through the range of the 'end of range' as a grade IV and fit in either side of it a plus (+) or a minus (−) sign allows the depiction of the force with which this 'end of range' point is approached (A. Edwards, unpublished observations).

> Point A, the starting position of the movement, is variable and is chosen by the therapist depending on the desired effect of the technique

Point A, the starting position of the movement, is also variable; its position may be the extreme of range opposite B or somewhere in mid-range, whichever is most suitable for the diagram. For example, if cervical rotation is the movement being represented and the pain or limitation occurs only in the last 10° of the range, the diagram will more clearly demonstrate the behaviour of the three factors if the base line represents the last 20° rather than 90° of cervical rotation. For the purpose of clarity, position A is defined by stating the range represented by the base line AB. In the above example, if the base line represents 90°, A must be at the position with the head facing straight forwards; similarly, if the base line represents 20°, position A is with the head turned 70° to the left (assuming of course that the normal average range of rotation is 90° to each side).

> Point B represents the extreme of passive movement, and lies variably beyond the extreme of active movement

As the movement diagram is used to depict what can be felt when examining passive movement, it must be clearly understood that point B represents the extreme of PASSIVE MOVEMENT, and that this lies variably, but very importantly, beyond the extreme of active movement.

The vertical axis AC represents the quality or intensity of the factors being plotted; point A represents complete absence of the factor and point C represents the maximum quality or intensity of the factor to which the examiner is prepared to subject the person. The word 'maximum' in relation to 'intensity' is obvious; it means point C is the maximum intensity of pain the examiner is prepared to provoke. 'Maximum' in relation to 'quality' refers to two other essential parts. They are:

1. *Irritability* – when the examiner would stop the testing movement if the pain was not necessarily intense but she assessed that if she continued the movement into greater pain there would be an exacerbation or latent reaction.

2. *Nature* – when $P_1$ represents the onset of, say, buttock pain, but as the movement is continued the pain spreads down the leg, the examiner may decide to stop when the provoked pain reaches the lower hamstring of upper calf area.

This meaning of 'maximum' in relation to each component is discussed again later. The basic diagram is completed by vertical and horizontal lines drawn from B and C to meet at D (*Figure A1.2*).

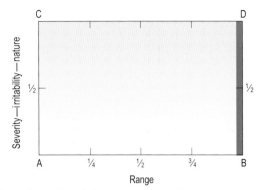

**Figure A1.2**   Completion of a movement diagram

Other variations of the base line AB are described on page 459–460.

## PAIN

$P_1$

The initial fact to be established is whether the patient has any pain at all and, if so, whether it is present at rest or only on movement. To begin the exercise it is assumed he only has pain on movement.

The first step is to move the joint slowly and carefully into the range being tested, asking the patient to report immediately when he feels any discomfort at all. The position at which this is first felt is noted.

The second step consists of several small oscillatory movements in different parts of the pain-free range, gradually moving further into the range up to the point where pain is first felt, thus establishing the exact position of the onset of the pain. There is no danger of exacerbation if sufficient care is used and if the examiner bears in mind that it is the very first provocation of pain that is being sought. The point at which this occurs is called $P_1$, and is marked on the base line of the diagram (*Figure A1.3*).

Thus there are two steps to establishing $P_1$:

1. A single slow movement first.
2. Small oscillatory movements.

If the pain is reasonably severe, then the point found with the first single slow movement will be deeper in the range than that found with oscillatory movements. Having thus found where the pain is first felt with a slow movement, the oscillatory test movements will be carried out in a part of the range that will not provoke exacerbation.

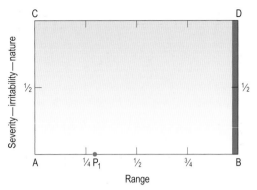

**Figure A1.3** Onset of pain

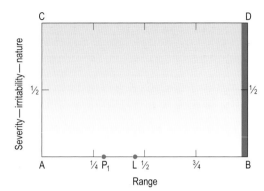

**Figure A1.4** Limit of the range

## L (A) WHERE

The next step is to determine the available range of movement. This is done by slowly moving the joint beyond $P_1$ until the limit of the range is reached. This point is marked on the base line as L (*Figure A1.4*).

## L (B) WHAT

The next step is to determine what component it is that prevents or inhibits further movement. As we are only discussing pain at this stage, $P_2$ is then marked vertically above L at maximum quality or intensity (*Figure A1.5*). The intensity or quality of pain in any one position is assessed as lying somewhere on the vertical axis of the graph (i.e. between A and C) between no pain at all (i.e. A) and the limit (i.e. C). It is important to realize that maximum intensity or quality of pain in the diagram represents the maximum the physiotherapist is prepared to provoke. This point is well within, and quite different from, a level representing intolerable pain for the patient. Estimation of 'maximum' in this way is, of course, entirely subjective, and varies from person to person. Though this may seem to some readers a grave weakness of the movement diagram, IT IS IN FACT ITS STRENGTH. When the student compares her 'L' and '$P_2$' with her instructor's, the differences that may exist will teach her that she has been too heavy handed or too 'kind-and-gentle'.

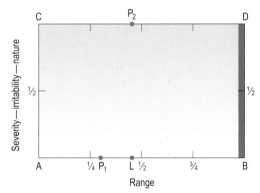

**Figure A1.5** Maximum quality or intensity of pain

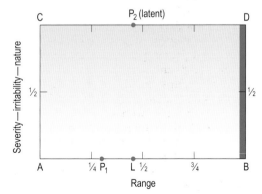

**Figure A1.6** Latent reaction of maximum quality or intensity of pain

## L (C) QUALIFY

Having decided to stop the movement at L because of the pain's 'maximum' quality or intensity and therefore drawn in point $P_2$ on the line CD, it becomes necessary to qualify what $P_2$ represents; if it is the

intensity of the pain that is the reason for stopping at L, then $P_2$ should be qualified thus: '$P_2$ (intensity)'.

If, however, the examiner believes that there may be some latent reaction if she moves the joint further even though the pain is not severe, then $P_2$ should be qualified thus: '$P_2$ (latent)' (*Figure A1.6*).

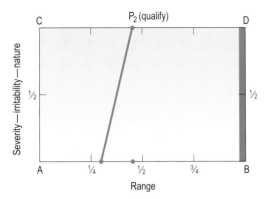

**Figure A1.7**    Pain increasing evenly with movement.
— = Pain

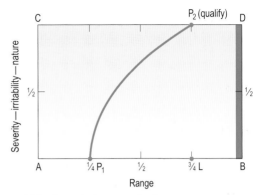

**Figure A1.8**    Irregular increase of pain

## P₁ P₂

The next step is to depict the behaviour of the pain during the movement between P₁ and P₂. If pain increases evenly with movement into the painful range, the line joining P₁ and P₂ is a straight line (*Figure A1.7*). However, pain may not increase evenly in this way; its build-up may be irregular, calling for a graph that is curved or angular. Pain may be first felt at about quarter range and may initially change quickly, then the movement can be taken further until a limit at three-quarter range is reached (*Figure A1.8*).

In another example, pain may be first felt at quarter range and remain at a low level until suddenly it changes, reaching P₂ at three-quarter range (*Figure A1.9*).

The examples given demonstrate pain that prevents a full range of movement of the joint, but there are instances where pain may never reach a limiting intensity. *Figure A1.10* is an example where a little pain may be felt at half range, but the pain scarcely changes beyond this point in the range and the end of normal range may be reached without provoking anything approaching a limit to full range of movement. There is thus no point L, and P′ (P′ means P prime) appears on the vertical line BD to indicate the relative significance of the pain at that point (*Figure A1.10*). The mathematical use of 'prime' in this context is that it represents 'a numerical value which has itself and unity as its only factors' (*Concise Oxford Dictionary*).

If we now return to an example where the joint is painful at rest, mentioned at the beginning of this appendix, an estimate must be made of the amount or quality of pain present at rest and this appears as P on the vertical axis AC (*Figure A1.11*). Movement is then begun slowly and carefully until the original level of pain begins to increase (P₁ in *Figure A1.12*). The behaviour of pain beyond this point is plotted in the manner

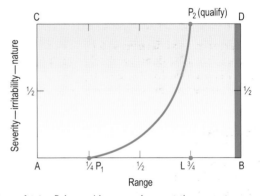

**Figure A1.9**    Pain reaching a maximum at three-quarter range

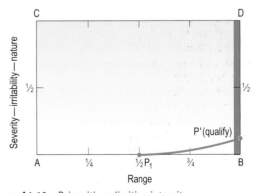

**Figure A1.10**    Pain with no limiting intensity

already described, and an example of such a graph is given in *Figure A1.13*. When the joint is painful at rest, the symptoms are easily exacerbated by poor handling. However, if examination is carried out with care and skill, no difficulty is encountered.

Again it must be emphasized that this evaluation of pain is purely subjective. Nevertheless, it presents an

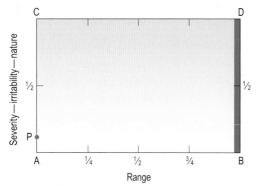

Figure A1.11  Pain at rest

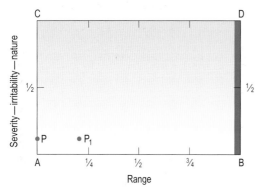

Figure A1.12  Level where pain begins to increase

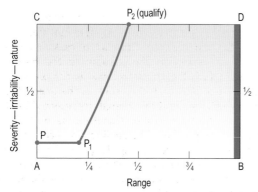

Figure A1.13  Pain due to subsequent movement

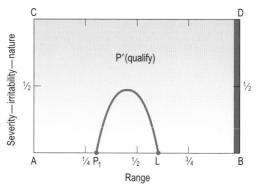

Figure A1.14  Arc of pain

An arc of pain provoked on passive movement might be depicted as shown in *Figure A1.14*.

## RESISTANCE (FREE OF MUSCLE SPASM)

These resistances may be due to adaptive shortening of muscles or capsules, scar tissue, arthritic joint changes and many other non-muscle spasm situations.

A normal joint, when completely relaxed and moved passively, has the feel of being well oiled and friction free (Maitland, 1980). It can be likened to wet soap sliding on wet glass. It is important for the physiotherapist using passive movement as a form of treatment to appreciate the difference between a free-running, friction-free movement and one that, although being full range, has minor resistance within the range of movement.

When depicting a compliance diagram of the forces applied to stretching a ligament from start to breaking point, the graph includes a 'toe region', a 'linear region' and a 'plastic region': the plastic region ends at the 'break point' (*Figure A1.15*).

When a physiotherapist assesses abnormal resistance present in joint movement, physical laws state that there must be a degree of resistance at the immediate moment that movement commences. The resistance is in the opposite direction to the direction of movement being assessed, and it may be so minimal as to be imperceptible to the physiotherapist. This is the 'toe region' of the compliance diagram, and it is omitted from the movement diagram as used by the manipulative physiotherapist.

The section of the compliance graph that forms the movement diagram represents the clinical findings of the behaviour of resistance when examining a patient's movement in the linear region only (*Figure A1.16*).

invaluable method whereby students can learn to perceive different behaviours of pain, and their appreciation of these variations of pain patterns will mature as this type of assessment is practised from patient to patient and checked against the judgement of a more experienced physiotherapist.

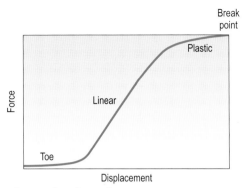

Figure A1.15    Compliance diagram

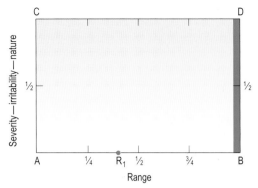

**Figure A1.17**    Positioning of R₁

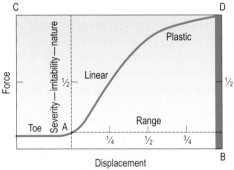

**Figure A1.16**    Movement diagram (ABCD) within compliance diagram. The dotted rectangular area (ABCD) is that part of the compliance diagram that is the basis of the movement diagram used for representing abnormal resistance (R₁R₂ or R₁R')

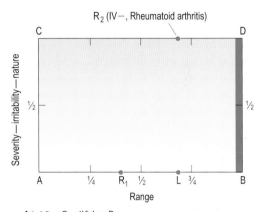

**Figure A1.18**    Qualifying R₂

## R₁

When assessing for resistance, the best way to appreciate the free running of a joint is to support and hold around the joint with one hand while the other hand produces an oscillatory movement back and forth through the chosen path of the range. If this movement is felt to be friction free, then the oscillatory movement can be moved more deeply into the range. In this way the total available range can be assessed. With experience, by comparing two patients, and also by comparing a patient's right side with his left side, the physiotherapist will quickly learn to appreciate minor resistance to movement. Point R₁ is then established and marked on the base line AB (*Figure A1.17*).

## L – WHERE, L – WHAT

The joint movement is then taken to the limit of the range. If resistance limits movement, the range is assessed and marked by L on the base line. Vertically

above L, R₂ is drawn on CD to indicate that it is resistance that limited the range. R₂ does not necessarily mean that the physiotherapist is too weak to push any harder; it represents the strength of the resistance beyond which the physiotherapist is not prepared to push. There may be factors such as rheumatoid arthritis, which will limit the strength represented by R₂ to being moderately gentle. Therefore, as with P₂, R₂ needs to be qualified. The qualification needs to be of two kinds if it is gentle (e.g. R₂ (IV−, RA)), the first indicating its strength and the second indicating the reason why the movement is stopped even though the strength is weak. When R₂ is a strong resistance (e.g. R₂ (IV++)), its strength only needs to be indicated (*Figure A1.18*).

## R₁ R₂

The next step is to determine the behaviour of the resistance between R₁ and L, that is between R₁ and R₂. The behaviour of the resistance between R₁ and R₂ is

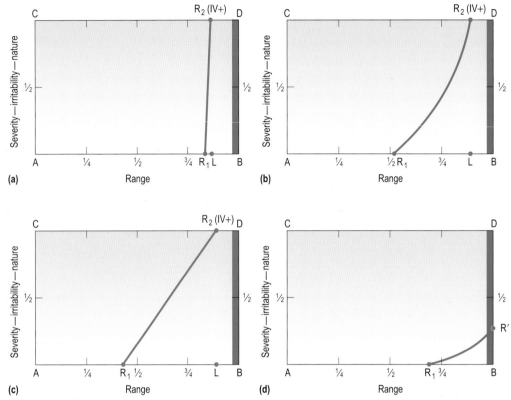

**Figure A1.19** Spasm-free resistance

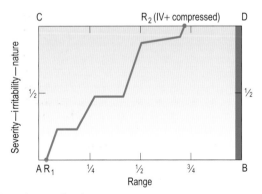

**Figure A1.20** Crepitus

assessed by movements back and forth in the range between $R_1$ and L, and the line depicting the behaviour of the resistance is drawn on the diagram (*Figure A1.19*). As with pain, resistance can vary in its behaviour, and examples are shown in *Figure A1.19*.

The foregoing resistances have been related to extra-articular structures. However, if the joint is held in such a way as to compress the surfaces, intra-articular resistance may be felt. Such resistance might be depicted as in *Figure A1.20*.

## MUSCLE SPASM

There are only two kinds of muscle spasm that will be considered here; one that always limits range and occupies a small part of it, and the other that occurs as a quick contraction to prevent a painful movement.

Whether it is spasm or stiffness that is limiting the range can frequently only be accurately assessed by repeated movement (1) taken somewhat beyond the point at which resistance is first encountered, and (2) performed at different speeds. Muscle spasm shows a power of active recoil. In contrast, resistance that is free of muscle activity does not have this quality; rather it is constant in strength at any given point in the range.

The following examples may help to clarify the point. If a resistance to passive movement is felt between $Z_1$ and $Z_2$ on the base line AB of the movement diagram (*Figure A1.21*), and if this block is 'resistance free of muscle spasm', at point 'O' between $Z_1$ and $Z_2$ (A $Z_1$ O $Z_2$ B (*Figure A1.22*)), the strength of the resistance

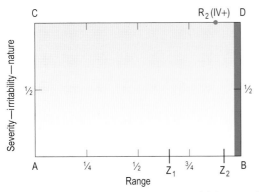

**Figure A1.21** Resistance to passive movement felt between $Z_1$ and $Z_2$

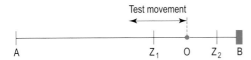

**Figure A1.22** Differentiating resistance from spasm

will be exactly the same irrespective of how fast or slowly a movement is oscillated up to it. However, if the block is a muscle spasm and test movements are taken up to a point 'O' at different speeds, the strength of the resistance will increase and be greater, with increases in speed (*Figure A1.22*).

Also, any increase in strength will be directly proportional to the depth in range, regardless of the speed with which the movement is carried out; that is, the resistance felt at one point in movement will always be less than that felt at a point deeper in the range.

The first of the two kinds of muscle spasm will feel like a steel spring and will push back against the testing movement, particularly if the test movement is varied in speed and in position in the range.

## $S_1$

Testing this kind of spasm is done by moving the joint to the point at which spasm is first elicited, and this point is noted on the base line as $S_1$. Further movement is then attempted. If maximum intensity is reached before the end of range, spasm thus becomes a limiting factor.

## L – WHERE, L – WHAT

This limit is noted by L on the base line, and $S_2$ is marked vertically above L on the line CD. As with $P_2$ and $R_2$, $S_2$ needs to be qualified in terms of strength and quality (e.g. $S_2$ IV−, very sharp).

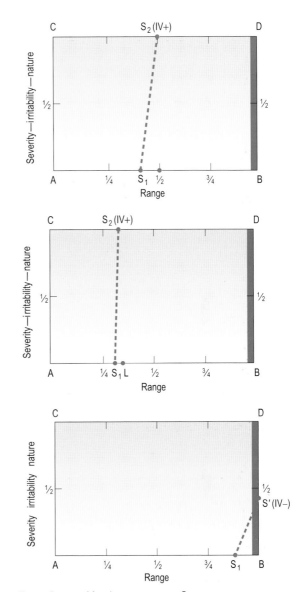

**Figure A1.23** Muscle spasm. —— = Spasm

## $S_1 S_2$

The graph for the behaviour of spasm is plotted between $S_1$ and $S_2$ (*Figure A1.23*). It will be found that when muscle spasm limits range it always reaches its maximum quickly, and thus occupies only a small part of the range. Therefore it will always be depicted as a near-vertical line (*Figure A1.23a and b*). In some cases when the joint disorder is less severe, a little spasm that increases slightly but never prohibits full movement may be felt just before the end of range (*Figure A1.23c*).

The second kind of muscle spasm is directly proportional to the severity of the patient's pain: movement of the joint in varying parts of the range causes sharply limiting quick muscular contraction. This usually occurs when a very painful joint is moved without adequate care, and can be completely avoided if the joint is well supported and moved gently. This spasm is reflex in type, coming into action very rapidly during the test movement. A very similar kind of muscular contraction can occur as a voluntary action by the patient, indicating a sharp increase in pain. If the physiotherapist varies the speed of her test movements, she will be able to distinguish quickly between the reflex spasm and the voluntary spasm because of the speed with which the spasm occurs – reflex spasm occurs more quickly in response to a provoking movement than does voluntary spasm. This second kind of spasm, which does not limit a range of movement, can usually be avoided by careful handling during the test.

To represent this kind of spasm a near-vertical line is drawn from above the base line; its height and position on the base line will signify whether the spasm is easy to provoke, and will also give some indication of its strength. Two examples are drawn of the extremes that may be found (*Figure A1.24a* and *b*).

## MODIFICATION

There is a modification of the base line AB that can be used when the significant range to be depicted occupies only say 10°, yet it is 50° short of B. The movement diagram would be as shown in *Figure A1.25*, and when used to depict a movement the range between L and B must be stated. The base line AB for the hypermobile joint movement to be depicted would be the same as that shown on page 175, where grades of movement are discussed, and the frame of the movement diagram would be as in *Figure A1.26*.

Having discussed at length the graphing of the separate elements of a movement diagram, it is now necessary to put them together as a whole.

## COMPILING A MOVEMENT DIAGRAM

This book places great emphasis on the kinds and behaviours of pain as they present with the different movements of disordered joints. Pain is of major importance to the patient, and therefore takes priority

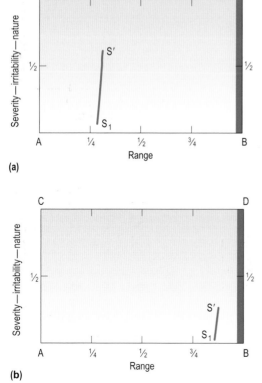

(a)

(b)

Figure A1.24   Spasm that does not limit range of movement

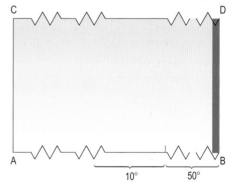

Figure A1.25   Modified movement diagram

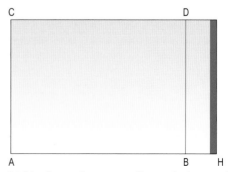

Figure A1.26   Frame of movement diagram for hypermobile joint in the examination of joint movement. The following demonstrates how the diagram is formulated. When testing the C3/4 joint by postero-anterior pressure on the spinous process of C3 (for example), the routine is as follows.

## STEP 1. $P_1$

Gentle, increasing pressure is applied very slowly to the spinous process of C3 in a postero-anterior direction, and the patient is asked to report when he first feels pain. This point in the range is noted, and the physiotherapist then releases some of the pressure from the spinous process and performs small oscillatory movements. Again she asks the patient if he feels any pain. If he does not, the oscillation should then be carried out slightly deeper into the range. Conversely, if he does feel pain, the oscillatory movement should be withdrawn in the range. By these oscillatory movements in different parts of the range, the point at which pain is first felt with movements can be identified and is then recorded on the base line of the movement diagram as $P_1$ (*Figure A1.27*). The estimation of the position in the range of $P_1$ is best achieved by performing the oscillations at what the physiotherapist feels is quarter range, then at one-third range and then at half range. By this means $P_1$ can be very accurately assessed. Therefore there are two steps to establishing $P_1$:

1. A single slow movement.
2. Small oscillatory movements.

## STEP 2. L – WHERE

Having found $P_1$, the physiotherapist should continue further into the range with the postero-anterior movements until she reaches the limit of the range. She identifies where that position is in relation to the normal range, and records it on the base line of the movement diagram as point L (*Figure A1.28*).

## STEP 3. L – WHAT

For the hypomobile joint, the next step is to decide *why* the movement was stopped at point L. This means that the examiner has moved the joint as far as she is willing to go, but she has not made it reach B. Having decided WHERE L is, the examiner has to decide why she chose to stop at L; WHAT was it that prevented her reaching B? If we assume, for the purpose of this example, that it was physical resistance free of muscle spasm that prevented movement beyond L, the point where the vertical line above L meets the horizontal projection CD is marked as $R_2$ (*Figure A1.29*). The $R_2$ needs to be qualified using words or symbols to indicate what it was about the resistance that prevented the examiner stretching it further, for example the

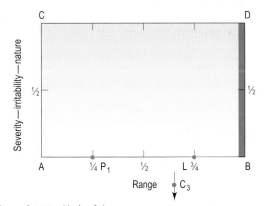

Figure A1.28    Limit of the range

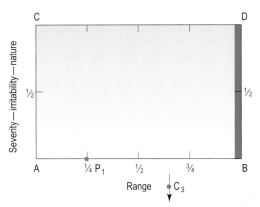

Figure A1.27    Point at which pain is first felt

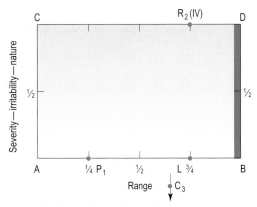

Figure A1.29    Spasm-free resistance limiting movement

patient may have rheumatoid arthritis and she may not be prepared to go further (*Figure A1.29*).

## STEP 4. P' AND DEFINED

The physiotherapist then decides the quality or the intensity of the pain at the limit of the range. This can be estimated in relation to two values: (1) what maximum would feel like, and (2) what halfway (50 per cent) between no pain and maximum would feel like. By this means the intensity of the pain is fairly easily decided, thus enabling the physiotherapist to put P' on the vertical above L in its accurately estimated position (*Figure A1.30*). If the limiting factor at L were $P_2$, then Step 4 would be estimating the quality or intensity of R' and defining it (*Figure A1.31*).

## STEP 5. BEHAVIOUR OF PAIN $P_1$ $P_2$ OR $P_1$ P'

The C3/4 joint is then moved in a postero-anterior direction between $P_1$ and L to determine, both by

watching the patient's hands and face and also by asking him, how the pain behaves between $P_1$ and $P_2$ or between $P_1$ and P'. In fact, it is better to think of pain between $P_1$ and L, because at L pain is going to be represented as $P_2$ or P'. The line representing the behaviour of pain is then drawn on the movement diagram, that is, the line $P_1$ $P_2$ or between $P_1$ and P' is completed (*Figure A1.32*).

## STEP 6. $R_1$

Having completed the representation of pain, resistance must be considered. This is achieved by receding further back in the range than $P_1$, where, with carefully applied and carefully felt oscillatory movements, the presence or otherwise of any resistance is ascertained. Where it commences is noted and marked on the base line AB as $R_1$ (*Figure A1.33*).

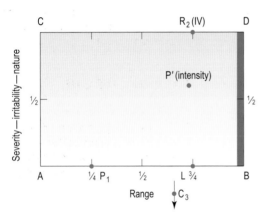

**Figure A1.30**  Quality or intensity of pain at L

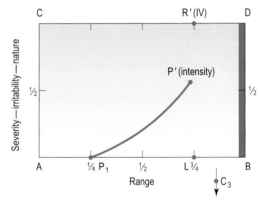

**Figure A1.32**  Behaviour of the pain

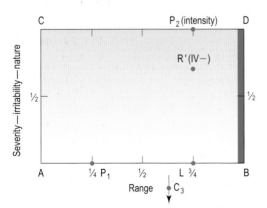

**Figure A1.31**  Quality or intensity of spasm-free resistance

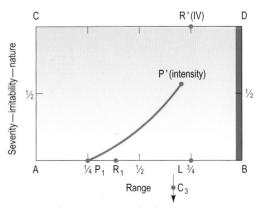

**Figure A1.33**  Commencement of resistance

## STEP 7. BEHAVIOUR OF RESISTANCE $R_1$ $R_2$

By moving the joint between $R_1$ and L the behaviour of the resistance can be determined and plotted on the graph between the joints $R_1$ and $R_2$ (*Figure A1.34*). It is also necessary to qualify or define $R_2$.

## STEP 8. $S_1$ $S'$

If no muscle spasm has been felt during this examination and if the patient's pain is not excessive, the physiotherapist should continue the oscillatory postero-anterior movements on C3, but perform them more sharply and quickly to determine whether any spasm can be provoked. If no spasm can be provoked, then there is nothing to record on the movement diagram. However, if with quick, sharper movements a reflex type of muscle spasm is elicited to protect the movement, this should be drawn on the movement diagram in a manner that indicates how easy or difficult it is to provoke. This can be done by placing the spasm line

towards A if it is easy to provoke, and towards B if it is difficult to provoke. The strength of the spasm so provoked is indicated by the height of the spasm line, $S'$ (*Figure A1.35*).

Thus the diagram for that movement is compiled, showing the behaviour of all elements. It is then possible to assess any relationships between the factors found on the examination. The relationships give a distinct guide as to the treatment that should be given, particularly in relation to the 'grade' of the treatment movements – that is, whether 'pain' is going to be treated or whether the treatment will be directed at the resistance.

## SUMMARY OF STEPS

Compiling a movement diagram may seem complicated, but it is not. It is a very important part of training in manipulative physiotherapy, because it forces the physiotherapist to understand clearly what it is she is feeling when moving the joint passively. Committing those thoughts to paper thwarts any guesswork, or any 'hit-and-miss' approach to treatment. *Table A1.1* summarizes the steps taken in compiling a movement diagram where resistance limits movement, and the steps when pain limits movement.

## MODIFIED DIAGRAM BASE LINE

> Where the limit of available range is very restricted and when the elements of the movement diagram occupy only a very small percentage of the full range, the movement diagram can be modified by breaking the base line

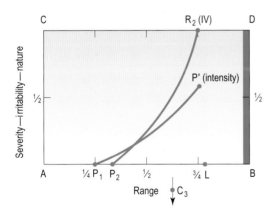

**Figure A1.34**    Behaviour of resistance

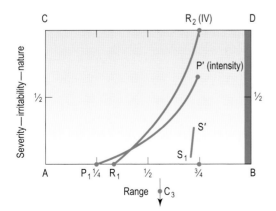

**Figure A1.35**    Strength of spasm

**Table A1.1**    Steps taken in compiling a movement diagram

| Where resistance limits movement | Where pain limits movement |
|---|---|
| 1.  $P_1$ (a) slow     (b) oscillatory | 1.  $P_1$ (a) slow     (b) oscillatory |
| 2.  L – where | 2.  L – where |
| 3.  L – what (and define) | 3.  L – what (and define) |
| 4.  $P'$ (define) | 4.  $P_1 P_2$ (behaviour) |
| 5.  $P_1$ $P'$ (behaviour) | 5.  $R_1$ |
| 6.  $R_1$ | 6.  $R'$ (and define) |
| 7.  $R_1 R_2$ (behaviour) | 7.  $R_1$ $R'$ (behaviour) |
| 8.  S (defined) | 8.  S (defined) |

When either the limit of available range is very restricted (i.e. L is a long way from B), or when the elements of the movement diagram occupy only a very small percentage of the full range, the basis of the movement diagram needs modification. This is achieved by breaking the base line as in *Figure A1.36*. The centre section can then be identified to represent any length, in any part of the minimal full range. When the examination findings are only to be found in the last, say, 5° of a full range, point A in the range is changed and the line AB is suitably identified as in *Figure A1.37*. This example demonstrates that from A to B is 8°, and A to 1/4 is 2°, and so on.

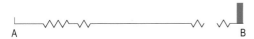

**Figure A1.36** Modified diagram base line

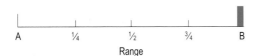

Range

**Figure A1.37** The last 8° of knee extension

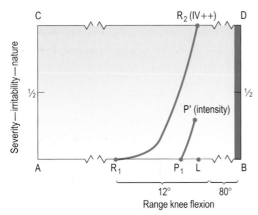

**Figure A1.38** Using a modified diagram

## EXAMPLE – RANGE LIMITED BY 50 PER CENT

Marked stiffness with L is a large distance before B necessitates a modified format of the movement diagram. The example will be restricted knee flexion, a condition of long standing following a fracture. The first element is $R_1$, and the distance between $R_1$ and L is only 12°. Pain is provoked only by stretching (*Figure A1.38*). If the movement diagram were drawn on an unmodified format, it would be as in *Figure A1.39*.

It is clear that the diagram in *Figure A1.39* wastes considerable diagram space, and it is difficult to interpret. With the same joint movement findings represented on the modified format of the movement diagram, it becomes clearer and much more useful. The modified format of the base line of the diagram (*Figure A1.38*) requires only two extra measurements to be stated:

1. The measurement between L and B.
2. The measurement between $R_1$ and L.

Knowing that $R_1$ to L equals 12° makes it easy to see that $R_1$ is approximately 7° before $P_1$. Because of the increased space allowed to represent the elements of the movement, the *behaviour* also is far easier to demonstrate.

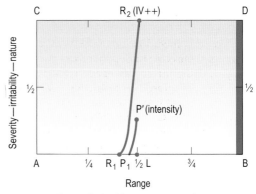

**Figure A1.39** Range limited by 50 per cent, shown on an unmodified diagram (160° knee flexion)

# Appendix 2

# Clinical examples of movement diagrams

## HYPERMOBILITY

This example is included for the express purpose of clarifying the misconceptions that exist about hypermobility, and the direct influence that some authors and practitioners afford it in restricting treatment.

If the movement (using the same C3/4 joint being tested with PAs on C3, pages 467–469), before having become painful, were hypermobile, the basic format of the movement diagram would be as shown in *Figure A2.1*.

## STEP 1. P$_1$

The method is the same as in Example 1 (p. 467; *see Figure A2.2*).

## STEP 2. L – WHERE

The method is the same as in Example 1 (pp. 471–472; *see Figure A2.3*).

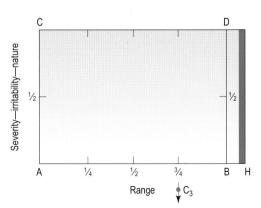

Figure A2.1   Movement diagram for hypermobile range

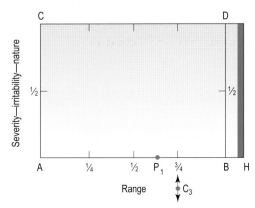

Figure A2.2   P$_1$, hypermobile joint

## STEP 3. L – WHAT (AND DEFINE)

The method is the same as in Example 1 (pp. 471–472; *see Figure A2.4*).

## STEP 4. P′ DEFINE (FIGURE A2.5)

## STEP 5. P₁P′ BEHAVIOUR (FIGURE A2.6)

## STEP 6. R1 (FIGURE A2.7)

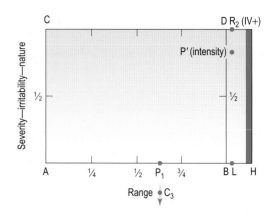

**Figure A2.5**  P′ – define, hypermobile joint

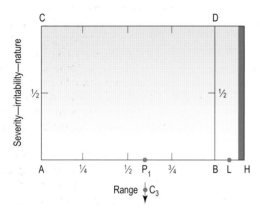

**Figure A2.3**  L – where, hypermobile joint

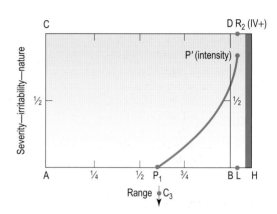

**Figure A2.6**  P₁P′ behaviour, hypermobile joint

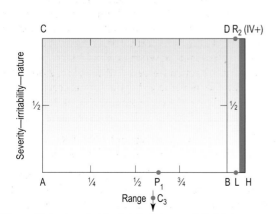

**Figure A2.4**  L – what (and define), hypermobile joint

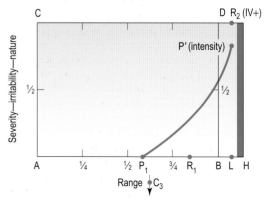

**Figure A2.7**  R₁, hypermobile joint

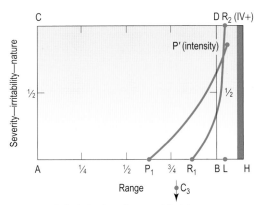

Figure A2.8    $R_1R_2$ behaviour, hypermobile joint

## STEP 7. $R_1R_2$ BEHAVIOUR (FIGURE A2.8)

### Treatment

Hypermobility is not a contraindication to manipulation. Most patients with hypermobile joints, one of which becomes painful, have a hypomobile situation at that joint. They are therefore treated on the same basis as is used for hypomobility. It makes no difference whether the limit (L) of the range, on examination, is found to be beyond the end of the average–normal range (as in the example above, L being beyond B) or before it (L being on the side of B).

## SCHEUERMANN'S DISEASE

Manipulative physiotherapists are frequently asked to treat patients who have back pain related to the stiffness resulting from old, inactive Scheuermann's disease. The purpose of presenting this series of movement diagrams is to emphasize the 'end-feel' characteristic of postero-anterior central vertebral pressures on a Scheuermann's spine.

These movement diagrams only represent the resistance (free of muscle spasm) element. It is assumed that the peak of the characteristic kyphosis is at L1, and that the patient is lying prone, which puts the main vertebra(e) involved at the limit of their range of extension and postero-anterior movement (point A on the base line of the diagram) (*Figure A2.9*).

It may be of interest to comment that in the young adolescent it is possible to know, by the feel of resistance to postero-anterior pressures over five adjacent vertebrae, that osteochondritis ('Scheuermann's disease') is present even before the radiological evidence is obvious. Of the five vertebrae referred to, the top and bottom ones will have a normal range, and the middle one of the five will have a slightly prominent spinous process and will be resistant to the postero-anterior pressures. The adjacent vertebrae to the central prominent and stiff one will have a degree of resistance to the pressures that is equal at the two vertebrae, and a degree of stiffness that is halfway between that of the two normal vertebrae.

## THE SPONDYLITIC CERVICAL SPINE

Many or most of the elderly patients referred for treatment of local cervical symptoms have underlying wear-and-tear degenerative changes. These changes of themselves are not necessarily responsible for the present problem, although they may account for some restriction of movement and a degree of discomfort which the patient considers to be normal. This being so, the manipulative physiotherapist does not have as her goal the restoration of a FULL pain-free range of movement. The goal is a 'compromise goal', which infers that the range of movement will be restored to what it was before it became symptomatic, and the symptoms will have either been cleared or restored to what the patient had considered to be his normal.

Such circumstances occur so often that they are worthy of description in terms of the movement diagram.

The example will be of an elderly man who has sought treatment because he is having increasing discomfort in the right mid-cervical area, which he notices with turning his head to the right, particularly when trying to reverse his car.

Prior to seeking treatment he believed he could turn his head equally to left and right, and the movements were painless. As is so often the case, his normal range of cervical rotation was only approximately 35–40°. Representing this on a movement diagram (that is, as rotation for the whole cervical spine rather than for one particular intervertebral level) at a time when he considered that he was normal, the diagram would be something like that shown in *Figure A2.10*.

At the time when he had had his right-sided cervical pain, the movement diagram of his cervical rotation to the right differed in small but significant ways from the above (*Figure A2.11*). The differences are:

1. $P_1P'$ (a significant change in the pain sensation).
2. $R_1R_2$ (the altered behaviour of the resistance).

The $P_1$ of *Figure A2.11* will only return to his 'normal' if the new curved first part (encircled) of the $R_1R_2$ behaviour of the resistance is cleared. If treatment is successful, the $R_1R_2$ line will change so that the behaviour

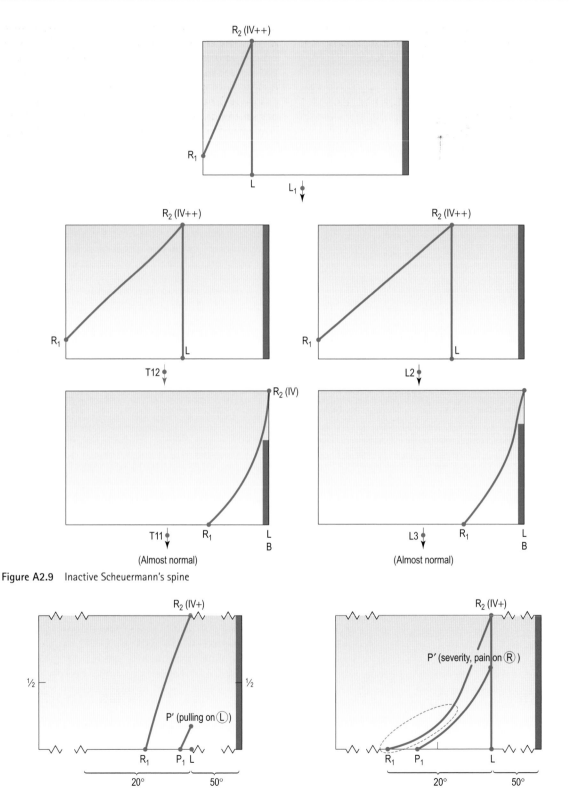

**Figure A2.9** Inactive Scheuermann's spine

**Figure A2.10** Cervical rotation right, normal movement diagram (spondylitic spine)

**Figure A2.11** Cervical rotation right, symptomatic movement diagram (spondylitic spine)

of resistance will return to its original straight line ($R_1R_2$ in *Figure A2.10*). $P_1P'$ of *Figure A2.11* will also resume to being the $P_1P'$ of *Figure A2.10*.

> It is surprising how precise a judgement of small changes in resistance can be

Readers may believe that it is impossible to assess such small changes in resistance (encircled part in *Figure A2.11*). However, if they apply themselves to the discipline required for compiling movement diagrams – that is, doing passive movements critically and analysing what they feel, rather than doing passive movements by instinct – they will be surprised at just how precise their judgements can become (Evans, 1982).

# Appendix 3

# Examination refinements and movement diagrams

## VARIED INCLINATIONS AND CONTACT POINTS

> The aim of varying the angle of inclination and point of contact is to find the movement that provokes the symptoms which are comparable with those of the patient

On pages 158–161 it was stated that palpation examination techniques need to be varied (1) in their angle of inclination by amounts even as small as 1–2°; and (2) in their contact points, which similarly may be as little as 1 mm or less apart. The aim of this examination technique is to find the movement that provokes symptoms comparable with the patient's symptoms. If postero-anterior central vertebral pressure is the movement being examined, the sagittal direction can be inclined:

1. Cephalad/caudad.
2. Left/right.
3. In various combinations of these.

The point of contact on each spinous process can be changed from the standard two bifid processes to:

1. One process.
2. Higher/lower on the one process.

3. Medially/laterally on the one process.
4. Various combinations of these.
5. The same variations (1)–(4) in contact with both processes (when (3) would read'left/right').

As an example of this, a patient may have an area of general mid-cervical pain spreading across the top of the trapezius on the right and reaching to the top of the right shoulder. On examination by palpation, moving the spinous process of C5 in variations of inclinations and contact points, the movement diagrams may be as follows:

1. The exact sagittal postero-anterior movement with each thumb contacting each bifid spinous process of C5 (*Figure A3.1*).

2. When the sagittal postero-anterior movement is emphasized onto the right bifid process the diagram changes in its pain response and is closer to being 'comparable' than in (1) above (*Figure A3.2*).

3. When the contact point is changed to the lateral side of the left bifid process and directed 10° towards the right, a quite different response results (*Figure A3.3*). Obviously this test movement is insignificant compared with the preceding two tests.

4. If the examination has been carried out in the sequence represented here, the thought may be: 'Well, pushing on the right bifid process is the

most limited movement so far, and the pain response does produce some spread of pain to the supraspinous fossa. I wonder what the pain response will be if I move my contact point to the lateral side of the right bifid process and incline the PA say 20° towards the left? (*Figure A3.4*). This pain response is much more comparable with his symptoms, and the movement is both stiffer and has a more similar behaviour to that of the pain than have any of the preceding movements.

5.  'I wonder if this is sufficiently comparable to be used as the treatment technique? I think I'll just try adding a bit of caudad inclination through the same contact point.' (*Figure A3.5*). This pain response, being such a clear 'reproduced pain', is very favourable. Another element indicating good comparability with the patient's symptoms is the similarity of the behaviour of the resistance element to the pain element.

This discussion can be carried one stage further, but in a somewhat different direction. If the manipulative physiotherapist chooses to use her thumb palpation

movement as her treatment technique, she has to choose between the following:

1.  Avoiding the patient's pain and therefore using *Figure A3.3* as the treatment technique.
2.  Reproducing his symptoms and therefore using *Figure A3.5*.

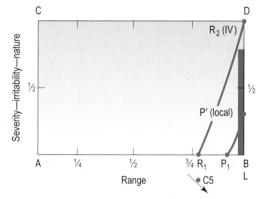

**Figure A3.3** Sagittal postero-anterior movement, contact point on lateral side of left bifid spinous process of C5 and directed 10° to the right

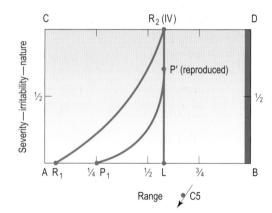

**Figure A3.4**

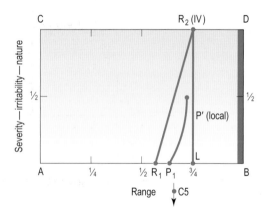

**Figure A3.1** Exact sagittal postero-anterior movement, thumbs contacting each of C5's bifid spinous processes

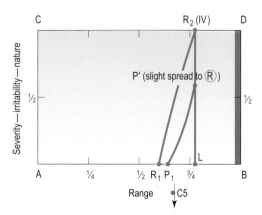

**Figure A3.2** Sagittal postero-anterior movement, emphasized on to right bifid spinous process of C5

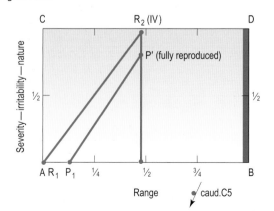

**Figure A3.5**

3. Taking a reasonably safe pathway by using *Figure A3.4* but doing it as a grade IV movement, or even grade IV–, so that a lesser degree of pain is provoked.

## SAGITTAL POSTERO–ANTERIOR MOVEMENTS IN COMBINED POSITIONS

> Postero-anterior movements in combined positions are valuable as a means of finding the movement which provokes the patient's symptoms. This can then be used as a treatment technique or progression of treatment

The value of combined movements in examination and treatment has been emphasized in this edition. Imagine a patient who has left suprascapular symptoms that are provoked by compressing type movements, such as extension, lateral flexion left, rotation left, and central postero-anterior movements on the left articular pillar of C5:

1. If the central postero-anterior movements are performed with the patient's head straight, the movement diagram may be as in *Figure A3.6*.

2. If the same sagittal postero-anterior movement is performed with the head rotated to the left, the diagram will be different, as shown in *Figure A3.7*.

3. Sagittal postero-anterior movements performed with the head in lateral flexion to the left may have the movement diagram shown in *Figure A3.8*.

4. If the patient's head is first laterally flexed to the left and then while in this position is rotated to the left, postero-anterior movements in this combination might be as shown in *Figure A3.9*.

Because the computations are endless, the manipulative physiotherapist should be aware of the possibilities available to her and be capable of exploiting them if progress is not up to the expectations.

## DIAGRAMS OF DIFFERENT MOVEMENTS ON A PATIENT WITH ONE DISORDER

> To draw diagrams for different movement directions in a patient with one disorder will help to determine which of these directions is likely to be more effective as a treatment technique. Furthermore, reassessment will determine the relationship between the patient's signs and symptoms and the movement diagram

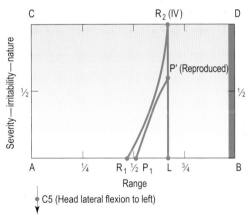

**Figure A3.7**  The same movements as in *Figure A3.6*, with head in lateral flexion to the left

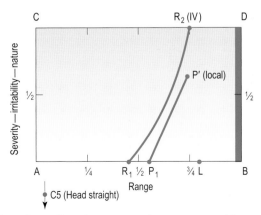

**Figure A3.6**  Central postero-anterior movements, with patient's head straight

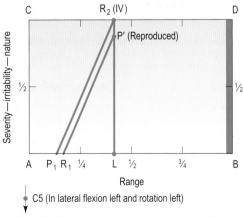

**Figure A3.8**  Sagittal postero-anterior movements, with patient's head first laterally flexed to the left and rotated to the left

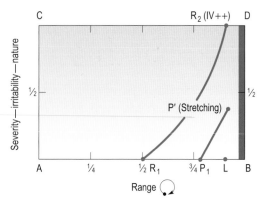

**Figure A3.10**   Cervical rotation to the right in the same patient as in *Figure A3.10*

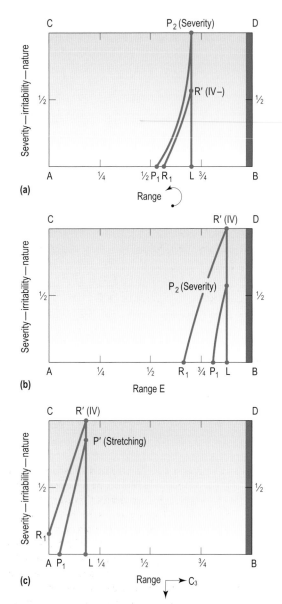

**Figure A3.9**   Movements provoking left mid-cervical pain. (*a*) Cervical rotation to the left. (*b*) Extension. (*c*) Postero-anterior unilateral vertebral pressure on left side of C3 (4 mm)

When examining a patient's movements, there may be three main movements that provoke his (say) left mid-cervical pain. Assume that the movements are cervical rotation to the left, extension, and postero-anterior unilateral vertebral pressure on the left side of C3. The movement diagrams of each movement might be as in *Figure A3.10*.

The three movement diagrams are different from each other, and seeing that they are different helps in determining which will be used (if any of them are) as a treatment technique. Also, if one *is* chosen, and it is successful, it would be hoped that all three diagrams would show the same kind of improvement. If, however, two of them did improve and the third did not, and also if the patient did not feel he was getting better, then perhaps the unchanged movement diagram would then be used as the treatment technique.

There is one other important aspect to bear in mind. As well as the three diagrams depicted, cervical rotation to the right might prove a useful diagram, and be useful as a treatment technique (*Figure A3.11*).

*Figures A3.10* and *A3.11* are related to the standard physiological and accessory movements. It becomes more complicated when combined movements are introduced. However, when combined movements are used as part of the examination, diagrams can be used for them in the same way as described earlier in this appendix.

# Appendix 4

# Clinical tips

The contents of this appendix are not strictly related to vertebral manipulative treatment. They are, however, factors that are related to the total management of spinal disorders, and yet they do not seem to be given sufficient credence or to be adequately appreciated by some authors and practitioners. The points to be mentioned are not necessarily related to each other and so are presented as short separate statements, some of which may be provocative.

## MUSCLE SPASM

> Protective lists of the lumbar spine are caused, at least in part, by the muscles

Articles and books have been written about muscle spasm as seen in spinal problems, particularly those involving the low lumbar spine. Some patients with lumbar pain undoubtedly have an accompanying protective list. This list is caused, at least in part, by

muscles, and despite the fact that it has been stated that there is no EMG response from the extensor muscles, most clinicians have no doubt that muscle spasm is present. Some authors have said that when the patient lies down, the spasm goes. This is no more true than is the interpretation of the lack of EMG response. The problem seems to lie in the fact that the spasm that goes on lying is related to the long back muscle extensors, and not enough importance is given to the intrinsic intrasegmental muscles between adjacent vertebrae. These muscles remain in spasm to protect the joint from being in a painful position.

> Intersegmental muscle spasm can be felt by palpation even when the patient is lying prone

The intersegmental muscle spasm can be felt by palpation even when the patient is lying prone. Although the load through the joint is less when the patient is lying, and therefore the joint's need for muscle spasm is less, it does not totally disappear as suggested by the EMG responses so far recorded.

## DISORDERS

There are three points to be made under this heading:

1. Components.
2. Effects of draughts.
3. Jointy people.

## COMPONENTS

> It is possible for a joint disorder to have a subclinical active degenerative process in conjunction with a mechanical component

Many musculoskeletal disorders that the manipulative physiotherapist is asked to treat are not solely mechanical disorders. They have a subclinical component that is inflammatory in nature. This subclinical component may be an active degenerative process of the intervertebral disc or an osteoarthritic process of the zygapophyseal joints. In other words, a joint disorder may have a subclinical active degenerative process in conjunction with a mechanical component.

The manipulative physiotherapist can improve the symptoms arising from the mechanical component, but can do little or nothing for the active subclinical component. Instruction in exercises and 'back care' play an important part in this area.

## EFFECTS OF DRAUGHT

> Believe patients who say that their neck pain began as a result of sleeping in a draught

Not all people treating musculoskeletal disorders are prepared to take much notice of a patient who says that his neck or back disorder is aggravated or provoked by sitting or lying in a draught. Some patients will even say that they are affected by the cold air from an air conditioner. Most clinicians have heard a patient say that the current episode of low back pain began as a result of sleeping in a draught. This is to be believed.

The feature is typical of a group of patients whose symptoms are easy to help but difficult to prevent recurring. If the problem lies in the cervical spine the use of a scarf is extremely valuable, irrespective of whether the weather is hot or cold.

Relative to the lumbar spine, there is an 'old wives' tale' that such people should wear a 'red flannel belt', and there are patients who have worn such a belt to advantage. The important points are that:

1. The belt does not have to be red.
2. The flannel should not go right around the person's body.
3. The warm flannel should cover the lumbar area alone, such that it keeps that area warmer than the area immediately above and below the belt.

## JOINTY PEOPLE

> People who have symptoms from many joints are considered to be 'jointy'

This title refers to patients who fit into one of three categories. The title itself means nothing more than that there are groups of people who have symptoms from many joints. One rheumatologist refers to these people as having 'acute joint awareness'.

The first group consists of patients who seek treatment for pain in, say, their lower cervical area. The symptoms are usually locally situated, though they may spread around the immediate area. When these patients gain improvement from the initial mobilization treatments, they comment about pain in the mid-thoracic area. If this area is treated as well, and it improves, the patients then comment about symptoms in the lower lumbar area. These patients are never totally free of some awareness of symptoms in one or more of the three areas. Mobilization helps to lower the level of symptoms at the time of an exacerbation, but they are patients for whom it is valuable to teach another member of the household how to mobilize gently specific sections of the spine (swimming is also a useful exercise).

The second group of people have intermittent joint symptoms in many peripheral joints. These symptoms do not form any regular pattern of joint involvement. They too can be helped by mobilization, and again instruction in home treatment by another member of the family has a place in the total management of the symptoms.

The third group includes patients who have a combination of the first two groups; that is, they have involvement both of the spine and of the peripheral joints. It is the least common of the groups.

## RECORDING

> The pattern of recording applies to any form of physiotherapy intervention

It has been clearly established that there is a need for a pattern of recording treatment. The pattern used in this book for recording manipulative treatment can also be used for any other physiotherapy treatment that may be given. For example, if ultra-sound is to be added as part of the treatment session, it should be recorded in the same manner as the manipulative techniques, including all of the symptomatic response during and after its application (*Table A4.1*). When exercises are to be part of the treatment management, the effect of each type should also be similarly assessed for pain response and recorded. It is even more important with the recording of exercises than of the ultrasound. The choice and effect of an exercise should be assessed at the treatment session, and the same assessments should be carried out by the patient when he performs the exercises at home. He should record the symptoms and ranges of movement at his home exercise session; first before, then during and after the session, in the same way as the physiotherapist. It is only by using this strict routine that their effect can be assessed.

## ASSESSMENT

> Patients with low back pain find their own way of getting up and down from and to the lying position. This can be an invaluable assessment asterisk

During a treatment session for patients with low back symptoms, some physiotherapists believe that patients must be taught a routine way to lie down and get up from the treatment couch. For example, they insist that when a patient is asked to get up from the lying position, he should turn on to his side, flex his hips and knees to a right angle and then lower his legs towards

**Table A4.1**   Example of recording ultrasound treatment

| Constant US 1 Watt cm$^2$ over articular pillar C2–4. Local warmth. 'Soothing'. | C/O much more comfortable. O/E Rot$^n$ Ⓡ. Same range but no P. now. |
|---|---|

the floor as he pushes his body upright with his arms. The reverse of this procedure is the method the patient would be taught to use to reach the lying position from sitting. The following statements are relevant to this:

1. When a patient has considerable pain in his lower back and has difficulty getting up from the lying position, he will usually find his own method for getting up that economizes on pain. If he is unable to find a satisfactory method, then – and only then – should the above instructions be given to help him.

2. The patient's method and degree of difficulty exhibited while getting on or off the treatment couch is an invaluable assessment 'asterisk'. Patients will not cause harm by their struggles to get off the treatment couch, no matter what means they use, and the assessment value cannot be over-emphasized.

## EXERCISES

> Exercises should be introduced singly, and reassessed during the treatment session

There are five main categories of exercises for vertebral problems. They consist of:

1. Stabilizing exercises.
2. Mobilizing exercises.
3. Exercises to increase muscle power.
4. Exercises to increase the speed of action of muscles.
5. Exercises to increase the endurance of muscle action.

For the lumbar spine, there are two other factors in relation to exercise: the use of flexion exercises as compared with extension exercises; and exercising the intersegmental muscles as compared with the longer muscles, which spread over many segments. Four points need to be made:

- In principle, exercises should be introduced singly and they should be performed at a treatment session so that a complete record of the effect during and after their performance can be assessed. If the patient performs the exercises at home, he should be taught to make the same assessments.

- To increase strength or repetitions in exercises, allow 48 hours minimum between increments.

- If mobilizing exercises are to be given to retain the range of movement of painful arthritic or spondylitic joints, they should be performed in a non-weight bearing or pendular position. They should be performed freely, slowly and painlessly.

- Under most circumstances it does not matter if exercises cause local pain while doing them, but it is essential that the symptoms should subside very quickly once the exercises are finished. If increased symptoms continue for more than half an hour after the exercise programme, the exercises may be reduced, modified or discontinued until a later stage.

Swimming is excellent as it uses all five categories of exercises. Caution must be used initially so the patient doesn't overdo it. For someone unaccustomed to general exercising, 10–15 minutes is sufficient for the first session.

## RECURRENCES

Many articles, books and pamphlets have been written on this subject, and the only purpose in making the following points is to raise some issues that do not seem to be adequately considered.

## EXERCISES

Not every patient with a vertebral disorder, once relieved of the symptoms, should be taught an exercise programme intended to be carried out on a regular long-term basis. If *every* patient is asked to do exercises to prevent recurrences, our judgement is poor. We may find later that the patient only did the exercises for 2 weeks and then forgot them, yet he did not have any trouble with his back for 5 years. The percentage of people who will continue with exercises on a long-term basis is small; most will give up within the first month.

Assessment of the need to do exercises is better determined if it is explained to the patient that exercises may provoke an exacerbation, therefore it may be better for him to be taught 'back care', and to leave exercises until it can be seen that he is susceptible to recurrences. If he has a recurrence in a short space of time as the result of a minor incident, then not only is it more purposeful to do prophylactic exercises, but it is more likely that he will continue the exercises because he is convinced of their possible value. The word 'possible' is especially included because the state of the pathology may be such as to prevent them.

The part that exercises can play to prevent recurrences in low lumbar discogenic disorders needs careful thought. Exercises should not be given routinely for all such disorders. The state of disc damage, the stage of progression of the pathology or the presence of a continuing subclinical active process may prohibit an exercise programme. At least we should be aware that exercises can be harmful, and their introduction should therefore be progressive and carefully monitored.

The question is often asked, should flexion exercises or extension exercises be used in particular situations of low lumbar disc disorder? The ideal end-result of a treatment programme for the patient is that he should be able to perform strong exercises for both the flexors and the extensors. Isometric exercises in either direction are less harmful than isotonic exercises because they involve very little joint movement; nevertheless, intradiscal pressure does increase during the exercise. Therefore, when disc pathology causes pain, any introduction of flexion demands caution.

## PILLOWS

> Wherever possible, recommend feather pillows for patients with neck pain

Some patients have cervical disorders in which their pillow is a source of irritation and of continuing symptoms or recurrences. In relation to the pillow, the two most important aspects are:

1. Its size relative to the patient's posture.
2. Its content relative to the irritability of the patient's disorder.

The pillow height should support the head and the neck fully and in a neutral position. The content of the pillow should be such that, if a hollow is made in the pillow with a fist, once the fist is removed the hollow should remain. The quicker the hollow disappears, because of the nature of its springy content, the worse is its effect on a neck that is easily disturbed. Patients should not sleep prone, because in this position the cervical intervertebral joints are put on full stretch in one direction.

## BEDS

Under normal circumstances, the rather firm, flat bed is the best choice. However, patients' requirements are very individual. If a patient has a very broad pelvis and narrow thorax and chooses to sleep on his side, he may be more comfortable lying on a softer bed than on a hard bed.

When a patient has low lumbar symptoms, it is common that either flexion will be comfortable and extension uncomfortable, or the reverse. The lumbar spine can be flexed or extended while the patient lies supine by (1) having the legs out straight with a small support under the lumbar spine (extension); or (2) with the hips and knees flexed without lumbar support (flexion). However, it is *far* better for the patient to lie on whichever side he finds most comfortable and to position the degree of hip and knee flexion that enables his lumbar spine to rest in the suited extended or flexed position.

As with the cervical spine, the prone position is commonly a bad position for a patient with low lumbar symptoms. Although there are some patients who are more comfortable in the prone position, the majority have great difficulty in turning over if they have been asleep in the prone position.

## DRAUGHTS

This has been discussed above, but the point is an important consideration and is worthy of reiteration.

## WEAK LINK

It is important for a person to know that if he has had symptoms of sufficient severity to require treatment, then, no matter how successful treatment may be, he will always have a 'weak link', even if it is asymptomatic. It should be pointed out that if the chain (the spine) is given too much work to do, it will be the weak link (the intervertebral joint) that breaks down first.

## CAPACITY TO ACCUMULATE

It should also be explained that the weakened structure that has caused the disorder has the capacity to accumulate damage asymptomatically until it reaches the stage when something minor becomes 'the last straw to break the camel's back'. These patients should therefore realize that even when they do a vigorous activity that does not cause any trouble, they should not feel that this means that their problem is cured and that they can go ahead and repeat it again and again.

It should be explained to them that the things most likely to cause a recurrence are those that involve:

- Heavy lifting, etc.
- Sustained activities in a position near or at the limit of a range.
- Sudden, unexpected, unguarded movements.
- A virus. A virus can cause the 'weak link' to be more vulnerable to injury. The injuring movement may be trivial but preceded by a virus. More

infrequently, the spinal stiffness and aching continues after the virus has resolved. These signs and symptoms can mimic an episode, and may respond to manual treatment.

Patients should also be told that their weak link is more subject to damage by the three events listed above at times when they are overtired, generally unwell, or under physical or mental stress.

## NEVER CLEARED

Many patients have recurring cervical or lumbar symptoms that some manipulators can free in one or two treatments. When these patients come to the manipulative physiotherapist, a clear assessment should be made of all the test movements, particularly those involving palpation of the verte brae. A very high percentage of these patients have their recurrences because treatment is discontinued once the patient is asymptomatic, yet the intervertebral joint is not totally clear of joint signs. With such patients, the joint signs should be demonstrated to them and it should be explained that *if* it is possible to 'clear' these joint signs, recurrences will be more widely spaced and less severe. It should be understood that not all joints can be made clear because of the state of the disorder, but if they can it is to the patient's advantage. In trying to prevent recurrences, this is one of the most important points. It is a point often neglected by those who treat vertebral disorders.

## MAINTENANCE TREATMENT

People who have disorders of the kind referred to above as 'subclinical' and 'acute joint awareness' are patients who do gain benefit from maintenance treatment. This treatment may be done in one of two ways:

1. As mentioned before, other members of the household can be taught techniques that can be performed on a regular basis to keep the symptoms at a reasonable level for the patient. The manipulative physiotherapist need only see the patient when an exacerbation cannot be cleared.

2. There are other patients for whom one treatment session every 4–8 weeks keeps their symptoms at a better level than would be the case if they were not given maintenance treatment.

In balancing out whether home treatment or maintenance treatment should be instituted, the manipulative physiotherapist must keep in mind the reality of the oft-quoted phrase, 'let sleeping dogs lie'.

# Appendix 5

# Physiotherapy for animals

## (with a contribution by T. J. Ahern, BVSc, MRCVS)

This chapter, including the contribution by TJ Ahern, aims to highlight the potential scope of the disciplines advocated within this concept rather than providing a comprehensive text of animal physiotherapy. The skills of non-verbal communication, assessment, re-assessment and manipulation techniques are readily transferable from the human to the animal world.

The treatment of animals, therefore within the field of physiotherapy is no different from the treatment of people. Not all physiotherapists, however, are good at non-verbal communication in its simplest form. When treating animals, it is important to almost instantly establish a caring rapport with the dog, cat, chimpanzee, horse, etc.

It is for this reason that the photograph of Amanda Sutton and the horse (*Figure A5.1*), with the generous approval of Amanda and the CSP *Frontline* Editor, Jane Tonkin, has been included in this text (Sutton, 1996). *Frontline* is the magazine of the Chartered Society of Physiotherapy, and Amanda Sutton worthily won the Frontline Excellence Award. There are several reasons for wanting to include the photograph. Having said that, what strikes you most?

Look at Amanda's eyes. They are semi-closed and looking downwards, giving the whole of her face the appearance of being deeply concentrating. Now look at what you can see of her left forearm, wrist and hand, and you will see how they are resting comfortingly, wrapped in a gentle, stabilizing manner over the horse's mane. Her right hand is in a similar stabilizing, comforting spread over the horse's forehead. If you look at the fingers of Amanda's right hand you will see the same wrapping, surrounding feature of an ideal physiotherapist's hand, and the particular emphasis is again the comforting, resting, wrapping around that gives the horse a feeling of confidence and comfort. Have a look at her right thumb and you can see how Amanda was lucky enough to have been born with a thumb ideally shaped (the distal phalanx of the thumb) for a physiotherapist. Even her forearms are very comfortingly enveloping the lucky horse's head and neck. Her face is full of concentration and care for the animal, and it is perfectly obvious from the horse's expression that it is full of safety and confidence in whatever Amanda is endeavouring to achieve.

If every person who starts on a physiotherapy training course as a student has these qualities in both hands and mind, he or she will finish training with as many of the ideal qualities as it is possible to have.

The horse, using non-verbal communication, could be saying 'go ahead, Amanda, whatever it is you have to do, I have confidence in the way you are going about everything'. This photograph shows so many of the qualities that are ideal for a hands-on therapist that it had to be included in this chapter.

To treat animals effectively with manual treatment it is essential to gain their confidence. The speed of

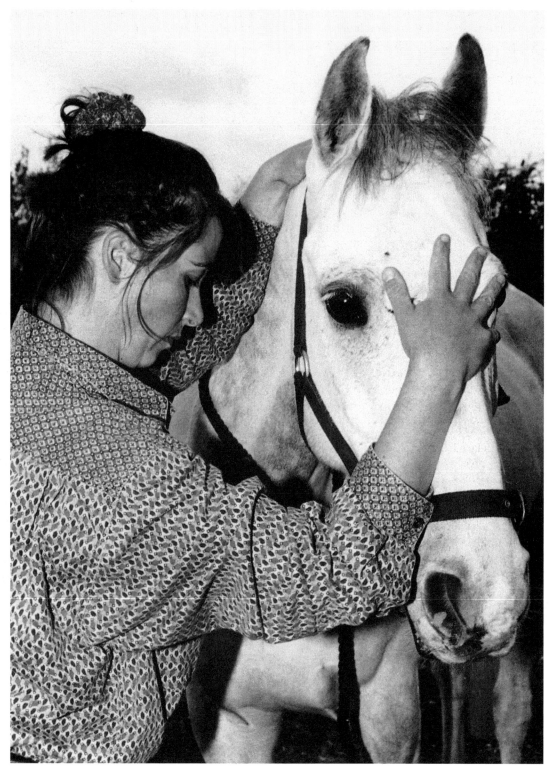

**Figure A5.1** Amanda Sutton and horse

movements undertaken must be slow, steady and gentle, and the therapist needs to respond immediately to any non-verbal message the animal is conveying.

## TRAINING

In many countries there is no need for a specialized training course for animal physiotherapists. They may also need an assistant or an anaesthetist. Assistance is not required for smaller animals such as dogs, but under these circumstances it is extremely helpful if the owner is present as the animal's confidence can be gained more quickly.

The thing that I have found most interesting in my work with Dr Tom Ahern is his use of mobilizing (manipulating) horses. The changes resulting from the manipulation happen as quickly and dramatically as they do when treating the same variety of disorders in humans. Ahern is in the process of writing his own book, *Passive Motion Therapy*, regarding repair in non-spinal joints and soft tissue (tendon and ligament) injury.

The thoraco/lumbar spine of the horse is a relatively immobile structure: the greatest range of movement is present in the lumbosacral joint. This area lends itself to standing techniques. Ahern directs most of his attention to the cervical vertebral region as this is the area of the spine of the horse which has the greatest inherent range of movement.

With the use of anaesthesia in the procedure, the horse is more relaxed and more stable. Ahern chooses to repeat the procedure after an interval of 10–12 weeks, but it may be possible to produce a 2–5 per cent favourable difference by treating horses in a shorter period of time. There have been no harmful effects by treating horses at shorter intervals.

The following quotation is from personal correspondence (Ahern, 1996) with kind permission:

*At present I have a case of a horse that had been continually lame and sore, with a 'distal forelimb vasculitis or similar' for a period of two years. When first presented nine weeks ago, the horse was 'acutely sore' and euthanasia was one option. Because of concurrent cervical spine tension we decided to utilize CVMUA. Eight weeks after the first CVMUA the condition had improved by 80%. A second was then performed, and two weeks later the horse now appears clinically normal.*

*I assume there must have been abnormal pressure or tension in the vicinity of the cervical vertebrae.*

Ahern (1994) wrote an article, which was reviewed in the *Journal of Equine Veterinary Science*, on mobilization of the cervical spine under anaesthesia. I am grateful to the author and the publisher for their permission to include it in full in this chapter.

## CASE HISTORY

A 6-year-old thoroughbred stallion had been intermittently lame in both forelegs over a 3-year period.

### Diagnosis and treatment
Hoof soreness and suspected navicular disease were diagnosed, though no lesions were detected. Intra-articular coffin joint injections of cortisone failed to give a clinical response. An attempt to increase the horse's body weight with increased availability of grain feed had resulted in the onset of laminitis 8 weeks prior to examination by the author. The horse presented with a typical 'caudal lean', and was constantly shifting its weight from one foreleg to the other. Just the sight of hoof testers was enough to render the horse violent; hence, response to lateral digital pressure was not gauged at the time, though the results were seen to be predictable. This attitude had resulted from repeated hoof examinations over the previous 3 years. The cervical joints were palpated, and a significant pain response was elicited in the region of C1, C2 and the lower cervical joints. A cervical manipulation under anaesthesia was performed. No other form of medication was administered, and there were no feed or environmental changes instituted.

The horse's condition improved gradually, and by week 3 a distinct unilateral (right-sided) lameness was present. By week 8 the lameness was mild in comparison to that at week 3. At this time a second manipulation under anaesthesia was performed.

The following day the horse's condition had regressed to one of a severe (reluctant to walk) bilateral forelimb lameness. The reversion dissipated gradually over the following 6 days, and by day seven the horse's condition was similar to that prior to the second manipulation under anaesthesia. By day 14 there was no evidence of the overt lameness, and the horse returned to the racing stables 2 weeks later. Associated with the regression of lameness was an increased willingness to exercise in the paddock.

The horse went on to race, and was described by both trainer and rider as being at his best as regards lack of lameness since he was first ridden as a 2-year-old. As an early 3-year-old, the horse had been involved in a mishap. He had become inverted and entangled, and extreme efforts had been necessary to extricate the animal (Ahern, 1995).

### Discussion
Lameness that appears to defy diagnosis is not uncommonly encountered in equine veterinary medicine.

In five instances, repeated diagnostic workups failed to elucidate the cause of lameness. On examination, all five cases presented with significant cervico-spinal pain, chronic lameness and demonstrable laminar corial hyperaesthesia of one or both fore hooves. A negative response to anti-inflammatory medication suggested that the origin of the lameness was not an inflammatory condition. The exception would have been case 1 at presentation.

Hyperaesthesia, hypoaesthesia and allodynia to cold and mechanical stimulation are some of the clinical findings associated with sympathetic disorders. Hyperaesthesia, rather than allodynia to mechanical stimuli, was chosen to describe the response to hoof tester pressure, as this pressure was being applied across the insensitive horn and not directly to the sensitive laminar corium. Much of the pressure was then being absorbed by the horn.

Many suggestions as to the cause of SMP involve the idea of a vicious cycle of events. The cycle is thought to be set up when peripheral trauma involving afferent nerve terminals occurs. The afferent activity arising from the damaged nerve is transmitted to the spinal cord, where it is proposed that it distorts normal somatosensory processes, leading to excessive activity in ascending spinal systems concerned with the transmission of nociceptive information.

However, the possibility also exists of a more centrally occurring disruption to somatic and autonomic pathways. This could occur either by direct neuropathology or via disturbances in neural biomechanics of the sympathetic chain secondary to cervico-spinal pain and reduced spinal mobility. There has been clear documentation of widespread patho-anatomical changes in and around the sympathetic trunk and ganglia in humans. Cervical sympathetic trunks are also exposed to mechanical trauma. In whiplash incidents in monkeys, damage to the cervical sympathetic plexus had been observed. In the five cases investigated here, cervical manipulation under anaesthetic was the only form of treatment utilized. Slater and co-workers (1991) considered it impossible to mobilize the vertebral column without mechanically affecting the sympathetic tract or sympathetic neurons in the neuraxis. In cases 1 and 3, the temporary return of overt lameness after the second cervical manipulation under anaesthesia may well have been a product of this consideration.

Recent studies of the innervation of arteriovenous anastomoses in the equine foot were useful in further understanding the function of sympathetic neural end transmission.

**Conclusion**

The elimination of chronic forelimb lameness by a two treatment cervical manipulation under anaesthesia protocol strongly suggested a more direct link between cervico-spinal pain, reduced spinal mobility and the lameness being investigated. The reduction in laminar corial hyperaesthesia which accompanied the recoveries appeared to explain the lower limb component of the lameness. The sympathetic nervous system was the most probable link between the higher and lower components of the lameness and the altered gaits observed. Peripheral trauma and hence peripheral neural trauma had not been recorded in the histories obtained. However, examination suggested that cervico-spinal neural trauma and/or altered cervico-spinal neural biomechanics, with direct or indirect involvement of sympathetic trunks, was more likely to be the source of altered neural transmission.

# SPINAL MOBILIZATION THERAPY: WITH PARTICULAR REFERENCE TO CERVICAL VERTEBRAL MOBILIZATION UNDER ANAESTHETIC

T. J. Ahern is one of the prime movers in the introduction of vertebral mobilization to the veterinary world. What follows, with his kind permission, are excerpts from a paper he was preparing for publication in 1997.

This was one of the techniques used to attempt to restore the mobility of a joint and neurological complex. It was a form of active motion therapy, i.e. where motion was initiated by and was under the control of the therapist. Slow movements were performed with direction, amplitude and pressures being selected by the therapist. Because the therapist was at all times in control of these movements, inappropriate forces were not applied. Movements could be maintained at the end of the available range of movement for extended periods of time. Joints were never taken past the limits.

Therapists using high velocity thrusts, which were typical of manipulative procedures, were less able to control the amplitude of joint movements. Thrusts initiating movements past the inherent range could have created rather than treated spinal trauma.

Mobilization was achieved by initiating movement in a single joint complex or by applying pressures through a series of adjacent complexes. The size of the animal and the ability to locate and palpate individual structures tended to dictate which approach was used. Small animals often provided the opportunity for the therapist to localize and treat individual spinal joints,

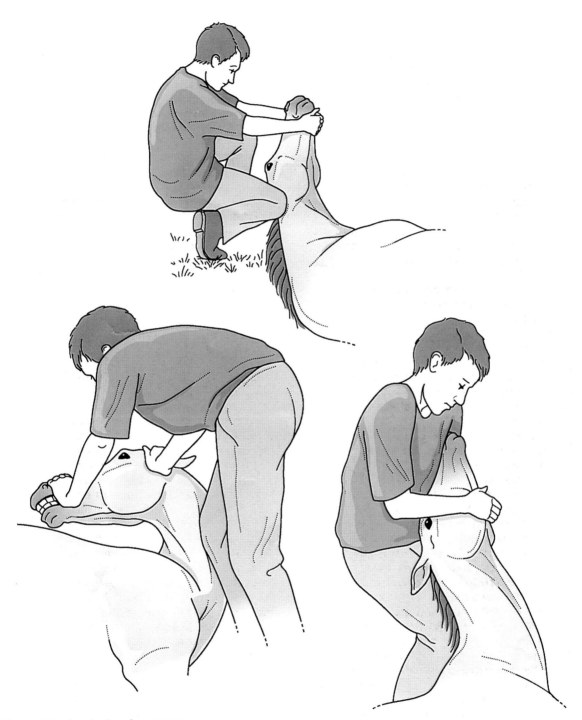

**Figure A5.2**  Examination of movement

whilst the same form of therapy was difficult to achieve in large animals. With small animals the therapist would often initiate movement by applying pressure through the dorsal spinous processes, particularly in the thoracolumbar spine. Both dorsal and lateral movements were possible in cervical and lumbar regions.

Two major contradictions with this form of therapy were those common to most forms of spinal therapy.

These were vertebral fractures, particularly in cases of non-union, and vertebral instability secondary to trauma or degenerative bone or joint disease. Vascular disease of the vertebral arteries was a major concern in the human species, but appeared to be of less significance in animals.

## CERVICAL VERTEBRAL MOBILIZATION UNDER ANAESTHETIC (FIGURE A5.2)

This procedure, which utilized anaesthesia, was designed specifically for horses. Some significant changes, mostly as a direct result of improved spinal mobility, were reported as early as 1–2 weeks after a single treatment. Problems included:

1. Reduced cervico-spinal ROM, resulting in altered gaits and a reduced ability to under-flex, bend laterally, collect or change gaits smoothly, occurred as a direct consequence of reduced spinal mobility.

2. Behavioural changes occurred, mostly due to exaggerated responses to touch (hyperaesthesia) and pressure (mechano-allodynia). The horses would resent saddle, girth or bridle pressure, grooming, general handling (especially by the louder and more aggressive handler or rider). Bucking and rearing were a few more dangerous acquired traits. Symptoms of claustrophobia (unwillingness to load into a van or starting gates) occurred, with apprehension prior to rushing through doorways, etc. There was avoidance of contact with other horses (ears back or hindquarters raised to warn others away); these animals were often found on the outside of the herd or on their own and were unwilling to race between other runners.

Recognition of the existence within the animal kingdom of abnormal conditions that result in varying degrees of spinal and reduced spinal mobility has provided the necessary stimulus to more thoroughly investigate spinal and associated anomalies. Australian human researchers in the field of manipulative therapy were regarded as world leaders, and with the benefit of their experience and research, a base for the veterinary application of such principles has been laid.

# Bibliography

References can be chosen and used like statistics; that is, they can be selected to say what you want them to say.

Some writers of reviews place emphasis not only on the *number* of references quoted, but also on the proximity in time which they bear to the article or book being reviewed. Such people, on reviewing the 6th edition of this book, may make such comments. However, this book should be read as a clinical text based on more than 50 years of clinical experience bound by regimented self-criticism and teaching. It is not an academic exercise, the text of which is justified by a long list of modern references. The references have been selected for their clinical relationship. The year of publication is unimportant, but the clinical significance is.

One of the best books on backache has been written by a world-respected author on the subject. The book is *Backache* by Ian Macnab, and has no bibliography.

AGNOLI, A. L. (1976). Anomale wurzelabgange im Lumbrosacralen Bereich und ihre klinische Bedeutung. *Journal of Neurology*, **211**, 217–228.

AHERN, T. J. (1992). Pain of spinal origin (PSO). *Centaur*, **IX**, 6–17.

AHERN, T. J. (1994). Cervical vertebral mobilization under anaesthetic (CVMUA); physical therapy for the treatment of cervico-spinal pain and stiffness. *Journal of Equine Veterinary Science*, **14**, 540–545.

AHERN, T. J. (1996). Reflex sympathetic dystrophy syndrome (RSDS). Complex regional pain syndromes – type 1, neuropathic pain: equine perspectives. Journal of Equine Veterinary Science, **16**, 463–468.

ARGYLE, M. (1975). *Bodily Communication*. London: Methuen.

BANDLER, R. and GRINDER, J. (1975a). *Patterns of Hypnotic Techniques*, Vol. 1, pp. 15–17. California: Meta Publications.

BANDLER, R. and GRINDER, J. (1975b). *The Structure of Magic*, Vol. 1, Ch. 2. Palo Alto, CA: Science and Behaviour Books.

BATESON, G. (1980). *Mind and Nature, A Necessary Unity*, pp. 37, 38, 122. London: Fontana.

BERNINI, P., WIESEL, S. W. and ROTHMAN, R. H. (1980). Metrizamide myelography and the identification of anomalous lumbosacral nerve roots. A report of two cases and review of the literature. *Journal of Bone and Joint Surgery*, **62A**, 1203–1208.

BLADIN, P. and MERORY, J. (1975). Mechanisms in cerebral lesions in trauma to high cervical portion of the vertebral artery – rotation injury. *Proceedings of the Australian Association of Neurology*, **12**, 35.

BOGDUK, N. (1978). The lumbar zygapophyseal joints. Their anatomy and clinical significance. *Proceedings of Symposium on Low Back Pain, Sydney, Australia.*

BOGDUK, N. (1980a). Lumbar dorsal ramus syndrome. *Medical Journal of Australia*, **ii**, 537–541.

BOGDUK, N. (1980b). The anatomy and pathology of lumbar back disability. *Bulletin of the Post-Graduate Committee on Medicine*, **36**, 2–17.

BOGDUK, N. (1987). Innervation, pain patterns and mechanisms of pain production. In: *Physical Therapy of the Low Back* (L. T. Twomey and J. Taylor, eds), Ch. 3. Edinburgh: Churchill Livingstone.

BOGDUK, N. (1994a). Cervical causes of headache and dizziness. In: *Grieve's Modern Manual Therapy*, 2nd edn., pp. 317–332. Edinburgh: Churchill Livingstone.

BOGDUK, N. (1994b). The innervation of the intervertebral discs. In: *Modern Manual Therapy of the Vertebral Column*, 2nd edn. (J. Boyling and N. Palastanga, eds), pp. 149–161. Edinburgh: Churchill Livingstone.

BOGDUK, N. (1997). *Clinical Anatomy of the Lumbar Spine and Sacrum*, 3rd edn. Edinburgh: Churchill Livingstone.

BOGDUK, N. and TWOMEY, L. T. (1991). *Clinical Anatomy of the Lumbar Spine*, 2nd edn. Edinburgh: Churchill Livingstone.

BOGDUK, W., WILSON, A. S. and TYNAN, W. (1982). The human lumbar dorsal rami. *Journal of Anatomy*, **134**, 383–387.

BRAIN, R. (1957). The treatment of pain. *South African Medical Journal*, **31**, 973.

BRAIN, L. and WILKINSON, M. (1967). *Cervical Spondylosis and Other Disorders of the Cervical Spine*. London: William Heinemann.

BREIG, A. (1978). *Adverse Tension in the Central Nervous System: An Analysis of Cause and Effect. Relief by Functional Neurosurgery*. Stockholm: Almqvist and Wilksell; London: Churchill Livingstone.

BREMNER, R. A. (1958). Manipulation in the management of chronic low backache due to lumbosacral strain. *Lancet*, **i**, 20.

BREMNER, R. A. and SIMPSON, M. (1959). Management of lumbosacral strain. *Lancet*, **ii**, 949.

BREWERTON, D. A. (1964). Conservative treatment of the painful neck. *Proceedings of the Royal Society of Medicine*, **57**, 163–165.

BREWERTON, D. A. (1986). The Doctor's Role in Diagnosis and Prescribing Vertebral Manipulation. In: *Vertebral Manipulation*, 5th edn. (G. D. Maitland, ed.), Ch. 2. London: Butterworth-Heinemann.

BUTLER, D. S. (1991). *Mobilisation of the Nervous System*, pp. 3–30. Edinburgh: Churchill Livingstone.

BUTLER, D. S. (1999). *The Dynamic Nervous System*. Adelaide: NOI Press.

CHARNLEY, J. (1951). Orthopaedic signs in the diagnosis of disc protrusion. *Lancet*, **i**, 186.

CLOWARD, R. B. (1958). Cervical discography; technique, indications and use in diagnosis of ruptured cervical discs. *American Journal of Roentgenology*, **79**, 563.

CLOWARD, R. B. (1959). Cervical discography. A contribution to the aetiology and mechanism of neck, shoulder and arm pain. *Annals of Surgery*, **150**, 1052–1064.

CLOWARD, R. B. (1960). The clinical significance of the sinu-vertebral nerve in relation to the cervical disc syndrome. *Journal of Neurology, Neurosurgery and Psychiatry*, **23**, 312–326.

COPE, S. and RYAN, G. M. S. (1959). Cervical and otolith vertigo. *Journal of Laryngology and Otolaryngology*, **73**, 113.

CORRIGAN, B. and MAITLAND, G. D. (1983). *Practical Orthopaedic Medicine*. London: Butterworths.

CRISP, E. J. (1960). *Disc Lesions and Other Intervertebral Derangements Treated by Manipulation, Traction and Other Conservative Methods*. London: Livingstone.

CSAG (1996). *Clinical Guidelines for the Management of Acute Low Back Pain*. London: HMSO.

CYRIAX, J. (1975). *Textbook of Orthopaedic Medicine*. Vol. 1, 8th edn., London Baillière Tindall.

CYRIAX, J. (1978a). *Textbook of Orthopaedic Medicine*. Vol. 1, 7th edn., p. 747. London: Baillière Tindall.

CYRIAX, J. (1978b). *Textbook of Orthopaedic Medicine*. Vol. 1, 6th edn., p. 709. London: Baillière Tindall.

CYRIAX, J. (1980). *Textbook of Orthopaedic Medicine*, Vol. 2, 10th edn. London: Baillière Tindall.

CYRIAX, J. (1982). *Textbook of Orthopaedic Medicine*, Vol. 2, 8th edn., p. 281. London: Baillière Tindall.

CYRIAX, J. H. and CYRIAX, P. J. (1993). *Cyriax's Illustrated Manual of Orthopaedic Medicine*, 2nd edn. London: Butterworth-Heinemann.

DEBONO, E. (1980). *Lateral Thinking*. Harmondsworth: Pelican Books.

DE KLEYN, A. and NIEUWENHUYSE, A. (1927). Schwindelanfalle und Nystagmus bei einer bestimmten Stellung des Kopfes. *Acta Otolaryngologica*, **VII**, 155–157.

DE PALMA, A. F. and ROTHMAN, R. H. (1970). *The Intervertebral Disc*. Philadelphia: Saunders.

DE SEZE, S. (1955). Les attitudes antalgiques dans la sciatique discoradiculaire commune. *Seminare Hôpital Paris*, **31**, 2291.

DREYFUSS, P., MICHAELSON, M. and FLETCHER, D. (1994). Atlanto-occipital and lateral atlanto-axial joint pain patterns. *Spine*, **19(10)**, 1125–1131.

DURRELL, S. (1996). Expanding the scope of physiotherapy: clinical physiotherapy specialists in consultant's clinics. *Manual Therapy*, **1(4)**, 210–213.

DWYER, A., APRILL, C. and BODGUK, N. (1990). Cervical zygapophyseal joint pain patterns 1: a study in normal volunteers. *Spine*, **15(6)**, 453–457.

EDGAR, M. A. and PARK, W. M. (1974). Induced pain patterns on passive straight-leg raising in lower lumbar disc protrusion. *Journal of Bone and Joint Surgery*, **56B**, 658–667.

EDWARDS, B.C. (1979). Combined movements of the lumbar spine, examination and clinical significance. *Australian Journal of Physiotherapy*, **25**, 4.

EDWARDS, B.C. (1980). Combined movements in the cervical spine (C2–7). Their value in examination and technique choice. *Australian Journal of Physiotherapy*, **26**, 5.

EDWARDS, B. (1992). *Manual of Combined Movements*. London: Churchill Livingstone.

ELVEY, R. L. (1979). Brachial plexus tension tests and the patho-anatomical origin of arm pain. *Proceedings of Multi-Disciplinary International Conference on Manipulative Therapy, Melbourne, Australia*, pp. 105–111.

ETHELBERG, S. and RÜSHEDE, J. (1952). Malformation of lumbar spinal roots and sheaths in the causation of low backache and sciatica. *Journal of Bone and Joint Surgery*, **34B**, 442–446.

EVANS, D. H. (1982). *Accuracy of Palpation Skills*. Unpublished thesis, South Australian Institute of Technology.

EVANS, D. H. (1994). The reliability of assessment parameter: accuracy and palpation technique. In: *Grieve's Modern Manual Therapy*, 2nd edn. (J. Boyling and N. Palastanga, eds). Edinburgh: Churchill Livingstone, pp. 539–546.

EVANS, P. (1997). The T4 syndrome. Some basic clinical aspects. *Physiotherapy*, **83(4)**, 186–189.

FARFAN, H. F. (1973). *Mechanical Disorders of the Low Back*, p. 54. Philadelphia: Lea & Febiger.

FARFAN, H. F. (1975). Muscular mechanism of the lumbar spine and the position of power and efficiency. *Orthopedic Clinics of North America*, **6**, 135–144.

FEINSTEIN, B., LANGTON, J., JAMESON, R. and SCHILLER, F. (1954). Experiments on pain referred from deep somatic tissues. *Journal of Bone and Joint Surgery*, **36A**, 981–997.

FRYMOYER, J. W., POPE, N. H., COSTANZA, M. C. *et al.* (1980). Epidemiologic studies of low-back pain. *Spine*, **5**, 419–423.

GLOVER, J. R. (1960). Back pain and hyperaesthesia. *Lancet*, **i**, 1165.

GLOVER, J. R. (1977). Characterization of localized pain. In: *Approaches to the Validation of Manipulation Therapy* (A. A. Buerger and J. S. Tobis, eds), p. 175. Springfield, IL: Charles C. Thomas.

GOGGIN, J. E. and WILDER, D. G. (1980). Epidemiologic studies of low-back pain. *Spine*, **5**, 419–423.

GOWERS, E. (1979). *The Complete Plain Words*. Harmondsworth: Penguin Books.

GRANT, R. (ed.) (1988). *Clinics in Physical Theory of the Cervical and Thoracic Spine*. New York: Churchill Livingstone.

GRANT, R. (1994). Vertebral artery insufficiency: a clinical protocol for pre-manipulation testing of the cervical spine. In: *Modern Manual Therapy of the Vertebral Column*, 2nd edn. (J. Boyling and N. Palastanga, eds), pp. 71–180. Edinburgh: Churchill Livingstone.

*Gray's Anatomy* (1981). 36th edn., p. 438. Edinburgh: Longman.

GREEN, D. and JOYNT, R. (1959). Vascular accidents to the brain stem associated with neck manipulation. *Journal of the American Medical Association*, **170**, 5.

GREEN, G. J., BALJET, B. and DRUKKER, J. (1990). Nerves and nerve plexuses of the human vertebral column. *American Journal of Anatomy*, **188**, 282–296.

GREGERSON, G. C. and LUCAS, D. B. (1967). An in-vivo study of the axial rotation of the human thoraco-lumbar spine. *Journal of Bone and Joint Surgery*, **49A**, 247–262.

GRIEVE, G. P. (1980). *Common Vertebral Joint Problems*. London: Livingstone.

GRIEVE, G. P. (1981). *Common Vertebral Joint Problems*. Edinburgh: Churchill Livingstone.

GRIEVE, G. P. (1988a). *Common Vertebral Joint Problems*, 2nd edn. Edinburgh: Churchill Livingstone.

GRIEVE, G. P. (1988b). Diagnosis. *Physiotherapy Practice*, **4**, 73–77.

GRIEVE, G. P. (1989). *Common Vertebral Problems*, 2nd edn. Edinburgh: Churchill Livingstone, p. 473.

GRIEVE, G. P. (1997). Letters to the Editor. *Manual Therapy*, **2(2)**, 106–107.

GROEN, G. J., BALJET, B. and DRUKKER, J. (1990). Nerves and nerve plexuses of the human vertebral column. *American Journal of Anatomy*, **188**, 282–293.

HARRIS, R. I. and MACNAB, I. (1954). Structural changes in the lumbar intervertebral discs. *Journal of Bone and Joint Surgery*, **36B**, 304–322.

HIRSCH, C., INGLEMARK, B. and MILLER, M. (1963). The anatomical basis for low back pain. *Acta Orthopaedica Scandinavica*, **33**, 1–17.

HOCKADAY, J. M. and WHITTY, C. W. M. (1967). Patterns of referred pain in the normal subject. *Brain*, **90**, 481–495.

INMAN, V. T. and SAUNDERS, J. B. de C. M. (1944). Referred pain from skeletal structures. *Journal of Nervous and Mental Diseases*, **99**, 660–667.

JEFFREYS, E. (1991). *Prognosis in Musculoskeletal Injury: A Handbook for Doctors and Lawyers*. London: Butterworth-Heinemann.

JUDOVICH, B. and NOBEL, G. R. (1957). Traction therapy, a study of resistance forces, preliminary report on a new method of lumbar traction. *American Journal of Surgery*, **93**, 108.

JULL, G., (1984). The sensitivity of manual examination. A preliminary report. *Proceedings MTAA on Low Back Pain*.

JULL, G., BOGDUK, N. and MARSLAND, A. (1988). The accuracy of manual diagnosis for cervical zygapophyseal joint pain syndrome. *Medical Journal of Australia*, **148**, 233–236.

JULL, G., TRELEAVEN, J. and VERSACE, G. (1993). Manual examination of spinal joints: is pain provocation a major diagnostic cue for dysfunction? *Proceedings of the Eighth Biennial Conference of the Manipulative Physiotherapists, Association of Australia, Perth*, pp. 40–42.

KAKAMURA, S., KAZUHISA, T., TAKAHASHI, Y. *et al.* (1996). The apparent pathways of discogenic low-back pain. *Journal of Bone and Joint Surgery*, **78B**, 606–612.

KAPANDJI, A. J. (1974). *Trunk and Vertebral Column. The Physiology of the Joints*. Vol. 3, 2nd edn. London: Churchill-Livingstone.

KEELE, K. E. (1967). Discussion on research into pain. *Practitioner*, **198**, 287.

KELLGREN, J. H. (1939). On the distribution of pain arising from deep somatic structures. *Clinical Science*, **4**, 35–46.

KELSEY, J. L. and HARDY, R. J. (1975). Driving of motor vehicles as a risk factor for acute herniated lumbar intervertebral disc. *American Journal of Epidemiology*, **102**, 63–73.

KENNEALLY, M., RUBENACH, H. and ELVEY, R. (1988). The upper limb tension test: the SLR of the arm. In: *Clinics in Physical Therapy of the Cervical and Thoracic Spine*, Vol. 17 (R. Grant, ed.). Edinburgh: Churchill Livingstone.

KEON-COHEN, B. (1968). Abnormal arrangement of the lower lumbar and first sacral nerves within the spinal canal. *Journal of Bone and Joint Surgery*, **50B**, 261–265.

KRUEGER, B. and OKAZAKI, H. (1980). Vertebral-basil distribution infarction following chiropractic cervical manipulation. *Mayo Clinic Proceedings*, **55**, 322.

LANCE, J. W. (1993). *Mechanisms and Management of Headache*, 5th edn. London: Butterworth-Heinemann.

LANDO, A. (1994). Temperature testing by manipulative physiotherapists in spinal examination. In: *Grieve's Modern Manual of the Vertebral Column*, 2nd edn. (J. Bayling and N. Palastanga, eds), pp. 547–554. Edinburgh: Churchill Livingstone.

LEHMANN, J. F. and BRUNNER, G. D. (1958). A device for the application of heavy lumbar traction. *Archives of Physical Medicine*, **39**, 696.

LEWIS, J., RAMOT, R. and GREEN, A. (1998). Changes in mechanical tension in the median nerve: possible implications for the upper limb tension test. *Physiotherapy*, **84(6)**, 254–261.

LEWITT, K., KRAFT, G. L. and LEVINTHAL, D. H. (1951). Facet synovial impingement – a new concept in the etiology of lumbar vertebral derangement. *Surgery, Gynaecology and Obstetrics*, **93**, 439.

LICHT, S. (1960). *Massage, Manipulation and Traction.* Connecticut: Licht.

LISS, L. (1965). Fatal cervical cord injury in a swimmer. *Neurology*, **15**, 675.

LOEBL, W. Y. (1973). Regional rotation of the spine. *Rheumatology and Rehabilitation*, **12**, 223.

LYSELL, E. (1969). Motion of the cervical spine. *Acta Orthopaedica Scandinavica*, Supplement 123.

MACDONALD, R. (1970). *Black Money*, p. 74. London: Collins-Fontana Books.

MACNAB, I. (1971). Negative disc exploration. An analysis of the causes of nerve root involvement in 68 patients. *Journal of Bone and Joint Surgery*, **53A**, 891–903.

MACNAB, I. (1977) *Backache*. Baltimore: Williams & Wilkins.

MAITLAND, G. D. (1957). Low back pain and allied symptoms, and treatment results. *Medical Journal of Australia*, **ii**, 851.

MAITLAND, G. D. (1961). Some observations on 'sciatic scoliosis'. *Australian Journal of Physiotherapy*, **7**, 84–87.

MAITLAND, G. D. (1966). Manipulation–mobilization. *Physiotherapy*, **52**, 382–385.

MAITLAND, G. D. (1970a). *Peripheral Manipulation*, 2nd edn. London: Butterworths.

MAITLAND, G. D. (1970b). Application of manipulation. *Physiotherapy*, **56**, 1–7.

MAITLAND, G. D. (1978). Acute locking of the cervical spine. *Australian Journal of Physiotherapy*, **24**, 103–109.

MAITLAND, G. D. (1980a). The hypothesis of adding compression when examining and treating synovial joints. *Journal of Orthopaedics and Sports Physical Therapy*, **2**, 7–14.

MAITLAND, G. D. (1980b). Movement of pain-sensitive structures in the vertebral canal in a group of physiotherapy students. *South African Journal of Physiotherapy*, **36**, 4–12.

MAITLAND, G. D. (1982a). Examination of the cervical spine. *Australian Journal of Physiotherapy*, **28**, 6.

MAITLAND, G. D. (1982b). Palpating examination of the posterior cervical spine: the ideal, average and abnormal. *Australian Journal of Physiotherapy*, **28**, 3.

MAITLAND, G. D. (1984). Canal signs and their significance in treatment. *Clinical Proceedings of the Low Back Pain Manipulative Therapists' Association of Australia, Melbourne*, pp. 119–133.

MAITLAND, G. D. (1986). *Vertebral Manipulation*, 5th edn. Oxford: Butterworth-Heinemann.

MAITLAND, G. D. (1990). *Peripheral Manipulation*, 3rd edn., pp. 155–156. London: Butterworths.

MAGAREY, M. E. (1986). The first treatment session. In: *Modern Manual Therapy of the Vertebral Column* (G. Grieve, ed.), pp. 661–672. Edinburgh: Churchill Livingstone.

MCCALL, I. W., PARK, W. M. and O'BRIEN, J. P. (1979). Induced pain referral from posterior lumbar elements in normal subjects. *Spine*, **4**, 441–446.

MCKENZIE, R. A. (1981). *The Lumbar Spine. Mechanical Diagnosis and Therapy.* New Zealand: Spinal Publications.

MELZACK, R. and WALL, P. (1984). *The Challenge of Pain.* Harmondsworth: Penguin Books.

MENNELL, J. McM. (1960). *Back Pain. Diagnosis and Treatment Using Manipulative Techniques.* London: Churchill.

MESDAGH, H. (1976). Morphological aspects and biomechanical properties of vertebro-axial joint (C2–3). *Acta Morphologica Neurologica Scandinavica* **14(1)**: 19–30.

MILLER, J. (1978). *The Body in Question.* London: Jonathan Cape.

MOONEY, V. and ROBERTSON, J. (1976). The facet syndrome. *Clinical Orthopaedics and Related Research*, **15**, 149–156.

NACHEMSON, A. and MORRIS, J. M. (1964). In vivo measurements of intradiscal pressure. *Journal of Bone and Joint Surgery*, **46A**, 1077.

NAKAMURA, S., TAKAKASHI, K., TAKANASH, Y. *et al.* (1996). The apparent pathways of discogenic low-back pain evaluation of L2 spinal nerve infiltration. *Journal of Bone and Joint Surgery*, **78B**, 606–612.

NATHAN, H. and FEUERSTEIN, M. (1970). Angulated course of spinal nerve roots. *Journal of Neurosurgery*, **2**, 349–352.

Original article (1966). Pain in the neck and arm: a multicentre trial of the effects of physiotherapy. *British Medical Journal*, **i**, 253.

PAINTAL, A. S. (1960). Functional analysis of group III afferent fibres of mammalian muscles. *Journal of Physiology (London)*, **152**, 250–270.

PARKE, W. A. (1975). *Applied Anatomy of the Spine. The Spine Vol. 1.* Philadelphia: Saunders, pp. 19–47.

PENNING, L. (1978). Normal movements of cervical spine. *American Journal of Roentgenology* **130(2)**: 317–326.

PHILLIPS, D. and TWOMEY, L. (1993). Comparison of manual diagnosis with a diagnosis established by a unilevel lumbar spinal block procedure. *8th Biennial Conference of MPAA Proceedings*, pp. 55–61.

PHILLIPS, D. R. and TWOMEY, L. T. (1996). A comparison of manual diagnosis with a diagnosis established by a uni-level spinal block procedure, *Manual Therapy*, **1(2)**, 82–87.

PHILLIPS, H. and GRIEVE, G. P. (1986). The thoracic outlet syndrome. In: *Modern Manual Therapy* (G. Grieve, ed.), Ch. 35. Edinburgh: Churchill Livingstone.

PRATT-THOMAS, H. and BERGER, K. (1947). Cerebellar and spinal injuries after chiropractic manipulation. *Journal of the American Medical Association*, **133**, 9.

QUINTNER, J. (1989). A study of upper limb pain and paraesthesiae following neck injury in motor vehicle accidents: assessment of the brachial plexus tension test of Elvey. *British Journal of Rheumatology*, **28**, 528–533.

RECAMIER, M. (1838). *Revue Medecine France*, **1**, 74.

ROLANDER, S. D. (1966). Motion of the lumbar spine with special reference to the stabilizing effect of posterior fusion. *Acta Orthopaedica Scandinavica*, Supplement 90.

RYAN, G. M. S. and COPE, S. (1955). Cervical vertigo. *Lancet*, **ii**, 1355.

RYAN, G. and COPE, S. (1959). Cervical and otolith vertigo. *Journal of Laryngology and Otology*, **73**, 113.

SCHEENAN, S., BAUER, R. and MEYER, J. (1969). Vertebral artery compressions in cervical spondylosis. *Neurology*, **10**, 968.

SCHWARTZ, G. and GEIGER, J. (1956). Posterior inferior cerebellar artery syndrome of Wellenburg after chiropractic manipulation. *Archives of Australian Medicine*, **97**, 352.

SCHWARTZER, A., APALL, C. and BOGDUK, N. (1995). The sacroiliac joint and chronic low back pain. *Spine*, **20(1)**, 31–37.

SCOTT, B. O. (1955). A universal traction frame and lumbar harness. *Annals of Physical Medicine*, **2**, 258.

SHELLHAS, K., LATCHAW, R., WENDLING, L. and GOLD, L. (1980). Vertebrobasilar injuries following cervical manipulation. *Journal of the American Medical Association*, **244**, 13.

*Shorter Oxford Dictionary on Historical Principles*, 3rd edn. Oxford: Oxford University Press.

SINCLAIR, D. C., FEINDEL, W. H. and FALCONER, M. A. (1948). The intervertebral ligaments as a source of segmental pain. *Journal of Bone and Joint Surgery*, **30B**, 515–521.

SLATER, H. (1991). Adverse neural tension in the sympathetic trunk and sympathetic maintained pain syndromes. *Proceedings of the Conference of Manipulative Physiotherapists Association, Australia*, p. 214–219.

SMITH, R. A. and ESTRIDGE, M. N. (1962). Neurological complications of head and neck manipulation. *Journal of the American Medical Association*, **182**, 528.

SMYTH, M. J. and WRIGHT, V. (1958). Sciatica and the intervertebral disc. An experimental study. *Journal of Bone and Joint Surgery*, **40A**, 1401.

SNOW, C. P. (1965). *Strangers and Brothers*, p. 67. London: Penguin Books.

STODDARD, A. (1959). *Manual of Osteopathic Technique*. London: Hutchinson.

STODDARD, A. (1969). *Manual of Osteopathic Practice*. London: Hutchinson Medical Publications.

SUTTON, A. (1966). Animal therapists run to victory. *Frontline*, Nov. 20, p. 16.

TAYLOR, J. R. and TWOMEY, L. T. (1993). Acute injuries to cervical joints: an autopsy study of neck sprain. *Spine*, **18**, 1115–1122.

TAYLOR, J. R. and TWOMEY, L. T. (1994). Anatomy of injuries. In: *Physical Therapy of the Cervical and Thoracic Spine*, 2nd edn. (R. Grant, ed.), p. 21. New York: Churchill Livingstone.

*The Age*. (1982). 21 August.

TROUP, J. D. G. (1978). Driver's back pain and its prevention. A review of the postural, vibratory and muscular factors, together with the problem of transmitted road-shock. *Applied Ergonomics*, **9**, 207–214.

TROUP, J. D. G., HOOD, C. A. and CHAPMAN, A. E. (1968). Measurements of the sagittal mobility of the lumbar spine and hips. *Annals of Physical Medicine*, **9**, 308–321.

TULSI, R. S. and PERRETT, L. V. (1975). The anatomy and radiology of the cervical vertebrae and the tortuous vertebral artery. *Australian Radiology*, **19**, 258–264.

TWOMEY, L. and TAYLOR, J. (1994) The lumbar spine; structure, function, age changes and physiotherapy. *Australian Journal of Physiotherapy*, **Jubilee issue**, 19–31.

TWOMEY L. (1992) Anatomy of the cervical spine. *Proceedings of the International Federation of Orthopaedic Manipulative Therapists* (S. Paris, ed.). Vail, USA: IFOMT.

TWOMEY, L. T. and TAYLOR, J. R. (1987). The lumbar spine, low back pain and physical therapy. In: *Physical Therapy of the Low Back* (L. T. Twomey and J. R. Taylor, eds), p. 303. New York: Churchill Livingstone.

TWOMEY, L. T. and TAYLOR, J. R. (1992). Pathology of whiplash. *Proceedings of the International Federation of Orthopaedic Manipulative Therapists* (S. Paris, ed.), p. 84. Vail, USA: IFOMT.

TWOMEY, L. T. and TAYLOR, J. R. (eds) (1994). *Physical Therapy of the Low Back*, 2nd edn. New York: Churchill Livingstone.

VAN BAAR, M. E., DEKKER, J. and BOSVELD, W. (1998). A survey of physical therapy goals and interventions for patients with back and knee pain. *Physical Therapy*, **78**, 33–42.

WEBER, H. (1994). Spine update. The natural history of disc herniation and the influence of intervention. *Spine*, **19(19)**, 2234–2238.

WELLS, P. E. (1986). Examination of the pelvic joints. In: *Modern Manual Therapy of the Vertebral Column* (G. Grieve, ed.), pp. 590–604. Edinburgh: Churchill Livingstone.

WHITE, A. A. and PANJABI, M. M. (1978). *Clinical Biomechanics of the Spine*. Philadelphia: Lippincott.

WORLD HEALTH ORGANIZATION (1980). *The International Classification of Impairments, Disabilities and Handicaps*. Geneva: WHO.

World Health Organization (1997). *ICIDH2, International Classification of Impairments, Activities and Participation. Beta-1 Draft for Field Trials*. Geneva: WHO.

WRIGHT, A. (1995). Hypoalgesia post-manipulative therapy: a review of potential neurophysiological mechanisms. *Manual Therapy*, **1(5)**, 11–16.

WYKE, B. (1976). The lumbar spine and back pain. In: *Neurological Aspects of Low Back Pain* (M. Jayson, ed.), pp. 189–256. New York: Grune & Stratton.

ZEIG, J. (ed.) (1980). *A Teaching Seminar with Milton H. Erickson*, p. 159. New York: Brunner-Mazel.

ZUSMAN, M. (1985). Reappraisal of a proposed neurophysiological mechanism for the relief of joint pain with passive joint movements. *Physiotherapy Practice*, **1**, 64–70.

# Index

References to major mentions of topics are in **bold**, whilst references to non-textual matter such as Figures or Tables are in *italic* print

# ELSEVIER CD-ROM LICENCE AGREEMENT

PLEASE READ THE FOLLOWING AGREEMENT CAREFULLY BEFORE USING THIS PRODUCT. THIS PRODUCT IS LICENSED UNDER THE TERMS CONTAINED IN THIS LICENCE AGREEMENT ("Agreement"). BY USING THIS PRODUCT, YOU, AN INDIVIDUAL OR ENTITY INCLUDING EMPLOYEES, AGENTS AND REPRESENTATIVES ("You" or "Your"), ACKNOWLEDGE THAT YOU HAVE READ THIS AGREEMENT, THAT YOU UNDERSTAND IT, AND THAT YOU AGREE TO BE BOUND BY THE TERMS AND CONDITIONS OF THIS AGREEMENT. ELSEVIER LIMITED ("Elsevier") EXPRESSLY DOES NOT AGREE TO LICENSE THIS PRODUCT TO YOU UNLESS YOU ASSENT TO THIS AGREEMENT. IF YOU DO NOT AGREE WITH ANY OF THE FOLLOWING TERMS, YOU MAY, WITHIN THIRTY (30) DAYS AFTER YOUR RECEIPT OF THIS PRODUCT RETURN THE UNUSED PRODUCT AND ALL ACCOMPANYING DOCUMENTATION TO ELSEVIER FOR A FULL REFUND.

**DEFINITIONS** As used in this Agreement, these terms shall have the following meanings:

"Proprietary Material" means the valuable and proprietary information content of this Product including without limitation all indexes and graphic materials and software used to access, index, search and retrieve the information content from this Product developed or licensed by Elsevier and/or its affiliates, suppliers and licensors.

"Product" means the copy of the Proprietary Material and any other material delivered on CD-ROM and any other human readable or machine-readable materials enclosed with this Agreement, including without limitation documentation relating to the same.

**OWNERSHIP** This Product has been supplied by and is proprietary to Elsevier and/or its affiliates, suppliers and licensors. The copyright in the Product belongs to Elsevier and/or its affiliates, suppliers and licensors and is protected by the copyright, trademark, trade secret and other intellectual property laws of the United Kingdom and international treaty provisions, including without limitation the Universal Copyright Convention and the Berne Copyright Convention. You have no ownership rights in this Product. Except as expressly set forth herein, no part of this Product, including without limitation the Proprietary Material, may be modified, copied or distributed in hardcopy or machine-readable form without prior written consent from Elsevier. All rights not expressly granted to You herein are expressly reserved. Any other use of this Product by any person or entity is strictly prohibited and a violation of this Agreement.

**SCOPE OF RIGHTS LICENSED (PERMITTED USES)** Elsevier is granting to You a limited, non-exclusive, non-transferable licence to use this Product in accordance with the terms of this Agreement. You may use or provide access to this Product on a single computer or terminal physically located at Your premises and in a secure network or move this Product to and use it on another single computer or terminal at the same location for personal use only, but under no circumstances may You use or provide access to any part or parts of this Product on more than one computer or terminal simultaneously.

You shall not (a) copy, download, or otherwise reproduce the Product or any part(s) thereof in any medium, including, without limitation, online transmissions, local area networks, wide area networks, intranets, extranets and the Internet, or in any way, in whole or in part, except for printing out or downloading nonsubstantial portions of the text and images in the Product for Your own personal use; (b) alter, modify, or adapt the Product or any part(s) thereof, including but not limited to decompiling, disassembling, reverse engineering, or creating derivative works, without the prior written approval of Elsevier; (c) sell, license or otherwise distribute to third parties the Product or any part(s) thereof; or (d) alter, remove, obscure or obstruct the display of any copyright, trademark or other proprietary notice on or in the Product or on any printout or download of portions of the Proprietary Materials.

**RESTRICTIONS ON TRANSFER** This Licence is personal to You, and neither Your rights hereunder nor the tangible embodiments of this Product, including without limitation the Proprietary Material, may be sold, assigned, transferred or sublicensed to any other person, including without limitation by operation of law, without the prior written consent of Elsevier. Any purported sale, assignment, transfer or sublicense without the prior written consent of Elsevier will be void and will automatically terminate the Licence granted hereunder.

**TERM** This Agreement will remain in effect until terminated pursuant to the terms of this Agreement. You may terminate this Agreement at any time by removing from Your system and destroying the Product and any copies of the Proprietary Material. Unauthorized copying of the Product, including without limitation, the Proprietary Material and documentation, or otherwise failing to comply with the terms and conditions of this Agreement shall result in automatic termination of this licence and will make available to Elsevier legal remedies. Upon termination of this Agreement, the licence granted herein will terminate and You must immediately destroy the Product and all copies of the Product and of the Proprietary Material, together with any and all accompanying documentation. All provisions relating to proprietary rights shall survive termination of this Agreement.

**LIMITED WARRANTY AND LIMITATION OF LIABILITY** Elsevier warrants that the software embodied in this Product will perform in substantial compliance with the documentation supplied in this Product, unless the performance problems are the result of hardware failure or improper use. If You report a significant defect in performance in writing to Elsevier within ninety (90) calendar days of your having purchased the Product, and Elsevier is not able to correct same within sixty (60) days after its receipt of Your notification, You may return this Product, including all copies and documentation, to Elsevier and Elsevier will refund Your money. In order to apply for a refund on your purchased Product, please contact the return address on the invoice to obtain the refund request form ("Refund Request Form"), and either fax or mail your signed request and your proof of purchase to the address indicated on the Refund Request Form. Incomplete forms will not be processed. Defined terms in the Refund Request Form shall have the same meaning as in this Agreement.

YOU UNDERSTAND THAT, EXCEPT FOR THE LIMITED WARRANTY RECITED ABOVE, ELSEVIER, ITS AFFILIATES, LICENSORS, THIRD PARTY SUPPLIERS AND AGENTS (TOGETHER "THE SUPPLIERS") MAKE NO REPRESENTATIONS OR WARRANTIES, WITH RESPECT TO THE PRODUCT, INCLUDING, WITHOUT LIMITATION THE PROPRIETARY MATERIAL. ALL OTHER REPRESENTATIONS, WARRANTIES, CONDITIONS OR OTHER TERMS, WHETHER EXPRESS OR IMPLIED BY STATUTE OR COMMON LAW, ARE HEREBY EXCLUDED TO THE FULLEST EXTENT PERMITTED BY LAW.

IN PARTICULAR BUT WITHOUT LIMITATION TO THE FOREGOING NONE OF THE SUPPLIERS MAKE ANY REPRESENTATIONS OR WARRANTIES (WHETHER EXPRESS OR IMPLIED) REGARDING THE PERFORMANCE OF YOUR PAD, NETWORK OR COMPUTER SYSTEM WHEN USED IN CONJUNCTION WITH THE PRODUCT, NOR THAT THE PRODUCT WILL MEET YOUR REQUIREMENTS OR THAT ITS OPERATION WILL BE UNINTERRUPTED OR ERROR-FREE.

EXCEPT IN RESPECT OF DEATH OR PERSONAL INJURY CAUSED BY THE SUPPLIERS' NEGLIGENCE AND TO THE FULLEST EXTENT PERMITTED BY LAW, IN NO EVENT (AND REGARDLESS OF WHETHER SUCH DAMAGES ARE FORESEEABLE AND OF WHETHER SUCH LIABILITY IS BASED IN TORT, CONTRACT OR OTHERWISE) WILL ANY OF THE SUPPLIERS BE LIABLE TO YOU FOR ANY DAMAGES (INCLUDING, WITHOUT LIMITATION, ANY LOST PROFITS, LOST SAVINGS OR OTHER SPECIAL, INDIRECT, INCIDENTAL OR CONSEQUENTIAL DAMAGES ARISING OUT OF OR RESULTING FROM: (I) YOUR USE OF, OR INABILITY TO USE, THE PRODUCT; (II) DATA LOSS OR CORRUPTION; AND/OR (III) ERRORS OR OMISSIONS IN THE PROPRIETARY MATERIAL.

IF THE FOREGOING LIMITATION IS HELD TO BE UNENFORCEABLE, OUR MAXIMUM LIABILITY TO YOU IN RESPECT THEREOF SHALL NOT EXCEED THE AMOUNT OF THE LICENCE FEE PAID BY YOU FOR THE PRODUCT. THE REMEDIES AVAILABLE TO YOU AGAINST ELSEVIER AND THE LICENSORS OF MATERIALS INCLUDED IN THE PRODUCT ARE EXCLUSIVE.

If the information provided In the Product contains medical or health sciences information, it is intended for professional use within the medical field. Information about medical treatment or drug dosages is intended strictly for professional use, and because of rapid advances in the medical sciences, independent verification of diagnosis and drug dosages should be made. The provisions of this Agreement shall be severable, and in the event that any provision of this Agreement is found to be legally unenforceable, such unenforceability shall not prevent the enforcement or any other provision of this Agreement.

**GOVERNING LAW** This Agreement shall be governed by the laws of England and Wales. In any dispute arising out of this Agreement, you and Elsevier each consent to the exclusive personal jurisdiction and venue in the courts of England and Wales.

## Minimum System Requirements

To function properly, the computer utilizing this collection should support at least an 1024 × 768 pixels screen resolution, millions of colors, 128 MB RAM and operate on the Windows 98, 2000, NT, ME or XP operating system or the MAC OS 9.1+ operating system. Also the computer must have a CD-ROM drive. To use this CD, QuickTime 6 is required to view the video clips. If not already installed, please install the appropriate version for your operating system, which you can find by browsing the software folder on the CD.

## Technical Support

Technical support for this product is available between 7.30 a.m. and 7.00 p.m. CST, 8.00 a.m. and 1.00 a.m. UK, Monday through Friday.

Before calling, be sure that your computer meets the minimum system requirements to run this software.

Inside the United States and Canada, call 1-800-692-9010.

Inside the United Kingdom, call 00800-6929-0100.

Outside North America, call +1-314-872-8370.

You may also fax your questions to +1-314-997-5080,

or contact Technical Support through e-mail: technical.support@elsevier.com.